LIPPINCOTT'S

Pathology

POCKET

LIPPINCOTT'S Pathology

Donna E. Hansel, MD, PhD
Resident, Department of Pathology
Johns Hopkins University School of Medicine
Baltimore, Maryland

Renee Z. Dintzis, PhD
Associate Professor of Cell Biology
Director of Organ Histology
Johns Hopkins University School of Medicine
Baltimore, Maryland

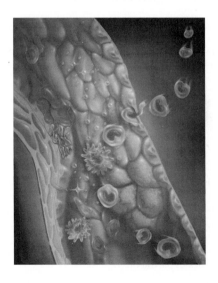

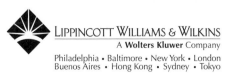

LIPPINCOTT WILLIAMS & WILKINS
A **Wolters Kluwer** Company
Philadelphia • Baltimore • New York • London
Buenos Aires • Hong Kong • Sydney • Tokyo

Acquisitions Editor: Betty Sun
Developmental Editor: Elena Coler
Marketing Manager: Emilie Linkins
Production Manager: Kevin Johnson
Compositor: Maryland Composition Co., Inc.
Printer: RR Donnelley & Sons / Crawfordsville

351 West Camden Street
Baltimore, Maryland 21201-2436 USA

530 Walnut Street
Philadelphia, Pennsylvania, 19106-3621

The publisher is not responsible (as a matter of product liability, negligence or otherwise) for an injury resulting from any material contained herein. This publication contains information relating to general principles of medical care which should not be constructed as specific instruction for individual patients. Manufacturer's product information should be reviewed for current information, including contraindications, dosages, and precautions.

Printed in the United States of America

Library of Congress Cataloging-in-Publication Data

Hansel, Donna E.
  Lippincott's pocket pathology / Donna E. Hansel, Renee Z. Dintzis.
     p. ; cm.
  Includes index.
  Abridged version of: Rubin's pathology. 4th ed. c2004.
  ISBN 0-7817-7127-7
  1. Pathology—Outlines, syllabi, etc.
  [DNLM: 1. Pathology. QZ 4 H2485L 2006] I. Dintzis, Renee Z. II. Rubin's pathology. III. Title. IV. Title: Pocket pathology. V. Title: Pathology.
RB120.H36 2006
616.07—dc22

                                     2005026311

The publishers have made every effort to trace copyright holders for borrowed material. If they have inadvertently overlooked any, they will be pleased to make necessary arrangements at the first oppurtunity.

To purchase additional copies of this book, call our curtomer service department at (800) 638-3030 or fax orders to (301) 223-2320. For other book services, including chapter reprints and large quantity sales, ask for the Special Sales department.

For all other calls originating outside of the United States, please call (301) 223-2300.

Visit Lippincott Williams & Wilkins on the Internet: http:// www.lww.com. Lippincott Williams & Wilkins custumer service representatives are available from 8:30 am to 6:30 pm, EST, Monday through Friday, for telephone access.

Preface

Lippincott's Pocket Pathology is designed to serve as an adjunct learning tool for medical students in the study of pathology. The material contained within this text is meant to present a concise, clear, and directed application of the material contained within the full-text version, with emphasis placed on the extraction of high-yield concepts.

The content of the condensed version presents key elements of the full-text version as text, bullets, tables, and diagrams. The diagrams have been extracted from the original text or created in order to present added information in a concise format. The disease entities are described with emphasis on demographics, clinical presentation, and pathologic findings. The authors have attempted to make the layout systematic and easy to follow.

Donna E. Hansel, MD, PhD
Renee Z. Dintzis, PhD

Table of Contents

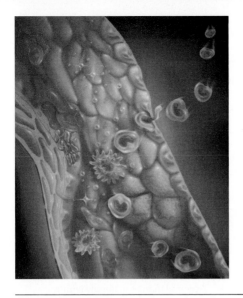

CHAPTER *1*

Cell Injury

Chapter Outline

Response to Stress and Injury

To function normally, living cells must maintain the plasma membrane as a barrier between the internal and external environment,

Table 1-1

Major Adaptive Responses to Stress and Injury

Type of Response	Characteristic
Responses Inside of Cells	
Atrophy	Decrease in size or function
Hypertrophy	Increase in size and functional capacity
Hyperplasia	Increase in number of cells in an organ or tissue
Metaplasia	Change of one differentiated cell type to another
Dysplasia	Disordered and irregular growth and arrangement
Intracellular Storage	Accumulation of materials within the cell
Responses Outside of Cells	
Dystrophic Calcification	Deposits of calcium salts in tissues
Hyaline	Reddish, homogeneous material in diverse lesions

store hereditary information in the DNA of the nucleus, and maintain the proper structure and function of the various intracellular organelles. Cells encounter many stresses as a result of changes in their internal and external environment, and they must have the capacity to adapt to these stresses (Table 1-1). The patterns of response to these stresses constitute the cellular bases of disease.

Responses within Cells

Atrophy

Causes of atrophy include:

- Reduced functional demand such as occurs in prolonged bed rest or limb immobilization
- Reduced blood circulation (ischemia), which can result in reduced oxygen supply and nutrients
- Interruption of trophic signals such as occurs with reduced hormone levels or muscle denervation
- Persistent cell injury caused by chronic inflammation
- Aging

Hypertrophy

Causes of hypertrophy include:

- Response to physiological or abnormal increases in hormone levels
- Increased functional demand. For example:
  - ➤ An increase in exercise may lead to an increase in muscle size.
  - ➤ In drug detoxification, an increase in liver cell size may be due to an augmentation of smooth endoplasmic reticulum containing detoxifying enzymes (Fig. 1-1).
  - ➤ Systemic hypertension may lead to an increase in heart size.
  - ➤ Removal of one kidney may lead to an increase in the size of the contralateral kidney.

Hyperplasia

Causes of hyperplasia include:

- Hormonal stimulation, whether physiological or pathological. For example:

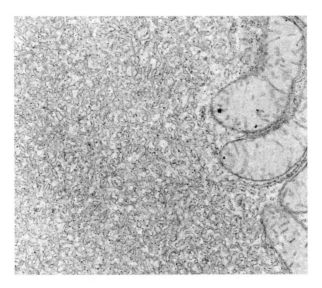

FIGURE   1-1
Proliferation of smooth endoplasmic reticulum in a liver cell in response to phenobarbital administration. (From Rubin E, Gorstein F, Rubin R, et al. Rubin's Pathology, 4th ed. Philadelphia: Lippincott Williams & Wilkins, 2005, p. 7.)

➤ An increase in estrogens at puberty leads to an increase in the size of the uterus.
➤ Decreased inactivation of estrogen by a diseased liver, leads to increased estrogen levels.

- Increased functional demand. For example:

➤ Residence at high altitude leads to an increase in red blood cell precursors to compensate for the low oxygen content of the air.
➤ Bacterial infection or transplant rejection can lead to increased lymphocyte numbers.

- Chronic cell injury (e.g., pressure from ill-fitting shoes can cause chronic cell injury, leading to hyperplasia of skin [corns or calluses]).

Metaplasia

Causes of metaplasia include:

- Tobacco smoke, which may lead to conversion of pseudostratified ciliated columnar epithelium to stratified squamous epithelium in the bronchi
- Chronic infection of the endocervix, which may cause conversion of simple columnar epithelium to stratified squamous epithelium
- Chronic reflux of gastric acid into the esophagus, which may lead to replacement of the stratified squamous epithelium of the esophagus with simple columnar surface mucous cells of the stomach (Barrett epithelium); Barrett's also includes columnar cells of the intestinal type
- Chronic gastritis, which may cause replacement of the surface mucous cells of the stomach by simple columnar absorptive and goblet cells of the small intestine (intestinal metaplasia)
- Chronic inflammation of the bladder, which may cause conversion of transitional epithelium to simple columnar epithelium (cystitis glandularis)

Dysplasia

Dysplasia most commonly occurs in stratified squamous epithelium (e.g., sunlight exposure may lead to actinic keratosis of the skin). Dysplasia may also occur in areas of squamous metaplasia in the bronchi or in the cervix. In addition, dysplastic lesions can occur in the simple columnar epithelium of large intestine (ulcerative colitis).

Dysplastic lesions can be preneoplastic but can regress with removal of the underlying cause. Dysplasia is included in the staging of intraepithelial neoplasia, because severe dysplasia shares many cytological features with cancer; thus, severe dysplasia should be treated aggressively.

Intracellular Storage

Substances that accumulate inside the cell may be normal and stored for future recycling, or they may be abnormal and consist of mutated proteins; substances that cannot be metabolized; or overloads of iron, copper, or cholesterol.

Fat Accumulation: most often in the liver, heart, and kidney

- In diabetes, increased fatty acids are delivered to the liver.
- Alcoholism can lead to a disturbance of lipid metabolism and an accumulation of fat in liver cells.
- Obesity itself can be a cause of fatty liver.

Glycogen Accumulation: most often in liver, heart, and skeletal muscle

- In inborn errors of metabolism, enzyme deficiencies in glycogen degradation lead to abnormal accumulation of glycogen, mainly in liver or muscle. There are now at least ten known inherited glycogen storage diseases (see "Glycogenoses" in Chapter 6)
- Uncontrolled diabetes can lead to excess glycogen in hepatocytes and kidney proximal tubule cells

Inherited Lysosomal Storage Diseases: defects in lysosomal degradative enzymes

- Accumulation of cerebrosides (Gaucher disease)
- Accumulation of gangliosides (Tay-Sachs disease)
- Defect in polysaccharide catabolism: Hurler and Hunter syndromes (accumulation of mucopolysaccharides; see Chapter 6)

Cholesterol Accumulation
- Atherosclerosis: occurs in macrophages of the arterial intima. In advanced lesions, cholesterol accumulates in and outside of smooth muscle cells of the tunica media.
- Familial hypercholesterolemia and primary biliary cirrhosis: occurs in macrophages. Clusters of macrophages in subcutaneous tissues lead to the formation of xanthomas.

Abnormal Proteins: altered amino acid sequences or a defect in protein folding. Chaperone proteins in the endoplasmic reticulum monitor nascent polypeptides and shepherd incorrectly folded

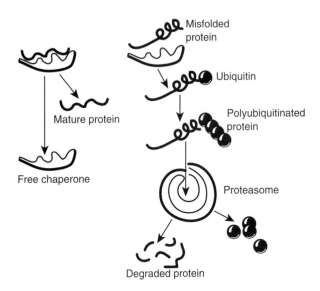

FIGURE 1-2
Quality control of correct protein folding. Differential handling of correctly (left) and incorrectly (right) folded protein. Correctly folded proteins are chaperoned to their proper cellular position. Ubiquitin binds to incorrectly folded proteins, and multiple ubiquitins are added. The complex is shepherded to the proteasome, where the incorrect protein is degraded and ubiquitins are liberated.

ones to the intracellular ubiquitin-proteasome machinery, where they are degraded (Fig. 1-2); numerous hereditary and acquired diseases are caused by evasion of this quality control system.

- In α_1- antitrypsin deficiency, the mutant protein accumulates intracellularly causing cell injury and cirrhosis in the liver. α_1 Antitrypsin is an antiprotease; thus, its deficiency in connective tissue (particularly in lung) leads to proteolysis of alveolar elastin, causing emphysema.
- Prion diseases cause neurodegenerative disorders due to the accumulation of abnormal prion proteins in neurons.
- Parkinson disease is characterized by the accumulation of Lewy bodies (α-synuclein) in neurons.
- Alzheimer disease is characterized by neurofibrillary tangles of amyloid beta protein that accumulate in cortical neurons.
- Alcoholic liver injury is characterized by the accumulation of Mallory bodies (intermediate filaments) in liver cells.

- In cystic fibrosis, mutated ion channel protein fails to reach the cell membrane, leading to defects in epithelial chloride transport.
- Certain types of hypercholesterolemia are caused by mutations in the LDL receptor.

Lipofuscin: golden-brown lipofuscin granules in infrequently dividing cells that are believed to result from the normal turnover of cell constituents. They increase with age and seem to cause little interference with cell function.

Melanin: insoluble, intracellular, brown-black pigment that is synthesized by melanocytes and distributed principally to epidermal cells of the skin. Melanin, which is also found in the eye and other organs, serves to protect cells from damaging effects of ultraviolet light. Melanin is a marker for melanoma, a cancer that arises in melanocytes.

Exogenous Pigments

- Inhaled carbon particles can be taken up by the macrophages of the lungs and can be carried by them to nearby lymph nodes.
- Tattoos consist of insoluble metallic and vegetable pigments taken up by dermal macrophages.

Iron, Lead, and Copper

- Iron: 25% of body iron is stored in iron-storage proteins, ferritin (in liver and bone marrow), and hemosiderin (in spleen, bone marrow, Kupffer cells of liver). Excess iron storage is associated with hepatocellular carcinoma. In hemosiderosis, the excess iron storage in skin, pancreas, heart, kidneys, and endocrine glands can damage vital organs. Hereditary hemochromatosis is a genetic abnormality in iron absorption.
- Lead: excess accumulation, particularly in children, can cause mental retardation.
- Copper: Wilson disease is characterized by the storage of excess copper in liver and brain.

Responses Outside of Cells
Dystrophic Calcification
Dystrophic calcification is characterized by the macroscopic deposition of calcium in injured tissues. In locations such as the aortic or mitral valves, it can impede blood flow. Mammography detects calcification of breast cancers. Congenital toxoplasmosis, which is an infection involving the central nervous system (CNS), is visualized as calcification in the infant brain. Metastatic calcification is associated with hypercalcemia leading to inappropriate calcification in lung alveolar septa, renal tubules, and blood vessels. Cal-

cium carbonate stones can form in gallbladder, renal pelvis, bladder and pancreatic duct.

Hyaline Deposits

Hyaline refers to a homogeneous eosinophilic deposit in diverse and unrelated lesions. Conditions using the term "hyaline" include hyaline arteriosclerosis, alcoholic hyaline of liver, and lung hyaline membranes.

Mechanisms of Cell Injury

Acute cell injury can occur when the cell is challenged by environmental changes to which it cannot readily adapt. If the stress is removed in time, or if the cell has time to adapt, the injury is reversible. Subcellular changes in reversibly injured cells (Fig. 1-3) may include:

- Hydropic swelling: a reversible increase in cell volume. Cell injury from varied causes can lead to a decrease in ATP synthesis, which in turn interferes with the efficiency of the plasma membrane Na^+/K^+-ATPase pump. The resultant leakage of Na^+ into the cell is followed by an increase in intracellular water (cell swelling).

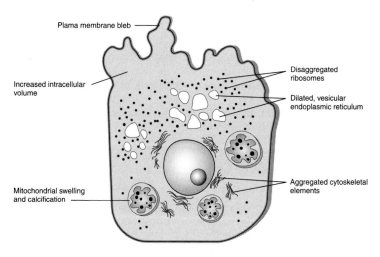

FIGURE 1-3
Ultrastructural features of reversible cell injury. (From Rubin E, Gorstein F, Rubin R, et al. Rubin's Pathology, 4th ed. Philadelphia: Lippincott Williams & Wilkins, 2005, p. 17.)

- Other morphological changes such as dilated cisternae of the endoplasmic reticulum, formation of plasma membrane blebs, mitochondrial swelling and calcification, disaggregation of membrane-bound polysomes, and aggregated cytoskeletal proteins.

Generation of Reactive Oxygen Species

Obstruction of blood flow may lead to ischemic cell injury. This leads to a decrease in ATP synthesis as well as chemical and pH imbalances accompanied by enhanced generation of injurious free radicals. Reactive oxygen species (ROS) have been identified as the likely cause of cell injury in many diseases (Fig. 1-4). Oxygen is

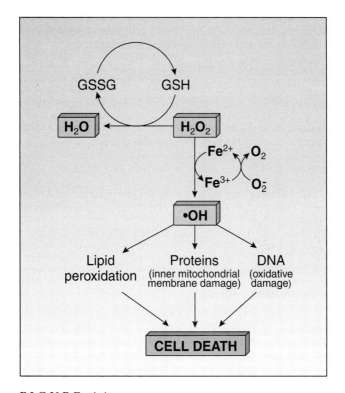

FIGURE 1-4
Mechanisms of cell injury by activated oxygen species. (From Rubin E, Gorstein F, Rubin R, et al. Rubin's Pathology, 4th ed. Philadelphia: Lippincott Williams & Wilkins, 2005, p. 20.)

essential for life, but its metabolism can produce partially reduced oxygen species, which may lead to cell injury in many organs.

Three potentially damaging ROS are formed in small amounts within tissues:

- Superoxide (O_2^-): produced principally by leaks in mitochondrial electron transport
- Hydrogen peroxide (H_2O_2): produced by a number of oxidases in intracellular peroxisomes
- Hydroxyl radical ($\bullet OH$): formed as the result of reactions with H_2O_2. Hydroxyl radical is the most reactive molecule of ROS.

ROS may be generated as the result of neutrophil phagocytosis of bacteria (Fig. 1-5). These primary ROS cause damage by reacting with lipids, proteins, nucleic acids, or metabolites to form secondary damaging ROS, such as peroxynitrite ($ONOO\bullet$), lipid peroxide radicals ($RCOO\bullet$), and hypochlorous acid (HOCl).

It is not surprising that the body has mechanisms to protect against ROS, because they are so potentially damaging to cells. Enzymes detoxify the damaging substances and include:

- Superoxide dismutase (SOD): converts superoxide to H_2O_2 and O_2
- Catalase (mainly in peroxisomes): converts H_2O_2 to H_2O and O_2
- Glutathione peroxidase: catalyzes the reduction of H_2O_2 and lipid peroxides in mitochondria and the cytosol

Scavengers of ROS offer some protection and include:

- Vitamin E: protects lipid membranes against lipid peroxidation
- Vitamin C: reacts directly with O_2, OH, and some products of lipid peroxidation
- Retinoids (precursors of vitamin A): function as chain-breaking antioxidants

Ischemia/Reperfusion Injury

Conditions such as infection or shock may lead to a transient ischemia, followed by the reestablishment of blood flow (reperfusion). The ischemic damage may generate free radicals, and the reperfusion may provide O_2 to combine with free radicals to form ROS. Ischemia/reperfusion injury activates neutrophils to release ROS and hydrolytic enzymes, and formation of NO is induced. This in turn causes an increase in injurious peroxynitrite ($ONOO^-$) formation. Inflammatory mediators such as tumor necrosis factor-α (TNF-α), interleukin-1, and platelet-activating factor may also be released.

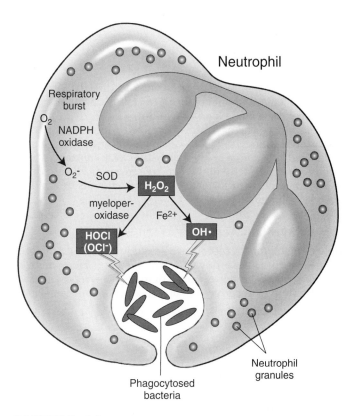

FIGURE 1-5
Generation of reactive oxygen species in neutrophils as a result of phagocytosis of bacteria. SOD, superoxide dismutase. (From Rubin E, Gorstein F, Rubin R, et al. Rubin's Pathology, 4th ed. Philadelphia: Lippincott Williams & Wilkins, 2005, p. 19.)

Injury by Ionizing Radiation

Ionizing radiation can cause formation of damaging hydroxyl radicals. High doses of ionizing radiation can lead to necrosis of both proliferating and quiescent cells.

Viral Cytotoxicity

- Direct injury: disruption of the normal homeostatic mechanisms of the cell by the virus
- Immunologic injury: recognition of viral antigens expressed by the virus-infected cell by the immune system, resulting in

apoptosis or necrosis of the cell via complement or cytotoxic T-cell–mediated pathways.

Chemical Injury

- Direct injury: Toxic chemicals may interact directly with cellular constituents without requiring metabolic activation (e.g., heavy metals, cyanide, and phalloidin).
- Indirect injury: The action of the mixed function oxygenase system in hepatocytes (P450) can metabolize ingested or administered substances to highly reactive toxic substances (e.g., carbon tetrachloride → highly reactive free radical; high doses of acetaminophen → formation of toxic amounts of a highly reactive quinone).

Abnormal G Protein Activity

A variety of membrane receptors are linked to intracellular G proteins that in turn activate downstream signaling. Hereditary or acquired defects in G protein subunits or in ligand-receptor interactions can interfere with correct signal transduction and can lead to significant cellular dysfunction.

Cell Death

Physiological cell death involves the activation of an internal suicide program, which results in cell killing by a process termed apoptosis. It is important in development, and is often activated for the detection and removal of damaged or infected cells. In contrast, necrosis, or pathological cell death, is not regulated, is invariably injurious to the organism, and is caused by exogenous stress (Table 1-2).

Necrosis

Types of Necrosis

- **Coagulative necrosis** refers to the changes visible in a dying cell when viewed under light microscopy. In general, cell and tissue outlines are preserved. Coagulative necrosis is characterized by cytoplasmic eosinophilia and darkly stained or fragmented nuclei. In tissue, coagulative necrosis appears as a pink or reddish area; over time, macrophages consume the necrotic cells and the tissue is replaced by a pale, collagenous scar.
- **Liquefactive necrosis** is characterized by dissolution of tissue, which may result from an acute inflammatory reaction. Hydrolase release from polymorphonuclear leukocytes can cause abscess formation. Liquefactive necrosis in the brain may result in a persistent CNS cavity or cyst.

Table 1-2

Characteristics of Necrosis versus Apoptosis

Necrosis	Apoptosis
No involvement of gene activation or protein signaling	Engages signaling cascades of cell
Usually involves large area of tissue or organ	Usually involves individual or small groups of cells
Cell and organelle swelling	Nuclear fragmentation and pyknosis
Usually elicits inflammatory response	Inflammatory response not usual
Invariably injurious to organism	Important in organismal development
Cell death results in pathology	Cell death crucial in cell number regulation
DNA fragmented irregularly	DNA cleaved into regular nucleosomal fragments (laddering)

- **Fat necrosis** most commonly results from the extracellular release of lipolytic enzymes in adipose tissue. In pancreatitis, fatty acids may be precipitated as calcium soaps which accumulate as amorphous basophilic deposits. In tissue with a high fat content, such as breast tissue, traumatic injury may result in the appearance of an irregular, chalky-white area.
- **Caseous necrosis** is a lesion characteristic of tuberculosis. Tuberculous granulomas contain dead mycobacteria engulfed by necrotic macrophages; they persist as coarse eosinophilic debris resembling clumpy cheese.
- **Fibrinoid necrosis** is characterized by the fibrinlike accumulation of eosinophilic plasma proteins in the walls of injured blood vessels and may be associated with immune-mediated arteritis.

Ischemia Leading to Necrosis

Processes by which ischemia leads to necrosis (Fig. 1-6) are:

- Anoxia from ischemia or blood loss leads to decreased delivery of oxygen, which in turn leads to decreased delivery of oxygen, decreased ATP synthesis, increased lactate accumulation, and lowering of pH. This causes cell injury.
- The decreased **ATP** levels also lead to distortion of the plasma membrane ion pump activities which eventually cause accu-

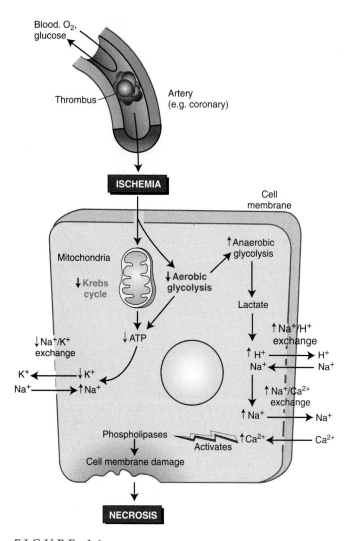

FIGURE 1-6

Mechanisms by which ischemia leads to cell death. (From Rubin E, Gorstein F, Rubin R, et al. Rubin's Pathology, 4th ed. Philadelphia: Lippincott Williams & Wilkins, 2005, p. 28.)

mulation of intracellular Ca^{++}. The accumulation of intracellular Ca^{++} activates phospholipase A_2, leading to cell membrane damage and inflammation.

- Increase of intracellular Ca^{++} also disrupts cytoskeletal/membrane interactions and results in cell shape changes.
- Impaired mitochondrial electron transport leads to the formation of ROS, peroxidation of mitochondrial membrane cardiolipin, and further decrease in ATP synthesis.
- Mitochondrial damage in the form of sustained opening of the mitochondrial permeability transition pore (MPTP) results in the release of cytochrome c into the cell cytosol. This is a trigger for irreversible apoptotic cell death.

Apoptosis

Apoptosis, known as programmed cell death, is a prearranged pathway of cell death whereby the cell commits suicide for the benefit of the organism. The process is important in many of the following developmental and physiological processes:

- Causes regression of anatomical structures in fetal development
- Eliminates self-recognizing lymphocyte clones in immunologic processes (Fig. 1-7)
- Prevents overpopulation in continuously renewing tissues
- Maintains the balance of cellularity in the response of tissues to hormones
- Deletes mutant cells or those with DNA damage
- Eliminates cells infected by viruses

Morphology of Apoptosis

Cells that die by necrosis swell and burst; their contents often cause a damaging inflammatory response in surrounding tissues. In contrast, cells that die by apoptosis do not damage their neighbors.

Apoptotic cells shrink, their nuclei condense, and the nuclear DNA breaks into fragments (Fig. 1-8). A recognition molecule exposed on the surface of apoptotic cells stimulates their rapid phagocytosis by macrophages and neighboring cells, thus avoiding leakage of cell contents and subsequent damaging consequences.

Apoptosis: Induction Mechanisms

- Apoptosis may be initiated by receptor-ligand interactions at the cell membrane. When transmembrane receptors for TNF-α and Fas are activated, "death domain" sequences in the receptors' cytoplasmic tails serve as docks for proteins that lead to a cascade of caspase proteases that initiate apoptosis.

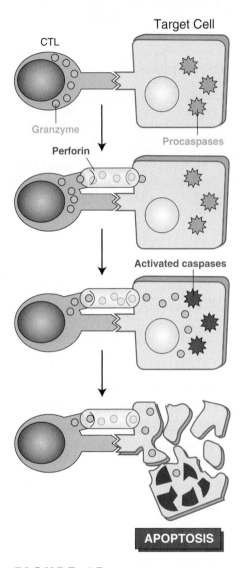

CTL

Target Cell

Granzyme

Procaspases

Perforin

Activated caspases

APOPTOSIS

FIGURE 1-7
A virus-infected cell (target cell) is recognized by a cytotoxic T cell (CTL), which secretes perforin into the target cell; this forms trans-membrane pores into which the protease, granzyme, is introduced, resulting in the activation of caspases. Activated caspases lead to apoptosis. (From Rubin E, Gorstein F, Rubin R, et al. Rubin's Pathology, 4th ed. Philadelphia: Lippincott Williams & Wilkins, 2005, p. 23.)

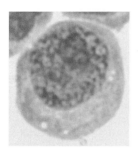 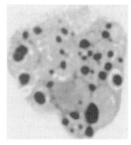

FIGURE 1-8

Apoptosis. A viable leukemic cell *(left)* **contrasts with an apoptotic cell** *(right)* **in which the nucleus has undergone condensation and fragmentation. (From Rubin E, Gorstein F, Rubin R, et al. Rubin's Pathology, 4th ed. Philadelphia: Lippincott Williams & Wilkins, 2005, p. 29.)**

- Apoptosis may be mediated by mitochondria. ROS and/or the nitric oxide radical can cause opening of MPTP. This in turn leads to the leakage of cytochrome c into the cytoplasm. Leakage of cytochrome c into the cytoplasm induces apoptosis.
- Apoptosis can be activated by p53. Several forms of stress (hypoxia, ribonucleotide depletion, loss of cell-cell adhesion) lead to accumulation of p53. When DNA damage is reparable, p53 causes an arrest in the cell cycle to allow for DNA repair. However, when DNA damage is irreparable, p53 activates apoptosis by downregulating transcription of Bcl-2 (an anti-apoptotic protein) and upregulating transcription and translocation to the cytosol of proapoptotic proteins.

Apoptosis: Detection Assays

Assays for detection of apoptosis make use of the fact that DNA is fragmented in apoptosis.

- Electrophoretic separation of cellular DNA fragments reveals a pattern of regularly spaced bands, called "laddering."
- The TUNEL assay (terminal deoxynucleotidyl transferase-mediated dUTP nick end labeling): a fluorescent nucleotide is transferred to DNA breakpoints leading to fluorescence of apoptotic cells.

Process of Biological Aging

The maximum human life span (~100 years) is not significantly altered by a protected environment. Functional and structural

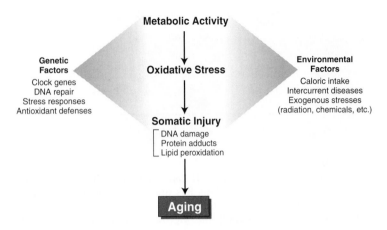

FIGURE 1-9
Factors that influence the development of biological aging. (From Rubin E, Gorstein F, Rubin R, et al. Rubin's Pathology, 4th ed. Philadelphia: Lippincott Williams & Wilkins, 2005, p. 38.)

changes accompany aging. These are evidenced by decreases in the velocity of nerve conduction, in the glomerular filtration rate, in cardiac contractility, and in a general decrease in vitality. Current evidence supports the notion that a combination of genetic and environmental factors contributes to aging (Fig. 1-9).

Cellular Basis of Aging

Normal cells in culture do not have an unrestrained capacity to replicate; however, if cells are exposed to an oncogenic virus, they continue to replicate and become "immortalized." Hybrids between normal human cells and immortalized cells do undergo senescence. This supports the concept of a genetically programmed lifespan.

Telomeres

The study of telomeres, the genetic elements at the tips of chromosomes, may reveal some explanations for cell senescence. Telomeres prevent the ends of chromosomes from accidentally becoming attached to each other and prevent chromosomes from losing base pair sequences at their ends. Properties of telomeres include:

- Each time a cell divides, some of the telomere is lost.
- When the telomere becomes too short, the chromosome can no longer replicate, and the cell becomes senescent and dies by apoptosis.

- Telomere shrinkage might be a clock that determines the longevity of a cell lineage.
- Senescence due to telomere shrinkage might be a tumor-suppressing mechanism; tumor suppressor genes (such as p53) are activated by telomere shortening.

Telomerase

Telomerase is a polymerase consisting of protein and an RNA molecule, which is used as a template for telomere synthesis. Telomerase compensates for telomere shortening by elongating telomeres. Properties of telomerase include:

- Telomerase is active in fetal tissues, germ line cells, some cells of the immune system, and cancer cells but has an almost undetectable activity in somatic cells.
- Telomerase influences cellular senescence; ectopic expression of telomerase reverses the senescent phenotype.
- Telomerase might have a use in cancer therapy. Inhibition of telomerase in cancer cells could lead to cancer cell senescence

Influence of Genetic Factors on Aging

In humans there is a modest correlation in longevity between related persons but an excellent concordance of life span among identical twins. Heritable human diseases are associated with accelerated aging:

- In Hutchinson-Guilford progeria, the aging process is compressed into a short life span. The biological basis of this disease is yet to be elucidated.
- Werner syndrome is a rare autosomal recessive disease characterized by very premature aging. The gene for Werner syndrome codes for DNA helicase, an enzyme that unwinds DNA duplexes to provide access to DNA-binding proteins. Cells from Werner syndrome patients display chromosomal deletions, inversions, and reciprocal translocations.

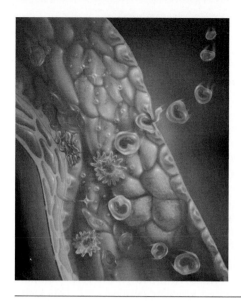

CHAPTER *2*

Inflammation

Chapter Outline

Inflammation is a protective action of the body to a variety of damaging stimuli, including trauma and infection. The body's response to inflammation brings fluid, proteins and cells from the blood into the damaged tissues where they are needed.

- One of the earliest reactions in the inflammatory response occurs in the vascular connective tissues, with vasodilatation, accompanied by increased vascular permeability. This facilitates recruitment of blood cells to the damaged site.
- Factors generated by vascular endothelial cells mediate recruitment of inflammatory cells. In acute inflammation, the neutrophils are especially active in early recruitment. Inflammatory cells release mediators such as cytokines, vasoactive amines, prostanoids, and reactive oxygen intermediates, all of which participate in the response to damage.
- Cytokine release by inflammatory cells such as macrophages activate the liver to increase its production of acute phase proteins such as protease inhibitors, coagulation proteins, complement proteins, transport proteins, and C-reactive protein. All these proteins play active host-defensive roles.
- If the mediators summoned in the inflammatory response are successful, invading and infectious agents will be removed, damaged tissues will be disposed of, new tissue will be induced to form, and a new blood supply to the area will be established.

The primary function of acute inflammation is elimination of the pathogenic insult, removal of injured tissue components, and restoration or replacement of the damaged tissue within a few days. When this cannot be achieved, chronic inflammation results, with persistence of inflammatory cells, tissue scarring, and organ dysfunction (Table 2-1). Inflammatory edema is one of the earliest responses to tissue injury.

Vascular Changes in Inflammation

The interchange of fluid between the vascular and the extravascular space results from a balance of forces that draw fluid into the vascular space or out into the tissues. These forces include:

Table 2-1

Characteristics of Acute versus Chronic Inflammation

Acute Inflammation	Chronic Inflammation
Endothelial cell damage → fluid leakage from vessels Mast cell activation	Accumulation and persistence of lymphocytes, plasma cells and macrophages
Activation of plasma-derived and cell derived inflammation mediators	Granulation and fibrosis of affected tissues
Neutrophils accumulate to "clean up" inflamed tissue	Tissue damage often aberrantly repaired → dysfunction and altered architecture

- Hydrostatic pressure: blood pressure within the capillary walls, which tends to force fluid out into the tissues
- Oncotic pressure: reflects the plasma protein concentration, which tends to draw fluid into vessels
- Osmotic pressure: proportional to the difference in concentration of solute molecules between the vascular and tissue spaces; fluid moves from areas of low osmotic pressure to areas of high osmotic pressure.
- Lymph flow: tissue fluid is drained into lymphatic capillaries and is eventually returned to the circulatory system via the thoracic duct and the right lymphatic duct.

Edema

Edema refers to fluid accumulation in the interstitial spaces; it may be noninflammatory, characterized by a transudate of low protein content, or inflammatory, characterized by a protein-rich exudate.

Noninflammatory Edema

Causes include:

- Increase in hydrostatic pressure due to thrombosis or congestive heart failure
- Reduction of plasma osmotic pressure caused by albumin loss due to kidney disease or decreased albumin synthesis due to a diseased liver or malnutrition
- Alteration of osmotic pressure due to abnormalities of sodium and/or water retention
- Obstruction of lymphatic flow

Inflammatory Edema

In the inflammatory response, increased vascular permeability is important in enabling cells and factors to reach the site of injury, and some edema can occur. Tissue injury leads to the characteristic "triple response" of acute inflammation.

- Red line (transient vasoconstriction of arterioles; rubor)
- Flare (vasodilation of arterioles→ redness and warmth; calor)
- Wheal (increase in endothelial cell permeability→ edema; swelling; tumor)

  Pain (dolor) is often added as a fourth sign of inflammation.

Terms Used to Describe the Pathology of Edema

- Effusion: excess fluid in body cavities (e.g., peritoneum or pleura)
- Transudate: edema fluid with low protein content
- Exudate: edema fluid with high protein content; appears early in mild injuries; may contain inflammatory cells
- Serous exudate or effusion: has a strawlike color; contains few cells
- Serosanguinous exudate: contains red blood cells and has a reddish tinge
- Fibrinous exudate: contains large amounts of fibrin as result of coagulation activation
- Purulent exudate or effusion: often associated with pyogenic bacterial infections and contains large numbers of neutrophils (polymorphonuclear leukocytes)
- Suppurative inflammation: purulent exudate with significant liquefactive necrosis (pus accumulation)

Plasma-derived Mediators of Inflammation

Plasma contains several enzyme cascades involved in mediating inflammation, which are composed of a series of sequentially activated proteases. They are characterized by a small starting number of proteins that are amplified by each successive enzymatic reaction. The cascade system rapidly produces a large response.

Hageman Factor Cascade

Hageman factor (clotting factor XII) is a protein produced by the liver and circulating in the blood; it is activated by agents associated with injury, such as basement membrane exposure, bacterial lipopolysaccharide, urate crystals (gout), and proteolytic enzymes.

  Activation of the Hageman factor results in the activation of additional plasma proteases, which leads to:

- Plasmin generation, which causes increases in vascular permeability and generation of anaphylatoxins
- Kinin production, which ultimately results in the formation of bradykinin, a potent vasodilator
- Activation of the alternative complement pathway
- Activation of the coagulation system (see Chapter 10)

Complement Cascade

This system consists of a set of some 30 plasma proteins that act together to attack pathogens and induce inflammatory responses that help to fight infection. Several complement precursor proteins are proteases that can themselves be activated by proteolytic cleavage. The complement precursors are widely distributed in body fluids and tissues and remain inert unless activated at sites of infection.

In complement nomenclature, native complement components are designated by a simple number (e.g., C1, C2), and cleavage products are designated by lower case letters (e.g., C3a)

Three Pathways of Complement Activation

All three pathways lead to the ultimate formation of the **MAC (membrane attack complex)**, which is instrumental in the killing of pathogens (Fig. 2-1).

Classical Complement Pathway

This pathway is often triggered by the binding of antibody to its antigen. Triggering can occur in solution or when antibodies have bound to antigens on a microbe surface.

- Activation of molecular complex, **C1**, leads (via a series of reactions) to the formation of **C3 convertase**, which catalyzes the cleavage of **C3**, the most abundant protein of the complement system, to **C3a** and **C3b**.
- **C3a (an anaphylatoxin)** can bind to receptors on basophils and mast cells triggering them to release their vasoactive contents (e.g., histamine); because of the role of these materials in anaphylaxis, C3a is called an anaphylatoxin (Fig. 2-2).
- **C3b (an opsonin)**: Macrophages and neutrophils have receptors for C3b and can bind the C3b-coated cell preparatory to phagocytosis, an effect called opsonization (Fig. 2-3).
- Some **C3b** activates a **C5 convertase** that cleaves **C5** to **C5a** and **C5b.**
- **C5a** is a potent anaphylatoxin (like C3a) and is also chemotactic for neutrophils.
- **C5b** initiates the assembly of a set of complement proteins that make up the **MAC.**

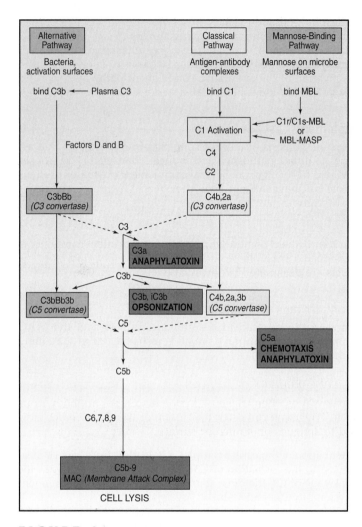

FIGURE 2-1

Complement activation. The alternative, classical, and mannose-binding pathways lead to generation of the complement cascade of inflammatory mediators and cell lysis by the membrane-attack complex. (From Rubin E, Gorstein F, Rubin R, et al. Rubin's Pathology, 4th ed. Philadelphia: Lippincott Williams & Wilkins, 2005, p. 49.)

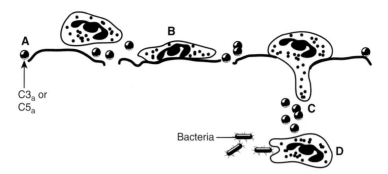

F I G U R E   2-2
Anaphylatoxin functions. A: Vessel permeability is increased by anaphylatoxins, such as complement components $C3_a$ and C5a. B: Anaphylatoxins increase neutrophil adhesion. C: Neutrophils follow the
chemotactic gradient established by the anaphylatoxins. D: Anaphylatoxins stimulate phagocytosis of bacteria and degranulation by the
neutrophils.

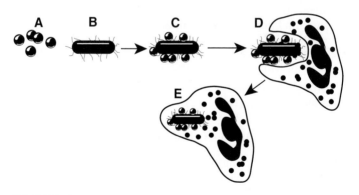

F I G U R E   2-3
Opsonization of a bacterium. A: Opsonins such as complement components C3b. B: Bacterium. C: Opsonins coat the bacterium. D: A
neutrophil has receptors for opsonized bacterium. E: Opsonized bacterium is phagocytosed by the neutrophil.

- The **MAC** results in the killing of the initiating pathogen. It forms a pore allowing free passage of water and solutes across the membrane, killing the cell. The MAC also activates phagocytic cells to generate oxidants and cytokines, which implement cell killing.

Alternative Pathway

This pathway is triggered by bacteria and other foreign materials, which cause spontaneous cleavage of C3 to **C3a** and **C3b.** When **C3b** binds to microbial cell surfaces, it forms **C3 convertase**. By a series of successive cleavages, **C5a** and **C5b** are formed, leading to **MAC** assembly.

Mannose-binding Pathway

This pathway is triggered by the binding of microbes bearing terminal mannose groups to mannose-binding lectin (**MBL**). Activation of the MBL pathway eventually results in the assembly of the classical complement pathway **C3 convertase**, and **MAC** is generated.

Regulation of the Complement System

A system that can activate so many proteolytic enzymatic components must be regulated. Complement components may be degraded by a number of mechanisms:

- Active components gradually decrease in quantity due to spontaneous decay.
- Plasma inhibitors bind to components to form inactive complexes.
- Cell-membrane-associated molecules bind to and inactivate some complement components.

When regulating mechanism do not function properly, disease or tissue injury occurs (Table 2-2).

Cell-derived Mediators of Inflammation

In addition to the inflammatory mediators in plasma, many inflammatory mediators are secreted by cells or are released from cell membrane phospholipids. These mediators interact with other cells in the following ways:

- **Paracrine**: Signals are released into the extracellular medium and act locally.
- **Endocrine**: Signals are released into the bloodstream and affect distant cells.
- **Juxtacrine**: The signaling cell is in direct contact with the cell containing the appropriate receptor.
- **Autocrine:** Cells affect themselves.

Table 2-2
Hereditary Complement Deficiencies

Complement Deficiency	Clinical Association
C3b, iC3b, C5, mannose-binding lectin	Pyogenic bacterial infections Membranoproliferative glomerulonephritis
C3, properdin, membrane-attack complex proteins	Neisserial infection
C1 inhibitor	Hereditary angioedema
CD59	Hemolysis, thrombosis
C1q, C1r and C1s, C4, C2	Systemic lupus erythematosus
Factor H and factor I	Hemolytic-uremic syndrome Membranoproliferative glomerulonephritis

From Rubin E, Gorstein F, Rubin R, et al. Rubin's Pathology, 4th ed. Philadelphia: Lippincott Williams & Wilkins, 2005, p. 51.

Inflammatory Factors Derived from Cell Membrane Phospholipids

Arachidonic Acid

Tissue damage leads to the activation of a membrane enzyme, phospholipase A_2, which, in turn, acts on a membrane phospholipid that contains arachidonic acid (Fig. 2-4). The arachidonic acid released from the phospholipid is now the substrate for one of two enzymes, cyclooxygenase (COX) or lipoxygenase (LOX). COX action gives rise to prostaglandins and thromboxane. LOX action gives rise to leukotrienes, hydroxyeicosatetraenoic acids (HETEs), and lipoxins.

Eicosanoids

The bioactivities of the eicosanoids are listed in Table 2-3.

- The products of COX and LOX activities are collectively called the eicosanoids (from the Greek *eikosi*, meaning 20, because they contain 20 carbon atoms).
- Eicosanoids are synthesized by many cells, especially the leukocytes, and have a wide range of actions linked to defense against damage and pathogens.

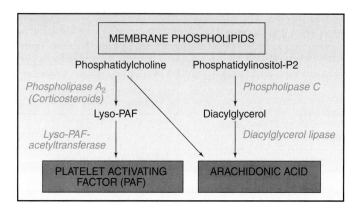

F I G U R E   2-4
The biological response of inflammatory cells is modulated by activating and inhibitory cyclic nucleotides. *TxA*, thromboxane A_2; *Ach*, acetylcholine. **(From Rubin E, Gorstein F, Rubin R, et al. Rubin's Pathology, 4th ed. Philadelphia: Lippincott Williams & Wilkins, 2005, p. 53.)**

- Eicosanoids act locally as paracrines, because they are degraded too rapidly to move about the body through the circulatory system.

Cyclooxygenases
COX-1
- Expressed constantly as a normal part of body functioning
- Found widely in the body
- Especially common in the digestive tract; in the stomach, COX-1 produces prostaglandins that inhibit secretions of stomach acid

COX-2
- Is released mainly by special inflammatory cells
- Expression is induced by various inflammatory paracrines.

Therapeutic Applications
Nonsteroidal Anti-inflammatory Drugs (NSAIDS): inhibitors of COX-1 and COX-2

- Inhibition of COX-1 can produce toxic side effects (erosive gastritis, renal toxicity).
- Inhibition of COX-2 leads to anti-inflammatory effects.

Acetaminophen (an NSAID)

Table 2-3
Bioactivities of the Eicosanoids

Vasodilation	Vaso-constriction	Broncho-dilation	Broncho-constriction	Vascular Permeability	Chemotactic for Neutrophils, Macrophages	Smooth Muscle Contraction
PGE$_2$	TXA$_2$	PGE$_2$	PGF$_{2a}$	LTB$_4$	LTB$_4$	LTC$_4$
PGD$_2$	LTC$_4$	PGD$_2$	TXA$_2$	LTC$_4$	12 HETE	LTD$_4$
PGI$_2$	LTD$_4$	PGI$_2$	LTC$_4$	LTD$_4$	LX (inhibits chemotaxis of neutrophils and eosinophils, but promotes chemotaxis of macrophages)	LTE$_4$
PGF$_2$	LTE$_4$		LTD$_4$	LTE$_4$		TXA$_2$
	12 HETE		LTE$_4$	PGE, PGF		PGH$_2$

HETEs, hydroxyeicosatetraenoic acids; LT, leukotrienes; PG, prostaglandins; PGI$_2$, prostacyclin; SRS-A, slow-reacting substance of anaphylaxis—a mixture of LTs; TX, thromboxanes.; PG and TX are prostanoids.

- Suppresses pain and fever
- Has relatively little effect on inflammation and the secretion of stomach acid

Aspirin

- Initiates the synthesis of aspirin-triggered lipoxins (15-epi-LXs), which are anti-inflammatory, and inhibits COX enzymes
- Low doses can inhibit platelet blood clotting.

Glucocorticoids

- Often used as powerful anti-inflammatory drugs
- Repress the expression of COX-2
- Induce synthesis of phospholipase A_2 inhibitor
- Block release of arachidonic acid

Polyunsaturated Fats (e.g., omega-3 fatty acids)

- Compete with linoleic acid in the arachidonic acid pathway
- Inhibit inflammation by reducing the metabolism of arachidonic acid

Platelet-activating Factor

As its name implies, platelet-activating factor (PAF) stimulates platelets and induces platelet aggregation and degranulation. It is a potent vasodilator, and its actions lead to increases in vascular permeability. PAF is synthesized by almost all activated inflammatory cells, endothelial cells, and injured tissue cells.

- As in arachidonic acid metabolism, the cell membrane enzyme initially involved in PAF formation is phospholipase A_2.
- PAF can function in a paracrine, endocrine, or juxtacrine fashion.

Cytokines

Cytokines are cell-derived polypeptides that affect the behavior of other cells. Most cells can produce cytokines, although they differ in their cytokine repertoire. Many cytokines are produced at inflammation sites.

- **Interleukins (ILs):** cytokines produced by leukocytes
- **Interferons (IFNs)**: cytokines that induce cells to resist viral replication
- **TNF**: produced by macrophages and T cells; may be cytotoxic
- **Granulocyte-macrophage colony stimulating factor:** growth factor for macrophages, granulocytes and endothelial cells
- **Chemokines**: small chemoattractant proteins that stimulate the migration and activation of granulocytes and lymphocytes

Cytokines and Macrophages

Macrophages are pivotal cells in controlling the inflammatory response in tissues. Activated macrophages produce an array of cytokines (Table 2-4). Macrophage activators include:

- Lipopolysaccharide (LPS), a molecule derived from the outer membrane of gram-negative bacteria, is one of the most potent stimuli of macrophages.
- IFN-γ, made by T lymphocytes and natural killer (NK) cells, is another macrophage activator.
- NK cells are lymphocyte-like cells with large cytoplasmic granules capable of lysing cells containing certain intracellular viruses. The production of IL-12 and TNF-α by macrophages stimulates NK cells to produce INF-γ, which stimulates the production of more macrophages.

Chemokines

Chemokines are a large family of cytokines that are the major mediators of leukocyte migration. Chemokines immobilized on activated vascular endothelial cells contribute to leukocyte adherence to the endothelial surface, whereas soluble chemokines in the extravascular tissue establish a gradient of increasing concentration facilitating leukocyte migration to the site of injury.

There are two major chemokine subfamilies:

- CC chemokines, in which the two amino terminal cysteine residues are adjacent
- CXC chemokines, in which the two amino terminal cysteine residues are separated by one amino acid.

Most CXC chemokines are chemoattractants for neutrophils, whereas CC chemokines generally attract monocytes, lymphocytes, basophils, and eosinophils.

Table 2-4	
Macrophage-derived Cytokines	
Cytokine	**Function**
TNF-α	Endothelial cell-leukocyte adhesion; can trigger or inhibit apoptosis
IL-8	Leukocyte recruitment
IL-6, IL-1	Acute phase response
IL-1, IL-6, IL-12	Immune functions

Chemokines are especially implicated in diseases with pronounced inflammatory components, such as rheumatoid arthritis, ulcerative colitis, Crohn disease, chronic bronchitis, asthma, multiple sclerosis, systemic lupus erythematosus, and vascular diseases such as atherosclerosis. In addition, chemokines may block entry of the AIDS virus (HIV-1) into cells. Receptors for some of the CC chemokines can act as coreceptors for the entry of the AIDS virus into human T cells; thus, chemokines might competitively block entry of HIV-1 by binding to the chemokine receptor, thus displacing HIV-1, and interfering with the cell-to-cell spread of the AIDS virus. For example, different HIV-1 viruses use either CCR5 or CXCR4 as chemokine co-receptors (along with CD4) to enter and infect T cells. People with mutations in these receptors have a very low risk of infection with HIV, because the virus cannot enter the T cells.

Reactive Oxygen Species

Reactive oxygen species (ROS) are chemically reactive molecules derived from oxygen. When generated inappropriately, they can activate pathways leading to oxidative stress (see Chapter 1).

Neurokinins and Injury at Nerve Terminals

Neurokinins are a family of peptides distributed throughout the central and peripheral nervous systems. They increase during inflammation, and can produce further mediators of inflammation. The family includes substance P, neurokinin A, and neurokinin B.

Stress Proteins That Protect against Inflammatory Injury

When cells are subjected to stress conditions, they increase production of a family of stress proteins called heat shock proteins. As molecular chaperones, heat shock proteins confer resistance to damaged and misfolded proteins by preventing protein denaturation and facilitating the refolding of already damaged proteins. Stress proteins are upregulated during inflammation, and are associated with protection against some of the damaging effects of inflammation. They suppress proinflammatory cytokines, increase nitric oxide-mediated cytoprotection, and enhance healing by stimulating collagen synthesis.

Extracellular Matrix Mediators

Body cells surround themselves with the extracellular matrix (ECM) specific to a given tissue. The structural components of the

ECM include glycoproteins, collagens, elastic fibers, and proteoglycans. Matricellular proteins do not function as structural components of the ECM but act as adaptors and modulators of cell-matrix interactions. Thus, they can regulate the tissue response to inflammation.

Matricellular proteins include:

- SPARC (secreted protein acidic and rich in cysteine): affects cell proliferation, migration, differentiation; acts as a counteradhesive, especially on endothelial cells.
- Thrombospondin: a secreted glycoprotein that modulates cell-matrix interactions, influences platelet aggregation, and supports neutrophil chemotaxis and adhesion
- Tenascins: counteradhesive proteins expressed during development, tissue injury, and wound healing
- Syndecans: transmembrane heparan sulfate proteoglycans, which mediate interactions of cells with their microenvironment
- Osteopontin (OPN): a phosphoprotein secreted by osteoblasts that is important in bone mineralization; a major cell- and hydroxyapatite-binding protein

Cellular Activity during Inflammation

Two major classes of cells interact in acute inflammation:

- Inflammatory cells derived from bone marrow progenitors, such as the leukocytes and platelets. Leukocytes most prominent in acute inflammation include neutrophils, monocytes, eosinophils, and basophils (Fig. 2-5).
- Tissue cells, such as endothelial cells, mast cells, and macrophages. Resident tissue macrophages are derived from monocytes that have migrated out of the blood.

Cells of Inflammation
Neutrophils
Hallmarks of acute inflammation:

- Originate in bone marrow from myelocyte progenitors
- Contain two main types of granules and a multilobed nucleus
- When activated, they migrate out of blood into the tissues, where they phagocytose invading microbes and dead tissue. They do not return to the blood.

Potentially damaging mediators are released from granules of activated neutrophils, and tissue injury may occur in the process of protection. Most neutrophil mediators function in the phagoly-

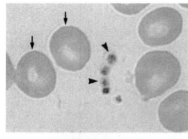

1. Red Blood Cells

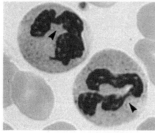

2. Neutrophils

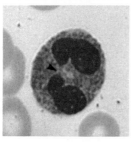

3. Eosinophils

FIGURE 2-5

Cells derived from bone marrow progenitors. (Pictured cells are human, X 1325.) (*1*) Red blood cells. Red blood cells (*arrows*) display a central clear region that represents the thinnest area of the biconcave disc. Platelets (*arrowheads*) possess a central dense region and a peripheral light region. (*2*) Neutrophils. Neutrophils display a somewhat granular cytoplasm and lobulated (arrowheads) nuclei. (*3*) Eosinophils. Eosinophils are recognized by their large pink granules and bilobed nucleus. The slender connecting link (*arrowhead*) between the two nuclear lobes can sometimes be distinguished. (*continues*)

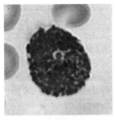

4. Basophils

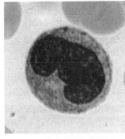

5. Monocytes

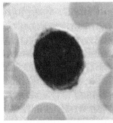

6. Lymphocytes

FIGURE 2-5

(*continued*) (*4*) *Basophils.* **Basophils are characterized by their dense, dark, large granules that often occlude the nucleus. (5) Monocytes. Monocytes are characterized by their large size, acentric, kidney-shaped nucleus, and pale cytoplasm with a "ground-glass" appearance. (6) Lymphocytes. Lymphocytes are small cells that possess a single, large nucleus and a narrow rim of light blue cytoplasm. (From Gartner, LP, and Hiatt, JL. Color Atlas of Histology, 3rd ed., Lippincott Williams & Wilkins, 2000, p. 95)**

sosomes; however, some can be released outside the cell to kill extracellular pathogens and also cause tissue damage (Fig. 2-6).

Monocyte/Macrophages

- Accumulate at sites of acute inflammation in response to inflammatory mediators; also important in maintenance of a chronic inflammatory state
- Have single-lobed and kidney-shaped nucleus

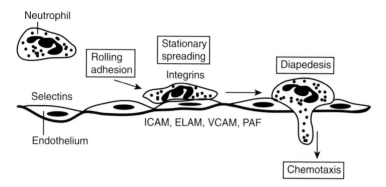

F I G U R E   2-6
Neutrophil recruitment from blood to injury site. Selectins on the surface of endothelial cells and neutrophils cause the leukocyte to slow down and be tethered to the endothelium. Integrins promote the binding of neutrophils to the ICAM, ELAM, VCAM, and PAF on endothelium. Eventually, neutrophils migrates into the tissue, guided to the injury site by chemotactic factors. (ELAM, endothelial-leukocyte CAM; ICAM, intercellular adhesion molecule; VCAM, vascular CAM.)

- Migrate out of blood to become resident tissue macrophages
- Activated tissue macrophages phagocytose microbes, debris
- Macrophages can process and present antigen to lymphocytes
- Produce bactericidal and proinflammatory mediators

Eosinophils

- Involved in defense against parasites; associated with allergic reactions
- Usually have a bilobed nucleus
- Contain large, eosinophilic granules, relatively uniform in size
- Circulate in blood; recruited to tissue in a manner similar to neutrophils
- Produce major basic protein and cationic proteins

Basophils

- Cellular sources of vasoactive mediators, particularly in response to allergens
- Rarest of blood leukocytes
- Contain large blue-staining granules of varying size
- Have receptors for IgE on their surface; binding of antigen specific to the surface IgE causes release of granules containing inflammatory mediators such as histamine and heparin; de-

granulation may also be induced by physical agonists, such as cold and trauma

Platelets

- Small, anucleate membrane-bounded cytoplasmic fragments derived from bone marrow megakaryocytes. They play a primary role in the initiation and regulation of clot formation. Platelets contain granules rich in serotonin, histamine, coagulation proteins, and platelet-derived growth factor (PDGF).
- Platelet adherence, aggregation, and degranulation occur following vascular injury exposing the ECM
- Activation of platelets results in increased vascular permeability

Mast Cells

- Tissue cells with appearance and functions similar to those of basophils
- Especially prevalent along mucosal surfaces of the lung, gastrointestinal tract, skin dermis, and microvasculature
- Products play an important role in vascular permeability and bronchial smooth muscle tone, especially in allergic hypersensitivity reactions

Endothelial Cells

- Flattened cells lining blood vessels and lymphatics
- Maintain vessel patency and blood flow by the production of antithrombotic agents
- Regulate vascular tone through the production of vasodilators and vasoconstrictors
- Injured endothelium leads to a local procoagulant signal. Important inflammatory mediators of endothelium are:

  - ➤ Nitric oxide: vasodilation; inhibits platelet aggregation
  - ➤ Endothelins: induce prolonged vasoconstriction
  - ➤ Arachidonic acid-derived constriction and relaxing factors
  - ➤ Anticoagulants that inactivate the coagulation cascade (see Chapter 10)
  - ➤ Fibrinolytic factors such as tissue-type plasminogen activator
  - ➤ Prothrombic agents such as von Willebrand factor

Common Intracellular Pathways for Inflammatory Cell Activation

G Protein Pathway

Many inflammatory mediators use receptors of the G protein family (guanine nucleotide-binding family) to produce intracellular signaling.

Tumor Necrosis Factor Receptor Pathway

TNF is a cytokine produced primarily by macrophages. It reacts with cell surface receptors resulting in a multiprotein-signaling complex at the cell membrane. Depending on cell conditions, this complex can either lead to or inhibit apoptosis.

Janus Kinase-signal Transducer and Activator of Transcription (JAK-STAT) Pathway

Binding of cytokines to their cognate receptor activates specific JAK tyrosine kinases. The activated JAK proteins phosphorylate and activate specific STAT transcription factors. The activated STAT proteins translocate into the nucleus and activate a specific set of genes.

Interactions between Leukocytes and Endothelial Cells

- Inflammatory signals activate endothelial cells to move vesicle-sequestered **selectins** to the cell surface.
- Carbohydrate ligands on the leukocyte surface bind loosely to the exposed endothelial selectins. This slows, but does not stop, leukocyte movement.
- Activated endothelium also expresses **PAF** and immunoglobulin (superfamily)/intercellular adhesion molecule (**ICAM)** on its surface.
- PAF activates leukocyte **integrins** that then bind tightly to endothelial ICAMs.
- Integrin/ICAM binding→firm adhesion of the leukocyte to the endothelial surface (leukocyte stops rolling).
- Leukocyte migrates out of the blood into the surrounding tissue, and chemotactic factors lead it along a chemical gradient to the injury site (Fig. 2-7).

Adhesion Molecules

Selectins

Bind carbohydrates; initiate leukocyte-endothelial interaction

- P-selectin: in platelet α-granules and endothelium Weibel-Palade bodies
- E-selectin: on activated endothelium
- L-selectin: lymphocyte "homing receptor" also on other leukocytes

Integrins

Integrins bind strongly to cell adhesion molecules and to the ECM; they can be found on a variety of leukocytes.

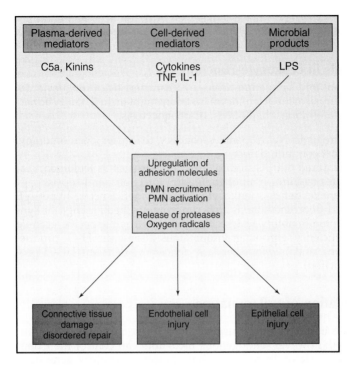

F I G U R E   2-7
**Leukocyte-mediated inflammatory injury, showing polymorphonu-
clear leukocyte activation. (From Rubin E, Gorstein F, Rubin R, et
al. Rubin's Pathology, 4th ed. Philadelphia: Lippincott Williams &
Wilkins, 2005, p. 72.)**

Addressins

- Mucinlike glycoproteins with the sialyl-Lewis X moiety; bind
  the lectin domain of selectins
- Expressed on surface of leukocytes and specific endothelial
  cells
- Addressins such as GlyCAM are expressed mainly on endothelium and bind selectins. The interactions of GlyCAM and L-
  selectin are involved in the exit of lymphocytes from the blood
  into lymphoid tissues,

Immunoglobulin Superfamily Cell Adhesion Molecules

- ICAM-1: on activated endothelium
- ICAM-2: on resting endothelium
- VCAM-1 (vascular CAM): on activated endothelium

- ELAM-1 (endothelial-leukocyte CAM): on activated endothelium

Defects in Leukocyte Function

Frequent and severe infections are characteristic of leukocyte defects. Impairment of leukocyte function might include faulty adherence, emigration, chemotaxis, or phagocytosis.

- Iatrogenic Neutropenia secondary to cancer chemotherapy; most common defect
- Acquired defects: accompany diseases such as leukemia, diabetes mellitus, malnutrition, viral infections, and sepsis
- Genetic defects: leukocyte adhesion deficiencies, hyper-IgE and poor chemotaxis (Job syndrome), Chediak-Higashi syndrome (inability to lyse bacteria), neutrophil-specific granule deficiency, chronic granulomatous disease (no H_2O_2 production), and myeloperoxidase deficiency (deficient HOCl production)

Regulation of Inflammation

Intense inflammatory injury can lead to organ failure if left unchecked; however, endogenous mediators can control the extent of injury. Many do so by inhibiting proinflammatory gene transcription.

- Interleukins (6,10,11,12,13): reduce production of TNF-α (a powerful proinflammatory cytokine)
- Protease inhibitors decrease connective tissue damage.
- Lipoxins (especially aspirin-triggered lipoxins) inhibit leukotriene biosynthesis.
- Secretion of glucocorticoids can have immunosuppressive effects.
- Kininases degrade bradykinin (a potent pro-inflammatory mediator).
- Phosphatases can play a role in preventing inflammatory cell activation because protein phosphorylation is important in signal transduction.

Outcomes of Acute Inflammation

- **Resolution:** Ideally, the inflammatory state is resolved by elimination of the injury source and restoration of normal tissue structure and function. Leukocyte influx stops, cell and tissue debris is removed, blood vessels, epithelium and ECM repaired.

- **Abscess:** When tissue destroyed by neutrophil products is walled off, an abscess is formed, containing dead tissue cells and neutrophils (pus).
- **Scar:** Irreversible tissue injury can result in replacement of normal tissue by a scar.
- **Lymphadenitis:** Lymph nodes draining the injured area can become enlarged with increased numbers of cortical follicles and sinus phagocytes.
- **Resolution failure:** Persistence of the inflammatory reaction can result in a prolonged acute response or more commonly in chronic inflammation.

Chronic Inflammation

Chronic inflammation may be due to a failure to completely eliminate the pathological insult, or it may result from an immune response to a foreign antigen. The events leading to chronic inflammation resemble those of acute inflammation and include injurious triggers, activation of complement and coagulation cascades, recruitment of inflammatory cells, and varying degrees of fibrosis.

Cells Involved in Chronic Inflammation

Monocyte/Macrophages

Monocytes exit the blood and differentiate into tissue macrophages which function as sources of inflammatory and immunological mediators. They generate enzymes, which are active in tissue destruction. For example, in emphysema, resident macrophages generate elastases, which destroy alveolar walls (Fig. 2-8).

T Lymphocytes and B Lymphocytes

T and B cells perform vital functions in both humoral and cell-mediated immune responses. T cells produce a large variety of lymphokines, some of which are proinflammatory. B cells, when stimulated by antigen, differentiate into plasma cells that produce antibodies to specific antigens at sites of chronic inflammation (see Chapter 4).

Dendritic Cells

These cells can phagocytose and present antigen to T cells, resulting in T-cell activation. They are present in inflamed tissue during chronic inflammation.

Fibroblasts

Although mainly involved in maintaining normal connective tissue environment, fibroblasts can be activated to produce inflammatory

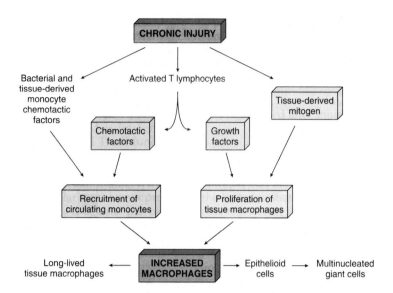

F I G U R E   2-8
Accumulation of macrophages in chronic inflammation. (From Rubin E, Gorstein F, Rubin R, et al. Rubin's Pathology, 4th ed. Philadelphia: Lippincott Williams & Wilkins, 2005, p. 76.)

mediators. In chronic inflammation, fibroblast activity can result in overabundant and disordered connective tissue and ECM.

Acute Inflammatory Cells

Although neutrophils are the prominent players in acute inflammation, they can be present in chronic inflammation in response to ongoing infection and tissue damage. Eosinophils are particularly conspicuous in chronic inflammation involving allergic-type reactions and parasitic infections.

Injury and Repair in Chronic Inflammation

Although the ultimate ideal outcome of inflammation is a restoration of normal architecture and function of the injured tissue, substances produced during a prolonged inflammatory response can lead to altered tissue architecture and tissue disfunction. Altered repair mechanisms that prevent resolution include:

- Ongoing proliferation of epithelial cells can result in metaplasia (e.g., goblet cell metaplasia in the bronchi of smokers and asthmatics).

- Fibroblast proliferation can lead to displacement of functional tissue cells.
- Elastin degradation of ECM components can lead to emphysema.
- Altered ECM can be chemoattractant to inflammatory cells.

Granulomatous Inflammation

Granulomatous inflammation is a mechanism whereby the body deals with certain "indigestible" bacteria, fungi, or foreign particles (Fig. 2-9). Principal cells involved in granulomatous inflammation are discussed in the following text.

Macrophages

Macrophages can sequester noxious agents intracellularly for relatively long periods. They are recruited and activated by local chemotactic factors and lymphokines. When recruited and filled with indigestible material, they lose motility and transform into epithelioid histiocytes (large tissue macrophages). Nodular collections of histiocytes form granulomas. Eventually, the cytoplasmic fusion of macrophages forms multinucleated giant cells:

- Langhans giant cell: peripheral nuclei arranged in a horseshoe pattern
- Foreign body giant cell: a term used when an ingested agent is identified in a histiocyte

Lymphocytes

- Activated lymphocytes secrete lymphokines that regulate macrophage activity
- Frequently surround granulomas
- May mount a cell-mediated immune response to the noxious agent

Eosinophils and Fibroblasts

These may also be associated with granulomas.

Chronic Inflammation and Malignancy

Several infectious diseases are associated with the development of malignancy. The environment created by chronic inflammation is conducive to the promotion of malignant tumors.

- HIV-AIDS is associated with lymphomas and Kaposi sarcoma.
- Schistosomiasis can lead to cancer of the urinary bladder.
- Chronic viral hepatitis is associated with liver cancer.

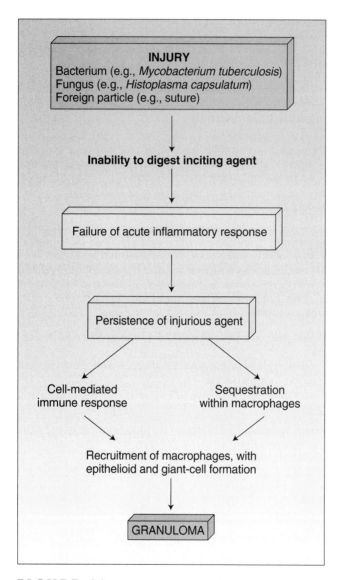

FIGURE 2-9
Mechanism of granuloma formation. (From Rubin E, Gorstein F, Rubin R, et al. Rubin's Pathology, 4th ed. Philadelphia: Lippincott Williams & Wilkins, 2005, p. 79.)

- Noninfectious inflammation (e.g., chronic bronchitis, emphysema, esophagitis, inflammatory bowel disease) often leads to an increased incidence of cancer.

Systemic Manifestations of Inflammation

- **Leukocytosis** is manifested by an increase in the number of circulating leukocytes.
- **Leukopenia** is manifested by a decrease in the circulating white cell count; it is especially encountered in chronic debilitation.
- **Acute phase response** is a physiological response characterized by changes in the plasma levels of acute phase proteins. These proteins are mostly made by the liver and released in large numbers during an acute inflammatory challenge (Table 2-5).
- **Fever** is the clinical hallmark of inflammation. It can be caused by exogenous pyrogens released by bacteria, viruses, or injured cells. Endogenous pyrogens, namely the cytokines and interferons released mainly by macrophages, can also cause fever.
- **Pain** receptors (nociceptors) are stimulated by mediators of inflammation, especially bradykinin, and cytokines such as TNF-α, IL-1, IL-6, and IL-8.

Table 2-5
Acute Phase Proteins

Protein	Function
Mannose-binding protein	Opsonization/complement activation
C-reactive protein	Opsonization
α_1-Antitrypsin	Serine protease inhibitor
Haptoglobin	Binds hemoglobin
Ceruloplasmin	Antioxidant, binds copper
Fibrinogen	Coagulation
Serum amyloid A protein	Apolipoprotein
α_2-Macroglobulin	Antiprotease
Cysteine protease inhibitor	Antiprotease

From Rubin E, Gorstein F, Rubin R, et al. Rubin's Pathology, 4th ed. Philadelphia: Lippincott Williams & Wilkins, 2005, p. 81.

- **Shock** is characterized by an acute disruption of circulatory function leading to inadequate delivery of nutrients to the tissues. It is a most severe systemic manifestation of inflammation. It may occur as the result of massive tissue injury or infection that has spread to the blood (sepsis). In shock, significant quantities of inflammatory mediators may be generated in the circulation. These have effects on the heart and peripheral vascular system causing cardiovascular decompensation.

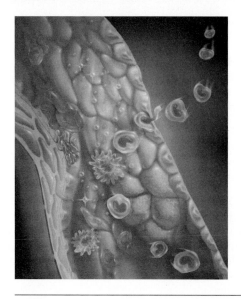

CHAPTER 3

Repair, Regeneration, and Fibrosis

Chapter Outline

Basic Processes of Wound Healing

Three key cellular mechanisms are necessary for wound healing:

- Cell migration
- Extracellular matrix organization and remodeling
- Cell proliferation

Cell Migration

Cell migration is initiated and facilitated when chemical and cytokine mediators increase small vessel permeability. Factors such as kinins, prostaglandins, cytokines, and platelet-derived growth factor cause the release of cellular chemoattractants (Fig. 3-1). Neutrophils arrive first at the injury site. They ingest and kill bacteria, and their released granule contents degrade and destroy damaged tissue.

- Macrophages arrive after neutrophils and remain longer at the site. They also phagocytose debris and dead bacteria. In addition, they release cytokines and chemoattractants for later cell arrivals.
- Later arrivals, such as fibroblasts, myofibroblasts and pericytes, arrive for synthesis of connective tissue matrix as well as tissue remodeling. T lymphocytes also appear and contribute to the healing process.
- Endothelial cells, released from their basement membranes and responding to growth factors, proceed to form new capillaries at the wound site.
- Lastly, epithelial cells detach themselves from the wound borders to bridge the break in the wound surface.

Extracellular Matrix Organization and Remodeling

The extracellular matrix (ECM) is modified in wound healing and consists of basement membranes and the stromal matrix (underlying connective tissue). At injury sites, a provisional matrix forms and associates with the preexisting stromal matrix to stop blood and fluid loss. The preexisting extracellular stromal matrix includes several substances.

Collagen

Collagen is the major protein of the ECM. Collagen molecules are trimers composed of α chains arranged as triple-stranded helixes. The amino acids have a repeating sequence: Gly-X-Y, where the X is most often proline and the Y is most often hydroxyproline. About 25 different α chains have been identified, each encoded by a different gene; different combinations of these genes are expressed in different tissues (Table 3-1). After being secreted, collagen triple helices are assembled into fibrils, which can then aggregate into cable-like collagen fibers.

Reduced, or abnormal collagen synthesis results in failed wound healing. Excess collagen deposition leads to fibrosis, which is the basis of connective tissue diseases such as:

- Scleroderma (autoimmune disease)
- Keloids (collagenous nodules)
- Chronic liver and kidney damage

1. Leukocyte migration

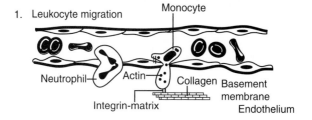

2. Migrating fibroblasts

Integrin-ICAM

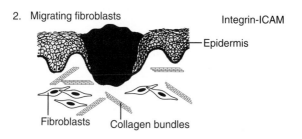

3. Endothelial migration-Angiogenesis

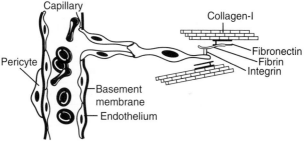

4. Reepithelialization-migrating epithelium

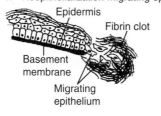

FIGURE 3-1
Cell migrations during repair. (Modified from Rubin E, Gorstein F, Rubin R, et al. Rubin's Pathology, 4th ed. Philadephia: Lippincott Williams & Wilkins, 2005, p. 87.)

Table 3-1
Distribution of Collagen Families

Type	Family	Distribution
Fibrillar: Triple helices self-associate to form banded fibrils		
	I	Bone, tendons ligaments, skin, dentin
	II	Hyaline cartilage, vitreous body
	III	Skin, blood vessels
	V	Placenta, synovial membranes
	XI	Hyaline cartilage
Sheet-forming: Polymerize into sheets		
	IV	Basement membranes
	VIII	Corneal membrane
	X	Hypertrophic cartilage
Connecting and anchoring		
	VI	Vessels, skin, intervertebral disks
	VII	Epidermal-dermal junction
	IX	Hyaline cartilage, vitreous body
	XII	Fetal tendon, skin
	XIV	Fetal tendon, skin
	XVIII	Basal lamina

- Inherited disorders of collagen synthesis, secretion and degradation (Ehlers-Danlos syndromes and osteogenesis imperfecta (see Chapter 6)

Elastin

Elastin allows tissues to bend, stretch, and recoil. It is the main component of elastic fibers. Elastic fibers have an elastin core decorated by microfibrillar proteins; mutations in the gene for one of these proteins, fibrillin, result in Marfan's syndrome.

Elastic fibers are particularly prominent in the connective tissue of the skin, artery walls, and lung. Elastin is not well repaired in skin and lung tissue, but in injured arterial walls, it can be repaired with rapid reformation of the elastic lamellae.

Matrix Glycoproteins

Matrix glycoproteins act as mediators between cells and the ECM, and have binding sites for components of the ECM as well as for cell surface receptors such as the integrins.

- Laminin: important constituent of basement membranes; binds to epithelial integrin and collagen VII; mutations in laminin, integrin or collagen VII ⇒ epidermolysis bullosa (a skin blistering disease)
- Fibronectin: an extracellular protein that exists in two forms:
  1. An insoluble dimer made by a number of ECM cells that serves to link matrix molecules to each other and to cells
  2. A soluble plasma dimer synthesized by hepatocytes. The major cell-binding domain contains an RGD motif (arg-gly-asp), which binds to integrins. This motif is also found in other adhesive glycoproteins.

Glycosaminoglycans and Proteoglycans

Glycosaminoglycans (GAGs) are long polysaccharides made up of repeating disaccharide units. Except for hyaluronan, GAGs are posttranslational modifications of proteoglycans. Proteoglycans are long polysaccharide chains linked to a protein core. Hyaluronan (formerly called hyaluronic acid) differs from other GAGs in that it is not a posttranslational modification of a protein nor modified postsynthetically.

Functions of GAGs and proteoglycans:

- May promote or inhibit cell motility or adhesion
- May provide signals for organizing connective tissue fibers
- Modulate the availability and actions of growth factors

Remodeling

Remodeling takes place in the later stages of repair and is carried out by digestive enzymes, which cleave components of the extracellular matrix, thus allowing cells to migrate into the provisional matrix. The metalloproteinases (**MMPs**), which are Zn-dependent endopeptidases, are the main degradative enzymes important in wound healing.

Cell Proliferation

Following the initial cell migration and matrix remodeling, the proliferative phase of wound healing begins. It is characterized by the formation of granulation tissue, which includes cells such as fibroblasts and myofibroblasts as well as new capillaries, all embedded in a loose extracellular matrix. The cellular components of granulation tissue are derived from the proliferation and differentiation of nearby cells, as well as from cells, which have migrated into the area. All this activity results from autocrine and paracrine signals from growth factors and chemokines in the granulation tissue. The key cellular receptors responding to these signals include:

- Protein tyrosine kinase receptors for peptide growth factors
- G protein–coupled receptors for chemokines
- Integrin receptors for extracellular matrix factors

Capillary buds sprout from nearby blood vessels, begin to branch, and eventually form a plexus through which blood will flow.

Repair

The sequence of wound healing in the skin generally parallels healing within hollow viscera and is used here as a model of repair (see Fig. 3-1).

- In the early stage of repair, a thrombus forms from plasma fibrin; the fibronectin within is soon cross-linked. The clot serves as a growth-factor–rich barrier with significant tensile strength. Neutrophils appear and remove necrotic debris and bacteria. Macrophages soon follow and process cell remnants and damaged extracellular matrix. Their activities generate chemoattractants to recruit a variety of cells to the wound site. Proteolytic enzymes loosen matrix proteins, facilitating the migration of epidermal cells to the margin of the wound. Keratinocytes form a confluent layer over the wound site, attach to the basement membrane, and resume their normal phenotype. Epithelium is thus newly formed.
- Granulation tissue forms in the mid-stages of repair. It is rich in proteoglycans, glycoproteins, and type III collagen, and it is highly vascular and edematous. Contraction of the wound site is mediated by fibroblasts and actin-containing myofibroblasts which link to collagen and to each other.
- In the late stage of repair, type I collagen replaces type III collagen, and its cross-linking results in permanent tensile strength of the tissue. Finally, the wound site devascularizes and conforms to stress lines n the skin.
- Numerous factors from numerous sources effect wound repair (Table 3-2).

Conditions That Affect Repair

Location of a wound, blood supply to the wound, and systemic factors such as coagulation defects or anemia, all affect the extent and effectiveness of wound repair.

Table 3-2

Signals in Wound Repair

Phase	Factor(s)	Sources	Effects
Coagulation	XIIIA TGF-α, TGF-β, PDGF, ECGF	Plasma Platelets	Thrombosis Chemoattraction of subsequently involved cells
Inflammation	TGF-β	Neutrophil	Attracts monocyte/macrophages and fibroblasts, differentiates fibroblasts
Granulation tissue formation	Basic FGF, TGF-β	Monocyte/ macrocyte, then fibroblasts	Various factors are bound to proteoglycan matrix
Angiogenesis	VEGFs	Monocyte/ macrocyte	Development of blood vessels
Contraction	TGF-β_1, TGF-β_2	Various	Myofibroblasts appear, bind to each other and collagen, and contract
Maturation-arrest of proliferation	TGF-β_1	Platelets, monocyte/macrophages	Accumulation of extracellular matrix
	Heparin sulfate proteoglycan, decorin	Secretory fibroblasts	Capture of TGF-β and basic FGF
	Interferon	Plasma monocytes	Suppresses proliferation of fibroblasts and accumulation of collagen
	Increased local oxygen	Repair process	Suppresses release of cytokines
Remodeling	PDGF-FGF	Platelets, fibroblasts	Induction of MMPs
	Matrix metallo- proteinases, t-PAs, u-PAs	Sprouted capillaries, epithelial cells	Remodeling by permitting ingrowth of vessels and restructuring of extracellular matrix
	Tissue inhibitors of metallopro- teinases	Local, not further defined	Balance the effects of MMPs in the evolving repair site

- Skin: A wound with closely apposed edges results in formation of a small scar and the repair process is termed **"healing by primary intention."** However, a gouged wound with substantial tissue loss results in a large scar and **"healing by secondary intention."**
- Liver: Although mitotic figures are rarely seen in individual hepatocytes, the organ itself, when not too severely scarred (cirrhotic) has remarkable regenerative capacity. In human liver transplants, partial donation of the right lobe of the liver is followed by complete regeneration of normal liver in both the recipient and the donor.
- Kidney: Regenerative capacity of renal tissue is maximal in cortical tubules, less in medullary tubules, and nonexistent in glomeruli.
- Lung: The degree of cell necrosis and the extent of damage to the ECM determine the outcome. Superficial injury to the trachea and bronchi heal by regeneration from adjacent epithelium. If the basement membrane of alveoli is relatively undamaged, regeneration mediated by type II pneumocytes occurs. Extensive damage to alveolar basement membrane, such as occurs in emphysema, leads to ineffective replacement of elastin and destruction of alveolar walls.
- Heart: Recent studies indicate that cardiac myocytes can regenerate from stem cells. However, myocardial injury usually results in replacement of myocytes by scar tissue.
- Nervous system: The cell bodies of mature neurons do not regenerate; however, regrowth and reorganization of nerve cell axons can occur after injury.
- Fetus: When corrective surgery is performed in utero, fetal wounds heal without scarring.

Suboptimal Wound Repair

- Deficient scar formation, such as in wound dehiscence (scar splitting open), incisional hernia, and ulceration, can occur because of inadequate blood supply.
- Excessive scar formation can occur, such as keloid, in which scarring progresses beyond the site of original injury. Dark-skinned persons are more frequently affected.
- Excessive contraction can occur, resulting in deformity of the wound and surrounding tissues, such as in Dupuytren contracture (palmar), Pederhosen disease (plantar), and Peyronie disease (contracture of corpus cavernosum of penis).
- Excessive regeneration can occur. Pyogenic granulomas are characterized by persistent overgrowth of granulation tissue, which lacks nerves and can be trimmed without anesthesia. This may develop in gum tissue in pregnant women and the squamocolumnar junction of the uterine cervix.

Regeneration

The cells of the body can be classified by their proliferative potential. Some mature cells do not divide at all, whereas others complete a cell cycle every 16 to 24 hours.

- Labile cells: found in tissues that are constantly renewing, such as the epidermis, epithelial lining of the gastrointestinal, urinary, respiratory and genital tracts, the bone marrow and lymphoid organs
- Stable cells: found in tissues that normally renew very slowly but are capable of more rapid renewal after injury; examples are the liver, endocrine glands, endothelium, and proximal renal tubules
- Permanent cells: terminally differentiated and have lost the capacity to regenerate; examples are neurons, cardiac muscle cells, and cells of the lens.

Stem cells are constituents of labile tissues. One daughter cell of each division becomes a new stem cell while the other goes on to terminal differentiation. Regeneration can be mediated by stem cells, labile cells, or stable cells.

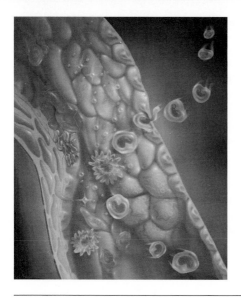

Immunopathology

Chapter Outline

Wiskott-Aldrich Syndrome
Acquired Immunodeficiency Syndrome (AIDS)

Autoimmunity
    Theories of Autoimmunity
    Tissue Injury and Autoimmune Disease
    Systemic Lupus Erythematosus (SLE)
    Lupuslike Diseases
    Sjögren Syndrome
    Scleroderma (Progressive Systemic Sclerosis)
    Polymyositis, Dermatomyositis, and Inclusion Body Myositis
      (IBM)
    Mixed Connective Tissue Disease (MCTD)

Biology of the Immune System

Cellular Components

The cellular components of the immune system are derived from pluripotent hematopoietic stem cells, which separate into two major cell lineages: lymphoid and myeloid. Lymphoid stem cells differentiate into T cells, B cells, and natural killer (NK) cells, whereas the myeloid line differentiates into colony-forming units (CFUs), which eventually give rise to neutrophils and monocytes, eosinophils, basophils, megakaryocytes, mast cells, and erythrocytes.

Lymphocytes

There are three major types of lymphocytes: T cells, B cells, and NK cells. T cells and B cells are central to the control and development of immune responses, and NK cells constitute a group of lymphocytes that have the intrinsic ability to destroy certain virally infected or tumor cells.

T Cells T-cell progenitors originate in the bone marrow but migrate to the thymus, where they acquire their specific receptors and surface markers. The two major classes of T-cell receptors are alpha/beta (α/β) and gamma/delta (γ/δ). These receptors specifically recognize and bind to various antigens. Both receptors are associated with the CD3 complex and together form the T-cell–receptor complex. T cells with the α/β receptor account for 95% of T cells in the circulation and belong to one of two major subsets: the helper T cells (T_H), expressing the surface marker CD4, or the cytotoxic T cells, expressing the surface marker CD8.

- T_H1 cells: produce specific cytokines and function mainly in the activation of macrophages. They are often called inflammatory CD4 T cells.

- T_H2 cells also produce specific cytokines and function mainly in the stimulation of B-cell antibody production.
- CD8 cytotoxic T cells: can kill other cells and are important in host defense against cytosolic pathogens.

B Cells

B cells originate and mature in the adult bone marrow, where they acquire their specific surface antigen-binding receptor, namely, membrane immunoglobulin. This receptor has the same antigen specificity as the soluble immunoglobulin that will be secreted when the B cell encounters its specific antigen.

NK Cells

NK cells are believed to form and mature in both the thymus and the bone marrow. They recognize target cells mainly through antigen-independent mechanisms, although they can occasionally lyse target cells via an antigen-dependent cellular cytotoxicity (ADCC).

Antigen-presenting Cells (APCs)

APCs process antigen and then express it on their surface in a form recognizable by T cells. A variety of cells have the capability of "presenting" antigen to T cells. Typically, protein antigens are degraded intracellularly into peptides, which are then carried to the cell surface bound to major histocompatibility complex (MHC) molecules. T cells can respond to antigen when it is presented in this way. In fact, T-cell receptors recognize antigen only if complexed with self-MHC molecules. This is termed *MHC restriction.*

- Main APCs: tissue macrophages, dendritic cells, and B cells.
- Dendritic cells: spider-like cells found in lymphoid and non-lymphoid tissue. Those in nonlymphoid tissue must be activated by antigen before migrating to lymphoid tissue for T-cell contact. Examples of such cells are the epidermal Langerhans cells.

Lymphocyte Homing and Recirculation

Lymphocytes are motile cells. Mature T cells and B cells are unique among the leukocytes in that they can circulate in the blood, migrate into tissues, and reenter the circulation if they do not encounter their cognate antigen. This lymphocyte trafficking allows small numbers of antigen-specific lymphocytes to move to sites where their specific antigen might be encountered.

Major Histocompatibility Complex (MHC)

The MHC is a cluster of genes found in all mammals and located on human chromosome 6. It encodes a set of membrane glycoproteins known as the MHC antigens. These antigens are also referred to as human leukocyte antigens (HLAs), because they were first identified on leukocytes. The products of the MHC genes are chiefly responsible for the rapid rejection of grafts between individuals and have important functions in signaling between lymphocytes and APCs.

Class I and Class II Histocompatibility Molecules

Class I and Class II histocompatibility molecules are encoded by highly polymorphic genes in regions of the MHC (Fig. 4-1).

- MHC class I molecules: present on almost all cells and platelets; associate with peptides generated in the cytosol of the cell, which are usually viral products of a virally infected cell. The resulting peptide–MHC complex can be recognized by and activate cytotoxic (CD8) T cells, resulting in the killing of the infected cell.
- MHC class II molecules: usually present only on APCs; associate with peptides generated from exogenous proteins, which get subsequently degraded in intracellular vesicles of the APC. This resulting peptide–MHC complex can be recognized by and activate helper (CD4) T cells.

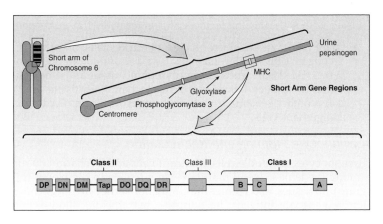

FIGURE 4-1
The highly polymorphic loci that encode Class I and Class II major histocompatibility antigens are located on the short arm of chromosome 6. (Modified from Rubin E, Gorstein F, Rubin R, et al. Rubin E, Gorstein F, Rubin R, et al. Rubin's Pathology, 4th ed. Philadelphia: Lippincott Williams & Wilkins, 2005, p. 128.)

To avoid serious rejection reactions, it is extremely important to predict a good match for a transplant between a donor and recipient. Clinical tissue typing (HLA typing) involves the genetic matching of the HLA (MHC) genes of prospective solid organ, bone marrow, or stem cell donors to recipient patients. Polymorphisms in the HLA genes are carefully compared between donor and recipient to determine the appropriateness of the transplant.

Immune Response

The prime purpose of an immune response is to protect the body against invasion by foreign material; however, in certain situations, the protective effects may give rise to tissue damage. An immune response that results in tissue injury is broadly referred to as a "hypersensitivity" reaction. Hypersensitivity reactions are classified according to the type of immune mechanism (Table 4-1). Type I, II, and III hypersensitivity reactions all involve the formation of a specific antibody against a foreign or self-antigen. Type IV reactions do not require the formation of an antibody but instead cause the release of injurious agents by cells that have been antigen activated.

Type I or Immediate Hypersensitivity

The initial causative mechanism in type I hypersensitivity is the formation, in sensitive individuals, of IgE antibody in response to exposure to an allergen (e.g., pollen, animal dander, dust mites). T_H2 cells mediate the formation of IgE antibodies, which bind avidly to receptors on mast cells and basophils. Subsequent exposure to the initiating allergen results in the binding of the allergen to its specific IgE, leading to the release of mast cell and basophil granules containing proinflammatory mediators (Fig. 4-2).

Because the basophil granules are preformed, their release causes immediate biological effects, hence the term "immediate hypersensitivity." However, leukotrienes C4, D4, and E4, known as the slow-reacting substances of anaphylaxis (SRS-As) are important in the second, delayed phase of the reaction, which can start hours after antigenic exposure and can last for days.

Basophils and mast cells can be activated by agents other than antibodies (e.g., certain drugs such as morphine, melittin from a bee sting, exposure to an ice cube, and physical urticaria). Also, as shown in Fig. 4-1, anaphylatoxins such as C3a and C5a can directly stimulate mast cells and basophils. Of the mast cell or basophil granule constituents, the biogenic amine, histamine is the most important effector.

Type II or Non-IgE Antibody-mediated Hypersensitivity Reactions

Type II (or cytotoxic type) hypersensitivity reactions are directly or indirectly cytotoxic through the action of antibodies (mainly

Table 4-1

Modified Gell and Coombs Classification of Hypersensitivity Reactions

Type	Mechanism	Examples
Type I (anaphylactic type): Immediate hypersensitivity	IgE antibody-mediated mast cell activation and degranulation	Hay fever, asthma, hives, anaphylaxis
Type II (cytotoxic type): Cytotoxic antibodies	Non-IgE-mediated Cytotoxic (IgG, IgM) antibodies formed against cell surface antigens' complement usually involved	Physical urticarias Autoimmune hemolytic anemias, Goodpasture disease
	Noncytotoxic antibodies against cell surface receptors	Graves disease
Type III (immune complex type): Immune complex disease	Antibodies (IgG, IgM, IgA) formed against exogenous or endogenous antigens; complement and leukocytes (neutrophils, macrophages) often involved	Autoimmune diseases (SLE, rheumatoid arthritis), many types of glomerulonephritis
Type IV (cell-mediated type): Delayed-type hypersensitivity	Mononuclear cells (T lymphocytes, macrophages) with interleukin and lymphokine production	Granulomatous disease (tuberculosis, sarcoidosis)

From Rubin E, Gorstein F, Rubin R, et al. Rubin's Pathology, 4th ed. Philadelphia: Lippincott Williams & Wilkins, 2005, p.130.

IgG and IgM) directed against fixed antigens on cell surfaces or in connective tissue. Complement participates in many of these cytotoxic events.

- Complement products can directly lyse target cells via the membrane attack complex (MAC; see Chapter 2).

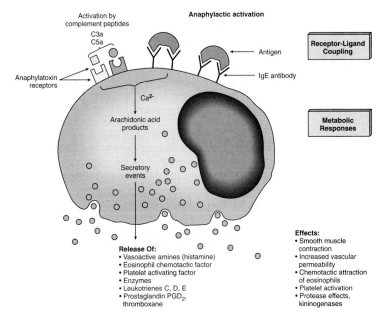

FIGURE 4-2

In a type I hypersensitivity reaction, allergen binds to cytophilic surface IgE antibody on a mast cell or basophil and triggers cell activation and the release of a cascade of proinflammatory mediators. These mediators are responsible for smooth muscle contraction, edema formation, and the recruitment of eosinophils. (From Rubin E, Gorstein F, Rubin R, et al. Rubin's Pathology, 4th ed. Philadelphia: Lippincott Williams & Wilkins, 2005, p. 131.)

- Complement activation can indirectly cause destruction of the target cell by formation of complement opsonin components, C3b or C5b, which coat the target, thus enhancing its phagocytosis.
- Complement can mediate the chemotactic attraction of phagocytic cells, which produce a large variety of tissue-damaging products.
- Some type II reactions are not complement mediated. Target cells may be killed by antibody-activated cytolytic leukocytes, a mechanism termed antibody-dependent cell-mediated cytotoxicity (ADCC).

Some type II reactions lead to impairment of function rather than killing of target cells. Antireceptor antibodies are examples of this:

- Graves disease: autoantibodies against the thyroid-stimulating hormone (TSH) receptor on thyroid follicle cells act as ligands, stimulate the follicle cells independently of TSH, and cause hyperthyroidism.
- Myasthenia gravis: autoantibodies bind to the acetylcholine receptors in the neuromuscular endplate, thus blocking acetyl-choline binding and muscle stimulation. This leads to the mus-cle weakness characteristic of the disease.

Some type II reactions result from formation of antibody against a structural connective tissue component. In Goodpasture syndrome, autoantibody against type IV collagen leads to damage to alveolar and glomerular basement membrane. The mechanism involves formation of complement chemotactic factors that recruit tissue-damaging inflammatory cells (Fig. 4-3).

Type III or Immune Complex Hypersensitivity

Antigen-antibody complexes formed in the circulation and depos-ited in tissues, or in the tissues themselves, are the mediators of injury in type III reactions. The immune complexes activate com-plement; this leads to recruitment and activation of neutrophils and monocytes, which release injurious inflammatory mediators. Immune complexes have been implicated in the pathogenesis of many human diseases.

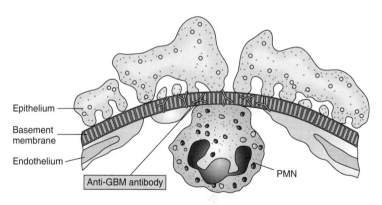

Epithelium

Basement membrane

Endothelium

Anti-GBM antibody

PMN

FIGURE 4-3

In a type II hypersensitivity reaction, antibody binds to a surface antigen, activates the complement system, and leads to the recruit-ment of tissue-damaging inflammatory cells. Several complement-derived peptides (e.g., C5a) are potent chemotactic factors. (From Rubin E, Gorstein F, Rubin R, et al. Rubin's Pathology, 4th ed. Phila-delphia: Lippincott Williams & Wilkins, 2005, p. 135.)

- Systemic lupus erythematosus (SLE): anti-double-stranded DNA deposits found in vasculitic lesions
- Cryoglobulinemic vasculitis: associated with hepatitis C infection
- Henoch-Schönlein purpura: IgA deposits found at vasculitis sites
- Rheumatoid arthritis
- Varieties of glomerulonephritis
- Serum sickness: caused by injection of a foreign protein and characterized by fever, arthralgias, vasculitis, and acute glomerulonephritis
- Arthus reaction: an experimental model of vasculitis in which a localized injury is induced by immune complexes

Type IV or Cell-mediated Hypersensitivity Reactions

Unlike other hypersensitivity reactions, type IV reactions are not antibody mediated. Rather, antigens are processed by macrophages and presented to antigen-specific T cells. The activated T cells then release a variety of mediators to activate additional T cells, as well as macrophages and fibroblasts. The resulting tissue damage is caused by T cells and macrophages. There are two major classes of type IV hypersensitivity reactions.

Delayed-type Hypersensitivity

This type of hypersensitivity peaks in 24 to 48 hours and can be summarized as follows:

- Foreign protein antigens are degraded into peptides by an APC (usually a macrophage) and presented on the cell surface along with class II HLA.
- $CD4^+$ T cells with receptors for the peptide–HLA complex are activated and secrete cytokines such as IL-2, IFN-γ, and TNF-α.
- Cytokines recruit and activate lymphocytes, monocytes, and other inflammatory cells, resulting in tissue damage.
- Elimination of antigenic stimulus results in resolution.
- Persistence of stimulus may lead to granulomatous reaction.

T-cell Cytotoxicity

$CD8^+$ cytotoxic T cells can kill virus-infected cells and tumor cells and play a key role in transplant rejection. This process can be summarized as follows:

- In the case of virus-infected or tumor cells, $CD8^+$ cytotoxic T cells are activated by foreign antigen/class I (self) HLA.
- In transplant rejection, foreign HLA on the transplant are potent activators of $CD8^+$ cytotoxic T cells.
- In both cases, cytotoxic T cells kill the target (Fig. 4-4).

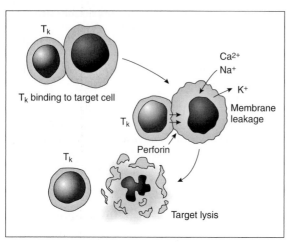

TARGET CELL KILLING
- T-cytotoxic/killer cells
  bind to target cell
- Killing signals perforin
  release and target cell
  loses membrane integrity
- Target cell undergoes
  lysis

FIGURE 4-4
Target cell killing. An activated T_k cell binds to the target cell and delivers perforin (and other lytic compounds). The target cell membrane loses integrity, and the target cell undergoes lysis. (Modified from Rubin E, Gorstein F, Rubin R, et al. Rubin's Pathology, 4th ed. Philadelphia: Lippincott Williams & Wilkins, 2005, p. 139.)

Immune Reactions to Transplanted Tissues

Transplantation of an organ or tissue almost always stimulates an immune response against the transplant. The antigens encoded by the MHC are most critical in stimulating transplant rejection. The greater the MHC difference, the more rapid and severe the rejection; therefore, "tissue typing" is performed before transplantation, in an attempt to match as closely as possible the MHC antigens of donor and recipient.

Transplant Rejection Reactions

There are three categories of transplant rejection reactions.

- Hyperacute rejection occurs within minutes to hours after transplantation and is characterized by a sudden cessation of function with vascular congestion, thrombi, edema, and neutrophilic infiltration. It necessitates prompt surgical removal of the transplant.

- Acute rejection occurs within the first few weeks or months after transplantation and is characterized by infiltrates of lymphocytes and macrophages, edema, and, in severe cases, vasculitis. If detected in its early stages, acute rejection can be reversed with immunosuppressive therapy.

- Chronic rejection occurs months to years after transplantation and is characterized by fibrosis, patchy mononuclear cell infiltrates, and thickened vascular walls. Severe transplant damage results from repeated episodes of rejection, and does not respond well to therapy.

Graft-versus-host Disease (GVHD)

Transplantation of bone marrow cells or stem cells from a donor into a patient who is immunodeficient, or whose immune system has been destroyed by chemotherapy, can result in the complication of graft-versus-host disease. In the tissue or organ transplant rejection reactions, rejection occurs because the recipient's immune system attacks the foreign tissue or organ of the donor. In bone marrow or stem cell transplants, the transplanted cells of the donor attack the "foreign" immune system of the recipient (i.e., the graft attacks the host), and GVHD ensues. GVHD may be acute, developing within the first 3 months and characterized by skin rashes, nausea, and diarrhea, or it may become chronic, affecting the mucous glands of the skin, stomach, and intestines. Treatment of GVHD requires immunosuppressive therapy.

Immune Status Evaluation

If there is clinical suspicion that an immune disorder exists, a number of tests may be performed to measure immune function:

- Electrophoretic measurement of immunoglobulin levels may detect deficiencies of immunoglobulins IgM, IgG, or IgA.
- Serological testing for antibodies against specific antigens can detect specific deficiencies in the B-cell system, even though B-cell levels are normal.
- Measurements of T-cell function

  ➤ Skin testing for delayed-type hypersensitivity to common antigens
  ➤ T-cell proliferative responses to mitogenic stimuli

- Flow cytometry quantitation of B and T cells in peripheral blood

Immunodeficiency Diseases

Deficiencies of B-cell Function
Bruton X-linked Agammaglobulinemia
- Persons affected: male infants at 5 to 8 months of age
- Genetic defect: on the X chromosome; an inactivating mutation in the gene for B-cell tyrosine kinase, an enzyme critical for B-cell maturation
- Characterstics: recurrent bacterial infections due to a lack of mature circulating B cells and plasma cells in tissues as well as very low levels of all immunoglobulin types.

Selective IgA Deficiency
- Persons affected: fairly common in Caucasians (1/700)
- Characteristics: inability to secrete certain IgA subclasses

  ➤ Patients may be asymptomatic or they may present with respiratory or gastrointestinal (GI) infections
  ➤ Patients display a strong predilection for allergies

Common Variable Immunodeficiency (CVID)
CVID consists of a heterogeneous group of disorders.

- Persons affected: both males and females at a mean age onset of 30 years of age
- Characteristics: low gammaglobulin levels, recurrent infections, and a high incidence of malignant disease, especially stomach cancer.

Transient Hypogammaglobulinemia of Infancy
- Characteristics: delayed synthesis of immunoglobulin by infants. Maternal antibodies protect newborns but wane at about 3 months. Due to this paucity of antibodies, some infants develop recurrent infections
- Clinical features: condition usually corrects itself, because infants eventually produce their own antibodies

Hyper-IgM Syndrome
- Pathogenesis: group of defects of immunoglobulin production of which 70% are X-linked. The most common X-linked form of the disease results in a failure to express CD40, a ligand necessary for B-cell isotype switching; hence, maturing B cells fail to class-switch from the more immature IgD/IgM isotypes to IgG and IgA.
- Clinical Features: infants with the X-linked form have an increased risk of infection and an increased tendency to develop

autoimmune hemolytic anemia, thrombocytopenic purpura, and recurrent neutropenia. Serum levels of IgM are high, whereas those of IgG and IgA are low.

Deficiencies of T-cell Function

DiGeorge Syndrome

- Cause: defective embryological development of the third and fourth pharyngeal pouches that give rise to the thymus and parathyroid glands
- Characteristics: cardiac defects, hypocalcemia (due to hypoparathyroidism), small or absent thymuses, and defective T-cell maturation. There is a lack of cell-mediated immunity (against intracellular bacteria and viruses). It may be treated with a thymic transplant.

Chronic Mucocutaneous Candidiasis

This type of candidiasis results from a congenital defect in T-cell function and is characterized by susceptibility to candidal infections. The precise cause of the defect is unknown. It is associated with hypoparathyroidism, Addison disease, and diabetes mellitus.

Combined Immunodeficiency Diseases: Severe Combined Immunodeficiency (SCID)

SCID is part of a heterogeneous group of diseases that reflect disorders of both B-cell and T-cell function. It occurs in both X-linked and autosomal recessive forms.

- X-linked form: the most common defect is due to a mutation of the γ-chain subunit of the IL-2 receptor. This same subunit is also part of receptors for other cytokines important in T-cell and B-cell development.
- Autosomal recessive form: the defect is due to a mutation in the gene which encodes a protein that associates with the same γ-chain subunit. Both mutations lead to defects in T-cell and B-cell development.

SCID is characterized by low immunoglobulin levels, with recurrent viral, bacterial, fungal, and protozoal infections. The thymus is small or absent, and blood lymphocyte counts are low.

Adenosine Deaminase (ADA) Deficiency is an autosomal recessive form of SCID due to mutations in the gene encoding the enzyme, adenosine deaminase. Defective or absent enzyme leads to the accumulation of metabolites toxic to T and B cells.

Purine Nucleoside Phosphorylase Deficiency

This rare immunodeficiency syndrome in which the T-cell count is very low, but B-cell numbers and functions are not affected.

Wiskott-Aldrich Syndrome

This rare X-linked recessive immunodeficiency syndrome is caused by numerous distinct mutations in a gene that encodes a protein, WASP (Wiskott-Aldrich syndrome protein), expressed in high levels in lymphocytes and megakaryocytesbinds to a family of enzymes that control numerous cellular processes.

Wiskott-Aldrich syndrome is characterized by eczema, low platelet count, low IgM levels with recurrent infections (especially by *Streptococcus. pneumoniae* and *Haemophilus influenzae*), and selective deficiencies in cell-mediated immunity. Bone marrow transplantation may be curative.

Acquired Immunodeficiency Syndrome (AIDS)

Human immunodeficiency virus (HIV) causes AIDS. There are two types: HIV-1 and HIV-2. Most patients in the U.S. and Europe are infected with HIV-1. HIV-2 is closely related and is endemic in West Africa. The fundamental lesion is infection of $CD4^+$ helper T cells by HIV, which leads to depletion of this cell population with consequent suppression of cell-mediated and humoral immunity. Other target cells of the AIDS virus (macrophages, dendritic cells, skin Langerhans cells, and neuroglia) all express CD4 on their surface. These cells may serve as storage depots of the virus.

Transmission

Transmission occurs mainly in the following ways:

- Sexual intercourse: both homosexual and heterosexual (heterosexual transmission occurs mainly from male to female rather than from female to male)
- Intravenous drug use
- Transfusion of HIV-infected blood or blood products
- Transmission from HIV infected mother to infant

Pathogenesis

HIV is an enveloped retrovirus containing a reverse transcriptase and two identical RNA strands. Two viral glycoproteins in the outer envelope, gp120 and gp41, are key in entry of the nucleocapsid (uncoated viral particle) into the CD4 T cell. Gp120 binds to the CD4 molecule on the T-cell membrane, allowing gp41 to insert into the membrane, thus promoting internalization of the virus.

The entry of HIV-1 into the target cell requires the viral binding to a coreceptor, β-chemokine receptor 5 (CCR-5). If this target cell chemokine receptor is defective, the virus cannot enter. Interestingly, about 1% of Caucasians are homozygous for major deletions in the *CCR-5* gene and remain uninfected with HIV even with extensive exposure to HIV. Even heterozygosity for the mutant *CCR-5* allele provides partial protection against HIV infection.

Inside the cell, the viral reverse transcriptase copies the viral RNA into double-stranded DNA, which is transported into the nucleus and integrated into the T-cell chromosomal DNA. This integrated viral DNA (provirus) is transcribed by the T-cell, generating genomic viral RNA and mRNA molecules. The T-cell machinery translates the mRNAs into viral glycoproteins and nucleocapsid proteins. Progeny virions then assemble and bud from the plasma membrane of the infected cell as free viruses, or infect another cell via a fusion event, thus disseminating the virus (Fig. 4-5).

Immunologic Response

CD4 helper T cells play critical roles in both the enabling of antibody production by B cells and in the activation of cytotoxic T cells and cell-mediated immunity. Thus, in AIDS, CD4 T-cells are destroyed, and the immune system is severely disabled.

Although antibody production in response to specific antigens is decreased, there is an increased production of nonspecific anti-

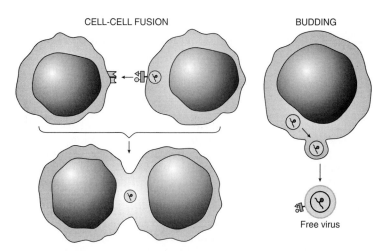

FIGURE   4-5
Viral dissemination to other target cells. To complete the life cycle, virus must spread to other cells and infect them. This is accomplished either by fusion of an infected cell with an uninfected cell (seen on the left) or by budding and release of free virus from the plasma membrane of the infect cell (seen on the right). (Modified From Rubin E, Gorstein F, Rubin R, et al. Rubin's Pathology, 4th ed. Philadelphia: Lippincott Williams & Wilkins, 2005, p. 149.)

bodies, possibly caused by concurrent infections with polyclonal B-cell–activating viruses such as Epstein-Barr virus. Cytotoxic T cells that normally would eliminate B cells infected with Epstein-Barr virus are markedly decreased in AIDS.

NK cell activity is severely decreased, and because NK cells kill virus-infected cells and tumor cells, this defect may contribute to the appearance of tumors and viral infections that plague patients with AIDS.

Some macrophages display surface CD4 and may be infected by HIV. Unlike T cells, macrophages are not killed by the virus but develop impaired phagocytosis and chemotaxis responses.

Defects in T-cell function are manifested by defective responses to skin testing (decreased delayed-type hypersensitivity) and by impaired proliferative response to mitogens and antigens.

Pathology and Clinical Features

A small fraction of Caucasians remain uninfected with HIV even with extensive exposure. This resistance has been ascribed to deletions in the chemokine receptor gene CCR-5, which functions as a coreceptor (along with CD4) for the entry of HIV into the T cell. When this receptor is defective, viral entry cannot occur.

When infection does occur in susceptible individuals, it can be divided into three phases:

- Acute early syndrome: occurs 2 to 3 weeks after exposure; symptoms such as fever, myalgia, enlarged lymph nodes, and rash correlate with viremia; initial symptoms may resolve, depending on the viral load and effectiveness of antiviral cytotoxic T-cell activity; seroconversion (antiviral antibodies) occurs 1 to 10 weeks after onset.
- Latent chronic phase: may last for years; persistent generalized lymphadenopathy may be present; viral replication continues at low level; individuals are infective although they may be asymptomatic; gradual decline in CD4 T-cell counts; as this phase approaches final phase, the CD4 declines to less than $400/mm^2$.
- Final severe phase (full-blown AIDS): associated with CD4 count of less than $200/mm^2$; phase is initiated by T-cell activation mediated by a variety of infectious agents; immune system destruction is characterized by opportunistic infections and neoplastic complications of AIDS (Fig. 4-6).

Treatment

Many goals of HIV therapy involve attempts to eliminate or inhibit proteins necessary for HIV replication, such as HIV reverse transcriptase and HIV protease. Combination chemotherapies to inhibit HIV are collectively termed *highly active antiretroviral therapy*

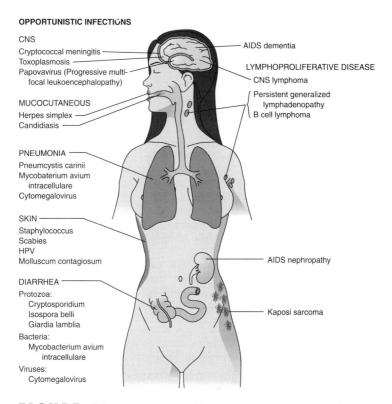

OPPORTUNISTIC INFECTIONS

CNS
Cryptococcal meningitis
Toxoplasmosis
Papovavirus (Progressive multi-
    focal leukoencephalopathy)

MUCOCUTANEOUS
Herpes simplex
Candidiasis

PNEUMONIA
Pneumcystis carinii
Mycobaterium avium
    intracellulare
Cytomegalovirus

SKIN
Staphylococcus
Scabies
HPV
Molluscum contagiosum

DIARRHEA
Protozoa:
    Cryptosporidium
    Isospora belli
    Giardia lamblia
Bacteria:
    Mycobacterium avium
        intracellulare
Viruses:
    Cytomegalovirus

AIDS dementia

LYMPHOPROLIFERATIVE DISEASE
CNS lymphoma

Persistent generalized
    lymphadenopathy
B cell lymphoma

AIDS nephropathy

Kaposi sarcoma

FIGURE 4-6
HIV-1–mediated destruction of the cellular immune system results in AIDS. The infectious and neoplastic complications of AIDS can affect nearly every organ system. (From Rubin E, Gorstein F, Rubin R, et al. Rubin's Pathology, 4th ed. Philadelphia: Lippincott Williams & Wilkins, 2005, p. 152.)

(HAART), and their use has greatly reduced AIDS-related mortality. Unfortunately, the high mutation rate of HIV generates mutations insensitive to HAART. The types of chemotherapy currently available do not eradicate the virus from the body, and even if they eliminate HIV-positive cells from the blood, temporary cessation of therapy allows reactivation of HIV from reservoirs outside of the circulation.

Autoimmunity

Immune tolerance is defined as the failure to respond to an antigen. Normally, the immune system is tolerant to self-antigens. B cells and T cells become tolerant to self-antigens mainly during their development to maturity. When tolerance is lost, the immune system can destroy self tissues, and autoimmune disease develops.

Theories of Autoimmunity

- Antigens that are normally inaccessible (e.g., lens tissue, spermatozoa, myelin) may be exposed or released after injury and recognized as foreign.
- Abnormal T-cell function can lead to autoimmunity, because most responses to antigen require T-cell participation and activation.
- Molecular mimicry: a bacterial antigen may contain an epitope similar to one on a protein of the body, so that the antibodies formed against the bacteria cross-react with the self antigen (e.g., in rheumatic heart disease, antibodies against streptococcal bacteria cross-react with antigens from cardiac muscle, causing cardiac damage).
- Polyclonal lymphocyte activation: polyclonal agents, such as LPS or bacterial "superantigens" can cause the proliferation of B or T cells in the absence of specific antigenic stimulation. Some of the resulting progeny of these cells may be autoreactive.

Tissue Injury and Autoimmune Disease

There are two types of autoimmune diseases: organ-specific and systemic. The parts of the immune system important in causing autoimmune disease, and tissue injury may vary. For example, in systemic lupus erythematosus (SLE), autoantibodies are believed to have a dominant role, whereas in other diseases, such as insulin-dependent diabetes mellitus (IDDM, or type 1 diabetes), T cells are thought to have a major destructive effect. Most autoimmune responses use the integrated immune system, and more than one immune effector can be involved in causing pathogenesis and tissue injury.

Systemic Lupus Erythematosus (SLE)

SLE is a chronic systemic autoimmune inflammatory disease that characteristically affects the kidneys, joints, serous membranes and skin. Eighty percent of patients are women of childbearing age. Autoantibodies are formed against a variety of self-antigens, but the most important diagnostic autoantibodies are:

- antinuclear antibodies (ANAs)
- antibodies against double-stranded DNA
- antibodies against a soluble nuclear antigen termed Sm (Smith) antigen.

Pathogenesis

SLE is considered the prototype of type III hypersensitivity reactions. because antigen-antibody complexes deposit in tissues, leading to the characteristic vasculitis, synovitis, and glomerulonephritis.

A variety of factors predispose to the development of SLE (Fig. 4-7). In addition, there is some genetic predisposition to SLE. The

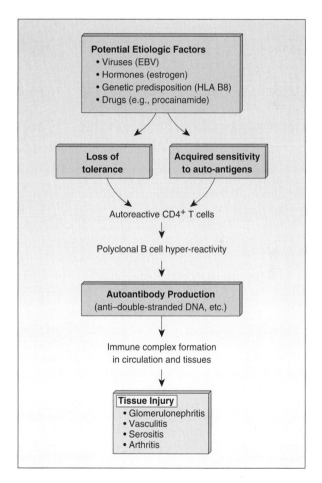

FIGURE 4-7
The pathogenesis of systemic lupus erythematosus is multifactorial. (From Rubin E, Gorstein F, Rubin R, et al. Rubin's Pathology, 4th ed. Philadelphia: Lippincott Williams & Wilkins, 2005, p. 155.)

HLA-B8 haplotype is often found in patients with SLE. It is associated with immunoregulatory disorders such as deficiency of certain complement components and antigen-driven B-cell hyperreactivity. Because CD4$^+$ helper T cells are intimately involved in B-cell activation, a defect in the functioning of this cell population is also probable.

Pathology and Clinical Features

- **Skin:** An erythematous malar "butterfly" rash is common. Microscopically, there is a basal cell degeneration. Immunofluorescence studies reveal deposition of immunoglobulin and complement at the dermal-epidermal junction (lupus band).
- **Joints:** most common manifestation of SLE. More than 90% of patients have polyarthralgia. Inflammatory synovitis occurs without joint destruction.
- **Kidneys:** Kidney disease afflicts 75% of patients, especially glomerulonephritis. There are four main histological types.

  1. *Mesangial lupus nephritis:* only slight increase in mesangial cells and matrix; immune complexes and complement found in mesangial regions; mild proteinuria and hematuria; prognosis, excellent
  2. *Focal proliferative nephritis:* increased cellularity in parts of some glomeruli with proliferation of endothelial and mesangial cells, and neutrophil and monocyte infiltration; necrosis and fibrin deposits may be present; prognosis, mixed
  3. *Diffuse proliferative lupus nephritis:* most serious type of renal disease, occurring in about 50% of patients with clinical renal involvement; increased cellularity, with fibrin deposition and necrosis; subendothelial and mesangial immune complex deposits; prognosis, may progress to renal failure
  4. *Membranous lupus nephritis:* associated with massive proteinuria and nephrotic syndrome, but minimal hypercellularity; deposition of immunoglobulin and complement on the subepithelial surface of the glomerular capillary cause diffusely thickened capillary loops

- **Respiratory Conditions:** Possible pneumonitis and pleuritis; progressive interstitial fibrosis may develop in some patients.
- **Cardiac Involvement:** Pericarditis may be encountered, although heart failure is rare.
- **Central Nervous System:** Vasculitis may lead to hemorrhage and infarction of the brain.
- **Other Conditions:** Presence of antiphospholipid antibodies can predispose patients with SLE to thromboembolic complications such as stroke, pulmonary embolism, and deep vein and portal vein thrombosis.

Clinical Course

The clinical course of SLE is highly variable, and like many autoimmune diseases has exacerbations and remissions. Before the advent of corticosteroids and other immunosuppressive therapies, SLE was frequently a fatal disease. At present, the overall 10-year survival approaches 90%.

Lupuslike Diseases

Drug-induced Lupus

This disease can occur following administration of drugs such as procainamide (arrhythmias), hydralazine (hypertension), and isoniazid (tuberculosis). Manifestations may range from an asymptomatic positive ANA test result to more SLE-like symptoms. Autoantibodies to histones, but not to double-stranded DNA or Sm antigen are found. Discontinuation of the offending drug is usually curative.

Chronic Discoid Lupus

In this cutaneous disease, erythematous plaques are found most commonly on face and scalp; there is deposition of immunoglobulins and complement at the dermal-epidermal interface. As many as 10% of patients eventually manifest other features of SLE.

Subacute Cutaneous Lupus

This disease is aggravated by sunlight exposure and characterized by papular and annular lesions on the trunk. Antibodies to a ribonucleoprotein complex are characteristic.

Sjögren Syndrome

Sjögren syndrome (SS) is an autoimmune disease characterized by keratoconjunctivitis sicca (dry eyes) and xerostomia (dry mouth). Salivary and lachrymal glands are targeted. SS is the second most common connective tissue disorder after SLE and affects 3% of population, occurring mostly in women, 30 to 65 years of age. SS is associated with a 40-fold increased risk of malignant lymphoma.

Pathogenesis

- Primary SS occurs alone, whereas secondary SS may occur in association with other autoimmune diseases, such as rheumatoid arthritis or SLE.
- Familial clustering occurs, afflicted families having a high prevalence of other autoimmune diseases.
- 50% of patients have autoantibodies to soluble nuclear nonhistone proteins.
- EBV (Epstein-Barr virus) and HTLV-1 (human T-cell leukemia virus-1) may play a role in a possible viral etiology of SS.

Clinical Manifestations

- Intense lymphocytic infiltrate (mostly with CD4 T cells) is seen in salivary and lacrimal glands, mostly around the ducts. Symptoms result mainly from the absence of saliva (atrophy, inflammation, cracking of oral mucosa) and the absence of tears (dry, fissured or ulcerated cornea).
- Submucosal glands in bronchi, esophagus, and GI tract may also be affected, as well as intrahepatic bile ducts and kidney tubules.

Scleroderma (Progressive Systemic Sclerosis)

Scleroderma is an autoimmune disease characterized by excessive collagen deposition and vasculopathy in the skin and internal organs such as the gastrointestinal tract, heart, lung, and kidneys. It occurs four times as often in women as in men, mostly in the 25 to 50 years age group. Scleroderma presents as (a) the generalized, progressive form and (b) the diffuse, cutaneous variant or CREST (**C**alcinosis, **R**aynaud syndrome, **E**sophageal dysfunction, **S**clerodactyly, and **T**elangiectasia). The progressive form of scleroderma includes all the symptoms of CREST, but is more severe, usually beginning with the Raynaud phenomenon, (intermittent episodes of ischemia of the fingers, marked by pallor, paresthesias, and pain). This is often followed by esophageal hypomotility and dysphagia. The antibody spectrum of the disease is marked by (a) antibodies to Scl-70, a topoisomerase, (in 30% of patients); (b) antibodies against RNA polymerase, and (c) anticentromere antibodies, which are associated with the CREST syndrome. Other clinical features include the following:

- Tightening of facial skin leads to the typical "stone facies" of afflicted patients.
- Interstitial pulmonary fibrosis with dyspnea occurs in 50% of patients.
- Vascular involvement of the kidneys may lead to malignant hypertension.

Polymyositis, Dermatomyositis, and Inclusion Body Myositis (IBM)

These diseases make up a group of rare autoimmune diseases of muscle that occur in children and adults.

- Polymyositis and IBM: muscle damage is mediated by activated CD8 T cells and macrophages
- Polymyositis and dermatomyositis: myositis-specific antibodies (MSAs) are found

- Dermatomyositis: deposition of immune complexes and complement leads to microangiopathy with a reduction in the number of capillaries in muscle fibers

Skin involvement may be manifested by a facial rash. Cancer frequency is many-fold higher than in general population.

Mixed Connective Tissue Disease (MCTD)

MCTD combines features of SLE, scleroderma, and dermatomyositis. There is controversy as to whether MCTD is actually a distinct disease entity or simply an overlap of symptoms in patients with other types of collagen vascular diseases. Between 80% and 90% of patients are adult females. Patients have high titers of an antibody to a ribonuclear protein. Symptoms may include those of SLE (rash, Raynaud phenomenon, arthritis, and arthralgias) and those of scleroderma (swollen hands, esophageal hypomotility, and pulmonary interstitial disease).

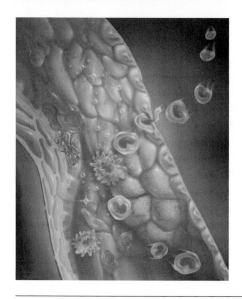

Neoplasia

Chapter Outline

Epidemiology of Cancer

Cancer accounts for one fifth of the total mortality in the United States and is the second leading cause of death after cardiovascular diseases and stroke. Overall, after decades of steady increases, the age-adjusted mortality due to all cancers has now reached a plateau. The most common tumor types in men and women in the United States are shown in Table 5-1. Geographic and ethnic differences in populations throughout the world influence the incidence of cancer, as shown in Table 5-2.

Benign versus Malignant Tumors

Benign Tumors

Benign tumors do not penetrate adjacent tissue borders nor spread to distant sites. The suffix "oma" for benign tumors is preceded by reference to the cell or tissue of origin. Examples of benign tumors include the following:

- Epithelioma: Benign tumor of squamous epithelium
- Papilloma: A neoplasm that grows outward from epithelium

Table 5-1
Most Common Tumor Types in Men and Women

Tumor Type	%
Men	
Prostate	33
Lung and bronchus	14
Colon and rectum	11
Urinary bladder	6
Melanoma	4
Non-Hodgkin lymphoma	4
Kidney	3
Oral cavity	3
Leukemia	3
Pancreas	2
All other sites	17
Women	
Breast	32
Lung and bronchus	12
Colon and rectum	11
Uterine corpus	6
Ovary	4
Non-Hodgkin lymphoma	4
Melanoma	3
Thyroid	3
Pancreas	2
Urinary bladder	2
All other sites	20

From Rubin E, Gorstein F, Rubin R, et al. Rubin's
Pathology, 4th ed. Philadelphia: Lippincott Williams &
Wilkins, 2005, p. 210.

Table 5-2

Geographic and Ethnic Differences in Cancer Incidence

Cancer	Higher Occurrence	Low or Rare Occurrence
Nasopharyngeal	Regions of China, Hong Kong, Singapore	Other world regions
Esophageal	Belt from Turkey to eastern China	Mormon women in Utah
Stomach	Japan, Chile	
Colorectal	United States	Japan, India, Africa
Liver	Regions where hepatitis B and C are endemic	
Skin	Northern Australia, south-western United States	Japanese, Chinese, Indians
Breast	United States, Europe	Africa, Asia
Cervix	Texas Hispanics	Israel Ashkenazi Jews
Choriocarcinoma	Pacific rim of Asia	
Prostate	African Americans	Japan
Testicular		African blacks
Penis	Parts of Africa and Asia	Circumcised men of any race
Burkitt lymphoma	Africa	Europe and America
Multiple myeloma	African Americans	Caucasian Americans
Chronic lymphocytic leukemia	Elderly Europeans and North Americans	Japan

- Adenoma: Benign tumor arising from glandular epithelium
- Polyp: Mass of tissue that bulges outward from a surface
- Teratoma: Arises from all three germ cell layers; may contain a variety of structures; occurs mainly in gonads, and may be benign or malignant. They do not penetrate adjacent tissue borders.
- Hamartoma: Disorganized caricature of normal tissue components
- Choristoma: Ectopic island of normal tissue

Malignant Tumors

Malignant tumors invade contiguous tissues and can metastasize to distant sites where subpopulations of malignant cells settle, grow and invade into new sites. Examples of malignant tumors include the following:

- Carcinoma: name applied to cancers of epithelial origin
- Sarcoma: name applied to cancers of mesenchymal origin

Malignant counterparts of benign tumors usually carry the same name, with the suffix carcinoma or sarcoma, depending on origin. For example, a malignant tumor of the stomach is a gastric adenocarcinoma, whereas a bone tumor composed of malignant chondrocytes is called a chondrosarcoma of bone.

Histological Diagnosis of Malignancy

The "gold standard" for diagnosis of cancer remains routine microscopy. The distinction between benign and malignant tumors is the most important diagnostic challenge.

Benign Tumors

Benign tumors resemble their parent tissue histologically and cytologically. The gross structure of a benign tumor may assume papillary or polyploid configurations, but the lining epithelium resembles that of normal tissue.

Malignant Tumors

Malignant tumors may differ from the parent tissue morphologically and functionally. Characteristics of malignant tumors include:

- Anaplasia (lack of differentiation) or atypical cells:
    - ➤ variation in size and shape of cells and cell nuclei
    - ➤ enlarged and darkly stained nuclei with prominent nucleoli
    - ➤ atypical and abundant mitoses
    - ➤ bizarre cells, including tumor giant cells

- Many of these features are preceded by a preneoplastic dysplastic epithelium, which may lead to carcinoma in situ (see Chapter 1).
- Mitotic activity: Abundant mitoses are a characteristic but not a necessary criterion of malignant tumors. For example, in the case of a leiomyosarcoma (sarcoma resembling smooth muscle cells), the diagnosis of malignancy is based on even a few mitoses.

- Growth pattern: Malignant tumors often have a disorganized and random spatial arrangement of cells. If they outgrow their blood supply, they may display ischemic necrosis.
- Invasion:
  - ➤ Malignant tumors infiltrate adjacent tissues, particularly blood vessels and lymphatics.
  - ➤ Unlike benign tumors, invading tumors have no well-defined capsule or cleavage plane to separate them from normal tissue.

- Metastases: A tumor is identified as malignant when invasion is followed by implantation of additional tumor masses to distal sites. The tissue or organ from which the tumor originated is not always apparent from its morphological properties. In such cases, electron microscopic examination or use of immunohistochemical tumor markers may aid in detecting the correct origin of a tumor.
  - ➤ Electron microscopic (EM) features: Because carcinomas are of epithelial origin, EM examination may reveal epithelial markers such as desmosomes or special junctional complexes. Presence of melanosomes signifies a melanoma. Membrane-bound granules with dense cores are features of endocrine neoplasms.
  - ➤ Immunohistochemical tumor markers are antigens that point to the origin of the neoplasm; immunoperoxidase stains and immunofluorescence are based on antibodies that bind to and stain specific antigens characteristic of a specific tissue or organ. Not all tumor markers are disease specific; however, they help determine the lineage of undifferentiated tumors. This is important because therapeutic decisions may be based on the appropriate identification.
  - ➤ DNA and genetic analyses are useful in diagnosis of lymphoid tumors, as well as in measurement of DNA content of tumor cells.
  - ➤ Some tumor-derived molecules (i.e., α-fetoprotein and carcinoembryonic antigen [CEA]) are normally expressed only in fetal tissues. When detected in adult body fluids, they may indicate undifferentiated neoplastic cells.

Table 5-3 lists markers that are frequently used to identify tumors originating in specific organs. Most lymphoid neoplasms express CD antigen markers.

Invasion and Metastasis

Invasion and metastasis are the two properties of cancer cells that are responsible for the majority of deaths from cancer.

Table 5-3

Frequently Used Markers to Identify Tumors

Marker	Target Cells
Epithelial cells	
Cytokeratins	Carcinomas, mesothelioma
CK7	Many adenocarcinomas
CK20	Gastrointestinal and ovarian carcinomas, bladder transitional cell carcinoma, Merkel cell tumor
Epithelial membrane antigen (EMA)	Carcinomas, mesothelioma, some large cell lymphomas
Ber-Ep4	Most adenocarcinomas, but not in mesothelioma
B72.3 (tumor-associated)	Many adenocarcinomas, but not in mesothelioma
CEA	Many adenocarcinomas, but not in mesothelioma
CD15	Many adenocarcinomas, but not in mesothelioma
Mesothelial cells	
Cytokeratins CH5/6	Mesothelioma
Vimentin	Mesothelioma
HBME	Mesothelioma
Calretinin	Mesothelioma
Melanocytes	
HMB-45	Malignant melanoma
S-100 protein	Malignant melanoma
MART-1	Malignant melanoma
Neuroendocrine and neural cells	
Chromogranins	Neuroendocrine carcinoma, carcinoid tumor
Synaptophysin	Neuroendocrine carcinoma, carcinoid tumor

(continues)

Table 5-3
(continued)

Marker	Target Cells
Neuron-specific enolase	Neuroendocrine carcinoma, carcinoid tumor
CD57	Neuroendocrine carcinoma
Neurofilament proteins	Neuroblastoma
Glial cells	
Glial fibrillary acidic protein (GFAP)	Astrocytoma and other glial tumors
Mesenchymal cells	
Vimentin	Most sarcomas
Desmin	Muscle tumors (myosarcomas)
Muscle-specific actin	Muscle tumors (myosarcomas)
CD99	Ewing sarcoma, peripheral neuroectodermal tumors (PNET)
Specific organs	
Prostate-specific antigen (PSA)	Prostatic cancer
Prostate-specific alkaline phosphatase (PSAP)	Prostatic cancer
Thyroglobulin	Thyroid cancer
α-Fetoprotein (AFP)	Hepatocellular carcinomas, yolk sac tumor
Carcinoembryonic antigen (CEA)	Gastrointestinal cancers
Placental alkaline phosphatase (PLAP)	Seminoma
Human chorionic gonadotropin (hCG)	Trophoblastic tumors
CA19.9	Pancreatic and gastrointestinal carcinomas
CA125	Ovarian carcinoma
Calcitonin	Medullary carcinoma of the thyroid

Modified from Rubin, Rubin's Pathology, 4th ed. Philadelphia: Lippincott Williams & Wilkins, 2005, p. 174.

Localized Growth: Carcinoma in Situ

Most carcinomas begin as localized growths confined to the epithelium in which they arise. As long as they do not penetrate the epithelial basement membrane, such tumors are termed carcinoma in situ. At this stage they are asymptomatic and curable.

Metastasis

Hematogenous Metastases

Capillaries and venules are more commonly invaded than are thicker-walled arterioles and arteries. Because the liver receives blood from the gastrointestinal (GI) tract, abdominal tumors can lead to hepatic metastases. Other tumors penetrate systemic veins that eventually drain into the vena cava and hence to the lungs. Some tumor cells pass through the microcirculation to reach the brain and the bones.

Lymphatic Metastases

Lymphatic capillaries lack a basement membrane; hence, tumor cells can penetrate them more readily than capillaries. Tumors arising in tissues that have a rich lymphatic network (e.g., the breast) often spread by this route. Cells that penetrate lymphatics are carried to the regional draining lymph nodes, where they lodge and grow. Lymph nodes bearing metastatic deposits may be enlarged many times their normal size, often becoming larger than the primary lesion.

Seeding of Body Cavities

Malignant tumors arising in organs adjacent to the peritoneal and pleural cavities may shed cells into these spaces. Tumors in these sites often produce large amounts of fluid (e.g., ascites, pleural fluid). Occasional seeding into the pericardial cavity, joint space, and subarachnoid space may occur as well.

Multistep Events in Invasion and Metastasis

A number of steps are required for malignant cells to establish a metastasis. Although most cancers originate from the malignant transformation of a single cell, subpopulations with diverse biological characteristics arise (tumor heterogeneity). In each step of the metastatic cascade, probably only the fittest cells survive:

1. Cell–cell adhesion molecules such as cadherins and catenins help to maintain cohesion of epithelial cells; expression of such molecules is reduced in most carcinomas. Epithelial tumor cells must detach from each other before they can invade the underlying basement membrane and extracellular matrix.

2. Proteolytic enzymes elaborated by the malignant cells enhance movement through the extracellular matrix.
3. The invading cancer penetrates vascular or lymphatic channels by the same mechanisms used to penetrate the extracellular matrix.
4. Survival and arrest within the circulating blood or lymph involves attachment of the tumor cells to endothelial cells, retraction of the endothelium, and binding to the underlying basement membrane. Clumps of tumor cells may grow within the vascular lumen.
5. Eventually, the tumor extravasates and exits from the circulation to a new tissue site.
6. The extravasated cancer cells grow in response to autocrine growth factors. A number of such growth factors (vascular endothelial growth factor, transforming growth factor-β, and platelet-derived growth factor) trigger and regulate angiogenesis, a process necessary to tumor survival.

Not all metastatic colonies enlarge immediately. Tumors may recur locally or at metastatic sites many years after the primary cancer has been surgically removed. The phenomenon is termed tumor *dormancy.*

Grading and Staging of Cancers

In an attempt to predict the behavior of a tumor, and to establish criteria for therapy, many cancers are classified by grade and stage. The choices of surgery and treatment are influenced by stage, which reflects the extent of spread, and grade, which reflects cellular characteristics.

Grading
Cytological and histological grading are based on the degree of anaplasia and on the number of proliferating cells. Grading schemes classify tumors into three or four grades. Low-grade tumors are well differentiated, and high-grade ones are anaplastic. The general correlation between grade and biological behavior is not invariable.

Staging
Commonly used criteria include (a) tumor size; (b) extent of local growth; (c) presence of lymph node metastases; and (d) presence of distant metastases. These criteria have been codified in the international TNM cancer staging system:

- **T**: refers to size of primary tumor
- **N**: regional node metastases
- **M**: presence and extent of distant metastases

Origin of Cancer

Clonal Origin

Studies of human and experimental tumors have provided strong evidence that most cancers arise from a single transformed cell. For example, a patient with multiple myeloma produces neoplastic plasma cells with a single immunoglobulin molecule unique to that patient.

Cancer as Altered Differentiation

In some cancers, there is evidence that malignant cells result from a maturation arrest in the sequence of development from a stem cell to a fully differentiated cell.

- Squamous cell carcinoma contains differentiated as well as undifferentiated cells. When transplanted into appropriate hosts, only the undifferentiated cells form tumors.
- When a single teratocarcinoma stem cell from a mouse is transplanted into an early mouse embryo, the entirely normal pup born at term is a mosaic composed of cells derived from both the embryo proper and the embryonal carcinoma. Thus, the progeny of the malignant cell, under the influence of normal developmental controls, differentiates into normal mature tissue elements.
- Studies of leukemias and lymphomas indicate that these cancers are not truly proliferative disorders but rather reflect an uncoupling of differentiation from proliferation. The malignant cells that accumulate are cells that have not attained terminal differentiation.
- Studies indicate that retinoids play a role in promoting the commitment of cancer cells to terminal differentiation. Members of this class of compounds have been reported to induce remission in certain leukemias.

Growth of Cancer

The major determinant of tumor growth is the fact that more cells are produced than die in a given time. Division time alone cannot account for tumor enlargement, because tumor cells do not necessarily divide more rapidly than normal cells. The various factors involved in tumor growth are described as follows:

- Tumor growth depends on the growth fraction (proportion of cycling cells) and the rate of cell death. The balance between cell renewal and cell death, which is strictly maintained in normal proliferating tissues, is defective in tumors.

- Tumor angiogenesis (the formation of new capillaries) is essential for the continued growth of tumors.
- Tumor dormancy accounts for the interval before the appearance of metastases. In tumors such as breast cancer and melanoma, metastases may remain dormant for many years. It is not known whether tumor cells in dormancy fail to grow because of interference with angiogenesis, unresponsiveness to growth factors, or the presence of immune growth restraints.

Molecular Genetics of Cancer

Cancer has a genetic basis. The properties of cancer that support this conclusion include the following:

- Genetic predisposition
- Presence of chromosomal abnormalities in neoplastic cells
- A correlation between impaired DNA repair and the occurrence of cancer
- The close association between carcinogenesis and mutagenesis

The growth of malignant cells results from the sequential acquisition of somatic mutations in genes that control cell growth, differentiation, apoptosis, and the maintenance of genome integrity. It is estimated that a minimum of four to seven mutated genes are required for the transformation of a normal cell into a malignant one, and this multistep process can take place over a period of years. Three main classes of genes are found to mutate in various cancers:

- Protooncogenes that regulate normal cell growth, differentiation, and survival
- Tumor suppressor genes whose products inhibit cellular proliferation
- DNA mismatch repair genes that maintain the fidelity of DNA replication

Oncogenes, Protooncogenes, and Cancer

Oncogenes are mutant versions of protooncogenes, the normal genes involved in growth regulation. The concept of oncogenes was originally derived from studies of animal tumor viruses (transforming retroviruses), which could impart a neoplastic phenotype to virally infected cells.

The transforming viral oncogenes were termed v-*onc* genes, and it was found that they had homology for eukaryotic DNA sequences called protooncogenes. Protooncogenes, which have been shown to mutate, are called cellular oncogenes and are designated by the prefix "c" (e.g., c-*myc*, c-*abl*).

Gene and Gene Product Nomenclature

The name of a gene is always printed in italics, whereas the protein product of the gene, although it may have the same name as the gene, is not printed in italics. For example, the protein product of the *p53* gene is p53.

Mechanisms of Activation of Cellular Oncogenes

Protooncogene may be converted to oncogenes, or activated, in the following ways:

- Point mutation: The first oncogene identified in a human bladder tumor was due to a point mutation (substitution of valine for glycine in codon 12) in the c-*ras* gene. Studies of other cancers have revealed point mutations involving other codons of the *ras* gene. Alterations in other growth-regulatory genes have also been described.
- Chromosomal translocation: The transfer of a portion of one chromosome to another has been implicated in the pathogenesis of several human leukemias and lymphomas. For example:

  - Philadelphia chromosome (found in 95% of myelogenous leukemia patients) is the result of a chromosomal translocation involving breaks at the ends of chromosomes 9 and 22. This creates a new hybrid gene, which generates mitogenic and antiapoptotic signals.
  - 75% of patients with Burkitt lymphoma have a translocation of the c-*myc* gene, a protooncogene involved in cell cycle progression. This translocation leads to the unregulated expression of the gene.

- Gene amplification: Chromosomal alterations that result in an increased number of copies of a gene have been found primarily in human solid tumors, and can lead to greatly increased expression of the gene. These alterations can be seen in as (a) homogeneous staining regions (HSRs); (b) abnormal banding regions; or (c) double minutes (extrachromosomal elements that appear as multiple small bodies).

  - Gene amplification of the *myc*-family has been demonstrated in lung small cell carcinoma, Wilms tumor, and hepatoblastoma.
  - Advanced neuroblastoma is associated with a 700-fold amplification of the N-*myc* gene.
  - The *erb B* protooncogene is amplified in up to one third of breast and ovarian cancers and is associated with poor overall survival.

Mechanisms of Oncogene Action

Oncogenes can be classified according to the roles of their normal counterparts (the protooncogenes). The protein products of oncogenes play important roles in cell growth and differentiation. These oncogene products perform their activities in a number of cellular compartments, some as extracellular growth factors, and others in cellular compartments ranging from membrane receptors to factors in the nucleus (Fig. 5-1).

Oncogenes and Growth Factors

When soluble extracellular growth factors bind to their specific cell surface receptors, a signaling cascade leads to entry of the cell into the mitotic cycle. Cancer cells can produce a mixture of growth factors with autocrine or paracrine activity. Examples of growth factors involved in neoplastic transformation include the following:

- Platelet-derived growth factor (PDGF) is encoded by the c-*sis* protooncogene and is a potent mitogen for fibroblasts, smooth muscle, and glial cells. Tumors such as sarcomas and glioblastomas produce PDGF-like polypeptides.

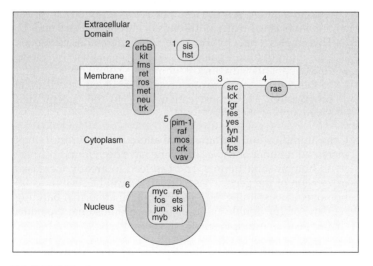

FIGURE 5-1
Cellular compartments in which oncogene or protooncogene products reside. (1) Growth factors, (2) transmembrane growth factor receptors (tyrosine kinase), (3) membrane associated kinases (4) *ras* GTPase family, (5) cytoplasmic kinases, (6) nuclear transcriptional regulators. (From Rubin E, Gorstein F, Rubin R, et al. Rubin's Pathology, 4th ed. Philadelphia: Lippincott Williams & Wilkins, 2005, p. 187.)

- A protein with homology to fibroblast growth factor (FGF) is produced by an oncogene, and has been identified in human stomach cancer and Kaposi sarcoma.

Oncogenes and Growth Factor Receptors

Certain mutations of growth factor receptors lead to unrestrained (constitutive) activation of the receptor, independent of ligand binding.

- Germline point mutations in c-*ret* lead to constitutive activation of the receptor, and are associated with the multiple endocrine neoplasia (MEN) syndromes and familial medullary thyroid carcinoma.
- Point mutations in the gene (c-*met*) that encodes the hepatocyte growth factor (HGF) receptor are associated with papillary renal cancers.
- Many growth factors stimulate cell proliferation by binding to membrane receptors with tyrosine kinase activity. An abnormal PDGF receptor with constitutive tyrosine kinase activity, generated as the result of a chromosomal translocation, has been found in patients with myelomonocytic leukemia.

Oncogenes and Nonreceptor Signaling Proteins

- Tyrosine kinases: A number of proteins with tyrosine kinase activity are not membrane-bound receptors and are coded by genes in the *src* family. The only *src* family member implicated in human tumorigenesis is c-*abl*, which codes for a cytoplasmic tyrosine kinase. In chronic myelogenous leukemia, c-*abl* is translocated from chromosome 9 to the *bcr* region of chromosome 22, forming a fusion gene (*bcr-abl*). The highly elevated tyrosine kinase activity resulting from the fusion gene activation leads to oncogenesis.
- c-*raf* gene: This gene codes for a soluble cytoplasmic oncoprotein that plays a role in signal transduction from cytoplasm to nucleus. Point mutations in this gene occur in as many as 10% of human cancers.
- *ras* oncogene: The *ras* protooncogene codes for a small ras protein that couples the activation of growth factor receptors to gene transcription in the nucleus.

  ➤ Ras is active when it binds GTP and inactive when it binds GDP. Ras has intrinsic GTPase activity, which can return activated ras to its inactive state.
  ➤ Mutations of the *ras* protooncogenes (H-*ras*, N-*ras*, and K-*ras*) are found in 25% of all human tumors. Most of the mutations causing malignant transformation have resulted in the abrogation of the normal GTPase activity of ras, causing it to remain in an unregulated stimulated state.

Oncogenes and Nuclear Regulatory Proteins

A number of nuclear proteins encoded by protooncogenes are intimately involved in the sequential expression of genes that regulate cellular proliferation and differentiation. The products of c-*myc*, c-*fos*, and c-*jun* are nuclear proteins that activate the expression of a variety of genes involved in cellular proliferation and differentiation. Mutation of these genes results in overexpression of their products. Overexpression of the c-*jun* protein has been described in lung and colorectal cancers. Overexpression of c-*myc* occurs in adenocarcinoma of lung and breast. As previously discussed, the translocation characteristic of Burkitt lymphoma constitutively activates c-*myc* expression.

Cell Cycle Control

Cells enter the mitotic cycle by progression from G_0 to G_1 in response to growth factors and cytokines. During G_1, a commitment to enter the S phase of DNA replication is termed the restriction, or R point. This checkpoint allows the cell to confirm that its DNA is intact before committing to replication of nuclear DNA in the S phase. The process is regulated by cyclins D and E, which in turn activate members of the cyclin-dependent protein kinases (Cdk) family. Cdk 2, 4, and 6 phosphorylate retinoblastoma protein (Rb), which then unleashes transcription factors of the E2F family. E2F has been identified as an important transcriptional activator playing a role in cell cycle control. E2F drives the cell past the R point and allows synthesis of genes involved in DNA replication. Cdk inhibitors are regulated by the tumor suppressor protein p53 (Fig. 5-2).

Cancer cells often display a loss of R point control through mechanisms such as overexpression of cyclin D1, loss of Cdk inhibitors, or inactivation of the phosphorylated Rb (pRb) or p53 proteins. Decreased levels of a Cdk inhibitor are associated with a poor prognosis in adenocarcinoma of the colon and certain cancers of the lung. Conversely, a number of malignant tumors have been shown to overexpress several cyclins and Cdks.

Bcl-2 and Apoptosis

Apoptosis, or programmed cell death, is an important regulatory pathway in eliminating cells that are no longer useful or that may be harmful to the body (see Chapter 1). Two major mechanisms trigger activation of the caspase cascade leading to apoptosis:

- Release of cytochrome c from mitochondria
- Binding of specific ligands to cell surface "death" receptors such as Fas and tumor necrosis factor (TNF)

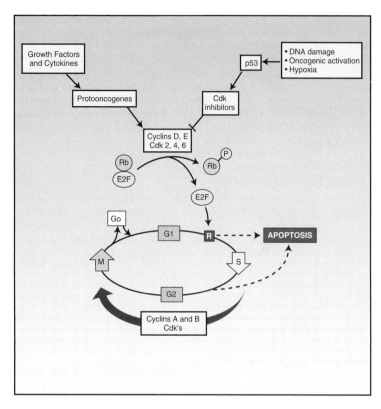

F I G U R E   5-2

Regulation of the cell cycle. Cells are stimulated to enter G_1 from G^0 by growth factors and cytokines via protooncogene activation. A critical juncture in the transition of cells from G_1 to S phase is the restriction point (R). A major regulatory event in this process is the phosphorylation of Rb by cyclin-dependent kinases (cdks), which causes the release of the transcriptional activator E2F. Cdks are suppressed by cdk inhibitors that are regulated by p53. Tumor suppressor proteins block cell cycle progression largely within G_1. Interruption of cell cycle progression during G_1 and G_2 may lead to apoptosis as a default pathway. S, G_2, and M phases are also regulated by cyclins, cdks, and cdk inhibitors. (From Rubin E, Gorstein F, Rubin R, et al. Rubin's Pathology, 4th ed. Philadelphia: Lippincott Williams & Wilkins, 2005, p. 190.)

For tumor cells to acquire malignancy, they must escape apoptosis by dismantling the apoptotic machinery. One mechanism is to cause overexpression of Bcl-2, an antiapoptosis protein. Bcl-2 prevents release of cytochrome c from mitochondria, thus suppressing apoptosis. Bcl-2 is overexpressed in follicular B-cell lymphomas, and *bcl-2* gene expression has been observed in a variety of other human cancers. Many human cancers show other abnormalities in the apoptotic cascade, including the overexpression of proteins that block caspase activation and the inactivating mutations of proapoptotic proteins.

Tumor Suppressor Genes

The previous discussion of oncogenes describes generation of malignancy via activation of genes that promote cell growth. However, malignancy may also result from inactivation of genes that normally suppress or negatively regulate cell growth. Two such tumor suppressor genes are the retinoblastoma (*Rb*) and *p53* genes.

Retinoblastoma (Rb) Gene

Rb is the protein product of the tumor suppressor gene *Rb*. As previously mentioned, when Rb is phosphorylated, it induces the release of E2F transcription factor, thereby allowing progression of the cell cycle from G_1 to S. Inactivating mutations in *Rb* permit unregulated cell proliferation.

Retinoblastoma is a rare childhood intraocular cancer attributed to the inactivation of the *Rb* gene. Approximately 40% of cases are associated with a germ line mutation (hereditary retinoblastoma). An affected child inherits one defective *Rb* allele and one normal gene. This heterozygous state is not associated with any observable changes in the retina, but if the remaining normal allele is inactivated by mutation or deletion, cancer develops (Fig. 5-3). Patients with hereditary retinoblastoma have a 200-fold increased risk of developing mesenchymal tumors later in life.

In sporadic (nonhereditary) cases, the child originally has two normal *Rb* genes, but both are inactivated by mutations in the retina. Incidence of sporadic retinoblastoma is very low (1/30,000).

p53 Gene

Mutations of *p53* are judged to be the most common genetic change in human cancer. The p53 molecule prevents cells from entering the S phase of the cell cycle if there is damage to DNA. It also augments repair of damaged DNA. If the DNA damage cannot be repaired, *p53* increases transcription of a gene that induces apoptosis of the cell with the damaged DNA.

Most human cancers display either inactivating mutations of *p53* or abnormalities in the proteins that regulate *p53* activity. The

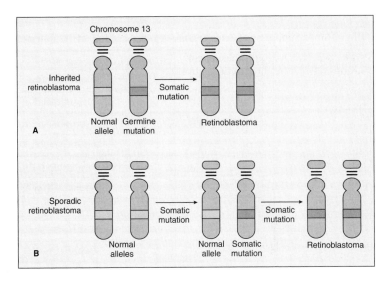

FIGURE 5-3

The "two-hit" origin of retinoblastoma. A. A child with the inherited form of retinoblastoma is born with a germ line mutation in one allele of the retinoblastoma gene located on the long arm of chromosome 13. A second somatic mutation in the retina leads to the inactivation of the functioning *Rb* allele and the subsequent development of a retinoblastoma. B. In sporadic cases of retinoblastoma, the child is born with two normal *Rb* alleles. It requires two independent somatic mutations to inactivate *Rb* gene function and allow the appearance of a neoplastic clone. (From Rubin E, Gorstein F, Rubin R, et al. Rubin's Pathology, 4th ed. Philadelphia: Lippincott Williams & Wilkins, 2005, p. 192.)

p53 gene is deleted or mutated in 75% of cases of colorectal cancer, and frequently in breast cancer, small-cell carcinoma of the lung, hepatocellular carcinoma, and astrocytoma. Li-Fraumeni syndrome refers to an inherited predisposition to develop cancers in many organs owing to germ-line mutations of *p53*.

Other Tumor Suppressor Genes

Most tumor suppressor genes inhibit unregulated cell growth by controlling cell cycle progression, repressing transcription of growth-promoting genes, or causing continual activation of growth factor receptors. Mutations in or deletions of tumor suppressor genes lead to removal of this suppression. Table 5-4 lists a number of tumor suppressor genes aside from *Rb* and *p53*.

Table 5-4
Other Tumor Suppressor Genes

Gene	Normal Gene or Product Function	Tumor
APC	Inhibits β-catenin, an activator of genes involved in cell cycle progression	Familial adenomatous polyposis coli
WT1	Is essential for normal development of urogenital tract and represses transcription of several growth-promoting genes	Wilms tumor, a cancerous tumor of the kidney occurring in children
NF1	Encodes neurofibromin, a negative regulator of *ras*	Neurofibroma type 1
VHL (von Hippel-Lindau)	Inhibits elongin, a molecule that promotes transcriptional elongation of growth-promoting genes	Renal carcinoma, hemangioblastoma of the brain, and pheochromocytoma
FHIT (fragile histidine triad)	FHIT protein is proapoptotic and growth suppressive	Cancers of the kidney, lung, and digestive tract
p15 and p16	Normal gene products are cdk inhibitors that serve as negative regulators of the cell cycle	Associated with breast, pancreas and prostate tumors
DPC4	Normal product is a transcriptional activator that mediates the growth inhibitory response to TGF-β.	90% of pancreatic carcinomas
BRCA1 and BRCA2	Tumor suppressors involved in checkpoint functions of the cell cycle; also function as DNA repair genes	Breast cancer susceptibility
PTEN (phosphatase and tensin)	Suppresses tumor growth by antagonizing tyrosine kinases	Prostate cancers, many gliomas, thyroid cancers

Epigenetic Factors in Cancer

Epigenetic factors are those that affect a cell's activity without directly altering the base sequence in its DNA. Unlike mutations, epigenetic modifications such as DNA methylation or histone acetylation are potentially reversible molecular events that can cause changes in gene expression. Histones are basic proteins associated with DNA in the chromosome, and histone acetylation is associated with enhanced transcriptional activity. Tumor suppressor genes can be targets of epigenetic factors, resulting in their inactivation by suppressing transcription or by blocking the binding of transcription factors.

DNA Repair Genes and Cancer

Errors may occur in DNA during synthesis, and the process of mismatch repair locates and removes mismatched base pairs. Environmental insults may also result in errors in DNA synthesis. DNA repair genes, sometimes called mutator or caretaker genes, are genes involved in mismatch repair. The loss of these gene functions renders the DNA susceptible to progressive accumulation of mutations; when these affect protooncogenes or tumor suppressor genes, cancer may result. Examples of cancers which have a defect of mismatch repair or a defective DNA repair:

- Hereditary nonpolyposis colon cancer (HNPCC): incidence of stomach and small bowel cancer is also increased in patients with HNPCC
- Ataxia Telangiectasia: a rare hereditary syndrome with predisposition to lymphomas, leukemias, and stomach and breast cancer
- Xeroderma Pigmentosum: autosomal recessive disease in which increased sensitivity to sunlight is accompanied by a high incidence of skin cancers
- Bloom Syndrome (BS): an autosomal recessive disease with predisposition to an array of cancers; cells from patients with BS show a high mutation frequency

Telomerase

Telomeres at the tips of chromosomes progressively shorten as the cells divide (see Chapter 1). Telomerase is an enzyme that adds repetitive telomeric sequences to maintain the length of the chromosome. Somatic cells do not normally express telomerase, but some cancer cells do. However, the role of telomerase in oncogenesis remains controversial.

Viruses and Human Cancer

It is estimated that viral infections are responsible for 15% of all human cancers. One RNA retrovirus and five DNA viruses are associated with human cancers.

RNA Retrovirus

- Human T-Cell Leukemia Virus-1 (HTLV-1) is an RNA retrovirus that has been firmly associated with a rare adult T-cell leukemia endemic in southern Japan and the Caribbean basin. Leukemia develops in less than 5% of infected persons and may have a latency of 40 years for its development.
- HTLV-1 has a tropism for $CD4^+$ lymphocytes.
- HTLV-1 genome contains no known oncogene, and does not integrate at a specific site in the host genome. Oncogenic stimulation is mediated by the viral transcriptional activation gene, *tax*, whose protein products promote the activity of genes involved in cell proliferation, such as the T-cell growth factor interleukin-2 (IL-2) and its receptor, granulocyte macrophage colony-stimulating factor (GM-CSF), and the protooncogenes c-*fos* and c-*sis*.

DNA Viruses

Human Papillomaviruses (HPVs)

HPVs induce lesions in humans that progress to squamous cell carcinoma.

- More than 80 distinct HPVs have been identified. Most are associated with benign lesions such as skin warts, genital warts, and laryngeal papillomas.
- At least 20 HPV types are associated with cancer of the uterine cervix, especially HPV 16 and 18.
- E6 and E7 are the major oncoproteins encoded by HPV. E6 targets p53 for degradation, and E7 inhibits Rb, thereby eliminating the tumor suppressing functions of these gene products.

Epstein-Barr Virus (EBV)

EBV is a widely disseminated herpesvirus; 95% of adults worldwide have antibodies to it. EBV infects B lymphocytes and gives them the ability to proliferate indefinitely in vitro (immortalizes them). EBV can cause infectious mononucleosis, a short-lived lymphoproliferative disease; however, it is also associated with the development of certain human cancers. EBV is also linked to the following conditions:

- Burkitt lymphoma, a childhood cancer localized mainly to equatorial Africa: Prolonged stimulation of the immune system, such as occurs in malarial infections in equatorial Africa, may result in uncontrolled B-cell proliferation, which may, in turn, lead to deregulation of the c-*myc* oncogene and uncontrolled proliferation of a malignant clone of B cells.
- Nasopharyngeal cancer: This variant of squamous cell carcinoma is endemic in southern China and parts of Africa. Seventy percent of patients are cured by radiation therapy alone.

- Polyclonal Lymphoproliferation in Immunodeficient States: Congenital or acquired immunodeficiency states can be complicated by the development of EBV-induced B-cell proliferative disorders. Lymphoid neoplasia is seen especially in immunosuppressed renal transplant recipients, and B-cell disorders are seen in patients with acquired immunodeficiency syndrome (AIDS).

Hepatitis Viruses
- Epidemiological studies have established an association between chronic infection with hepatitis B virus (chronic hepatitis and cirrhosis) and primary hepatocellular carcinoma.
- Chronic infection with a hepatotropic RNA virus (hepatitis C virus) also carries a high risk of hepatocellular carcinoma.

Human Herpesvirus 8 (HHV 8)
Kaposi sarcoma is a vascular neoplasm most commonly associated with AIDS, and the neoplastic cells contain sequences of the virus HHV 8. Like other DNA viruses, the HHV 8 genome encodes proteins that interfere with the *p53* and *Rb* tumor suppressor pathways.

Chemical Carcinogenesis

Pathogenesis
There are four stages of chemical carcinogenesis:

1. **Initiation:** A mutation in a single cell occurs.
2. **Promotion**: Clonal expansion of the initiated cell occurs, but the altered cells remain dependent on the promoting stimulus.
3. **Progression**: Growth is autonomous, and cells become immortalized.
4. **Cancer**: Cells acquire the capacity to invade and metastasize.

Screening Assays
Screening assays for potential carcinogenic activity have centered on the relationship between carcinogenicity and mutagenicity. A mutagen is an agent that can permanently alter the genetic constitution of a cell. Ninety percent of known carcinogens are mutagenic in the assay systems used.

- The Ames test uses the appearance of frameshift mutations and base-pair substitutions in a culture of *Salmonella typhimurium* bacteria to measure carcinogenicity.
- Animal cells such as rat hepatocytes and Chinese hamster ovary cells are observed for mutations, unscheduled DNA synthesis, and DNA strand breaks.

Table 5-5

Chemical Carcinogens Associated with Human Cancer

Carcinogen	Activation	Type of Malignancy
Polycyclic aromatic hydrocarbons (coal tar derivatives)	Depends on microsomal cytochrome P450-dependent mixed-function oxidases	Broad range of target organs; produce cancer at site of application; presence in cigarette smoke linked to lung cancer
Alkylating agents (many chemotherapeutic drugs are alkylating agents)	Are direct-acting carcinogens; transfer alkyl groups to DNA	Patients receiving this therapy have higher risk of future cancer development.
Aflatoxin B1 (a product of the fungus *Aspergillus flavus,* which grows on peanuts and grains)	Metabolized to an epoxide, which is either detoxified or binds to DNA	Among the most potent of liver carcinogens, especially in parts of Africa
Aromatic amines and azo dyes	Primarily metabolized in the liver; N-hydroxylation to form hydroxylamino derivatives	Occupational exposure to aromatic amines in the form of aniline dyes → bladder cancer
Nitrosamines (commonly added nitrite preservative in foods may react with other dietary components to form nitrosamines)	Hydroxylation, followed by formation of a reactive alkyl carbonium ion	Linked to esophageal and G.I. cancers
Miscellaneous agents; metals, asbestos, plastics, dextran polymers	Activation mechanisms obscure	Many cancers occur in occupational settings; association between lung cancer and asbestos exposure is clearly established in smokers

- Cultured human cells are now used increasingly for assays of mutagenicity.

Human Chemical Carcinogens

Direct-acting Carcinogens

- These chemicals (some alkylating and acylating agents) cause cancer directly, without having to be altered.
- They are inherently reactive enough to bind covalently to cellular macromolecules.

Indirect-acting Carcinogens

Most organic carcinogens require metabolic conversion to a more reactive compound. This conversion is enzymatic. Many body cells, particularly liver cells, possess enzyme systems that convert procarcinogens to their active forms. Genetically determined enzyme levels in different people can determine sensitivity to carcinogens. Table 5-5 lists some of the chemical carcinogens associated with human cancer.

Physical Carcinogenesis

Ultraviolet (UV) Radiation

- Cancers attributed to sun exposure, namely basal cell carcinoma, squamous carcinoma, and melanoma, occur predominantly in fair-skinned people. The effects of UV radiation on cells include enzyme inactivation, inhibition of cell division, mutagenesis, cell death, and cancer.
- Xeroderma pigmentosum, a disease with a high incidence of skin cancers resulting from sensitivity to sunlight, exemplifies the importance of DNA repair in protecting against the harmful effects of UV radiation. Both neoplastic and nonneoplastic skin disorders in xeroderma pigmentosum are attributed to impairment in the excision of UV-damaged DNA.

Asbestos and Mesothelioma

Mesothelioma, a cancer of the pleural and peritoneal cavities, occurs mainly in workers who have had heavy exposure to asbestos. There is a strong correlation between lung cancer and asbestos-exposed cigarette smokers.

Tumor Immunology

The theory of immune surveillance holds that mutant clones with neoplastic potential arise frequently but are eliminated by cell-mediated immune responses. However, evidence of this concept is highly controversial.

Mechanisms of Immunological Cytotoxicity

The contribution of any specific immunological mechanism to tumor cell destruction in vivo has not been clearly defined. A number of possible mechanisms are being actively studied (Fig. 5-4).

T-cell–mediated Cytotoxicity

Cytotoxic T cells (CD8+) can recognize and destroy a cell containing "foreign" antigens when peptides derived from those antigens

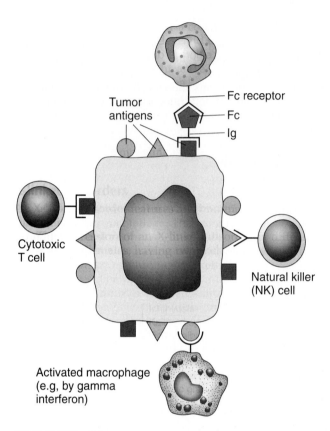

FIGURE 5-4
Possible mechanisms of immunological tumor cytotoxicity in animal studies. (From Rubin E, Gorstein F, Rubin R, et al. Rubin's Pathology, 4th ed. Philadelphia: Lippincott Williams & Wilkins, 2005, p. 206.)

are associated with class I major histocompatibility complex (MHC) molecules and displayed on the tumor cell surface. CD8+ T cells can be sensitized to tumors under the following circumstances:

- The tumor cell expresses an antigen specific to that tumor cell that is not present on normal body cells (tumor-specific antigen).
- The tumor cell expresses an antigen present on that tumor cell and also present on certain body cells (tumor-associated antigen).
- The tumor cell overexpresses an antigen.

- The tumor cell expresses a viral peptide encoded by an oncogenic virus.

Other Mechanisms

- **Natural killer (NK) cell-mediated cytotoxicity:** NK cells are lymphocyte-like cells with tumoricidal activity that does not depend on prior sensitization to tumor cell antigens.
- **Macrophage-mediated cytotoxicity:** Macrophages can kill tumor cells in a nonspecific manner; however, their role in control of malignant tumors is unclear.
- **Antibody-dependent cell-mediated cytotoxicity:** Antibodies directed against tumor-associated antigens do not kill the tumor cell but can act as a link between the appropriate effector (killer) and the tumor cell. Effectors can be macrophages, neutrophils, or lymphocytes.
- **Complement-mediated cytotoxicity:** Tumor cells that have been coated with specific antibodies can be lysed by the action of complement.

Evasion of Immunological Cytotoxicity

Conclusive proof that immunological tumor surveillance is a valid process is lacking. A number of tumor cell properties have been proposed for the failure of immune responses to limit tumor growth, including the following:

- Deficient (or lack of) expression of tumor-specific antigens
- Deficient histocompatibility (MHC, HLA) expression
- Deficient tumor antigen peptide processing
- Lack of costimulators needed for T-cell activation
- Expression of immunosuppressive factors

Systemic Effects of Cancer on the Host

Cancer may produce remote effects not attributable to tumor invasion or metastasis, which are collectively termed "paraneoplastic" syndromes. These may be the first manifestation of disease and may also provide a means of monitoring disease progression.

- Fever: most commonly occurs in Hodgkin disease, renal cell carcinoma, and osteogenic sarcoma
- Anorexia and weight loss: may be accompanied by an elevated metabolic rate; TNF-α (cachectin) may lead to cachexia.
- Endocrine syndromes: often manifest in the ectopic production of a number of peptide hormones not under normal regulatory control. Examples include Cushing syndrome caused by adrenocorticotropic hormone, sodium and water retention caused by inappropriate antidiuretic hormone, hypercalcemia caused

by parathormonelike peptide, hypocalcemia caused by calcito-nin-secreting medullary thyroid carcinoma, and hypoglycemia caused by excessive insulin production by islet cell tumors of the pancreas.

- Neurological syndromes: Subacute motor neuropathy, a spinal cord disorder, is strongly associated with cancer. Peripheral neuropathies may indicate occult tumors.
- Skeletal muscle syndromes: dermatomyositis and polymyositis are associated with cancer.
- Hematological syndromes: erythrocytosis, anemia, increase in granulocyte and platelet counts, and the hypercoagulable state may be indications of malignancy.
- GI syndromes: GI or liver damage (with depression of albumin synthesis) is possible.
- Nephritic syndrome: This may be a consequence of renal vein thrombosis.
- Cutaneous syndromes: acanthosis nigricans (a skin disorder marked by regional hyperpigmentation and hyperkeratosis) may occur.
- Amyloidosis: About 15% of cases occur in association with cancers.

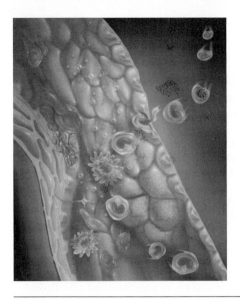

CHAPTER 6

Developmental and Genetic Diseases

Chapter Outline

Multifactorial Inheritance
Screening for Carriers of Genetic Disorders
Prenatal Diagnosis of Genetic Disorders
Prematurity and Intrauterine Growth Retardation
    Apgar Score
    Organ Immaturity as a Cause of Neonatal Problems
    Respiratory Distress Syndrome (RDS) of the Newborn
    Erythroblastosis Fetalis
    Birth Injuries
    Sudden Infant Death Syndrome (SIDS)
Neoplasms of Infancy and Childhood

Diseases that originate during prenatal development range from conditions caused solely by factors in the fetal environment to those that are exclusively determined by genomic abnormalities. Developmental and genetic disorders are classified as follows:

- Errors of morphogenesis
- Chromosomal abnormalities
- Single-gene defects
- Polygenic inherited diseases

Each year, about one quarter of a million infants are born in the United States with a birth defect. No more than 6% of all birth defects can be attributed to uterine factors, maternal disorders, and environmental hazards. Most of the remaining cases are caused by genomic defects and chromosomal abnormalities.

Teratology

Teratology is the discipline concerned with developmental anomalies, and teratogens are the chemical, physical, and biological agents that cause them.

- Susceptibility to teratogens is variable (e.g., fetal alcohol syndrome affects only some children of alcoholic mothers).
- Susceptibility to teratogens is specific for each developmental stage (e.g., maternal rubella infection causes fetal abnormalities only during the first 3 months of pregnancy).
- The mechanism of teratogenesis is specific for each teratogen.
- Teratogenesis is dose dependent.
- Teratogens produce death, growth retardation, malformation, or functional impairment.

Errors of Morphogenesis

- Exposure to adverse influences in the preimplantation and early postimplantation stages of development most often leads to prenatal death. This early stage of embryonic death often passes unnoticed or is perceived as heavy, delayed menstrual bleeding.

- Injury during the first 8 to 10 days after fertilization may result in an incomplete separation of blastomeres, which may lead to the formation of conjoined twins.
- Periods of maximal sensitivity to teratogens are those in which primordial organ systems are developing. These vary for different organ systems, but overall are limited to the first 8 weeks of pregnancy.
- After the third month of pregnancy, exposure to teratogenic influences rarely results in major errors of morphogenesis.

Terms Used to Describe Developmental Anomalies

- *Aplasia*: absence of an organ, or an undeveloped organ rudiment
- *Hypoplasia*: reduced size of an organ owing to incomplete development of all or part of it
- *Dystrophic anomalies*: defects caused by fusion failure (e.g., spina bifida [spinal canal and overlying bone and skin have not fused])
- *Involution failures*: persistence of embryonic or fetal structures
- *Division failures*: incomplete cleavage (e.g., incompletely separated fingers)
- *Atresia*: incomplete formation of a lumen
- *Dysplasia*: abnormal organization of cells into a tissue
- *Ectopia*: an organ is not in its normal anatomical site
- *Dystopia*: retention of an organ at early developmental site (e.g., failure of testes to descend into scrotum)
- *Polytopic effect*: one noxious stimulus affects several organs
- *Monotopic effect*: a single anomaly results in a cascade of pathogenic events
- *Developmental sequence anomaly*: a pattern of defects related to a single anomaly. For example, in the Potter complex, a number of congenital abnormalities are manifested (pulmonary hyperplasia, contractures of the limbs, urinary tract obstruction). These all result from a severely reduced amount of amniotic fluid (oligohydramnios), irrespective of the cause of the decreased volume of fluid.
- *Developmental syndrome*: refers to multiple anomalies that are pathogenetically related
- *Developmental association (syntropy)*: refers to multiple anomalies that are associated statistically but do not necessarily share the same pathogenetic mechanisms
- *Deformation*: abnormality of form, shape, or position of a body part. Most anatomical defects caused by adverse influences in the latter two trimesters of pregnancy fall into this category.

Neural Tube Defects

Incomplete fusion of the neural tube and overlying bone, soft tissues, or skin leads to several defects, varying from mild anomalies (e.g., spina bifida occulta) to severe anomalies (e.g., anencephaly). Neural tube defects are discussed in more detail in Chapter 28.

Folic acid supplied in the periconceptual period decreases the incidence of neural tube defects. Since 1998, the U.S. Food and Drug Administration mandate to manufacturers to supplement flour and bread with folate has led to a significant decrease in the incidence of neural tube defects.

Types of neural tube defects include the following:

- *Anencephaly* is a defect of neural tube closure, and refers to the congenital absence of the cranial vault, with cerebral hemispheres completely missing or reduced to small masses attached to the base of the skull.
- *Spina bifida* refers to the incomplete closure of the spinal cord or vertebral column or both, and represents the mildest abnormality of the central nervous system.
- *Craniorachischisis*: defective closure from the cranium into the spinal cord
- *Meningocele*: hernial protrusion of the meninges through the vertebral column
- *Myelomeningocele*: hernial protrusion of the spinal cord through the vertebral column

Defects Caused by Maternal Exposure to Drugs or Alcohol

Thalidomide-induced Malformations

Thalidomide, a derivative of glutamic acid, is teratogenic between the 28th and 50th days of pregnancy. In the 1960s, many children born to mothers who had taken thalidomide had skeletal deformities, such as short and malformed arms. Although the drug was subsequently banned from the market, an estimated 3,000 malformed children were born.

Fetal Hydantoin Syndrome

Ten percent of children born to mothers with epilepsy who were treated during pregnancy with antiepileptic drugs such as hydantoin show characteristic facial features such as a flat nasal bridge, epicanthic folds, a prominent upper lip and a small head. They also exhibit hypoplasia of nails and digits, and various congenital heart defects

Fetal Alcohol Syndrome

This complex of abnormalities induced by maternal alcohol abuse includes (a) growth retardation; (b) possible mental retardation and problems with development, learning, and behavior; and (c) characteristic facial dysmorphology, such as thin upper lip, short nose, short eye openings, and flat cheeks. Heavy alcohol consumption during the first trimester of pregnancy is particularly dangerous. The mechanism by which alcohol damages the developing fetus remains unknown.

Defects Caused by Fetal or Neonatal Infections

TORCH Complex

This acronym refers to a complex of similar symptoms produced by fetal or neonatal infection with a variety of microorganisms including **t**oxoplasma, **r**ubella, **c**ytomegalovirus, and **H**erpes simplex virus. Infections with TORCH agents occur in 1 to 5% of all liveborn infants in the U.S, and are among the major causes of neonatal morbidity and mortality. The specific organisms of the TORCH complex are discussed in detail in Chapter 9. Only a minority of newborns has the entire spectrum of abnormalities, but growth retardation, and abnormalities of the brain, eyes, liver, hematopoietic system, and heart are common (Fig. 6-1).

Congenital Syphilis

Treponema pallidum, the organism that causes syphilis, is transmitted by the infected mother to the fetus. Many infants are asymptomatic but develop symptoms in the first few years of life. Later symptoms reflect slowly evolving tissue destruction and repair and include the following:

- Rhinitis with edematous nasal mucosa and nosebleeds
- Maculopapular rash, especially of palms and soles
- Affected visceral organs: pale lungs (pneumonia alba), enlarged liver, spleen and lymph nodes, which become enlarged.
- Teeth: notched incisors and malformed molars (Hutchinson's teeth)
- Bones: inflammation of the periosteum
- Eyes: corneal vascularization and corneal scarring
- Nervous system: mental retardation, deafness

Penicillin is the drug of choice for treatment of both intrauterine and postnatal syphilis. If it is given for both these conditions, it prevents most symptoms.

Chromosomal Characteristics

Normal Chromosomes

The 46 chromosomes of human somatic cells consist of 23 pairs. Of those 23 pairs, 22 are alike in males and females and are called autosomes. The remaining pair are the sex chromosomes, XX in females and XY in males. Chromosomes can be isolated from mi-

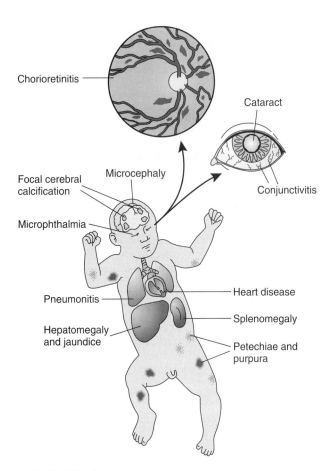

FIGURE 6-1
Toxoplasma, rubella, cytomegalovirus, and Herpes simplex virus (TORCH) complex. Children infected in utero with Toxoplasma, rubella virus cytomegalovirus, or herpes simplex virus show remarkably similar effects. (From Rubin E, Gorstein F, Rubin R, et al. Rubin's Pathology, 4th ed. Philadelphia: Lippincott Williams & Wilkins, 2005, p. 224.)

totic cell and stained and classified according to their length and positioning of the centromere (Fig. 6-2).

Techniques for Chromosome and Gene Identification

- *Fluorescence in situ hybridization (FISH)* uses fluorescently labeled DNA probes to identify small regions of chromosomes or individual genes.

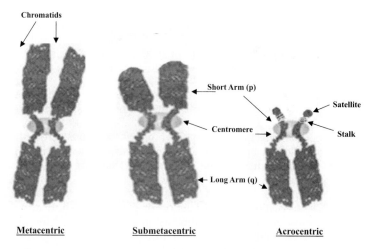

FIGURE 6-2
Chromosome types. Metacentric chromosomes show centromeres exactly in the middle; in submetacentric chromosomes, the centromere divides the chromosome into a short arm (*p*) and a long arm (*q*); acrocentric chromosomes display very short arms or stalks and satellites attached to an eccentrically located centromere.

- *Chromosomal banding* is a technique making use of special stains to delineate specific bands on chromosomes. The pattern of bands is unique to each chromosome and makes possible the identification of each chromosome, as well as defects in a segment of chromosome.

Chromosomal Abnormalities

Structural Chromosomal Abnormalities

Most structural chromosomal abnormalities that may arise when somatic cells divide are of little consequence to the whole organism because the individual cell with the abnormality either manages to function, or it dies. Under some circumstances, somatic structural abnormalities may involve protooncogenes and contribute to the pathogenesis of certain cancers (see Chapter 5).

However, structural chromosomal abnormalities that originate during gametogenesis are important because they are transmitted to all somatic cells of the offspring and may result in disease. During normal meiosis, homologous chromosomes pair and exchange genetic material. In an abnormal process called translocation, non-homologous chromosomes pair and exchange genetic material. In balanced translocations, there is no loss of genetic material; carriers are phenotypically normal but are at risk for producing offspring with unbalanced karyotypes and severe phenotypic abnormalities.

Some of the following types of structural rearrangements observed in human chromosomes are illustrated in Figure 6-3.

- Reciprocal Translocation: exchange of acentric chromosomal segments between two different (nonhomologous) chromosomes
- Robertsonian Translocation: Two nonhomologous acrocentric chromosomes break near the centromere to form one large metacentric chromosome composed of the long arms of the pair. The short arms are usually lost.
- Chromosomal Deletions: Loss of a portion of a chromosome; in *cri du chat syndrome* (deletion of part of the short arm of chromosome 5), some retinoblastomas (deletions of the long arm of chromosome 13), and Wilms tumor aniridia (deletions in short arm of chromosome 11)
- Chromosomal Inversion: Refers to (a) break of a chromosome at two points, (b) inversion of the segment between the breaks, and (c) rejoining of the two broken ends. This may lead to interference with pairing and crossover during meiosis.
- Ring Chromosome: Abnormally shaped chromosome may impede normal meiotic division, but normally of no consequence
- Isochromosomes: Metacentric chromosomes produced during meiosis or mitosis when the centromere splits transversely instead of longitudinally, resulting in one chromosome having the two long arms of the original chromosome and the other chromosome having the two short arms and no long arms; in *Turner syndrome* (15% of those affected have an isochromosome of the X chromosome)

Numerical Chromosome Abnormalities

Useful Terms

- Haploid: A single set (n) of each of the chromosomes (n = 23 in humans); only germ cells have a haploid number (n) of chromosomes
- Diploid: A double set (2n) of each of the chromosomes (2n = 46 in humans); most somatic cells are diploid.
- Euploid: Any multiple of the haploid number from n to 8n; many liver cells are euploid (4n). When the multiple is greater than diploid, the karyotype is said to be polyploid.
- Aneuploid: Karyotypes that are not exact multiples of the haploid number. Many cancer cells are aneuploid, a characteristic associated with aggressive biological behavior.

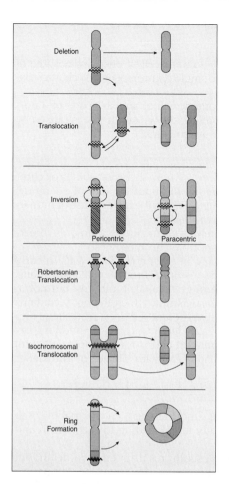

FIGURE 6-3

Structural abnormalities of human chromosomes. The deletion of a portion of a chromosome leads to the loss of genetic material and a shortened chromosome. A reciprocal translocation involves breaks on two nonhomologous chromosomes, with exchange of the acentric segments. An inversion requires two breaks in a single chromosome. If the breaks are on opposite sides of the centromere, the inversion is *pericentric*; it is *paracentric* if the breaks are on the same arm. A Robertsonian translocation occurs when two nonhomologous acrocentric chromosomes break near their centromeres, after which the long arms fuse to form one large metacentric chromosome. Isochromosomes arise from faulty centromere division, which leads to duplication of the long arm (iso q) and deletion of the short arm, or the reverse (iso p). Ring chromosomes involve breaks of both telomeric portions of a chromosome, deletion of the acentric fragments, and fusion of the remaining centric portion. (From Rubin E, Gorstein F, Rubin R, et al. Rubin's Pathology, 4th ed. Philadelphia: Lippincott Williams & Wilkins, 2005, p. 228.)

- Monosomy: Absence in a somatic cell of one chromosome of a homologous pair (e.g., a single X chromosome is characteristic of Turner syndrome)
- Trisomy: Presence in a somatic cell of an extra copy of a normally paired chromosome (e.g., Down syndrome is caused by the presence of three chromosomes 21)

Nondisjunction

- Nondisjunction is the failure of paired chromosomes or chromatids to separate and move to opposite poles at anaphase, either during mitosis or meiosis. It is the major cause of numerical chromosomal abnormalities.
- Nondisjunction during meiosis occurs more commonly in persons with structurally abnormal chromosomes.
- Mitotic nondisjunction may involve embryonic cells in early stages of development and result in chromosomal aberrations, which are transmitted through some cell lineages, but not in others. This results in **mosaicism** in which the body contains two or more karyotypically different cell lines. Autosomal mosaicism is rare and is probably lethal; mosaicism involving sex chromosomes is fairly common and is found in patients with gonadal dysgenesis who present with Turner or Klinefelter syndrome.

Effects of Chromosomal Aberrations

- Most major chromosomal abnormalities are incompatible with life. The defects are usually lethal leading to early death and abortions.
- Autosomal monosomies usually result in embryo death, but monosomy of the X chromosome (45X) may be compatible with life, although more than 95% of such embryos are lost during pregnancy.
- Absence of an X chromosome (45Y) results in early abortion.
- Approximately 0.3% of all liveborn infants have a chromosomal abnormality.
- Autosomal trisomies are usually lethal, except for trisomy 21 (Down syndrome)

Nomenclature of Chromosomal Aberrations

Table 6-1 shows chromosomal nomenclature.

Syndromes of Numerical or Structural Chromosomal Aberrations

Trisomy 21 (Down Syndrome)

Trisomy 21 is one of the most common causes of mental retardation. Two thirds of conceptuses with this defect are aborted spontaneously or die in utero.

Table 6-1

Chromosomal Nomenclature

Numerical designation of autosomes	1–22
Sex chromosomes	X, Y
Addition of a whole or part of a chromosome	+
Loss of a whole or part of a chromosome	−
Numerical mosaicism (e.g., 46/47)	/
Short arm of chromosome (petite)	p
Long arm of chromosome	q
Isochromosome	I
Ring chromosome	r
Deletion	del
Insertion	ins
Translocation	t
Derivative chromosome (carrying translocation)	der
Terminal	ter
Representative karyotypes	
Male with trisomy 21	47,XY, +21
Female carrier of fusion-type translocation between chromosomes 14 and 21	45,XX-14, −21,+t(14q21q)
Cri du chat syndrome (male) with deletion of a portion of the short arm of chromosome 5	46,XY,del(5p)
Male with ring chromosome 19	46,XY,r(!()
Turner syndrome with monosomy X	45,X
Mosaic Klinefelter syndrome	46,XY/47,XXY

Pathogenesis

The three mechanisms by which three copies of the genes on chromosome 21 may be present on somatic cells in Down syndrome are as follows:

- Nondisjunction during the first meiotic division, leading to the presence of a complete extra chromosome 21 (95% of cases)
- Translocation of an extra long arm of chromosome 21 to another acrocentric chromosome (5% of cases)
- Mosaicism for trisomy 21, caused by nondisjunction during mitosis of a somatic cell in early embryogenesis, with some cells having a normal number of chromosome 21 and others with an extra chromosome 21 (2% of cases)

Older mothers have a greater risk of giving birth to an infant with Down syndrome due to nondisjunction; the incidence reaches 1 in 30 at 45 years of age.

Pathology and Clinical Features

Diagnosis of Down syndrome is ordinarily made at the time of birth by observing the characteristic physical appearance of the infant and then confirmed by cytogenetic analysis. As the child develops, typical abnormalities appear (Fig. 6-4). The major determinant of survival in Down syndrome is the presence or absence of congenital heart disease.

Other Trisomies

Trisomy 18 is an order of magnitude less frequent than Down syndrome. Trisomies 13 and 22 occur but are even more rare. Affected infants with these trisomies usually die within the first 3 months of life.

Partial trisomies occur. For example, 9p-trisomy [translocation of the short arm of chromosome 9 to a number of different autosomes], and reciprocal translocation between the long arms of chromosomes 22 and 11.

Carriers of balanced translocations are usually asymptomatic, but their offspring may have a variety of defects.

Chromosomal Deletion Syndromes

Deletion of an entire autosomal chromosome is not compatible with life, but deletions of parts of chromosomes occur. All such deletions are indicated by chromosome number followed by p (short arm) or q (long arm). Almost all the resultant deletion syndromes are characterized by low birth weight, mental retardation, skeletal abnormalities, congenital heart disease, and urogenital abnormalities. These syndromes include the following:

- 5p-syndrome (cri du chat syndrome): high-pitched cry of an infant similar to that of a kitten; calls attention to the disorder

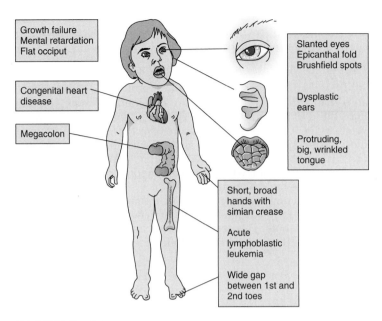

F I G U R E   6-4
Clinical features of Down syndrome. (From Rubin E, Gorstein F, Rubin R, et al. Rubin's Pathology, 4th ed. Philadelphia: Lippincott Williams & Wilkins, 2005, p. 234.)

- 11p-syndrome: results in absence of iris (aniridia) and is often accompanied by Wilms tumor.
- 13q-syndrome: associated with retinoblastoma and caused by the loss of the *Rb* tumor suppressor gene present on the long arm of chromosome 13

Other deletion syndromes involving deletions of material from chromosomes 18, 19, 20, 21, and 22 have been documented. Deletions and rearrangements of subtelomeric sequences have been reported and demonstrated to be a cause of mental retardation and dysmorphic features.

Chromosomal Breakage Syndromes

Some recessive syndromes associated with frequent chromosomal breakage and rearrangements are accompanied by a significant risk of leukemia and cancers. These disorders include xeroderma pigmentosum, Bloom syndrome, Fanconi anemia, and ataxia telangiectasia. Acquired chromosomal breaks and rearrangements (translocations) are associated with leukemias and lymphomas, the best documented of which are chronic myelogenous leukemia, t(9;22), and Burkitt lymphoma, mostly t(8;14). See Table 6-1 for review of chromosomal nomenclature.

Numerical Aberrations of Sex Chromosomes

Additional sex chromosomes seem to produce less genetic imbalance than extra autosomes and are considerably more common than those of the autosomes, with the exception of trisomy 21. Whereas the X chromosome has more than 1,300 genes, the Y chromosome is considerably smaller and has only about 200 genes, one of which is the sex-determining region Y (SRY). SRY encodes a small nuclear protein, which plays an important role in the development of the male phenotype.

Although males carry only one X chromosome, both males and females produce the same amounts of gene products encoded by the X chromosome. This seeming discrepancy has been explained by the **Lyon effect,** on which the following principles are based:

- In females, one X chromosome is irreversibly inactivated early in embryogenesis. The inactivated X chromosome is detectable in interphase nuclei as a dark clump of chromatin, termed the Barr body.
- Either the paternal or the maternal X chromosome is inactivated randomly, and the inactivation is transmitted to progeny cells. Thus, all females are mosaic for paternally and maternally derived X chromosomes.
- The inactivated X chromosome retains some functioning genes that are important in gametogenesis as well as normal growth and development.

Klinefelter Syndrome (47,XXY)

Klinefelter syndrome is related to the presence of one or more X chromosomes in excess of the normal XY complement. It is a prominent cause of male hypogonadism and infertility. Most males with this syndrome have a 47,XXY karyotype, but some are mosaics (e.g., 46,XY/47,XXY) or have more than two X chromosomes. Regardless of the number of X chromosomes, the presence of the Y chromosome ensures a male phenotype. The clinical features of Klinefelter syndrome are shown in Figure 6-5.

XYY Male

Characteristics of the XYY phenotype are tall stature, a tendency toward cystic acne, and some problems in motor and language development. Assertions of aggressive and antisocial behavior in XYY males have not been substantiated.

Turner Syndrome (45,X)

Turner syndrome refers to the spectrum of abnormalities that results from a complete or partial monosomy of the X chromosome

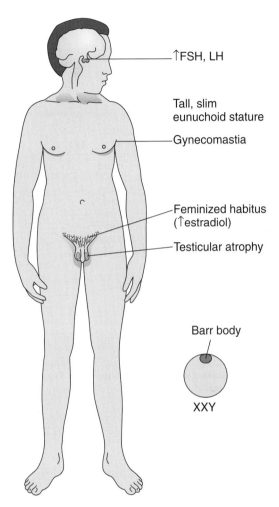

↑FSH, LH

Tall, slim
eunuchoid stature

Gynecomastia

Feminized habitus
(↑estradiol)

Testicular atrophy

Barr body

XXY

FIGURE 6-5
Clinical features of Klinefelter syndrome. (From Rubin E, Gorstein F, Rubin R, et al. Rubin's Pathology, 4th ed. Philadelphia: Lippincott Williams & Wilkins, 2005, p. 238.)

in a phenotypic female. The 45,X karyotype is one of the most common aneuploid abnormalities in human conceptuses, but almost all are aborted spontaneously. Clinical features of Turner syndrome are shown in Figure 6-6.

Only about half of women with Turner syndrome lack an entire X chromosome; the rest are mosaics or display structural aberra-

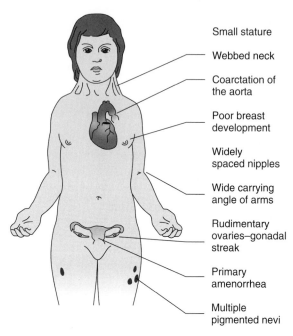

Small stature

Webbed neck

Coarctation of
the aorta

Poor breast
development

Widely
spaced nipples

Wide carrying
angle of arms

Rudimentary
ovaries–gonadal
streak

Primary
amenorrhea

Multiple
pigmented nevi

FIGURE   6-6
Clinical features of Turner syndrome. (From Rubin E, Gorstein F, Rubin R, et al. Rubin's Pathology, 4th ed. Philadelphia: Lippincott Williams & Wilkins, 2005, p. 239.)

tions of the X chromosome. Women with the 45,X/46,XX mosaic karyotype have milder phenotypic features and may even be fertile. Patients with the mosaic karyotype 45,X/46,XY, in which an original male zygote was modified by a mitotic nondisjunction, are at 20% risk of developing a germ cell cancer and should have prophylactic removal of the abnormal gonads.

Syndromes in Females with Multiple X Chromosomes

One extra X chromosome in a phenotypic female (47,XXX) is the most frequent abnormality of sex chromosomes in women. Most are fertile and of normal intelligence, although there is an increased incidence of congenital defects in their children.

Women with four and five X chromosomes are mentally retarded and do not mature sexually. All women with extra X chromosomes have additional Barr bodies, indicating inactivation of all but one X chromosome.

Single Gene Abnormalities (Mendelian Disorders)

Mendelian traits are classified as (a) autosomal dominant, (b) autosomal recessive, (c) sex-linked dominant, and (d) sex-linked recessive.

Mendelian Inheritance

The classic laws of mendelian inheritance are as follows:

- A mendelian trait is determined by two copies of the same gene (alleles) located at the same locus on two homologous chromosomes. In the case of the X and Y chromosomes in males, a trait is determined by just one allele.
- Autosomal genes are located on one of the 22 autosomes.
- Sex-linked traits are encoded by loci on the X chromosome.
- A dominant phenotypic trait requires the presence of only one allele of a gene pair, regardless of whether the alleles are homozygous or heterozygous.
- A recessive phenotypic trait requires that both alleles be identical (homozygous).
- In codominance, both alleles in a heterozygous pair are fully expressed.

Mutations

A mutation is a stable, heritable change in DNA, and a broad range of mutations accounts for the large number of genetic polymorphisms in the population. A polymorphism is a genetic variant that appears in at least 1% of a population. Some examples of well-known polymorphisms are the human ABO blood groups, the human Rh factor, and the human major histocompatibility complex (MHC).

The major types of mutations that are found in human genetic disorders are as follows:

- Point mutations: replacement of one base by another
- Frameshift mutation: In the genetic code, each set of three bases constitutes a codon specific for a particular amino acid; insertions or deletions of a number of bases, that is not a multiple of 3, into the coding region of DNA, changes the reading frame of the message. When this happens, every codon downstream from the mutation has a new sequence and codes for a different amino acid.
- Large deletions: deletion of an extensive segment of DNA
- Expansion of unstable trinucleotide repeat sequences: The human genome contains frequent tandem trinucleotide repeat sequences. When these are expanded above a threshold number, disease can ensue. Examples:

  ➤ Huntington disease: expansion of a CAG repeat within the coding sequence of the *huntingtin* gene.

➤ Fragile X syndrome: expansion of a CGG repeat in a noncoding region adjacent to the *FMRI* gene on the X chromosome
➤ Myotonic dystrophy: expansion of a CTG repeat in an untranslated region of the myotonic dystrophy gene
➤ Friedreich ataxia: expansion of a GAA repeat in the *frataxin* gene

Autosomal Dominant Disorders

Autosomal dominant disorders are expressed in heterozygotes. A dominant disease occurs when only one defective gene (i.e., mutant allele) is present, whereas the allele on the homologous chromosome is normal. Some salient features of autosomal dominant traits are as follows:

- The mutated gene determines phenotypic expression.
- Males and females are equally affected, and there can be transmission from either parent to progeny of either sex.
- The trait encoded by the mutant gene can be transmitted to successive generations (unless it interferes with reproductive capacity).
- Every person with the disease has an affected parent (unless the disorder results from a new mutation).
- These disorders may impair function and have some reduction in life expectancy, but most individuals survive to at least reproductive age.
- Homozygosity is generally fatal.

More than 1,000 human diseases are inherited as autosomal dominant traits. Examples are given in Table 6-2.

Biochemical Basis of Autosomal Dominant Disorders

There are several major mechanisms by which autosomal dominant disorders cause disease.

- *Haploinsufficiency*: If the gene product is a component of a complex network (e.g., a receptor or an enzyme), half of the normal amount of the gene product is not sufficient to maintain the normal state. Examples include β thalassemia and familial hypercholesterolemia.
- *Extra copy of the allele*: Duplication of the peripheral myelin protein-22 gene causes Charcot-Marie-Tooth disease type 1A.
- *Constitutive activation of a gene*: This is seen in familial cancer syndromes. For example, mutations in the RET protooncogene cause abnormally increased activity of a tyrosine kinase, which leads to increased cell proliferation in multiple endocrine neoplasia type 2.

Table 6-2

Representative Autosomal Dominant Disorders

Disease	Frequency	Chromosome
Familial hypercholesterolemia	1/500	19p
von Willebrand disease	1/8,000	12p
Hereditary spherocytosis (major forms)	1/5,000	14,8
Hereditary elliptocytosis (all forms)	1/2,500	1,1p,2q,14
Osteogenesis imperfecta (types I-IV)	1/10,000	17q,7q
Ehlers-Danlos syndrome, type III	1/5,000	?
Marfan syndrome	1/10,000	15q
Neurofibromatosis type 1	1/3,500	17q
Huntington chorea	1/15,000	4p
Retinoblastoma	1/14,000	13q
Wilms tumor	1/10,000	11p
Familial adenomatous polyposis	1/10,000	5q
Acute intermittent porphyria	1/15,000	11q
Hereditary amyloidosis	1/100,000	18q
Adult polycystic kidney disease	1/1,000	16p

From Rubin E, Gorstein F, Rubin R, et al. Rubin's Pathology, 4th ed. Philadelphia: Lippincott Williams & Wilkins, 2005, p. 243.

- *Disruption of normal morphological patterns*: Mutations in genes that encode structural proteins such as collagen and cytoskeletal components can result in abnormal molecular interactions. This is exemplified by diseases such as osteogenesis imperfecta and hereditary spherocytosis.

Autosomal Dominant Inherited Disorders of Connective Tissue

This discussion is limited to three of the most common and best-studied entities: Marfan syndrome, Ehlers-Danlos syndrome, and osteogenesis imperfecta.

Marfan Syndrome

Marfan syndrome is characterized by abnormalities in heart, aorta, skeleton, eyes and skin. The syndrome is caused by a missense mutation in the gene coding for fibrillin-1, a glycoprotein that is the major constitutive element of extracellular microfibrils and has widespread distribution in both elastic and nonelastic connective tissue throughout the body. The abnormal fibrillin coded by the defective gene has a dominant negative effect, interfering with the assembly of normal microfibrils. The gene (*FBN1*) has been mapped to the long arm of chromosome 15 (15q21.1).

Characteristics of Marfan syndrome include the following:

- Skeletal system: Patients are usually tall and thin, with long, spiderlike fingers and hyperextensible joints (double-jointedness).
- Cardiovascular system: The most important clinical cardiovascular defect is a weakness in the elastic tunica media of the aorta causing a susceptibility to dissecting aortic aneurisms. Aortic valve insufficiency and mitral valve prolapse also can occur.
- Eyes: Ocular changes reflect the intrinsic lesion in connective tissue and include dislocation of the lens (ectopia lentis), severe myopia and retinal detachment.

Ehlers-Danlos Syndromes

Ehlers-Danlos Syndrome (EDS) are a group of connective tissue disorders resulting from defects in collagen. EDS are clinically and genetically heterogeneous, and more than 10 varieties have been distinguished. The common feature in all syndromes is a generalized defect in collagen, including abnormalities in its molecular structure, synthesis, secretion and degradation. Depending on the type of EDS, the molecular collagen lesions are associated with conspicuous weakness in the supporting structures of the skin, joints, arteries, and visceral organs. Characteristic features include remarkable hyperelasticity and fragility of the skin, joint hypermobility, and easy bruising.

Osteogenesis Imperfecta

Osteogenesis imperfecta (OI), or brittle bone disease, is a group of disorders in which a generalized abnormality of connective tissue is expressed principally as fragility of bone. There are four types of OI, with heterogeneous genetic defects, but all affect the synthesis of type 1 collagen. In 90% of cases, mutations in the *pro-α1* and *pro-α2* collagen genes are present, resulting in the substitution of other amino acids for the obligate glycine at every third residue.

The most common variant is often accompanied by multiple childhood bone fractures, and blue sclerae resulting from the translucency of the thin connective tissue overlying the choroids.

Osteogenesis Imperfecta is discussed in further detail in Chapter 26.

Other Autosomal Dominant Disorders

Neurofibromatoses (NF)

Neurofibromatoses are autosomal dominant disorders characterized by the development of multiple neurofibromas (benign tumors of peripheral nerves).

There are two main forms of NF: NF type 1 (von Recklinghausen disease) and NF type 2 (central neurofibromatosis). NF1 and NF2 are caused by two separate abnormal genes; the gene for NF1 is located on chromosome 17, and the gene for NF2 is on chromosome 22. Both NF1 and NF2 genes are tumor suppressor genes; defects in these genes are believed to be responsible for the predisposition to the formation of nerve tumors.

Typical features of NF1 include the following:

- Cutaneous, subcutaneous, and plexiform neurofibromas Plexiform neurofibromas usually involve larger peripheral nerves, are often large and may cause disfigurement of face or extremity.
- Café au lait spots (numerous light brown skin patches)
- Lisch nodules (pigmented nodules of the iris, consisting of masses of melanocytes)
- Skeletal lesions, mild intellectual impairment, and the risk of malignant myeloid disorders also occur in the disease.

NF2 is characterized by bilateral tumors of the eighth cranial nerve (acoustic neuromas) and, commonly, meningiomas and gliomas. It is less common than NF1.

Achondroplastic Dwarfism

This hereditary disturbance of epiphyseal chondroblastic development leads to inadequate endochondral bone formation. This causes a form of dwarfism characterized by short limbs and normal head and trunk. Achondroplasia is discussed in Chapter 26.

Familial Hypercholesterolemia

This disorder is characterized by high levels of low-density lipoproteins (LDLs) in the blood. The disorder results from abnormalities in the gene that codes for the cell surface receptor that removes LDL from the blood. The gene is located on the short arm of chromosome 19. More than 150 different mutations in the LDL receptor gene have been described, including insertions, deletions, and nonsense and missense point mutations. Classes of genetic defects in a number of the steps involved in the synthesis and intracellular processing of the LDL receptor have been observed.

Familial hypercholesterolemia results in a decreased transport of LDL cholesterol into cells and conspicuous hypercholesterolemia. There is early onset of atherosclerosis, coronary heart disease, and tendon xanthomas.

Autosomal Recessive Disorders

Autosomal recessive disorders are associated with clinical symptoms when both alleles at a locus on homologous chromosomes are defective. Most genetic metabolic diseases exhibit an autosomal recessive mode of inheritance and are characteristically caused by deficiencies in enzymes rather than abnormalities in structural proteins. Some salient features of autosomal recessive traits are as follows:

- The more infrequent the mutant gene, the lower the probability that unrelated parents both carry the trait; therefore, rare autosomal recessive disorders are often the product of consanguineous marriages.
- Both parents are usually heterozygous for the trait and are clinically normal.
- Symptoms appear on average in one fourth of the offspring. One half of all offspring are heterozygous for the trait and are asymptomatic.
- Males and females are equally likely to be affected.
- Recessive traits are more commonly evident in childhood, whereas dominant disorders may initially appear in adults.
- Any specific autosomal recessive disease may vary in severity, age of onset, and existence of an acute or chronic form.

Some representative autosomal recessive disorders are shown in Table 6-3.

Cystic Fibrosis

Cystic fibrosis (CF) is the most common autosomal recessive disorder in Caucasian children. CF is rare in blacks and virtually unknown in Asians. CF is characterized by (a) chronic pulmonary disease, (b) deficient exocrine pancreatic function, and (c) other complications of increased mucous viscosity.

Pathogenesis

A mutation in the cystic fibrosis transmembrane conductance regulator (*CFTR*) gene, which has been localized to the long arm of chromosome 7, is the genetic defect in CF. Many mutations in the *CFTR* gene disrupt the synthesis, intracellular transport, binding domains, and channel pore structure of the transmembrane CFTR protein. The *CFTR* gene codes for an ATP-binding membrane transporter protein that facilitates the movement of chloride across epithelial membranes. Disease results from abnormal electrolyte transport caused by impaired function of the chloride channel of epithelial cells.

Secretion of chloride ions by mucus-secreting epithelial cells controls the parallel secretion of fluid, and, consequently, the viscosity of the mucus. All the pathological consequences of CF can

Table 6-3

Representative Autosomal Recessive Disorders

Disease	Frequency	Chromosome
Cystic fibrosis	1/2,500	7q
α-Thalassemia	High	16p
β-Thalassemia	High	11p
Sickle cell anemia	High	11p
Myeloperoxidase deficiency	1/2,000	17q
Phenylketonuria	1/10,000	12q
Gaucher disease	1/1,000	1q
Tay-Sachs disease	1/4,000	15q
Hurler syndrome	1/100,000	22p
Glycogen storage disease Ia (von Gierke disease)	1/100,000	17
Wilson disease	1/50,000	13q
Hereditary hemochromatosis	1/1,000	6p
α₁-Antitrypsin deficiency	1/15,000	11q
Oculocutaneous albinism	1/20,000	11q
Alkaptonuria	<1/100,000	3q
Metachromatic leukodystrophy	1,100,000	22q

From Rubin E, Gorstein F, Rubin R, et al. Rubin's Pathology, 4th ed. Philadelphia: Lippincott Williams & Wilkins, 2005, p. 248.

be attributed to the presence of abnormally thick mucus, which obstructs the lumina of airways, pancreatic and biliary ducts, and the fetal intestine.

Diagnosis

Diagnosis of CF is most reliably made by the "sweat test." These increased concentrations of electrolytes in the sweat are caused by failure of chloride reabsorption by the cells of the sweat gland ducts, leading to the accumulation of sodium chloride.

Pathology and Clinical Features

CF affects many organs that produce exocrine secretions (Figure 6-7).

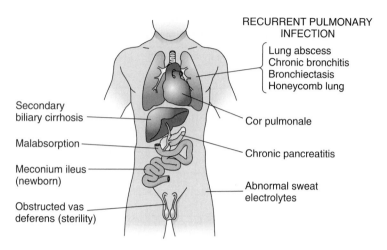

F I G U R E 6-7
Clinical features of cystic fibrosis. (From Rubin E, Gorstein F, Rubin R, et al. Rubin's Pathology, 4th ed. Philadelphia: Lippincott Williams & Wilkins, 2005, p. 251.)

- Respiratory tract: Pulmonary disease is responsible for most of the morbidity and mortality associated with CF. Recurrent obstructions and infections result in chronic bronchiolitis and bronchitis. *Pseudomonas* species are the most common organisms infecting the lungs of CF patients.
- Pancreas: A form of chronic pancreatitis with mucus-blocked dilated and cystic ducts affects 85% of patients with CF.
- Liver: Thick mucus obstructs bile flow leading to secondary biliary cirrhosis, chronic portal inflammation, and septal fibrosis.
- Gastrointestinal tract: Small bowel obstruction (meconium ileus) affects 5% to 10% of newborns with CF.
- Reproductive tract: Almost all males with CF exhibit obstructive atrophy or fibrosis of parts of the reproductive duct system, resulting in infertility. Most females with CF are infertile as well.

Lysosomal Storage Diseases

Lysosomal storage diseases are characterized by the accumulation of unmetabolized normal substrates in lysosomes because of deficiencies of specific acid hydrolases. Lysosomes are membranous sacs of hydrolytic enzymes that carry out intracellular digestion of materials both from outside and inside the cell; their many types of hydrolytic enzymes degrade virtually all types of biological molecules and are optimally active at an acidic pH of 3.5–5.5.

- Virtually all lysosomal storage diseases result from mutations in genes that encode lysosomal hydrolases.
- A deficiency in one of the more than 40 acid hydrolases can result in the accumulation of the undigested material in the lysosome, which will become engorged and expand to interfere with the normal functioning of the cell.
- Lysosomal storage diseases are classified according to the material abnormally retained within (e.g., in sphingolipidoses, sphingolipids accumulate within lysosomes).
- Phagocytic cells are rich in lysosomes, and organs such as the liver and spleen with high numbers of these cells become enlarged in several of the lysosomal storage diseases.

Gaucher Disease

Gaucher disease is characterized by the accumulation of glucosyl-ceramide, primarily in the lysosomes of macrophages, and is due to a deficiency of the enzyme, glucocerebrosidase, a type of lysosomal β-glucosidase. The deficiency can be traced to a variety of single base mutations in the *β-glucosidase* gene.

Pathology

The hallmark of Gaucher disease is the presence of Gaucher cells, which are lipid-laden macrophages in spleen red pulp, liver sinusoids, lymph nodes, lungs, and bone marrow. The Gaucher cell is large, PAS positive, and has a distinctive "wrinkled tissue paper" appearance. Enlargement of the spleen is virtually universal. The glucosylceramide of Gaucher cells in the brain is believed to originate from the turnover of plasma membrane gangliosides of cells in the central nervous system.

Classification and Clinical Features

There are three distinct forms of Gaucher disease:

- Type I (chronic nonneuropathic) is the most common form. It is found principally in adult Ashkenazi Jews and is characterized by a very enlarged spleen. There is some bone erosion, but no brain involvement. Life expectancy is normal. Type 1 is treated by the intravenous administration of modified acid glucose cerebrosidase.
- Type 2 (acute neuropathic) is a rare form of the disease with age of onset at about 3 months. It is not prevalent in any particular ethnic group. Infants exhibit hepatosplenomegaly and neurological deterioration. Death occurs before 1 year of age.
- Type 3 (subacute neuropathic) disease combines features of type 1 and type 2. It is less severe than type 2, with neurological deterioration presenting at an older age and progressing more slowly.

Tay-Sachs Disease (GM₂ Gangliosidosis, Type 1)

Tay-Sachs disease is the catastrophic infantile variant of a class of lysosomal storage diseases known as GM_2 gangliosidases, in which this ganglioside is deposited in neurons of the central nervous system, caused by a failure of lysosomal degradation. Tay-Sachs disease results from about 50 different mutations in the gene on chromosome 15 that codes the α subunit of hexosaminidase A, with a resulting defect in the synthesis of this enzyme. It is predominantly a disease of Ashkenazi Jews in whom the carrier rate is 1 in 30.

The symptomatology of Tay-Sachs disease appears between 6 and 10 months of age with progressive motor and mental deterioration as well as blindness. Involvement of the retinal ganglion cells is detected by ophthalmoscopy as a cherry-red spot in the macula. Most children with the disease die before the age of 4 years.

Niemann-Pick Disease

Niemann-Pick disease (NPD) refers to lipidoses that are characterized by the lysosomal storage of sphingomyelin in macrophages of many organs, hepatocytes, and brain. The characteristic storage cell in NPD is a foam cell, a large cell containing sphingomyelin and cholesterol; these are numerous in the spleen, lymph nodes and bone marrow. Ashkenazi Jews have a high frequency of NPD, but the disorder is present in other ethnic groups as well.

NPD may be classified as types A and B:

- Type A appears in infancy and is characterized by hepatosplenomegaly and progressive neurodegeneration, with death occurring by 3 years of age. There is a complete absence of sphingomyelinase activity.
- Type B is more variable with hepatosplenomegaly, minimal neurological involvement and survival to adulthood. In this type of NPD, 10% of normal enzyme activity can be detected.

Cystinosis

Cystinosis is a lysosomal storage disease that is unusual in that the defect is not due to a deficiency in an acid hydrolase within the lysosome, but rather an absence of the lysosomal transmembrane cystine transporter. This results in the trapping of cystine within the lysosome. If untreated, it results in renal failure often before adolescence. The use of cysteamine to decrease lysosomal cystine greatly slows progression of the disease.

Mucopolysaccharidoses

The mucopolysaccharidoses (MPS) comprise an assortment of lysosomal storage diseases characterized by the accumulation of glycosaminoglycans (mucopolysaccharides) in many organs. All types of MPS are autosomal recessive with the exception of Hunter syndrome, which is an X-linked recessive disorder. These rare diseases are caused by deficiencies in any one of the ten lysosomal enzymes involved in the sequential degradation of glycosaminoglycans (GAGs). GAGs are large polysaccharide chains synthesized by fibroblasts as normal constituents of many tissues.

Although the severity and location of the lesions in MPS vary with the specific enzyme deficiency, certain features are common to most of these syndromes:

- Undegraded GAGs tend to accumulate in lysosomes of macrophages, fibroblasts, endothelial cells, neurons, and hepatocytes.
- Affected cells are swollen and clear. By electron microscopy, many swollen lysosomes containing granular or striped material are noted.
- The central nervous system suffers loss of neurons and cortical atrophy. Skeletal deformities, cardiac lesions and hepatosplenomegaly develop.

Hurler syndrome is the most severe clinical form of MPS. The features of this and other varieties of MPS are summarized in Table 6-4.

Glycogenoses (Glycogen Storage Diseases)

The glycogenoses are a group of inherited diseases caused by defects in the metabolism of glycogen. They are characterized by the accumulation of glycogen principally in those organs that are normally rich in glycogen—the liver, skeletal muscle, and heart. With one rare exception (X-linked phosphorylase kinase deficiency), all types of glycogen storage diseases represent autosomal recessive traits. Only several representative examples will be discussed here:

- *Von Gierke Disease (type IA glycogenosis)* is characterized by accumulation of glycogen in the liver as the result of a deficiency in glucose-6-phosphatase. The defect results in hepatomegaly and hypoglycemia.
- *Pompe Disease (type II glycogenosis)* is caused by a deficiency in the lysosomal enzyme, α-glucosidase. This leads to the accumulation of glycogen in the lysosomes of many different cells. All organs are involved, and death results from heart failure before 2 years of age.
- *Andersen Disease (type IV glycogenosis)* is a very rare condition in which an abnormal form of glycogen (amylopectin) is deposited principally in the liver. The disorder results from a deficiency in the enzyme (amyloglucantransferase), which is responsible for creating the branch points in the normal glycogen

Table 6-4

Mucopolysaccharidoses

Type	Eponym	Location of Gene	Clinical Features
I H	Hurler	4p16.3	Organomegaly, cardiac lesions, dysostosis multiplex, corneal clouding, death in childhood
I S	Scheie	4p16.3	Stiff joints, corneal clouding, normal intelligence, longevity
II	Hunter	X	Organomegaly, dysostosis multiplex, mental retardation, death earlier than 15 years of age
III	Sanfilippo	12q14	Mental retardation
IV	Morquio	16q24	Skeletal deformities, corneal clouding
V	Obsolete	—	—
VI	Maroteaux Lamy	5q13–14	Dysostosis multiplex, corneal clouding, death in second decade
VII	Sly	7q21.1–22	Hepatosplenomegaly, dysostosis multiplex

From Rubin E, Gorstein F, Rubin R, et al. Rubin's Pathology, 4th ed. Philadelphia: Lippincott Williams & Wilkins, 2005, p. 255.

molecule. Children with the disease usually die from liver cirrhosis by 4 years of age.

- *McArdle Disease (type V glycogenosis)* is characterized by accumulation of glycogen in skeletal muscle owing to a deficiency of muscle phosphorylase, the enzyme responsible for the release of glucose-1-phosphate from glycogen. Symptoms consist of muscle cramps and spasms during and after exercise.

Inborn Errors of Amino Acid Metabolism

Certain heritable disorders involve the metabolism of many amino acids. The following discussion considers defects in the metabolism of phenylalanine and tyrosine.

Phenylketonuria (PKU)

This autosomal recessive disorder is characterized by progressive mental deterioration in the first few years of life because of high levels of circulating phenylalanine secondary to a deficiency of the hepatic enzyme phenylalanine hydroxylase.

Pathogenesis

Phenylalanine is an essential amino acid that is oxidized in the liver to tyrosine by phenylalanine hydroxylase. High serum concentrations of phenylalanine are neurotoxic. The deficiency in PAH also causes the formation of phenylketone, but this substance in not responsible for the neurological damage in PKU. Phenylketone is excreted in the urine, hence the name of the disease, phenylketonuria.

Clinical Features

The affected infant appears normal at birth but mental deterioration is usually pronounced by 1 year of age. Infants with PKU tend to have fair skin and blond hair because the inability to convert phenylalanine to tyrosine leads to reduced melanin synthesis.

Treatment

A phenylalanine-restricted diet is the treatment of choice. This usually requires a semisynthetic diet. About 10 million newborns worldwide are screened annually for hyperphenylalaninemia by a simple blood test, and most of the estimated 1,000 new cases are promptly treated.

Tyrosinemia

This rare autosomal recessive disease manifests as acute liver disease in infancy or as a more chronic disease of the liver, kidneys, and brain in children. Elevated levels of tyrosine and its metabolites are found in the blood. Both forms are caused by a deficiency of fumarylacetoacetate hydrolase, the last enzyme in the catabolic pathway that converts tyrosine to fumarate and acetoacetate. Cell injury is attributed to the formation of abnormal toxic metabolites.

Alkaptonuria (ochronosis)

This rare autosomal recessive disease is characterized by the excretion of homogentisic acid in the urine, generalized pigmentation, and arthritis. It is caused by a deficiency of homogentisic acid oxidase, which prevents the catabolism of homogentisic acid, an intermediate in the metabolism of phenylalanine and tyrosine.

Patients with alkaptonuria excrete urine that darkens rapidly on standing due to pigment formation by the oxidation of homogentisic acid. A similar pigment is deposited in numerous body tissues.

Albinism

Albinism refers to a heterogeneous group of at least 10 inherited disorders characterized by hypopigmentation as a result of absent or reduced synthesis of melanin. The most common type is oculocutaneous albinism (OCA), a family of closely related diseases. There is a deficiency or a complete absence of melanin pigment in the skin, hair follicles, and eyes. Persons with OCA have ophthalmic problems (photophobia, strabismus, nystagmus), a striking sensitivity to sunlight, and a greatly increased risk of developing squamous cell carcinoma.

Two major forms of OCA are distinguished by the presence (tyrosine-positive OCA) or absence (tyrosine-negative OCA) of tyrosinase. In tyrosine-positive OCA patients, a small amount of pigment accumulates with age, whereas tyrosine-negative patients have no detectable melanin.

X-linked Disorders

An X-linked disorder features an abnormal gene on the X chromosome (Fig. 6-8).

The expression of an X-linked disorder is different in males and females. Females, having two X chromosomes, may be homo-

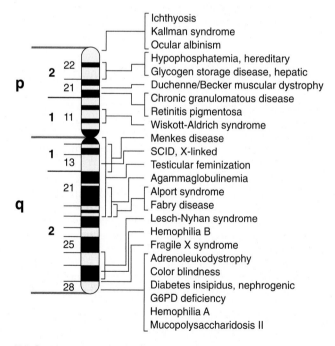

FIGURE 6-8
Localization of representative inherited diseases on the X chromosome. (From Rubin E, Gorstein F, Rubin R, et al. Rubin's Pathology, 4th ed. Philadelphia: Lippincott Williams & Wilkins, 2005, p. 261.)

zygous or heterozygous for a given trait, and the clinical expression of that trait is variable, depending on whether it is dominant or recessive. By contrast, males, having only one X chromosome are said to be *hemizygous* for the trait, so regardless of whether the trait is dominant or recessive, it is invariably expressed by the male.

X-linked Dominant Traits

Distinctive features include the following:

- Females are affected twice as frequently as males.
- A heterozygous female transmits the disorder to half her children, whether male or female.
- A male with a dominant X-linked disorder transmits the disease only to his daughters, never to his sons.
- The clinical expression of the disease tends to be less severe and more variable in heterozygous females than in hemizygous males. This is explained in part by the fact that in the female, the inactivation of one X chromosome is random, resulting in mosaicism for the mutant allele, a condition that may be associated with inconstant expression of the trait.

X-linked Recessive Traits

Distinctive features include the following:

- Most X-linked traits are recessive; that is, heterozygous females do not exhibit clinical disease.
- Sons of females who are carriers of the trait have a 50% chance of inheriting the disease; the daughters are not symptomatic.
- All daughters of affected males are asymptomatic carriers, but the sons are free of the trait and cannot transmit the disease to their children.
- Symptomatic homozygous females result only from the rare mating of an affected male and an asymptomatic heterozygous female.
- The trait tends to occur in maternal uncles and in male cousins descended from the mother's sisters.

Table 6-5 presents a list of X-linked recessive disorders.

X-linked Muscular Dystrophies (Duchenne and Becker Muscular Dystrophies)

The X-linked muscular dystrophies are among the most frequent human genetic diseases, occurring in 1 per 3,500 boys, an incidence approaching that of CF. *Duchenne muscular dystrophy (DMD),* the most common variant is a fatal progressive degeneration of muscle that appears before the age of 4 years. *Becker muscular dystrophy (BMD)* is allelic with DMD but is less frequent and milder.

Table 6-5
Representative X-linked Recessive Diseases

Disease	Frequency in Males
Fragile X syndrome	1/2,000
Hemophilia A (factor VIII deficiency)	1/10,000
Hemophilia B (factor IX deficiency)	1/70,000
Duchenne-Becker muscular dystrophy	1/3,500
Glucose-6-phosphate dehydrogenase deficiency	Up to 30%
Lesch-Nyhan syndrome (HPRT deficiency)	1/10,000
Chronic granulomatous disease	Not rare
X-linked agammaglobulinemia	Not rare
X-linked severe combined immunodeficiency	Rare
Fabry disease	1/40,000
Hunter syndrome	1/70,000
Adrenoleukodystrophy	1/100,000
Menke disease	1/100,000

From Rubin E, Gorstein F, Rubin R, et al. Rubin's Pathology, 4th ed.
Philadelphia: Lippincott Williams & Wilkins, 2005, p. 263.

Pathogenesis

Both DMD and BMD are caused by a deficiency of dystrophin, a cytoskeletal protein located on the cytoplasmic face of the plasma membrane of muscle cells, and linked to it by integral membrane glycoproteins. These, in turn are bound to extracellular laminin. Dystrophin molecules form a network connecting intracellular actin fibers to the extracellular matrix, a function that maintains the mechanical properties of the muscle cell. DMD patients have no detectable dystrophin, whereas BMD patients have a smaller than normal dystrophin molecule.

Clinical Features

The symptoms of DMD progress with age. In advanced disease, cardiomyopathy is a common cause of death. There is an overall decrease in intelligence. The mean age at death in boys with DMD is 17 years. BMD has a later onset and milder symptoms. In both variants, there are characteristic pathologic findings in a muscle biopsy (see Chapter 27).

Hemophilia A (Factor VIII Deficiency)

This disease is an X-linked disorder of blood clotting that results in spontaneous bleeding, particularly into joints, muscles, and internal organs. Classic hemophilia is actually two distinct diseases, one resulting from mutations in the gene encoding factor VIII (hemophilia A), and the other caused by defects in the gene for factor IX (hemophilia B). Hemophilia A is the most frequently encountered, and will be discussed here.

Pathogenesis

The gene encoding factor VIII is located at the tip of the long arm of the X chromosome; mutations in it include gene inversions, deletions, point mutations, and insertions. Each family with hemophilia in its history harbors a different mutation. In half the cases, de novo mutations are the cause of the disorder.

Pathology and Clinical Features

The severity of the bleeding tendency depends on the amount of factor VIII activity in the blood. Repeated bleeding into the joints causes a deforming arthritis. Hematuria as well as intestinal and respiratory obstruction may all occur, with bleeding into the lungs and gastrointestinal tract. Human recombinant factor VIII is now available for treatment, in addition to the more classical blood transfusions.

Fragile X Syndrome

This syndrome is the most common cause of inherited mental retardation; it is second only to Down syndrome ss a cause of mental retardation. The name refers to a cytogenetic marker, non-staining gaps in which the chromatin fails to condense during mitosis, caused by expansion of a trinucleotide CGG repeat on the X chromosome at Xq27.3. The syndrome afflicts both males and females.

Pathogenesis

In families who have a history of fragile X syndrome, later generations are more likely to be affected than earlier ones, probably because chromosomes with more than about 52 triplet repeats can expand the number of repeats, particularly during meiosis in females, leading to larger expansions (premutations) in successive generations. Expansions with more than 200 repeats are associated with mental retardation and represent full mutations. Males and females with premutations may be asymptomatic carriers.

Clinical Features

Newborn males with full mutations appear normal, but characteristic features appear (facial coarsening, enlarged testes, abnormalities of cardiac valves) during childhood. Mental retardation is profound. A significant proportion of autistic male children carry a fragile X chromosome. Females with full mutations may or may not exhibit mental retardation.

Fabry Disease

This X-linked syndrome is a lysosomal storage disease caused by a deficiency of α-galactosidase. Glycosphingolipids accumulate in the endothelium of body tissues. Skin lesions are characterized by a particular type of tumor (angiokeratoma). Affected persons die in early adulthood from progressive vascular insufficiency resulting in cerebral, renal, and cardiac infarcts.

Mitochondrial Diseases

Mitochondrial proteins are encoded by both nuclear and mitochondrial genomes. Most inherited defects in mitochondrial function result from mutations in the mitochondrial genome. Features of the unique genetics of the mitochondria include the following:

- Maternal inheritance: All vertebrate mitochondria are inherited from the mother. During fertilization, the sperm mitochondria in the sperm tail do not enter the oocyte; therefore, the fertilized ovum carries the female and male chromosomes, but only the female mitochondria.
- Variability of mitochondrial DNA (mtDNA) copies: The number of mitochondria and the number of copies of mtDNA per mitochondrion vary in different tissues. ATP is synthesized in the mitochondrion, and the DNA content per mitochondrion correlates with the need for ATP in a particular cell type.
- Threshold effect: Mutations in mtDNA lead to mixed populations of mutant and normal mitochondrial genomes in any given cell. The phenotype associated with mtDNA mutations reflects the severity of the mutation, the proportion of mutant genomes, and the demand of the tissue for ATP. Different tissues require minimum thresholds of ATP to sustain metabolic activity; brain, heart and skeletal muscle have particularly great demands for ATP, so diseases caused by mutations in the mitochondrial genome principally affect the nervous system, heart and skeletal muscle.
- High mutation rate: The rate of mutation of mtDNA is considerably higher than that of nuclear DNA, in part because of less DNA repair capacity.

All inherited mitochondrial diseases are rare and have variable clinical presentations. The first human disease recognized as being caused by an mtDNA point mutation was *Leber hereditary optic neuropathy*, a condition characterized by progressive loss of vision. Since then, various mitochondrial myopathies and encephalomyopathies have been described.

Genetic Imprinting

Genetic imprinting refers to the observation that the phenotype associated with some genes differs depending on whether the allele is inherited from the mother or the father. This phenomenon implies that in the case of imprinted genes, either the maternal or paternal allele is maintained in the inactive state. The nonimprinted (active) allele provides the biological function of the genetic locus. If the nonimprinted allele becomes disrupted through mutation, the imprinted (inactive) allele cannot compensate for the missing biological function. Imprinting occurs in meiosis during gametogenesis, and the pattern of imprinting is maintained to variable degrees in different tissues. It is reset during meiosis in the next generation, so the selection of a given allele for imprinting can vary from one generation to the next.

Genetic imprinting is illustrated by two rare syndromes in which the same deletion of the 15q11–13 chromosomal locus results in remarkably differing phenotypes in the progeny, depending on whether the deletions were transmitted maternally or paternally.

- Prader-Willi syndrome results from paternal transmission. It is characterized by hypotonia, obesity, hypogonadism and mental retardation.
- Angelman syndrome results from maternal transmission and is characterized by hyperactivity, inappropriate laughter, and seizures.

Multifactorial Inheritance

Multifactorial inheritance is a term that describes a process by which a disease results from the additive effects of a number of abnormal genes and environmental factors. For example, the formation of the lip and palate is under the control of a number of genes and occurs at about the 35th day of gestation. Rubella, anticonvulsants or chromosomal abnormalities can interfere with the fusion process and result in cleft lip or palate. Multifactorial inheritance has the following characteristics:

- The expression of symptoms is proportional to the number of mutant genes.
- Environmental factors influence the expression of the symptoms or trait.
- The risk of expression in parents, siblings, and children is the same (5%–10%).
- The probability of expression in later offspring is influenced by expression of the trait in earlier siblings.
- The more severe the defect, the greater the risk of transmitting it to offspring.
- Some abnormalities show a sex predilection.

Table 6-6

Representative Diseases Associated with Multifactorial Inheritance

Adults	Children
Hypertension	Pyloric stenosis
Atherosclerosis	Cleft lip and palate
Diabetes, type 2	Congenital heart disease
Allergic diathesis	Meningomyelocele
Psoriasis	Anencephaly
Schizophrenia	Hypospadias
Ankylosing spondylitis	Congenital hip dislocation
Gout	Hirschsprung disease

From Rubin E, Gorstein F, Rubin R, et al. Rubin's Pathology, 4th ed. Philadelphia: Lippincott Williams & Wilkins, 2005, p. 267.

Some representative diseases associated with multifactorial inheritance are shown in Table 6-6.

Screening for Carriers of Genetic Disorders

The objective of screening for genetic disorders is to identify couples in which both members are heterozygous carriers of a genetic disease and belong to an ethnic group with a high frequency of that disease. Such couples would have a 25% risk of having an affected offspring with each pregnancy. These couples can be offered prenatal diagnosis to determine the genetic status of the fetus. Some centers offer preimplantation genetic diagnosis to ensure that an implanted embryo will not have the disease.

Prenatal Diagnosis of Genetic Disorders

Amniocentesis and chorionic villus biopsy are the most important methods for diagnosis of a developmental or genetic disorder. Indications for performing prenatal diagnosis are: (a) age 35 years and older (woman), (b) previous chromosomal abnormality, (c) translocation carrier, (d) history of familial inborn error of metabolism, (e) identified heterozygotes, and (f) family history of X-linked disorders. New molecular techniques for carrier detection and early prenatal diagnosis are of ever increasing utility.

Prematurity and Intrauterine Growth Retardation

The duration of human pregnancy is normally $40(+/-2)$ weeks, and most newborns weigh $3,300(+/-600)$ g. Prematurity has been defined as a gestational age of less than 37 weeks, and a birth weight below 2,500 g. However, some full-term infants may weigh less than 2,500 g because of intrauterine growth retardation. Factors that predispose to premature birth are (a) maternal illness, (b) uterine incompetence, (c) fetal disorders, and (d) placental abnormalities. Factors that predispose to intrauterine growth retardation are (a) impaired maternal health and nutrition, (b) inadequate placental circulation, or (c) disturbed growth or development of the fetus.

Apgar Score

Clinical assessments of neonatal maturity are usually performed 1 and 5 minutes after delivery. Parameters such as heart rate, respiratory effort, muscle tone, color, and response to a catheter in the nostril are scored. The higher the Apgar score, the better the clinical condition of the infant; an infant in the best possible condition receives a maximum score of 10.

Organ Immaturity as a Cause of Neonatal Problems

- *Lungs*: Immaturity of the lungs poses one of the greatest threats to the viability of the low-birth-weight infant. Two factors contribute to the threat: (a) Sluggish respiratory movements of the immature infant may not rid the alveoli of amniotic fluid, and (b) a deficiency of surfactant—a secretion made by type II pneumocytes—which serves to keep alveoli expanded by reducing the surface tension.
- *Liver:* A deficiency in glucuronyl transferase and the resultant inability to conjugate and excrete bilirubin often lead to neonatal hyperbilirubinemia with jaundice and kernicterus (neuronal damage and possible severe neurologic sequelae).
- *Brain*: In premature infants, incomplete development of the central nervous system is often reflected in poor vasomotor control, hypothermia, feeding difficulties, and recurrent apnea.

Respiratory Distress Syndrome (RDS) of the Newborn

RDS is principally associated with prematurity and is the leading cause of morbidity and mortality among neonates. In addition to prematurity, other predisposing factors include maternal diabetes, delivery by cesarian section, and neonatal asphyxia. Pulmonary surfactant is released into the amniotic fluid and can be sampled before birth by amniocentesis to assess the maturity of the fetal lung.

Pathogenesis

Pathogenesis is linked to a deficiency of surfactant, a complex substance containing phospholipids, lecithin, and phosphatidylglycerol, secreted on to the alveolar surface by type II pneumocytes. Surfactant keeps the alveoli from collapsing when the infant exhales. The immature lung is deficient in both the amount and composition of surfactant. The resultant hypoxia leads to pulmonary ischemia, damage to pulmonary capillaries, and leakage of protein-rich fluid into the alveoli.

Pathology

Grossly, the lungs are dark red and airless. Microscopically, the alveoli are collapsed. The alveoli, ducts, and small bronchioles are lined by accumulated eosinophilic debris described as a hyaline membrane.

Clinical Features

RDS is characterized by increased respiratory effort and rate and cyanosis. The major complications of RDS relate to anoxia and acidosis and include the following:

- Intraventricular cerebral hemorrhage due to rupture of dilated thin-walled veins in this area
- Persistence of the patent ductus arteriosus with possible subsequent congestive heart failure
- Necrotizing enterocolitis related to ischemia of the intestinal mucosa
- Bronchopulmonary dysplasia, which is thought to result from oxygen toxicity resulting from positive pressure respirators

Treatment

Corticosteroids induce the formation of surfactant. Direct tracheal instillation of surfactant has been shown to reduce mortality and morbidity in infants with RDS.

Erythroblastosis Fetalis

This disorder is a hemolytic disease of the fetus caused by maternal antibodies against fetal red cell antigens such as Rh antigens and ABO blood group antigens. The maternal antibodies cause hemolysis of the fetal red blood cells and fetal anemia.

Pathogenesis

Rh Incompatibility

The Rh blood group system consists of 25 components. The cde/CDE alleles are the most significant in the disease; antibodies against D cause 90% of erythroblastosis fetalis cases. An Rh-negative mother can be sensitized by exposure to Rh-positive fetal erythrocytes at the time of delivery.

Erythroblastosis fetalis does not ordinarily occur during the first pregnancy, but if the mother again bears an Rh-positive fetus, a rising titer of antibodies against the fetal red blood cells may be detected. The severity of the disease tends to increase with each succeeding pregnancy. However, many Rh-negative women do not mount a substantial immune response against Rh-positive fetal blood; only 5% of Rh-negative women are ever delivered of infants with erythroblastosis fetalis.

ABO Incompatibility

Since the availability of RhoGAM prophylaxis of Rh-negative mothers, the incidence of Rh-incompatible erythroblastosis has drastically decreased. Today, ABO incompatibility is the principle cause of hemolytic disease of the newborn. It occurs mainly in newborns of blood group A with mothers of blood group O. Most infants suffer mild disease, and jaundice is the only clinical feature.

Pathology and Clinical Features

The severity of the erythroblastosis fetalis varies from mild hemolysis to fatal anemia, and the pathological findings are determined by the extent of the hemolytic disease.

- Death in utero occurs in the most severe form of the disease.
- Hydrops fetalis is characterized by severe edema secondary to congestive heart failure caused by severe anemia.
- Kernicterus (bilirubin encephalopathy) is characterized by bile staining of the brain, particularly of the basal ganglia, pontine nuclei, and dentate nuclei in the cerebellum. The excessive destruction of red blood cells in the disease leads to bilirubin formation. Because the immature fetal liver conjugates bilirubin poorly, it is released into the blood, causing jaundice, which, if severe, develops into kernicterus.

Prevention and Treatment

The use of human anti-D globulin (RhoGAM) administered to the mother within 72 hours of delivery suffices to neutralize antigenic fetal cells that may have entered maternal circulation during delivery, thus preventing maternal sensitization to the fetal blood.

Birth Injuries

Birth injury spans the spectrum from mechanical trauma to anoxic damage, and occurs in about 5 per 1,000 live births.

- *Cranial Injuries* can include skull fractures and intracranial hemorrhage. The latter is one of the most dangerous birth injuries, and can result in chronic neurological residuals.

- *Peripheral Nerve Injuries* can occur as brachial palsy, facial palsy, or phrenic nerve paralysis. Most of these conditions generally resolve within a few months. Prognosis depends on whether the nerves were lacerated or simply injured by pressure.
- *Fractures* may involve the clavicle and/or humerus. Immobilization of the arm and shoulder are required for complete healing.
- *Liver Rupture* may occur as the result of mechanical pressure during a difficult birth. Surgical repair may be needed if the laceration is large.

Sudden Infant Death Syndrome (SIDS)

SIDS is defined as "the sudden death of an infant or young child which is unexpected by history and in which a thorough postmortem examination fails to demonstrate an adequate cause of death." Most deaths occur during sleep. The recent decline in death rates for SIDS has been attributed to the encouragement of parents to place infants on their backs for sleeping. The pathogenesis of SIDS is poorly understood. Risk factors include low birth weight, prematurity, or an illness within 2 weeks before death.

Neoplasms of Infancy and Childhood

Cancer is the leading cause of death from disease in children from 1 to 15 years of age. In children, most malignant tumors arise from hematopoietic, nervous, and soft tissues, In children, most malignant tumors arise from hematopoietic, nervous, and soft tissues, unlike in adults, in whom most cancers are of epithelial origin (Fig. 6-9). Some neoplasms are apparent at birth and are obviously developmental tumors that have evolved in utero. In addition, abnormally developed organs, persistent organ primordial, and displaced organ rests are all vulnerable to neoplastic transformation.

Particular cancers of childhood are discussed in the chapters dealing with the organs involved. The basic principles of neoplasia and carcinogenesis are discussed in Chapter 5.

Benign tumors and tumorlike conditions in children include the following:

- *Hamartomas* are tumors that represent benign overgrowths of normal tissue, with the cells arranged in a highly irregular fashion.
- *Choristomas* are similar to hamartomas but are tiny aggregates of normal tissue components in aberrant locations (e.g., adrenal tissue in the renal cortex).
- *Hemangiomas* or tumors made up of blood vessels are frequently seen in children; most regress with age. A "port wine stain" is a congenital capillary hemangioma on the skin of the face or scalp, giving a dark purple color to the affected area.

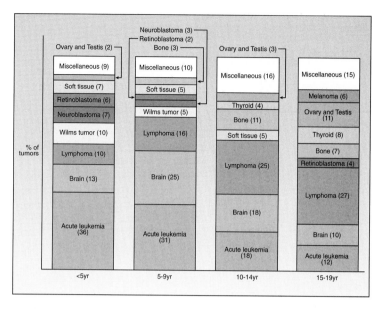

F I G U R E   6-9
Distribution of childhood tumors according to age and primary site.
(From Rubin E, Gorstein F, Rubin R, et al. Rubin's Pathology, 4th
ed. Philadelphia: Lippincott Williams & Wilkins, 2005, p. 277.)

- *Lymphangiomas* are swellings consisting of many dilated lymphatic channels separated by fibrous septa. Most occur on the head and neck, but the floor of the mouth, mediastinum and buttocks are not uncommon sites. They do not regress spontaneously and should be resected.
- *Sacrococcygeal teratomas* are large lobulated masses in the region of the sacrum or buttocks, composed of many tissues, particularly of neural origin. They occur most commonly in girls. Most are benign in the young infant but may become malignant later in life; they should be resected.

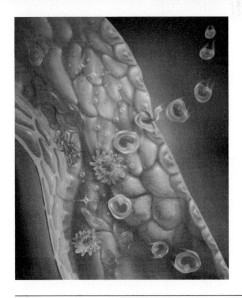

CHAPTER 7

Hemodynamic Disorders

Chapter Outline

Cerebral Edema
Fluid Accumulation in Body Cavities
Fluid Loss and Overload
Shock
    Pathogenesis
    Types of Shock
    Septic Shock and Systemic Inflammatory Response Syndrome
    Multiple Organ Dysfunction Syndrome as the End Result of
      Shock

Normal Circulation

The circulatory system has two functional components, the blood vascular system, and the lymphatic system. The blood vascular system is a circuit composed of a muscular pump (the heart) connected to vessels that either deliver blood to the organs and tissues of the body, or return blood to the heart to complete the circuit. In contrast, the lymphatic system is a passive drainage system for returning excess extravascular fluid (lymph) to the blood vascular system.

Disorders of Perfusion

Hyperemia

Hyperemia is an excess of blood in the capillaries and small vessels of an organ.

Active Hyperemia

Active hyperemia results from an increased supply of blood from the arterial system caused by arteriolar dilation and recruitment of more capillaries. It may be due to increased functional demand of heart and muscles during exercise, or it may occur along with inflammation, accompanied by increased capillary permeability and edema.

Passive Hyperemia

This congestion results from an impediment to the exit of blood through venous pathways. It may be acute or chronic. Acute passive congestion results in venous engorgement leading to an accumulation of transudate in the tissues (*interstitial edema*). Chronic passive hyperemia, which is typically due to left heart failure or mitral stenosis, results in slower blood flow to a number of organs, including lungs, liver, and spleen. Chronic passive hyperemia has the following manifestations:

- Lungs: Increased pressure in alveolar capillaries may cause three possible conditions: (a) microhemorrhages into the alveoli, which release red blood cells that are then phagocytosed by *"heart failure cells"* (macrophages laden with hemoglobin degradation products); (b) pulmonary edema resulting from accumulation of transudate in the alveoli; (c) fibroses containing macrophage debris in the lung interstitium (*brown induration*).
- Liver: Hepatic veins empty into the inferior vena cava, making the liver particularly vulnerable to passive congestion; this results in dilation of hepatic central veins and sinusoids and atrophy of centrilobular hepatocytes; because of these changes, a cut section of liver will have a speckled appearance (*nutmeg liver*).
- Spleen: Higher splenic vein pressure can lead to a congested and enlarged spleen with diffuse fibroses and calcified foci of old hemorrhage.

Hemorrhage

Hemorrhage is the escape of blood from the circulation into the surrounding tissues or to the exterior of the body. It can be caused by accidental trauma, surgical procedures, atherosclerosis, aneurism rupture, infection, or erosion of vessel walls by a neoplasm. Kinds of hemorrhage include the following:

- Hematoma; hemorrhage into soft tissue may be trivial (as in a muscle bruise) or fatal (if located in the brain)
- Hemothorax; hemorrhage into the pleural cavity
- Hemopericardium; hemorrhage into the pericardial space
- Hemoperitoneum; hemorrhage into the peritoneal cavity
- Hemarthrosis; bleeding into a joint space
- Purpura: diffuse superficial hemorrhage in the skin, up to 1 cm in diameter
- Ecchymosis; larger (>1–2 cm) superficial hemorrhage in the skin; may generate a "black and blue" mark, reflecting skin discoloration by products of heme degradation, resulting from release of hemoglobin from red blood cells
- Petechiae; pinpoint hemorrhages, usually in the skin or conjunctiva; represent the rupture of capillaries or arterioles and can occur in conjunction with *coagulopathies* or *vasculitis*

Thrombosis

Thrombosis refers to the formation of a thrombus—an aggregate of coagulated blood with platelets, fibrin, and entrapped cellular elements within the lumen of a blood vessel. A thrombus differs from a blood clot and a hematoma, as indicated by the following:

- Thrombus: Adheres to the vascular endothelium
- Blood clot: Reflects the result of activation of the coagulation cascade; can form in vitro or in situ in the postmortem state
- Hematoma: Results from hemorrhage and subsequent clotting outside the vascular system

Thrombus formation and the coagulation cascade are discussed in further detail in Chapters 10 and 20. This section presents the causes and consequences of thrombosis in different sites.

Thrombosis in the Arterial System
In the arterial system, thrombosis is usually due to atherosclerosis. The most common vessels involved are the coronary, cerebral, mesenteric, and renal arteries, as well as those of the lower extremities.

Pathogenesis
Pathogenesis involves three factors, known as *Virchow's Triad*:

1. Damage to the endothelium with platelet aggregation and fibrin formation
2. Alterations in blood flow from turbulence or at vessel branching points
3. Increased coagulability of the blood, as in *polycythemia vera* or in association with some cancers

Pathology
Initially, an arterial thrombus is soft, friable, and dark red with light-colored bands of platelets, leukocytes, and fibrin (lines of Zahn). When a thrombus has formed, it may have several possible outcomes. It may be lysed by fibrinolytic activity, it may increase in size, it may be invaded by connective tissue and become firmer, or it may travel and become lodged in a more distant vessel (*embolization*, discussed below). Occasionally, the endothelial cells lining the artery will proliferate and penetrate the thrombus, forming tiny canals through it (a process termed canalization).

Clinical Features
Arterial thrombosis as a consequence of atherosclerosis is the most common cause of death in Western industrialized countries. When thrombi occlude an artery, they often lead to ischemic necrosis of the tissue supplied by the artery (i.e., an *infarct*).

Thrombosis in the Heart
The inner lining of the heart, the endocardium, is analogous to the endothelium, the inner lining of the arteries; therefore, as in blood vessels, injury to the lining and changes in blood flow are associ-

ated with mural thrombosis (a thrombus adhering to the underlying wall of the heart).

Disorders such as *myocardial infarction, atrial fibrillation, or cardiomyopathy*, are all associated with mural thrombi. *Endocarditis* with bacterial infection of cardiac valves may cause small thrombi (vegetations) to develop. In patients with *systemic lupus erythematosus (SLE)* or with chronic wasting disease, valvular vegetations may form even in the absence of infection.

Thrombosis in the Venous System

The most common manifestation of venous thrombosis is thrombosis of the deep veins of the legs, termed *deep venous thrombosis*.

Pathogenesis and Pathology

The same factors that dispose toward arterial and cardiac thrombosis cause deep venous thrombosis, namely, stasis, injury, and hypercoagulability. Advanced age and sickle cell disease can also contribute to development of deep venous thrombosis. The potential outcomes of venous thrombi are similar to those of arterial thrombi.

Clinical Features

Occlusive thrombosis of iliofemoral veins may cause edema and cyanosis of the lower extremity. Thrombosis of mesenteric veins can cause hemorrhagic infarction of the small intestine. Thrombosis of cerebral veins may be fatal, whereas thrombosis of hepatic veins (*Budd-Chiari syndrome*) may destroy the liver.

Embolism

Embolism is the passage through the circulation of material capable of lodging in a blood vessel and obstructing its lumen. Most emboli arise from a thrombus that has formed in one location and traveled to a distant site. This is termed a thromboembolus.

Pulmonary Arterial Thromboembolism

Pulmonary embolism occurs in 1% to 2% of postoperative patients older than 40 years of age. Most pulmonary embolisms arise from deep veins of the lower extremity, whereas most of the fatal ones arise from the ileofemoral veins. Acute pulmonary embolism is divided into the following syndromes:

- Asymptomatic small pulmonary emboli
- Transient shortness of breath (*dyspnea*) and fast breathing (*tachypnea*) without other symptoms
- Pulmonary infarction, with pleuritic chest pain, coughing up blood (*hemoptysis*), and pleural effusion
- Cardiovascular collapse with sudden death

Massive Pulmonary Embolism

Massive pulmonary embolism is the most common cause of death after major orthopedic surgery. It is also common in patients subjected to prolonged immobilization for any reason. A large pulmonary embolus may lodge at the branching of the main pulmonary artery, obstructing blood flow to both lungs and outflow from the right ventricle. This can cause severe hypotension and death.

Pulmonary Embolism with and without Infarction

Pulmonary infarction is a hemorrhagic consolidation in an area of lung. It results from the lodging of small emboli in peripheral branches of the pulmonary artery. The infarct is hemorrhagic because the unobstructed bronchial artery pumps blood into the area. With time, the blood in the infarct can be resorbed, granulation tissue can form at the edges, and a fibrous scar will form.

Because the lung has a dual circulation, supplied by both the pulmonary and bronchial arteries, 75% of small emboli do not produce infarcts because of collateral circulation development. Rarely, recurrent pulmonary emboli produce pulmonary hypertension due to vasoconstriction and bronchial constriction resulting from vasoactive substance release near the emboli site. Small pulmonary emboli may completely resolve, or they may become organized and leave strings of fibrous tissue attached to the inner wall of pulmonary artery branches.

Systemic Thromboembolism

The heart is the most common source of arterial thromboemboli, which usually arise from mural thrombi or diseased valves. The thromboembolus may become a more severe obstruction, or it may fragment and lyse. Organs that suffer most from arterial thromboembolism include:

- Brain: Emboli cause ischemic necrosis of brain tissue (strokes).
- Intestine: Mesenteric emboli cause bowel infarction; ensuing acute abdomen necessitates immediate surgery.
- Lower extremity: Embolism of a leg artery leads to pain, absence of pulses, and a cold limb.
- Kidney: Renal artery embolism may infarct the entire kidney.

Air Embolism

Air may be introduced into veins through neck wounds or as a consequence of invasive procedures. Air bubbles in quantities of 100 ml or more may obstruct blood flow and cause ischemia.

- Decompression sickness (the bends): When divers descend to significant underwater depth, large amounts of nitrogen are dissolved in body fluids; this is then exhaled on ascent. However, if ascent is too rapid, gas bubbles form in the blood and in tissues, obstructing blood flow and injuring cells (air embolism). Involvement of cerebral blood vessels may be severe enough to cause coma or death.

- Caisson disease: This complication occurred in bridge and tunnel construction workers in diving bells (caissons). The disease refers to decompression sickness in which the vascular obstruction causes multiple foci of ischemic necrosis, mainly in bone.

Amniotic Fluid Embolism

This is a rare but serious complication of childbirth, and refers to the entry, into the maternal circulation, of amniotic fluid containing fetal cells and debris. This can cause maternal pulmonary emboli as well as coagulopathy resulting from the high thromboplastin activity of amniotic fluid. The clinical presentation of amniotic fluid embolism can be dramatic with sudden onset of cyanosis and shock, followed by coma and death.

Fat Embolism

Fat embolism describes the release of emboli of fatty marrow into damaged blood vessels following severe trauma to fat-containing tissue, particularly long bone fracture. In its most severe form, this syndrome is characterized by respiratory failure, mental changes, thrombocytopenia, and widespread petechiae. Some aspects of the fat embolism syndrome remain poorly understood, and disagreement about its etiology and pathophysiology persists.

Infarction

Pathogenesis

Infarction is defined as the process by which coagulative necrosis develops in an area distal to the occlusion of the arterial supply. Usually, thrombi or emboli are responsible for the occlusion. The ischemic necrotic zone is termed an infarct.

Pathology

The gross and microscopic appearance of an infarct depends on its location and age. Several types of infarcts are distinguishable by gross examination.

- Pale infarcts: typical in the heart, kidneys, and spleen. These are organs in which end-arteries supply specific areas with little or no overlap, (i.e., little collateral circulation). One or two days after the initial hyperemia, the infarct appears sharply delineated and light yellow.

- Red infarcts: may result from either arterial or venous occlusion and are distinguished by bleeding into the necrotic area from adjacent arteries or veins. These infarcts are typical of organs with a dual blood supply, or with extensive collateral circulation, such as the small intestine and brain.

Edema

Edema refers to the presence of excess fluid in the interstitial spaces of the body. Various terms define the body space involved: hydrothorax (pleural cavity), ascites (peritoneal cavity), hydropericardium (pericardium), and anasarca (severe generalized edema). Edema may be local or generalized.

Local edema occurs in the following situations:

- Often with inflammation (see Chapter 2)
- In a limb, resulting from venous or lymphatic obstruction
- In burns when permeability of local vessels is disrupted
- In type I hypersensitivity reactions (e.g., hives)

Generalized edema reflects a global disorder of fluid and electrolyte metabolism, and can occur in the following:

- Congestive heart failure
- Renal diseases with serum protein loss (e.g., nephrotic syndrome)
- Liver cirrhosis

The various causes of edema can be attributed to changes in capillary filtration and reabsorption, sodium and water metabolism, hydrostatic and oncotic pressure, and lymphatic flow (see Chapter 2). Table 7-1 lists disorders associated with edema.

Edema of Congestive Heart Failure

In the United States, congestive heart failure is most commonly associated with ischemic heart disease.

Pathogenesis

Both low cardiac output and venous congestion contribute to the pathogenesis of the edema of congestive heart failure:

- Low cardiac output→decreased glomerular filtration rate
- Decreased glomerular filtration rate→increased renin secretion
- Renin→release of aldosterone; in addition, reduced blood flow to the liver impairs the catabolism of aldosterone
- High aldosterone levels→sodium reabsorption and fluid retention

Table 7-1
Disorders Associated with Edema

Increased hydrostatic pressure	
Arteriolar dilation	Inflammation Heat
Increased venous pressure	Venous thrombosis Congestive heart failure Cirrhosis (ascites) Postural inactivity (e.g., prolonged standing)
Hypervolemia	Sodium retention
Decreased oncotic pressure	
Hypoproteinemia	Nephrotic syndrome Cirrhosis Protein-losing gastroenteropathy Malnutrition
Increased capillary permeability	Inflammation Burns Adult respiratory distress syndrome
Lymphatic obstruction	Cancer Postsurgical lymphedema Inflammation

From Rubin E, Gorstein F, Rubin R, et al. Rubin's Pathology, 4th ed. Philadelphia: Lippincott Williams & Wilkins, 2005, p. 299.

- Increased sodium reabsorption and fluid retention→increased plasma volume→increased pulmonary and systemic pressure
- Increased pulmonary and systemic pressure→increased capillary pressure in the respective capillary beds
- Increased capillary pressure→**generalized edema of congestive heart failure**

Pathology

Left ventricle failure is associated with lung congestion and pulmonary edema. When chronic, this leads to right ventricle failure, characterized by generalized subcutaneous edema and enlarged heart.

Clinical Features

Patients in left-sided congestive heart failure may have shortness of breath, distended jugular veins, and pulmonary edema. Patients in right-sided failure may have pitting edema of the lower extremities, and enlarged liver.

Pulmonary Edema

Pathogenesis and Pathology

Pulmonary edema features increased fluid in the alveolar spaces and interstitium of the lung. The most common cause of this condition is left ventricular failure, which serves to increase perfusion pressure in the pulmonary capillaries and block effective lymphatic drainage.

Edema of the fibrous and elastic visceral pleura and lobular septa represents the earliest phase of pulmonary edema; when the fluid can no longer be contained in the interstitial spaces, it spills into the alveoli, leading to the more advanced stage of the disease (alveolar edema). Microscopic examination of the edematous lung reveals congested capillaries and damaged alveoli with debris-containing films of proteinaceous material (hyaline membranes).

Clinical Features

Dyspnea and coughing may occur; in more severe cases, large amounts of frothy pink sputum are expectorated. Restricted pulmonary function results in hypoxia.

Edema in Cirrhosis of the Liver

Cirrhosis of the liver is often accompanied by ascites and peripheral edema. Cirrhosis is a chronic disease in which liver parenchyma deteriorates; the lobules become infiltrated with fat and dense connective tissue. This tends to block blood flow through the liver, and because the portal vein supplies 75% of the total blood flow to the liver, portal hypertension may occur. The increased hydrostatic pressure leads to peripheral edema and the accumulation of serous fluids in the peritoneal cavity (ascites). Clotting of blood in the hepatic vein, the major vein leaving the liver, can also lead to ascites. This is a symptom in the Budd-Chiari syndrome.

Edema and the Nephrotic Syndrome

The nephritic syndrome results from damage to the kidney glomeruli, and is marked by high levels of protein loss in the urine. The resultant low level of protein in the blood (lower oncotic pressure) leads to edema, especially around the eyes, feet and hands.

Cerebral Edema

Edema of the brain is dangerous because the confined cranial space allows little room for expansion. Increased intracranial pressure from edema compromises the blood supply, distorts brain structure, and interferes with the function of the central nervous system. Cerebral edema is divided into the following three categories:

- Vasogenic: excess fluid in the extracellular space
- Cytotoxic: cell swelling in response to cell injury
- Interstitial: fluid accumulation in the cerebral ventricles and periventricular white matter

Fluid Accumulation in Body Cavities

Accumulation of fluid in the body cavities represents extensions of the interstitial space and is an expression of a general tendency to form edema. It may collect in the pleural space, in the pericardial sac, or, as previously discussed, in the peritoneal cavity as ascites.

Fluid Loss and Overload

Dehydration is characterized by inadequate fluid to fill the body fluid compartments. It results from insufficient fluid intake, excessive fluid loss, or both. When patients suffer from burns, vomiting, excessive sweating, or diarrhea, they not only lose fluid but also have electrolyte imbalances. Severe fluid loss shifts water from within cells to extracellular space and can lead to drastic fall of blood pressure and death.

Overhydration is rare but may result from kidney injury or excessive secretion of antidiuretic hormone. It can also be caused by administration of excessive amounts of intravenous fluids.

Shock

Shock is a condition of profound hemodynamic and metabolic disturbance characterized by failure of the circulatory system to maintain an appropriate blood supply to the microcirculation with consequent inadequate perfusion of vital organs.

Pathogenesis

Shock is most commonly due to a decreased cardiac output resulting from either a defective cardiac pump or decreased blood volume caused by hemorrhage. Shock may also be due to widespread vasodilation resulting from microbial infections, anaphylaxis, or brain injury.

Decreased tissue perfusion leads to hypoxia and injury to the following:

- Endothelial cells, resulting in increased vascular permeability
- Kidney and skeletal muscle, leading to metabolic acidosis which further decreases cardiac output and tissue perfusion
- Myocardial cells, decreasing their ability to pump and further reducing cardiac output and tissue perfusion

Types of Shock

The classification of shock is shown in Figure 7-1 and listed in the following:

- Cardiogenic shock is caused by myocardial pump failure, usually as the result of a large myocardial infarction.
- Hypovolemic shock results from a decrease in blood or plasma volume caused by hemorrhage, fluid loss from severe burns, diarrhea, diuresis, perspiration, or severe trauma.

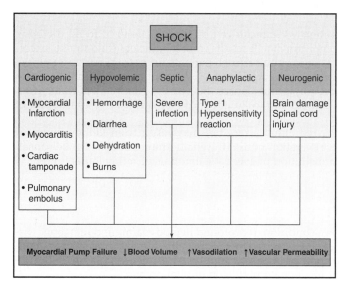

FIGURE   7-1

Classification of shock. Shock results from (1) an inability of the heart to pump adequately (cardiogenic shock); (2) decreased effective blood volume as a consequence of severely reduced blood or plasma volume (hypovolemic shock); or (3) widespread vasodilation (septic, anaphylactic, or neurogenic shock). Increased vascular permeability may complicate vasodilation by contributing to a reduced effective blood volume. (From Rubin E, Gorstein F, Rubin R, et al. Rubin's Pathology, 4th ed. Philadelphia: Lippincott Williams & Wilkins, 2005, p. 305.)

- Septic shock is caused by severe systemic microbial infections (discussed below).
- Anaphylactic shock occurs as the result of a systemic type I hypersensitivity reaction, which leads to widespread vasodilation and increased vascular permeability.
- Neurogenic shock is associated with injury to the brain or spinal cord. This impairs neural control of vasomotor tone and leads to generalized vasodilation.

Septic Shock and Systemic Inflammatory Response Syndrome

Systemic inflammatory response syndrome (SIRS) is an exaggerated and generalized manifestation of a local immune or inflammatory reaction, which is often fatal. Septicemia with gram-negative organisms is the most common cause of septic shock. The invading bacteria are responsible for the release of lipopolysaccharide (LPS; endotoxin). The pathophysiology involves the following:

- The LPS binds to a receptor molecule, CD14, on the surface of macrophages. CD14 presents the LPS to a signal-transducing receptor in the membrane, toll-like receptor.
- This binding activates the nuclear factor NF-κB, which triggers the release of large amounts of cytokines such as tumor necrosis factor (TNF), interleukin-1 (IL-1) IL-6, IL-8, IL-12, and platelet activating factor (PAF).
- The cytokines stimulate the production of inflammatory mediators such as prostaglandins and leukotrienes as well as activating both the complement pathways and the coagulation pathway.
- Coagulation activation can lead to disseminated intravascular coagulation (DIC).
- TNF also increases the expression of adhesion molecules on endothelial surfaces, thereby promoting leukocyte adhesion and leukostasis. Activated neutrophils in the pulmonary circulation damage alveoli and play a role in respiratory distress syndrome.
- This series of reactions causes the overwhelming cardiovascular collapse characteristic of septic shock.

Multiple Organ Dysfunction Syndrome as the End Result of Shock

Progressive deterioration of organ function is a serious consequence of septic shock. Multiple organ dysfunction syndrome (MODS) is seen in one third of cases of septic shock. Organ failure is the strongest predictor of death in the critically ill patient. Shock is associated with specific changes in a number of organs.

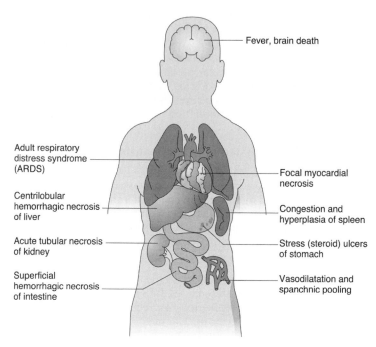

Fever, brain death

Adult respiratory
distress syndrome
(ARDS)

Focal myocardial
necrosis

Centrilobular
hemorrhagic necrosis
of liver

Congestion and
hyperplasia of spleen

Acute tubular necrosis
of kidney

Stress (steroid) ulcers
of stomach

Superficial
hemorrhagic necrosis
of intestine

Vasodilatation and
spanchnic pooling

FIGURE 7-2
Complications of shock. (From Rubin E, Gorstein F, Rubin R, et al. Rubin's Pathology, 4th ed. Philadelphia: Lippincott Williams & Wilkins, 2005, p. 308.)

- Heart: petechial hemorrhages in the epi- and endocardium; necrotic foci of varying sizes
- Kidney: swollen kidney; tubular necrosis; interstitial edema in cortex
- Lung: firm and congested; interstitial edema; hyaline membranes in the alveoli
- Gastrointestinal tract: erosions of the gastric mucosa; superficial intestinal ischemic necrosis
- Liver: enlarged and mottled liver; centrilobular congestion and necrosis
- Pancreas: ischemic damage leading to acute pancreatitis
- Brain: rare lesions; occasional microscopic hemorrhages
- Adrenals: hemorrhage in the inner cortex; Waterhouse-Friderichsen syndrome, associated with overwhelming meningococcal septicemia, can cause massive hemorrhagic necrosis of the entire gland.

The complications of shock involve many organs (Fig. 7-2).

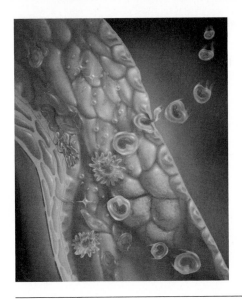

CHAPTER *8*

Environmental and Nutritional Pathology

Chapter Outline

Aromatic Halogenated Hydrocarbons
Cyanide
Air Pollutants
Metals

Thermal Regulatory Dysfunction
Hypothermia
Hyperthermia

Altitude-related Illnesses

Physical Injuries

Radiation
Whole-body Irradiation
Radiation Therapy for Tumors
Radiation and Cancer

Nutritional Disorders
Obesity
Protein-calorie Malnutrition
Vitamins
Essential Trace Minerals

Environmental pathology deals with the diseases caused by exposure to harmful external agents and deficiencies of vital substances. It encompasses all nutritional, infectious, chemical, and physical causes of illness.

Tobacco Smoking

Smoking tobacco is the single largest preventable cause of death in the United States. More than 400,000 deaths a year—about one sixth of the total mortality in the United States—occur prematurely because of smoking. The major diseases responsible for the excess mortality in cigarette smoking are, in order of frequency, coronary heart disease, cancer of the lung, and chronic obstructive pulmonary disease (Fig. 8-1).

Cardiovascular Disease

Cigarette smoking is a major independent risk factor for myocardial infarction and acts synergistically with other risk factors such as high blood pressure and elevated blood cholesterol. Atherosclerosis of the coronary arteries and aorta, as well as atherosclerotic peripheral vascular disease, is more severe among cigarette smokers, and the effect is related to the number of cigarettes smoked per day and the duration of the smoking habit. Other effects of smoking that may predispose to myocardial infarction include the pharmacological actions of nicotine, an alkaloid in cigarette smoke

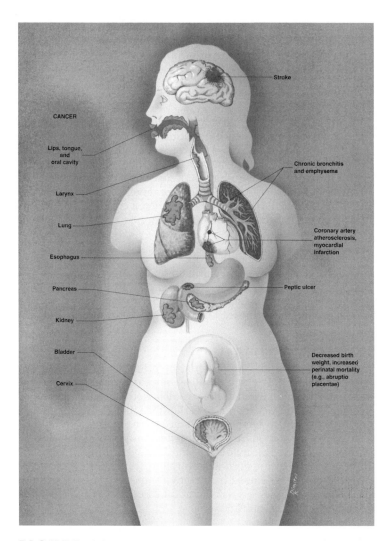

FIGURE 8-1
Diseases associated with cigarette smoking. The cancers whose incidences are known to be increased in cigarette smokers are shown on the left. The nonneoplastic diseases associated with cigarette smoking are shown on the right. (From Rubin E, Gorstein F, Rubin R, et al. Rubin's Pathology, 4th ed. Philadelphia: Lippincott Williams & Wilkins, 2005, p. 312.)

that is responsible for tobacco addiction. Nicotine acts primarily on the autonomic nervous system and mimics the effect of acetylcholine. Approximately 3 mg of nicotine is inhaled from one cigarette. This amount increases heart rate and constricts blood vessels.

Lung Cancer

Cigarette smoke is toxic and carcinogenic. Lung cancer is the single most common cause of death from cancer in both men and women in the United States, and more than 85% of deaths from lung cancer are attributed to cigarette smoking. Cigarette smoking and lung cancer are associated with certain occupational exposures, such as occurs in asbestos workers. The risk of developing lung cancer is increased as much as 50 to 90 times when a cigarette smoker has been exposed to asbestos in the workplace.

Other Cancers

Cancers of the oral cavity occur mainly in cigarette smokers. Adenocarcinoma of the kidney is increased 50% to 100% in smokers. Cancers of the larynx, esophagus, bladder, pancreas, and uterine cervix also have an increased frequency of occurrence in smokers.

Nonneoplastic Diseases

Chronic bronchitis and emphysema are primarily dose-related diseases of smokers. Peptic ulcer disease, osteoporosis, thyroid diseases, and macular degeneration are all linked to cigarette smoking. Women who smoke experience earlier menopause than nonsmokers. Infants born to women who smoke are small for gestational age, and perinatal mortality is higher among the offspring of women smokers. The children of mothers who smoke show deficiencies in growth, intellectual maturation, and emotional development. Exposure to smoke in the environment (passive smoking) has been considered as a risk factor for disease, particularly of the respiratory tract, in nonsmokers.

Alcoholism

There are about 12 million alcoholics in the United States. Chronic alcoholism may be defined as the regular intake of alcohol that is enough to injure a person socially, psychologically, or physically. For most persons, this would be a daily consumption of more than 45g alcohol (10 g alcohol = 1 oz, or 30 ml of 86 proof spirits). Levels greater than 100 mg/dL are considered legal evidence of driving while intoxicated. At levels greater than 300 mg/dL, most people become comatose, and at concentrations greater than 400 mg dL, death from respiratory failure is common.

The mechanism of inebriation is not understood. A few mechanisms have been proposed, but none has conclusively been verified.

- There is a substantial change in the intracellular redox potential during the oxidation of ethanol to acetaldehyde.
- Acetaldehyde, a product of alcohol metabolism is highly toxic.
- Alcohol like all anesthetics, disorders cell membranes by intercalating into the lipid bilayer of the membrane.

Organs and Tissues Affected by Alcohol Ingestion

In addition to the effects of alcohol on the organs and tissues listed below, the incidence of cancer of the oral cavity, larynx, and esophagus is higher in alcoholics than in the general population. Figure 8-2 illustrates some complications of chronic alcohol abuse.

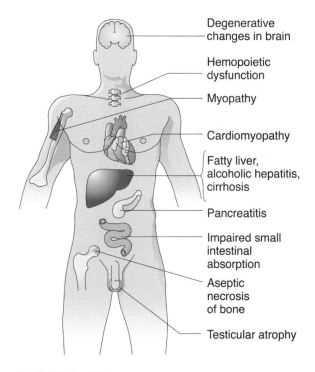

F I G U R E   8-2
Complications of chronic alcohol abuse. (From Rubin E, Gorstein F, Rubin R, et al. Rubin's Pathology, 4th ed. Philadelphia: Lippincott Williams & Wilkins, 2005, p. 320.)

- *Liver*: Alcoholic liver disease is the most common medical complication of alcoholism; this accounts for a large proportion of liver cirrhosis. The nature of the alcoholic beverage is irrelevant.
- *Nervous system:* Cerebral dysfunction is mediated by a thiamine deficiency (Wernicke encephalopathy) and is characterized by mental confusion, ataxia, and polyneuropathy. Retrograde amnesia and confabulation is characteristic of Korsakoff psychosis.
- *Pancreas:* Chronic calcifying pancreatitis is an unquestioned result of alcoholism and an important cause of pancreatic insufficiency.
- *Heart:* A toxic effect of alcohol is a form of dilated cardiomyopathy (alcoholic cardiomyopathy), which leads to low-output congestive heart failure. The alcoholic heart is also more susceptible to arrhythmias.
- *Skeletal muscle:* Muscle weakness is extremely common; a severe debilitating chronic myopathy occurs occasionally.
- *Endocrines:* Feminization and testicular atrophy can occur in males, and decreased fertility can occur in females.
- *Gastrointestinal tract:* Injury to the mucosa of the esophagus and stomach is a direct toxic effect of alcoholism. Alcohol inhibits the active transport of amino acids, thiamine, and vitamin B_{12}.
- *Blood:* Megaloblastic anemia secondary to a deficiency of folic acid is not uncommon in malnourished alcoholics.
- *Bone:* People with chronic alcoholism, particularly postmenopausal women, are at increased risk for osteoporosis.

Fetal Alcohol Syndrome

Infants born to mothers who consume excess alcohol during pregnancy may show a cluster of abnormalities, including growth retardation, microencephaly, facial dysmorphology, and neurological dysfunction. Only about 6% of the offspring are afflicted by the full fetal alcohol syndrome, but less severe abnormalities may appear.

Drug Abuse

The use of illicit drugs is estimated to cause about 20,000 deaths a year in the United States. Drug abuse involves agents that are used to alter mood and perception. These chemicals include (a) derivatives of opium (heroin, morphine); (b) depressants (barbiturates, tranquilizers, and alcohol); (c) stimulants (cocaine, amphetamines), marijuana, psychedelic drugs (LSD); and (d) inhalants (amyl nitrite, organic solvents such as those in glue).

Illicit Drugs

Illicit drugs account for many pathological syndromes, as described below.

Heroin

Heroin is a potent diacetyl derivative of morphine and is usually administered subcutaneously or intravenously. It produces euphoria and drowsiness. Overdoses may result in hypothermia, bradycardia, and respiratory depression. Other opiates subject to abuse include morphine, hydromorphone (Dilaudid), and oxycodone (OxyContin).

Cocaine and Amphetamines

Cocaine is an alkaloid that is commonly "cracked" into smaller pieces and smoked ("crack"). It produces euphoria and a sense of heightened sensitivity. Overdose leads to anxiety, delirium, and occasional seizures. Cardiac arrhythmias may cause sudden death in apparently healthy persons. Cardiac ischemia resulting from acute cocaine use may occur in the drug abusing population. The mechanism of action of cocaine is related to its interference with the reuptake of the neurotransmitter dopamine.

Amphetamines are sympathomimetic and resemble cocaine in their effects. The most serious complications of abuse are seizures, cardiac arrhythmias, and hyperthermia.

Hallucinogens

Hallucinogens include phencyclidine, or PCP, and lysergic acid diethylamide (LSD). Although chemically unrelated, they both alter perception and sensory experience. Overdoses of either can produce tachycardia, hypertension, coma, and convulsions.

Organic Solvents

The recreational inhalation of commercial preparations such as glues, plastic cements, and lighter fluid is widespread particularly among adolescents. Large doses may result in nausea, hallucinations, and eventually coma.

Medical Complications of Intravenous Drug Abuse

Apart from reactions related to the pharmacological or physiological effects of drug abuse, the most common complications are caused by bacterial and viral infections (Fig. 8-3). The most common infections are at the site of injection (e.g., abscesses, cellulitis, ulcers). Bacteremia can cause bacterial endocarditis, pulmonary, renal, and intracranial abscesses, meningitis, and osteomyelitis. Addicts who exchange needles are at risk for AIDS and viral hepatitis B and C.

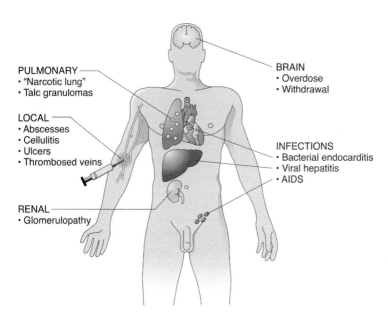

FIGURE 8-3
Complications of intravenous drug abuse. (From Rubin E, Gorstein F, Rubin R, et al. Rubin's Pathology, 4th ed. Philadelphia: Lippincott Williams & Wilkins, 2005, p. 324.)

Drug Addiction in Pregnant Women and Risks for the Fetus

Infants of drug-dependent mothers often exhibit a withdrawal syndrome, with symptoms such as tremors, irritability, seizures, and hyperactive reflexes. In utero, excessive fetal movements and oxygen demand increase the risk of intrapartum hypoxia and meconium aspiration. Drug addicted mothers experience higher rates of toxemia of pregnancy and premature labor.

Iatrogenic Drug Injury

Iatrogenic drug injury refers to the unintended side effects of therapeutic or diagnostic drugs prescribed by physicians. The typical hospitalized patient is given about 10 different medications; the risk of an adverse reaction increases proportionately with the number of different drugs. Adverse reactions are found in 2% to 5% of patients hospitalized on medical services; of these reactions, 2–12% are fatal. Untoward effects of drugs result from (a) overdose, (b) exaggerated physiological response, (c) hypersensitivity mechanisms, (d) a genetic predisposition, (e) interactions with other drugs, and (f) other unknown factors.

Sex Hormones

Oral Contraceptives

Hormonal preparations using synthetic estrogens and steroids with progesteronelike activity are now the most commonly used contraceptives in industrialized countries. They act either by preventing ovulation or by preventing implantation. They carry a small risk of complications:

- *Vascular:* Deep vein thrombosis risk is increased about threefold.
- *Neoplastic:* Risk of ovarian and endometrial cancer is decreased, while risk of breast cancer is slightly increased.
- *Benign liver adenomas:* Risk increases with duration of use.

Postmenopausal Hormone Replacement

Preparations containing combinations of estrogen and progesterone have proved effective in the treatment of postmenopausal symptoms and in mitigating osteoporosis. However, recent studies have found that hormone replacement treatment in postmenopausal women increases the risk of breast cancer, heart attacks, strokes, and blood clots, particularly after prolonged use.

Environmental Chemicals

Volatile Organic Solvents and Vapors

- *Chloroform ($CHCl_3$) and carbon tetrachloride (CCl_4):* These solvents exert anesthetic effects and are also hepatotoxins. Large doses lead to acute hepatic necrosis, fatty liver, and liver failure.
- *Trichloroethylene (C_2Hcl_3):* This industrial solvent depresses the central nervous system in large doses.
- *Methanol (CH_3OH):* The most characteristic lesion of methanol toxicity is necrosis of retinal ganglion cells with subsequent degeneration of the optic nerve.
- *Ethylene glycol ($HOCH_2CH_2OH$):* Commonly used as an antifreeze, the toxicity of ethylene glycol relates to acute kidney tubular necrosis.
- *Benzene (C_6H_6):* Benzene is a widely used solvent in industry. Almost all cases of acute and chronic benzene poisoning have resulted from industrial exposure. Acute benzene poisoning affects the central nervous system, and death comes from respi-

ratory failure. Long-term effects of exposure are on the bone marrow, causing aplastic anemia, acute myeloblastic leukemia, erythroleukemia, or multiple myeloma.

Agricultural Chemicals

Pesticides, fungicides, herbicides, and organic fertilizers are widely used in agriculture. Inadvertently contaminated food can cause severe acute illness. In the United States, 30 to 40 persons die annually of acute pesticide poisoning. Delayed neurotoxicity has been reported with triorthocresyl phosphate, a cooking oil contaminant. Acute poisoning with this compound leads to a peripheral neurotoxicity that progresses to motor weakness of limbs, which in some cases is only partially reversible. Certain types of hematopoietic malignancies have been reported in farmers who used large amounts of the herbicide, 2, 4-dichlorophenoxyacetic acid (2,4-D). Chronic toxicity of a number of agricultural chemicals in birds and fish has been well documented.

Aromatic Halogenated Hydrocarbons

Four aromatic halogenated hydrocarbons that have received considerable attention as possibly causing human disease are (a) the polychlorinated biphenyls (PCBs); (b) chlorophenols (pentachlorophenol used as a wood preservative); (c) hexachlorophene, used as an antibacterial in soaps; and (d) the dioxin TCDD, a byproduct of the synthesis of herbicides and hexachlorophene. Long-term animal toxicity of this class of substances is well documented.

Cyanide

Cyanide blocks cellular respiration by reversibly binding to cytochrome oxidase, thus producing acute anoxia. Human intestinal flora contain enzymes, which can liberate cyanide from amygdalin, a glucoside found in apricot (and other fruit) pits. In the past, extracts of apricot pits were used in the making of fraudulent anticancer nostrums, and resulted in cases of cyanide poisoning.

Air Pollutants

Studies have established a connection between air pollutants and chronic respiratory symptoms and mortality. Adverse effects mainly involve persons with existing respiratory ailments (asthma, chronic bronchitis, and emphysema) and cardiovascular disease. The most important air pollutants implicated in human disease are the following:

- *Sulfur dioxide*: This results from the combustion of sulfur-containing petroleum and coal in power plants, oil refineries, and industries such as paper mills and smelters.
- *Ozone and nitrogen oxides*: These do not derive principally from industrial activities, but rather from the action of sunlight on the products of vehicular internal combustion engines.
- *Carbon Monoxide (CO)*: CO is an odorless gas that results from the incomplete combustion of organic substances. Environmental CO is derived mainly from automobile exhaust emissions, fires, and in some cases, home heating systems.

  ➤ CO combines with hemoglobin with a 240× greater affinity than that of oxygen. Therefore, CO inhibits the function of hemoglobin as an oxygen carrier.
  ➤ Concentrations of CO greater than 50% cause coma and convulsions, and concentrations greater than 60% are usually fatal due to irreversible hypoxic injury.
  ➤ Severe CO poisoning is characterized by a cherry-red skin color. Recovery may be associated with brain damage.

Metals

Lead

Exposure

Occupational exposure to lead is a hazard in lead smelting and in the manufacture and recycling of automobile batteries. Leaded gasoline, before its manufacture was outlawed, was a source of lead contamination, and was linked to the deaths of employees working in tetraethyl lead gasoline plants. In addition, most homes built before 1940 were decorated with paint containing lead; accidental lead poisonings have occurred in the renovation of old homes. Children living in older homes heavily coated with flaking paint are at risk of developing chronic lead poisoning.

Metabolism and Toxicity

Lead is absorbed through either the lungs or the gastrointestinal tract and equilibrates in the blood. Lead inhibits incorporation of iron into heme, thus causing hypochromic anemia with a characteristic basophilic stippling of red blood cells. Classic lead toxicity is manifested in the dysfunction of the nervous system, kidneys, and hematopoietic system. Lead nephropathy is characterized by impaired proximal tubule reabsorption of amino acids, phosphate, and glucose. Toxic amounts of lead cause encephalopathy and peripheral neuropathy. Figure 8-4 illustrates the various manifestations of lead intoxification in different areas of the body.

Mercury

Mercury released into the environment from industrial wastes may be bioconcentrated and enter the food chain. Bacteria in the bottoms

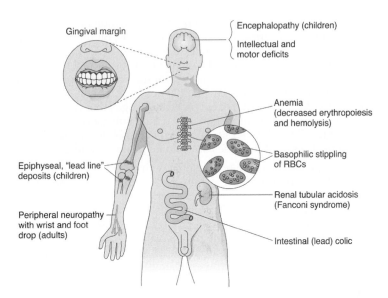

F I G U R E   8-4
Complications of lead intoxication. (From Rubin E, Gorstein F, Rubin R, et al. Rubin's Pathology, 4th ed. Philadelphia: Lippincott Williams & Wilkins, 2005, p. 331.)

of bays and oceans can convert mercury compounds into neurotoxic organomercurials. These are transferred up the food chain and are eventually concentrated in the large predatory fish that make up a large part of the diet of many countries.

Both inorganic and organic mercury are concentrated in the kidney. At present, chronic mercurial nephrotoxicity is almost always a consequence of long-term industrial exposure. Proteinuria is common, with a membranous glomerulonephritis. Methylmercury also distributes to the brain. Mercurial neurotoxicity is manifested as a constriction of visual fields, paresthesias, ataxia, and hearing loss.

Arsenic

Arsenic compounds contaminate the soil and drinking water as a result of naturally occurring arsenic-rich rock formations or from coal burning or the use of arsenical pesticides. Death from arsenic poisoning is due to central nervous system toxicity. Cancers of the skin and respiratory tract have been attributed to industrial and agricultural exposure to arsenic.

Cadmium

Cadmium is used in the manufacture of alloys, alkali storage batteries, and as a pigment. The lungs and kidneys are the principal target organs of chronic cadmium intoxication. Emphysema, pneumonitis, and proteinuria have been consistent findings in cadmium toxicity.

Nickel

Nickel is widely used in electronics, coins, steel alloys, batteries, and food processing. Dermatitis is the most frequent effect of overexposure. Exposed nickel workers have increased incidence of lung cancer, and cancer of the nasal cavities.

Iron

Ferrous sulfate is the easily absorbed form of iron present in pills. Acute poisoning occurs chiefly in young children who have eaten ferrous sulfate tablets, thinking them to be candy. Excess iron intake in adults is rare but has occurred in the Bantus of South Africa who cook and prepare alcoholic beverages in iron pots.

The body does not excrete iron. A small loss occurs in the desquamation of epithelium; a larger loss is in the menstrual blood. Excess accumulation of iron in the liver is known as siderosis; severe siderosis leads to liver cirrhosis.

Thermal Regulatory Dysfunction

Hypothermia

Generalized Hypothermia

Generalized hypothermia involves a decrease in body temperature below 35°C (95°F). If prolonged, several of the consequences of decreased body temperature are related to altered cerebrovascular function. When the body core temperature reaches 32°C (89.6°F), the cold person becomes lethargic, apathetic, and withdrawn. A further decline in temperature increases the lethargy to intermittent stupor and eventually coma. A core temperature below 28°C (82.4°F) results in bradycardia and atrial fibrillation.

Focal Thermal Alterations

Focal thermal alterations refer to local rather than systemic reduction in temperature, typically in the skin. Vasoconstriction occurs to reduce heat loss. In frostbite, ice crystals form within and between tissue cells causing physical disruption of cell membranes. The extent of tissue loss depends on the duration and depth of freezing. The most significant cellular damage occurs on thawing, when further mechanical disruption of membrane structures may occur.

Hyperthermia

Systemic Hyperthermia

This elevation in body core temperature can be caused by (a) increased heat production, (b) decreased elimination of heat from the body, or (c) thermal regulatory center disturbance. A body temperature above 42.5°C (108.5°F) leads to general vasodilation, inefficient cardiac function, and altered respiration; elevations above this are not compatible with life.

- *Fever:* Interleukin-1 and tumor necrosis factor are the chief factors responsible for resetting the body's "thermostat" during infection or inflammation to allow a higher body core temperature.
- *Heat stroke:* This form of hyperthermia is not mediated by endogenous pyrogens, but appears under high ambient temperatures and reflects impaired cooling responses (e.g., lack of sweating). People doing unusually vigorous exercise, very young children, the aged, and people with cardiovascular disease are especially vulnerable. External cooling and fluid and electrolyte replacement are effective therapy.
- *Malignant hyperthermia:* This hypermetabolic state occurs in genetically susceptible persons after exposure to certain anesthetics.

Cutaneous Burns

These forms of localized hyperthermia have been separated into three categories of severity:

- *First-degree burns (e.g., mild sunburn):* Mild endothelial injury produces vasodilation.
- *Second-degree burns:* Necrosis of the epithelium but the dermis is spared; blisters may form separating the epidermis from the dermis.
- *Third-degree burns:* Both epidermis and underlying dermis are charred. Re-epithelializatiion can occur if the skin appendages have been spared. Deeper burns require skin grafting. Loss of body water from the denuded areas is a serious systemic disturbance, which may result in hemoconcentration, shock, and acute tubular necrosis of the kidneys. Surface infections and sepsis are also serious concerns.

Inhalation and Electrical Burns

Persons trapped in burning buildings can suffer inhalation burns with damage to the oral cavity and all respiratory tract passages. Respiratory distress syndrome may ensue.

Electrical injury damages in two ways: (a) dysfunction of the cardiovascular conduction system, and (b) conversion of electrical energy to heat energy when the current meets the tissue resistance.

Altitude-related Illnesses

High-altitude illness can occur in persons ascending to 8,000 ft (2,500 m) or higher. The physiological modifications induced by high altitude are related to decreased atmospheric pressure and, therefore, to decreased oxygen availability. Acute mountain sickness is the most common form of altitude illness and may develop at 2,500 m. It is characterized by headache, lassitude, anorexia, weakness, and difficulty in sleeping. High-altitude systemic edema can occur at elevations above 3,000 m and results from an asymptomatic increase in vascular permeability. On return to lower elevations, a diuresis causes the edema to disappear. High-altitude retinal hemorrhage may develop at altitudes above 5,000 m. These usually resolve without sequelae.

More serious high-altitude illnesses at higher elevations involve pulmonary edema and hypertension. Encephalopathy with cerebral edema and hypoxia may also develop.

Physical Injuries

The effect of mechanical trauma is related to the force transmitted to the tissue, the rate at which the transfer occurs, the surface area to which the force is transferred, and the area of the body that is injured. Examples of various kinds of trauma include the following:

- A **contusion** is a localized mechanical injury with focal hemorrhage, but with no epidermal disruption. Blood cells that leak into the tissue space from damaged capillaries are ingested by macrophages; the degraded hemoglobin yields heme pigments, giving the area typical bruise discoloration.
- An **abrasion** is a skin defect caused by crushes or scrapes. Epithelium is disrupted.
- A **laceration** is a split or tear of the skin.

   Wounds are mechanical disruptions of tissue integrity.

Radiation

Radiation is the emission of energy in the form of electromagnetic waves (x-rays, gamma rays) or particles (alpha particles, beta particles, neutrons). Radiation is emitted by radioactive substances or comes from man-made sources such as x-ray and radiation therapy machines. Radiation may be quantitated in the following ways:

- A **roentgen** is a measure of the emission of radiant energy from a source. It refers to the amount of ionization produced in air.
- One **rad** equals 100 ergs of energy absorbed per gm of tissue
- One **gray** (Gy) equals one joule of energy absorbed per kilogram of tissue. A centigray (cGy) is equivalent to 1 rad.

- A **rem** is the amount of radiation producing the biological effect equal to 1 rad of x-rays or gamma rays.
- A **sievert** (Sv) is the dose in grays multiplied by an appropriate quality factor Q, so that 1 Sv of radiation is roughly equivalent in biological effectiveness to 1 Gy of gamma rays.

At the cellular level, radiation has two effects: (a) a somatic effect, associated with acute cell killing, and (b) the induction of genetic damage. There is a differential sensitivity of tissues to radiation. Organs and tissues in which cells are multiplying quickly, such as the intestines and bone marrow, are harmed more easily by radiation than those in which cells multiply more slowly, such as muscles and tendons.

Whole-body Irradiation

Except for unusual circumstances, as in the high-dose irradiation that precedes bone marrow transplantation, significant levels of whole-body irradiation result only from industrial accidents or from the explosion of nuclear weapons. In whole-body radiation, comparable doses of radiant energy are transmitted to all organs; therefore, the development of different acute radiation syndromes reflects the dissimilarities in vulnerability of the target tissues (Fig. 8-5). Whole-body irradiation of 2,000 rads or more causes death

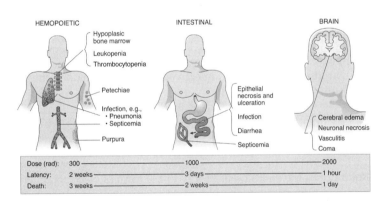

FIGURE 8-5

Acute radiation syndromes. At a dose of approximately 300 rads of whole body radiation, a syndrome characterized by hematopoietic failure develops within two weeks. In the vicinity of 1,000 rads, a gastrointestinal syndrome with a latency of only 3 days is seen. With doses of 2,000 rads or more, disease of the central nervous system appears within 1 hour, and death ensues rapidly. (From Rubin E, Gorstein F, Rubin R, et al. Rubin's Pathology, 4th ed. Philadelphia: Lippincott Williams & Wilkins, 2005, p. 340.)

within several hours due to central nervous system damage, whereas 300 rads leads to hematopoietic failure within 2 weeks. The resulting bleeding, anemia, and infection can cause death in 3 weeks.

After the nuclear blasts in Japan, teratogenic effects were observed in children who were exposed during fetal and embryonic stages of development; however, follow-up and long-term studies have found no evidence of genetic damage in the form of either congenital abnormalities or hereditary diseases in the later offspring of survivors of the nuclear blasts.

Radiation Therapy for Tumors

In the course of radiation therapy for malignant neoplasms, some normal tissue is inevitably included in the radiation field. Damage to radiation-exposed tissue can be attributed to (a) compromise of the vascular supply, and (b) a fibrotic repair reaction to acute necrosis and chronic ischemia. Although almost any organ can be damaged by radiation, the clinically important tissues are the skin, lungs, heart, kidney, bladder, and intestine (Fig. 8-6).

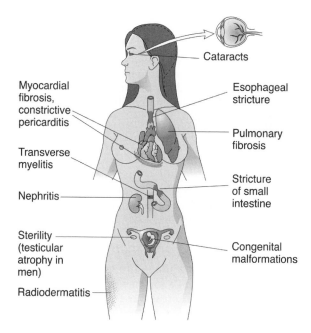

FIGURE 8-6

The nonneoplastic complications of radiation. (From Rubin E, Gorstein F, Rubin R, et al. Rubin's Pathology, 4th ed. Philadelphia: Lippincott Williams & Wilkins, 2005, p. 341.)

Radiation and Cancer

The evidence that radiation can lead to cancer is incontrovertible and comes from animal experiments and studies of the effects of occupational exposure, radiation therapy for nonneoplastic conditions, the diagnostic use of certain radioisotopes, and nuclear explosions. Examples include the following:

- High rate of lung cancer in uranium miners
- Thyroid cancer in adults who had received irradiation of the thymus as infants
- High breast cancer rate in women treated with thoracic radiation for childhood Hodgkin disease
- Development of aplastic anemia and myelogenous leukemia in persons treated for ankylosing spondylitis with low-dose spinal irradiation
- An increase in brain tumors in persons who received cranial irradiation for tinea capitis as children
- Survivors of the atom bomb explosions suffered from a number of cancers

Nutritional Disorders

Obesity

Obesity is the most common nutritional disorder in the industrialized countries, where it is far more common than all the nutritional deficiencies combined. Obesity is determined according to body mass index (BMI), calculated as weight (kg)/height (m^2). A BMI of 25 to 30 is classed as overweight, 30 to 40 as obesity, and above 40 as morbid obesity.

Pathogenesis

Obesity results from the excess storage of triglycerides in adipose tissue depots, and it is caused by excessive caloric intake, insufficient expenditure of energy, or both. Both genetic and environmental factors are important in the pathogenesis of obesity.

Hormones involved in the regulation of body weight have been described (Fig. 8-7).

- Thyroid hormone increases metabolic rate. Persons with a deficiency of thyroid hormone have lower basal metabolic rates and are heavier than normal whereas those with excess thyroid hormone have higher metabolic rates and are thinner.
- Melanocortins are a group of peptides derived by post-translational cleavage of the proopiomelanocortin gene product. α-Melanocyte stimulating hormone (α-MSH), one of these peptides, binds to receptors in the hypothalamus and regulates the intake of food by suppressing the appetite.

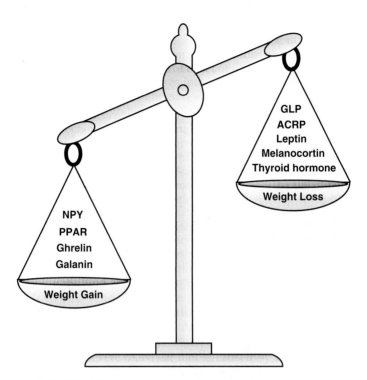

FIGURE 8-7
The balance of chemical mediators that promote fat accumulation (weight gain) and those that promote fat loss (weight loss). (From Rubin E, Gorstein F, Rubin R, et al. Rubin's Pathology, 4th ed. Philadelphia: Lippincott Williams & Wilkins, 2005, p. 345.)

- Leptin, the product of the *ob* (obese) gene, is produced by adipose tissue. High levels of leptin reflect greater adipocyte mass and lend to a feeling of satiety.
- Ghrelin is a peptide produced mainly by the stomach. It serves to provoke appetite and promote fat storage in adipocytes.
- Glucagon-like peptide (GLP-1) promotes a feeling of satiety, thereby decreasing food intake.
- Galanin is a peptide neurotransmitter that stimulates food intake.
- Adipocyte complement-related protein (ACRP30) is a peptide made by adipocytes and is inversely associated with body weight and insulin resistance. Its levels in the blood are lower in obese persons.

- Neuropeptide Y (NPY) is the peptide product of three different nuclei in the hypothalamus, and is a potent stimulator of appetite.
- Peroxisome proliferator-activated receptors (PPAR) are proteins belonging to a family of transcription factors. One isotype, PPARγ, is thought to be most involved in regulating obesity. It is present on adipocytes and when activated, increases uptake of fatty acids and glucose by adipocytes.

Pathology and Clinical Features

Obesity leads to an overall increase in mortality and morbidity (Fig. 8-8).

- Obese people are at risk for developing type II diabetes, with associated with high levels of circulating insulin and peripheral insulin resistance.
- Obesity is linked to atherosclerosis and myocardial infarction.
- Obesity is associated with hypercholesterolemia, low levels of HDL, and hypertension.

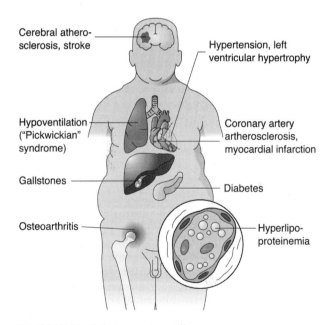

Cerebral athero-sclerosis, stroke

Hypertension, left ventricular hypertrophy

Hypoventilation ("Pickwickian" syndrome)

Coronary artery artherosclerosis, myocardial infarction

Gallstones

Diabetes

Osteoarthritis

Hyperlipo-proteinemia

FIGURE 8-8

Complications of obesity. (From Rubin E, Gorstein F, Rubin R, et al. Rubin's Pathology, 4th ed. Philadelphia: Lippincott Williams & Wilkins, 2005, p. 346.)

- Osteoarthritis and degenerative joint disease can result from the physical effect of excess body weight.
- In morbidly obese persons, the abdominal fat hinders chest expansion during inspiration (Pickwickian syndrome).

Protein-calorie Malnutrition

Marasmus and kwashiorkor are two common protein-calorie deficiencies in the nonindustrialized world.

Marasmus

Marasmus refers to a deficiency of calories from all sources. It is characterized by decreased body weight and growth failure, diminished subcutaneous fat, protuberant abdomen, and muscle wasting.

Kwashiorkor

Kwashiorkor is a form of malnutrition in children caused by a diet deficient in protein. Symptoms are similar to those of marasmus except there is edema and apathy. The abdomen is distended because of flaccid muscles, hepatomegaly, and ascites due to hypoalbuminemia (Fig. 8-9). Microscopically, hepatocytes contain fat, derived from the carbohydrate in the diet; however, the liver is fatty due to inadequate apoprotein to carry the lipid out of the hepatocytes. Fatty liver reverts to normal when sufficient protein is provided in the diet. The hair becomes a reddish color with a characteristic linear depigmentation (flag sign), providing evidence of particularly severe periods of protein deficiency.

Vitamins

The body depends totally on dietary sources for vitamins. They are necessary in trace amounts for metabolic functions.

Vitamin A

This fat-soluble vitamin is actually a family of substances. Two forms occur naturally as retinoids, which are abundant in liver and eggs. A precursor, β-carotene, found mainly in green, leafy vegetables, is converted in the intestinal mucosa to retinoids. Ninety percent of the body's vitamin A is stored in the perisinusoidal stellate cells of the liver.

- Vitamin A is a constituent of the photosensitive pigments in the retina and is important in the maintenance of skin, hair, and specialized epithelial linings. It also functions in skeletal maturation and in cell membrane structure.

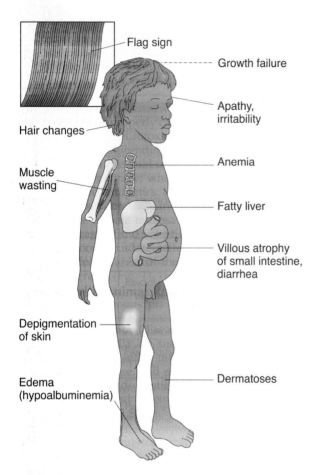

F I G U R E   8-9
Complications of kwashiorkor. (From Rubin E, Gorstein F, Rubin R, et al. Rubin's Pathology, 4th ed. Philadelphia: Lippincott Williams & Wilkins, 2005, p. 347.)

- The lack of vitamin A results in squamous metaplasia, especially in glandular epithelium (Fig. 8-10). The earliest sign of deficiency is often diminished vision in dim light. Vitamin A is a necessary component in the pigment of the retinal rods and is active in light transduction.

Vitamin B Complex

The members of this water-soluble group are vitamin B_1 (thiamine), niacin, vitamin B_2 (riboflavin), vitamin B_5 (pantothenic acid), vita-

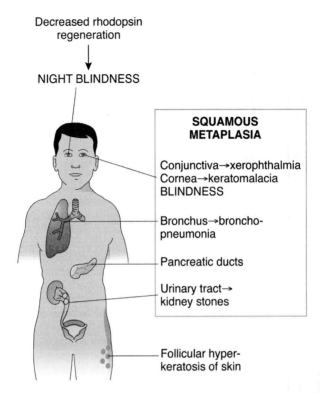

Decreased rhodopsin regeneration

NIGHT BLINDNESS

SQUAMOUS METAPLASIA

Conjunctiva→xerophthalmia
Cornea→keratomalacia
BLINDNESS

Bronchus→broncho-pneumonia

Pancreatic ducts

Urinary tract→kidney stones

Follicular hyper-keratosis of skin

FIGURE 8-10
Complications of vitamin A deficiency. (From Rubin E, Gorstein F, Rubin R, et al. Rubin's Pathology, 4th ed. Philadelphia: Lippincott Williams & Wilkins, 2005, p. 348.)

min B_6 (pyridoxine), and vitamin B_{12} (cyanocobalamin). With the exception of vitamin B_{12}, which is derived only from animal sources, the vitamins of the B complex are found mainly in leafy green vegetables, milk, and liver.

Vitamin B_1 Thiamine

The active form of thiamine is thiamine pyrophosphate is important in carbohydrate metabolism.

- Thiamine deficiency was classically seen in Asia, where people subsisted on highly polished rice, from which milling removed the thiamine-rich husk. In Western countries, deficiency occurs mainly in alcoholics and people with poor nutrition.

- The cardinal symptoms of thiamine deficiency are polyneuropathy, edema, and cardiac failure (Fig. 8-11). The deficiency syndrome is divided into "dry" beri-beri with symptoms referable to the neuromuscular system, and "wet" beri-beri, in which manifestations of cardiac failure predominate.
- In severe cases, the deficiency is manifested by involvement of the brain (Wernicke encephalopathy), with progressive dementia, ataxia, and paralysis of the extraocular muscles.

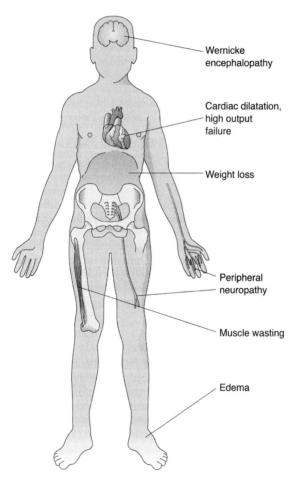

FIGURE 8-11
Complications of thiamine deficiency (beri-beri). (From Rubin E, Gorstein F, Rubin R, et al. Rubin's Pathology, 4th ed. Philadelphia: Lippincott Williams & Wilkins, 2005, p. 349.)

- The most reliable diagnostic test for thiamine deficiency is an immediate and dramatic response to parenteral administration of thiamine.

Niacin

Niacin refers to two chemically distinct compounds: nicotinic acid and nicotinamide. These components are derived from dietary niacin or are biosynthesized from available tryptophan.

- Niacin plays a major role in the formation of NAD and its phosphate, NADP. These compounds are important in intermediary metabolism. Animal protein and many types of grain are good sources.
- Pellagra (Italian meaning "rough skin") refers to clinical niacin deficiency and mainly is seen in patients weakened by other diseases, and in malnourished alcoholics.
- Pellagra is characterized by the three "Ds" of niacin deficiency: dermatitis, diarrhea, and dementia (Fig. 8-12). The skin is rough and scaly. In the mouth, inflammation and edema lead to a large, red tongue.

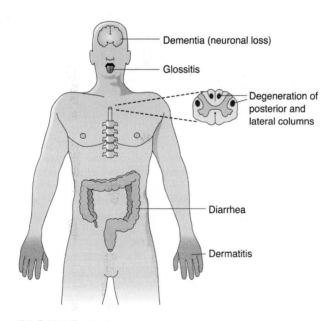

FIGURE 8-12
Complications of niacin deficiency (pellagra). (From Rubin E, Gorstein F, Rubin R, et al. Rubin's Pathology, 4th ed. Philadelphia: Lippincott Williams & Wilkins, 2005, p. 350.)

Vitamin B_2 Riboflavin

Riboflavin is derived from many plant and animal sources. It is a component of the flavin nucleotides, which play important roles in electron transport. Clinical symptoms of deficiency are usually seen only in debilitated patients or poorly nourished alcoholics. Complications of riboflavin deficiency are pictured in Figure 8-13. A characteristic feature is cheilosis, with fissures in the skin at the angles of the mouth.

Vitamin B_5 Pantothenic Acid

Pantothenic acid is an antioxidant vitamin utilized in the breakdown of carbohydrates, proteins and fats. It is needed for proper and healthy growth of hair. Vitamin B_5 is contained in foods such as whole grain cereals, legumes, eggs, and meat. Deficiency is rare, but may occur in the elderly with poor nutrition. Deficiency symptoms include allergies, adrenal insufficiency, and rheumatoid arthritis.

Vitamin B_6 Pyridoxine

Pyridoxine activity is found in three naturally occurring compounds: pyridoxine, pyridoxal, and pyridoxamine, and it is widely

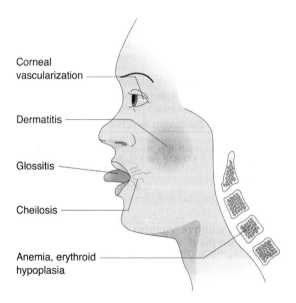

FIGURE   8-13
Complications of riboflavin deficiency. (From Rubin E, Gorstein F, Rubin R, et al. Rubin's Pathology, 4th ed. Philadelphia: Lippincott Williams & Wilkins, 2005, p. 351.)

distributed in vegetable and animal foods. Pyridoxine is converted to pyridoxal phosphate, a coenzyme for many enzymes including transaminases and carboxylases. The primary expression of deficiency is in the central nervous system, a feature consistent with its role in the formation of pyridoxal-dependent decarboxylase of the neurotransmitter γ-aminobutyric acid (GABA).

Vitamin B_{12} Cyanocobalamin

Cyanocobalamin is found in almost all animal protein, especially liver. Deficiencies are seen in cases of pernicious anemia, most of which result from a lack of secretion of intrinsic factor by the parietal cells of the stomach fundus. Intrinsic factor is necessary for absorption of vitamin B_{12} from the ileum.

Folic Acid

This vitamin is found in meats, nuts, beans, and green, leafy vegetables; however, excessive cooking destroys much of it in foods. In tissues, folic acid is enzymatically reduced to its active coenzyme form, which functions as an intermediate carrier of 1-carbon groups in a number of complex enzymatic reactions. Pregnancy increases the requirement for folic acid 5- to 10-fold. Importantly, it has been found that supplementation of the diet of pregnant women with folic acid prevents spina bifida and other dysraphic anomalies in the newborn. Deficiency is associated with megaloblastic anemia.

Vitamin C (Ascorbic Acid)

Vitamin C is abundant in citrus fruits and vegetables. It acts in the hydroxylation of procollagen and is thus important in the formation and maintenance of many types of connective tissue that depend on collagen for tensile strength. Vitamin C also has antioxidant properties and augments the absorption of iron from the intestine.

Vitamin C has long been known as the "anti-scurvy" vitamin. Scurvy is characterized in children by defects in the development of bones and teeth. Because collagen in blood vessel walls is abnormal, hemorrhages can occur, and wound healing is poor (Fig. 8-14).

Vitamin D

Vitamin D is a fat-soluble steroid hormone that is found in two forms: vitamin D_3 (cholecalciferol) and vitamin D_2 (ergocalciferol). Vitamin D_3 is produced in the skin, and vitamin D_2 is derived from plant ergosterol. Both forms have equal biological potency.

- To achieve biological potency, vitamin D (whether D_2 or D_3) must be hydroxylated to active metabolites in the liver and kidney.

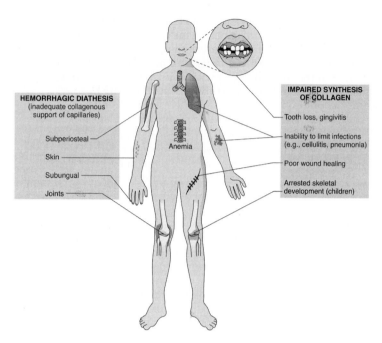

FIGURE 8-14
Complications of vitamin C deficiency (scurvy). (From Rubin E, Gorstein F, Rubin R, et al. Rubin's Pathology, 4th ed. Philadelphia: Lippincott Williams & Wilkins, 2005, p. 353.)

- The active form of the vitamin promotes calcium and phosphate absorption from the small intestine and may directly influences bone mineralization.
- Vitamin D deficiency results from (a) insufficient vitamin D in the diet, (b) insufficient production in the skin because of limited sunlight, (c) inadequate absorption from the diet, or (d) defect in conversion to its active form (as in liver disease or renal failure).
- In children, vitamin D deficiency causes rickets, a progressive weakening of bone structure; in adults, osteomalacia (adult rickets) occurs.

Vitamin E

Vitamin E is an antioxidant that is believed to protect membrane phospholipids from lipid peroxidation by free radicals formed by cellular metabolism. Corn and soybeans are rich in vitamin E. Because vitamin E is a fat-soluble vitamin, any defect in fat absorption results in low levels in the body.

Vitamin K

Vitamin K is a fat-soluble vitamin. Green leafy vegetables are rich in this vitamin. Deficiencies occur in conditions that interfere with fat absorption, such as sprue or biliary tract obstruction. Vitamin K confers calcium-binding properties to certain proteins; therefore, itis important for the activity of four clotting factors: prothrombin, factor VII, factor IX, and factor X. Deficiency can lead to serious hemorrhage; parenteral vitamin K therapy is rapidly effective.

Essential Trace Minerals

Essential trace minerals such as iron, copper, zinc, cobalt, iodine, and selenium are mostly components of enzymes and cofactors. Deficiencies in any trace mineral may result from malabsorption syndrome or during total parenteral nutrition. Dietary deficiencies of iron and iodine are discussed in Chapters 20 and 21.

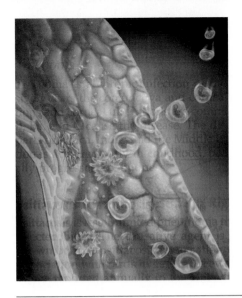

Infectious and Parasitic Diseases

Spirochetal Infections
   Syphilis
   Nonvenereal Treponematoses
   Lyme Disease
   Leptospirosis
   Relapsing Fever

Chlamydial Infections
   Psittacosis (Ornithosis)
   Chlamydia pneumoniae

Rickettsial Infections
   Rocky Mountain Spotted Fever
   Epidemic (Louse-borne) Typhus
   Endemic (Murine) Typhus
   Scrub Typhus
   Q Fever

Mycoplasmal Infections

Mycobacteria
   Tuberculosis
   Leprosy

Fungal Infections
   Candida
   Aspergillosis
   Mucormycosis (Zygomycosis)
   Cryptococcosis
   Histoplasmosis
   Coccidioidomycosis
   Blastomycosis
   Paracoccidioidomycosis (South American Blastomycosis)
   Sporotrichosis
   Chromomycosis
   Dermatophyte Infections
   Mycetoma

Protozoal Infections
   Malaria
   Babesiosis
   Toxoplasmosis
   Pneumocystis carinii (*jiroveci*) Pneumonia
   Amebiasis
   Cryptosporidiosis
   Giardiasis
   Leishmaniasis
   Chagas Disease (American Trypanosomiasis)

African Trypanosomiasis
Primary Amebic Meningoencephalitis
Helminthic Infection
Filarial Nematodes
Intestinal Nematodes
Tissue Nematodes
Flukes (Trematodes)
Intestinal Tapeworms (Cestodes)

Infectious diseases are disorders in which tissue damage or dysfunction is produced by a microorganism. The impact of infectious diseases is greatest in developing countries, where millions of people die of a treatable or preventable infectious disease. Even in the United States each year, infectious diseases cause more than 200,000 deaths.

General Considerations

Infectivity and Virulence

Virulence refers to the complex of properties that allows an organism to achieve infection and cause disease of different degrees of severity. Such properties include the ability of the organism to (a) gain access to the body, (b) avoid host defenses, (c) be able to grow in the human milieu, and (d) parasitize human resources.

Host Factors in Infections

The body's defense mechanisms against invading organisms include (a) anatomical barriers such as the skin and the aerodynamic filtration system of the upper airway, (b) the mucociliary airway blanket, (c) the acidity of the stomach, (d) the normal competing microbial flora of the gastrointestinal tract, and (e) secretions such as lysozyme with antimicrobial properties. Factors that affect susceptibility to infection include heritable differences, age, behavior (as in sexually transmitted diseases), and compromised host defenses (such as may result from trauma, burns, or immunosuppressive therapies).

Viral Infections

Viruses range in size from 20 to 300 nm and consist of RNA or DNA contained in a protein shell. Some viruses are enveloped in a lipid membrane. They are not capable of independent metabolism or reproduction and are thus obligate intracellular parasites, requiring living cells in which to replicate. After invading cells, viruses divert the cellular mechanisms to the synthesis of viral-encoded nucleic acids and proteins. Disease-causing viruses may function in the following ways:

- Viruses may cause disease by killing the infected cells.
- Viruses may interfere with a function of cells without killing them.
- Viruses may promote release of mediators that elicit inflammation.
- Viruses may persist in cells without interfering with cellular functions.
- Viruses may cause cells to proliferate and form tumors.

Respiratory Viruses

Respiratory infections caused by viruses are described in Table 9-1.

Common Cold (Coryza)

This most common of the respiratory diseases, is acute, self-limited, and caused by a variety of RNA viruses, including over 100 distinct rhinoviruses and several coronaviruses. Rhinoviruses and coro-

Table 9-1

Respiratory Infections Caused by Viruses

Respiratory Infection	Causative Agent	Pathology
Common cold	Rhinoviruses, coronaviruses	Self-limited, upper respiratory tract
Influenza	Types A, B, C (enveloped, single-stranded RNA)	Necrosis of ciliated epithelium; necrosis of alveolar lining
Parainfluenza	Enveloped, single-stranded RNA	Croup (laryngotracheo-bronchitis)
Respiratory syncytial virus	Enveloped, single-stranded RNA virus	Bronchiolitis and Pneumonia in infants
Adenovirus	Nonenveloped DNA virus	Pneumonia in military recruits; Smudge cells, Cowdry type A inclusions
Severe acute respiratory syndrome (SARS)	Coronavirus	Multinucleated syncytial cells; alveolar damage

naviruses have a tropism for upper respiratory tract epithelium and cause increased mucus production and edema. Rhinoviruses and coronaviruses do not destroy infected epithelium. Infected cells release mediators such as bradykinin, which produce most of the symptoms.

Influenza

Influenza is an acute, self-limited infection of the upper and lower airways, caused by strains of influenza virus. Types A, B, and C of influenza virus cause human disease; type A is the most common. Influenza viruses are enveloped and contain single-stranded RNA. A viral glycoprotein, hemagglutinin, binds to sialic acid residues on the respiratory epithelial cell, and enters the cell by fusion with the membrane. The virus kills the ciliated epithelium of the respiratory tract, crippling the mucociliary blanket, thus predisposing to bacterial pneumonia. Epidemics are accompanied by deaths both from the disease and its complications. Killed viral vaccines specific to epidemic strains are 75% effective in preventing influenza.

Parainfluenza Virus

The parainfluenza viruses cause acute upper and lower respiratory tract infections, particularly in young children. Parainfluenza viruses are enveloped, single-stranded RNA viruses; there are four antigenically distinct types. The viruses infect and kill respiratory epithelial cells, eliciting an inflammatory response. Parainfluenza virus are the most common cause of croup (laryngotracheobronchitis). Subglottic swelling, airway compression, and respiratory distress characterize croup. It evidenced by a characteristic barking cough and inspiratory stridor.

Respiratory Syncytial Virus (RSV)

Respiratory syncytial virus is an enveloped, single-stranded RNA virus and is the major cause of bronchiolitis and pneumonia in infants. Viral surface proteins interact with specific receptors on host cells to cause binding and fusion. producing necrosis and sloughing of bronchial, bronchiolar and alveolar epithelium. RSV is associated mainly with a lymphocytic inflammatory infiltrate and spreads in respiratory aerosols and secretions. Infants and young children present with wheezing, cough, and respiratory distress.

Multinucleated syncytial cells are sometimes seen in infected tissues.

Adenovirus

Adenoviruses are nonenveloped DNA viruses that cause necrotizing respiratory lesions. Certain serotypes are common causes of acute respiratory disease and pneumonia in military recruits. Some adenoviruses are important causes of chronic pulmonary disease in infants and young children. Pathological changes include necrotizing bronchitis and bronchiolitis.

Severe Acute Respiratory Syndrome (SARS)-associated Coronavirus

An epidemic of severe pneumonia, which originated in Guangdong province of China in 1993 and spread to other Asian countries, the U.S., Canada, and Europe. The World Health Organization now provides regular reports of SARS outbreaks when they occur anywhere on the globe. It is caused by a novel coronavirus, which has probably mutated from a nonhuman host. The mortality rate is as high as 15% in patients who are elderly or who have other respiratory disorders. At autopsy, the lungs disclosed diffuse alveolar damage. Multinucleated syncytial cells without viral inclusions have also been observed.

Viral Exanthems

A number of viral diseases are characterized by rashes and skin eruptions (Table 9-2).

Table 9-2

Viral Infections Causing Skin Eruptions

Viral Infection	Causative Agent	Pathology
Measles (rubeola)	Enveloped, single-stranded RNA	Necrosis of respiratory epithelium; small vessel vasculitis; lymphoid hyperplasia; Warthin-Finkeldey giant cells; Koplik spots on buccal mucosa
Rubella	Enveloped, single-stranded RNA (rubellavirus)	Rhinorrhea, conjunctivitis, postauricular lymphadenopathy
Human parvovirus B19	Single-stranded DNA	Interruption in red blood cell production
Smallpox (variola)	Poxviridae	Skin vesicles with reticular degeneration; eosinophilic intracytoplasmic inclusion bodies (Guarnieri bodies)

Measles (Rubeola)

Measles virus is an enveloped, single-stranded RNA virus that causes an acute, self-limited illness characterized by upper respiratory tract symptoms, fever, and a rash. The virus is transmitted in respiratory aerosols and secretions, and is primarily a disease of children. The initial infection site is the mucous membranes of the nasopharynx and bronchi. From there, the virus spreads to regional lymph nodes and the bloodstream and involves the skin and lymphoid tissues. Clinical features include the following:

- Rash results from the action of T lymphocytes on virally infected vascular endothelium. It begins on the face and spreads to the trunk and extremities. Mucosal lesions (Koplik spots) consist of gray dots on a red base, and appear on the posterior buccal mucosa.
- Necrosis of infected respiratory epithelium. In the skin, the virus produces a vasculitis of small blood vessels.
- Prominent lymphoid hyperplasia: Multinucleated giant cells (Warthin-Finkeldey giant cells) containing up to 100 nuclei, with both intracytoplasmic and intranuclear inclusions, may be present in infected tissue and are pathognomonic for measles.

Live, attenuated vaccines are highly effective in preventing measles and eliminating the spread of the virus. The disease is now uncommon in the United States.

Rubella

Rubella is an enveloped, single-stranded RNA virus that causes a mild, self-limited systemic disease, usually associated with a rash. In pregnant women, rubella is a destructive fetal pathogen that may cause congenital anomalies and even death of the fetus. Rubella infects the respiratory epithelium and then spreads through the blood and lymph. Fetal infection occurs through the placenta during the viremic phase of the maternal illness. Infection early in gestation can produce fetal deafness, cataracts, glaucoma, heart defects, and mental retardation.

A live, attenuated viral vaccine prevents rubella. The disease is now uncommon in the United States.

Human Parvovirus B19

Human parvovirus B19 is a single-stranded DNA virus that causes systemic infections characterized by rash, arthralgias, and transient interruption in erythrocyte production. The virus produces characteristic cytopathic effects in erythroid precursors; the enlarged nucleus of an infected cell contains an eosinophilic glassy material. The virus spreads by the respiratory route and is best known for causing the childhood skin eruption called "fifth disease."

Most persons suffer a mild illness, but the disease can be serious in two circumstances: (a) persons with chronic hemolytic anemia may suffer a potentially fatal transient aplastic crisis, and (b) an infected fetus may suffer severe anemia, hydrops fetalis, or even death in utero.

Smallpox (Variola)

Smallpox was a highly contagious exanthematous viral infection produced by the variola virus, a member of the family Poxviridae. Microscopic features of the skin vesicle of variola showed reticular degeneration. Eosinophilic intracytoplasmic inclusion bodies (Guarnieri bodies) had great diagnostic value.

Smallpox has been eradicated by successful vaccination campaigns. The last reported human cases were laboratory-acquired infections in 1978. In 1980, the World Health Organization declared that smallpox had been eradicated globally.

Mumps

Mumps virus is an enveloped, single-stranded RNA virus that causes an acute, self-limited, systemic illness. Mumps is primarily a disease of childhood and spreads through the respiratory route. The virus infects and causes swelling of the salivary glands, especially the parotid). Less commonly, the central nervous system, pancreas, and testes can be infected. Lesions are of a lymphocytic inflammatory infiltrate, with interstitial edema. Epididymoorchitis occurs in 30% of males infected after puberty. Orchitis is usually unilateral and so rarely causes sterility. A live attenuated mumps vaccine prevents mumps, and the disease has been largely eliminated in most developed countries.

Intestinal Virus Infections

Rotavirus Infection

This double-stranded RNA virus usually infects young children, and is the most common cause of severe diarrhea worldwide. It spreads by oral–fecal route. Rotavirus infects the enterocytes of the duodenum and jejunum, disrupting absorption and causing a loss of fluid into the bowel lumen; this leads to diarrhea and dehydration.

Norwalk Virus and Other Viral Diarrheas

In addition to rotavirus, there are numerous other viral causes of diarrhea, including adenoviruses, caliciviruses, and astroviruses. The Norwalk virus is the prototype of the group.

Viral Hemorrhagic Fevers

The hemorrhagic fevers encompass a group of at least 20 distinct viral infections that cause varying degrees of hemorrhage, shock, and sometimes death (Table 9-3).

Yellow Fever

Yellow fever is an acute hemorrhagic fever caused by a mosquito-borne flavivirus, an enveloped, single-stranded RNA virus. It is sometimes associated with extensive hepatic necrosis and jaundice. The virus has a tropism for liver cells, which it sometimes damages extensively; hence the jaundice of yellow fever. Hemorrhage and shock result from damage to the endothelium of small blood vessels. Midzonal necrosis of liver lobules can occur. Necrotic hepatocytes lose their nuclei and become intensely eosinophilic and apoptotic. Apoptotic liver cells that have dislodged from adjacent hepatocytes are known as Councilman bodies.

Ebola Hemorrhagic Fever

This severe and often fatal disease is caused by the Ebola virus, an RNA virus. It causes hemorrhagic disease in several regions of Africa. The virus can be transmitted via bodily secretions, blood, and used needles. The virus replicates in endothelial cells, mononuclear phagocytes, and hepatocytes.

Ebola virus causes the most widespread destructive tissue lesions of all viral hemorrhagic fever agents. In the liver, it causes hepatocellular necrosis and Kupffer cell hyperplasia, apoptotic bodies and fatty change.

Table 9-3

Properties of Viral Hemorrhagic Fevers

Infection	Causative Agent	Pathology
Yellow fever	Flaviviruses, enveloped, single-stranded RNA	Coagulative hepatocyte necrosis; eosinophilic, apoptotic liver cells prominent
Ebola	Filoviridae, RNA viruses	Widespread destruction of endothelial cells, phagocytes, and hepatocytes; necrosis in liver, kidneys, gonads, spleen, and lymph nodes
West Nile	West Nile virus	Mononuclear meningoencephalitis; brainstem involved extensively

West Nile Virus

This virus is spread between various mosquito vectors and birds. In 1937, it was first identified in the west Nile region of Uganda, and in 1999, it was identified in the Western Hemisphere. Most infections are subclinical; however, patients can develop a more severe illness with encephalitis and varying degrees of neuronal necrosis and brain stem involvement.

Herpesvirus

The virus family Herpesviridae includes a large number of enveloped DNA viruses. The most important pathogens among the herpes viruses cause chickenpox and shingles (varicella-zoster), cold sores (herpes simplex virus type 1), and genital sores (herpes simplex virus type 2). Other organs or tissues may be affected infrequently (Table 9-4).

Varicella-Zoster Infection

The first exposure to varicella-zoster virus (VZV) produces chickenpox whose dominant feature is a generalized vesicular eruption. The virus then becomes latent, and its reactivation causes herpes zoster (shingles), a localized, painful, vesicular skin eruption. The intraepidermal vesicle fills with neutrophils and erodes to become a shallow ulcer. Infected cells within the vesicle have large eosinophilic nuclear inclusions. Some cells form multinucleated giant cells. The vesicle eventually ruptures and heals.

In its latent stage, the virus resides in a dorsal root ganglion, where it remains dormant for many years. When latent VZV be-

Table 9-4
Herpes Simplex Viral Diseases

Viral Type	Common Presentations	Infrequent Presentations
HSV-1	Oral-labial herpes	Conjunctivits, keratitis Encephalitis Herpetic whitlow Esophagitis Pneumonia Disseminated infection
HSV-2	Genital herpes	Perinatal infection Disseminated infection

From Rubin E, Gorstein F, Rubin R, et al. Rubin's Pathology, 4th ed. Philadelphia: Lippincott Williams & Wilkins, 2005, p. 371.

comes reactivated, it spreads along the sensory nerves to the peripheral nerves of sensory dermatomes, causing shingles. The skin lesions of chickenpox and shingles are indistinguishable from each other.

Herpes Simplex Virus

Herpes simplex virus (HSV) produces recurrent painful vesicular eruptions of the skin and mucous membranes. HSV-1 causes oral, facial, and ocular lesions ("above the waist"), whereas HSV-2 causes genital ulcers and perinatal infection ("below the waist"). Perinatal herpes is acquired during passage of the newborn through an infected birth canal.

As with varicella-zoster, there is a primary and latent infection. Primary HSV disease occurs at the site of inoculation, such as the oropharynx, genital mucosa, or skin. In latent infection, the virus resides in sensory neurons of affected ganglia. When reactivated, HSV travels back down the nerve to the epithelial site served by the ganglion and again infects epithelial cells. Reactivation can be caused by intense sunlight, emotional stress, febrile illness, and menstruation.

Epstein-Barr Virus

Epstein-Barr virus (EBV) is a member of the herpesvirus family. In most instances, the infection is asymptomatic, but in some persons, it is the cause of infectious mononucleosis, a disease characterized by fever, pharyngitis, lymphadenopathy, and increased circulating lymphocytes. EBV invades and replicates within the salivary glands or pharyngeal epithelium and is shed into the saliva and respiratory secretions. EBV infects B lymphocytes, which undergo polyclonal activation. Some infected B cells are transformed into immature malignant lymphocytes of Burkitt lymphoma.

- Exposure in childhood leads to immunity; in unexposed adults, EBV causes infectious mononucleosis.
- In some persons, the virus transforms pharyngeal epithelial cells, leading to nasopharyngeal carcinoma.

In infectious mononucleosis, the following pathological changes are prominent in the lymph nodes and spleen:

- The lymph nodes are enlarged; germinal centers contain frequent mitoses. The nodes contain large hyperchromatic cells with polylobular nuclei that resemble Reed-Sternberg cells.
- The spleen has hyperplasia of the red pulp.
- Liver sinusoids contain atypical lymphocytes.
- The heterophile reaction (Paul Bunnell antibodies) is positive.

Cytomegalovirus

Cytomegalovirus (CMV), another herpesvirus, is an opportunistic pathogen that infects 50% to 85% of adults in the United States. However, it usually produces an asymptomatic infection, except in immunocompromised persons. Infectious CMV can be found in urine, saliva, blood, tears, semen, and breast milk. Once infected, a person can carry the usually dormant virus for life, although an infected pregnant woman can pass the virus to her fetus, who is particularly vulnerable to the destructive effects of the virus in the brain, inner ears, eyes, liver, and bone marrow. Severe disease can cause fetal death in utero.

Microscopically, the lesions of fetal CMV disease show cellular necrosis and a characteristic cytopathic effect, consisting of marked cellular enlargement and inclusions. The giant nucleus contains a large central inclusion surrounded by a clear zone.

Human Papillomavirus

Human papillomaviruses (HPVs) are nonenveloped, double-stranded DNA viruses that are members of the papovavirus group. HPVs cause proliferative lesions of squamous epithelium, including warts, especially of the hands, feet, and genitals. Some strains are associated with squamous cell carcinoma of the female genital tract. HPVs are now believed to be the major cause of cervical cancer. Some types of HPV infection are transmitted from person to person by direct contact, and the viruses that cause genital lesions are transmitted sexually.

Bacterial Infections

Bacterial Characteristics

Bacteria are the smallest living cells, ranging in size from 0.1 to 10 μm. They are prokaryotic organisms characterized by the lack of a membrane-bound nucleus and other organelles. Basic components are three: a nuclear body, cytosol, and envelope. The nuclear body consists of a single, coiled circular molecule of double-stranded DNA with associated RNA and proteins. The Gram stain is a staining technique used to classify bacteria.

- Gram-positive bacteria retain iodine-crystal violet complexes and appear dark blue when decolorized.
- Gram-negative bacteria lose the iodine-crystal violet stain, when decolorized, and appear red with a counterstain.

Bacteria are distinguished on the basis of shape.

- Round or oval bacteria are called *cocci*, and those that grow in pairs are called *diplococci*.

- Elongate bacteria are known as *rods* or *bacilli.*
- Curved ones are termed *vibrios.*
- Spiral-shaped bacteria may be called *spirochetes.*

Bacteria can cause disease in a number of ways:

- They may secrete toxins that damage cells.
- They may disturb the function of cells without killing them.
- Gram-negative bacteria have a structural element (lipopolysaccharide) in their outer membranes, known as endotoxin. Endotoxin can activate the complement, coagulation, fibrinolysis, and bradykinin systems. It also causes the release of inflammatory mediators such as tumor necrosis factor (TNF) and interleukin-1 (IL-1). The actions of endotoxin produce shock, complement depletion, and disseminated intravascular coagulation.

Pyogenic Gram-positive Cocci

Gram-positive staphylococci and streptococci cause a number of pyogenic infections (Table 9-5).

Staphylococcus aureus

S. aureus is a gram-positive coccus that grows in clusters and is one of the most common bacterial pathogens. It normally resides on the skin. When inoculated into deeper tissues, it can cause suppurative infections. Infections commonly involve the skin, joints and bones, and heart valves but may spread to other regions, as described in the following examples:

- Skin lesions include boils, styes, and carbuncles, as well as scalded skin syndrome. The syndrome affects infants and young children and is characterized by a sunburnlike rash.
- Osteomyelitis may follow skin infections with *S. aureus.*
- Infections of burns or surgical wounds may occur in susceptible people.
- Respiratory tract infections with *S. aureus* occur in infants and young children.
- Bacterial arthritis may afflict older people.
- Septicemia may occur in patients with low resistance.
- Bacterial endocarditis is a complication of *S. aureus* septicemia.
- Toxic shock syndrome most commonly afflicts menstruating women and has been associated with the use of tampons.
- Staphylococcal food poisoning is caused by preformed *S. aureus* toxin present in contaminated food.

Coagulase-negative Staphylococci

Coagulase is an enzyme that causes plasma to clot. This enzyme is elaborated by *S. aureus* but not by the coagulase-negative staphy-

Table 9-5

Infections Caused by Gram-positive Staphylococci and Streptococci

Causative Agent	Primary Infections	Secondary Infections	Complications
Staphylococcus aureus Coagulase positive	Purulent skin lesions Abscesses	Infective endocarditis Osteomyelitis	Toxins produced may cause systemic effects: Scalded skin syndrome; Toxic shock syndrome; Food poisoning
Staphylococcus epidermidis Coagulase negative	Infects prosthetic devices	Do not produce extensive tissue necrosis	
Streptococcus pyogenes (Group A streptococcus)	Pharyngitis (strep throat) Erysipelas rash Aphthous ulcer (canker sore) Impetigo of skin Puerperal sepsis Pneumonia Cellulitis	Meningitis Subacute bacterial endocarditis Septicemia	Scarlet fever Rheumatic fever Glomerulonephritis
Streptococcus pneumoniae	Major cause of lobar pneumonia; common cause of otitis media in children	Sinusitis Meningitis	
Group B streptococcus	Leading cause of neonatal pneumonia, meningitis	Sepsis	Acquired in passage through birth canal

lococci such as *Staphylococcus epidermidis* and *Staphylococcus saprophyticus*. Coagulase-negative staphylococci are the major cause of infections associated with the use of medical devices such as intravenous catheters, prosthetic heart valves, heart pacemakers, orthopedic prostheses, cerebrospinal fluid shunts, and peritoneal catheters. *Staphylococcus epidermidis* is the most frequent cause of infections associated with medical devices, whereas *S. saprophyticus* causes 10% to 20% of acute urinary infections in young women. In contrast to infections caused by *S. aureus*, coagulase-negative staphylococcal infections do not often produce extensive local tissue necrosis or large amounts of pus.

Streptococcus pyogenes

S. pyogenes is a gram-positive coccus also known as group A streptococcus. It is one of the most frequent bacterial pathogens of humans, causing diseases of many organ systems. The diseases caused by *S. pyogenes* are in two categories:

1. Suppurative diseases, including pneumonia, occur at sites where the bacteria invade and cause tissue necrosis and an acute inflammatory response.
2. Nonsuppurative diseases occur at sites remote from the site of bacterial invasion. Two major nonsuppurative diseases are rheumatic fever (see Chapter 11) and acute poststreptococcal glomerulonephritis (see Chapter 16).

Several suppurative *S. pyogenes–caused* diseases of note follow:

- *Streptococcal pharyngitis ("strep throat")* involves an acute inflammatory response, often producing an exudate of neutrophils. *S. pyogenes* attaches to epithelial cells by binding to fibronectin on their surface. It produces a battery of enzymes, which invade and damage tissue. Specific proteins on its cell wall protect it from phagocytosis. In a few cases, streptococcal pharyngitis leads to rheumatic fever and acute poststreptococcal glomerulonephritis.
- *Scarlet fever* is characterized by a punctate red rash on the skin and mucous membranes in some suppurative *S. pyogenes* infections, most commonly pharyngitis. The erythrogenic toxin produced by the lysogenic strain of the bacterium causes the disease.
- *Erysipelas* is an erythematous swelling of the skin. The inflammatory infiltrate is composed mainly of neutrophils and is most intense around vessels and adnexa of the skin.
- Impetigo is a localized intraepidermal infection of the skin, and is caused by an *S. pyogenes* strain antigenically distinct from the one causing pharyngitis. Skin lesions begin as erythematous papules that become pustules, which eventually erode. Impetigo may sometimes lead to poststreptococcal glomerulonephritis but not to rheumatic fever.
- *Streptococcal cellulitis* is an acute spreading infection of the deeper layers of the dermis. It appears as areas of redness, warmth, and swelling.
- *Puerperal sepsis* refers to postpartum infection of the uterine cavity by *S. pyogenes*. It originates from contaminated hands of attendants at delivery and is now rare in developed countries.

Streptococcus pneumoniae

S. pneumoniae is an aerobic, encapsulated, gram-positive diplococcus. Often called pneumococcus, it causes pyogenic infections involving the lungs (pneumonia), middle ear (otitis media), sinuses (sinusitis), and meninges (meningitis). *S. pneumoniae* is a commensal organism in the oropharynx, and virtually all persons are colonized at some time. The polysaccharide capsule of *S. pneumoniae* protects it from phagocytosis. The organisms elicit an acute inflammatory response and spread to involve one or many lobes of the lung. Pneumococcus infection is often preceded by an insult (cold, influenza, tobacco smoke) that injures the protective ciliated epithelium of the airways; the affected air spaces become filled with fluid conducive to the growth of the pneumococci.

Group B Streptococci

Group B streptococci are gram-positive bacteria that grow in short chains. They are the leading cause of neonatal pneumonia, meningitis, and sepsis. Thirty percent of women carry the streptococci as part of the normal vaginal flora; most newborns acquire the organism as they pass through the birth canal. Several thousand neonatal infections occur in the U.S. each year, and about 30% of infected infants die.

Bacterial Infections of Childhood

Diphtheria

Diphtheria is an acute infection caused by *Corynebacterium diphtheriae*, an aerobic, pleomorphic, gram-positive bacterium. The disease once had a high mortality rate but is now rare in developed countries where infants are vaccinated with inactivated *C. diphtheriae* toxin (toxoid).

    C. diphtheriae spreads in respiratory droplets and oral secretions, lodging in the mucous membranes of the upper respiratory tract. There it causes damage in two ways:

1. The toxin produced by the bacterium acts on tissues throughout the body; the heart, nerves, and kidneys being most susceptible to damage. The toxin inhibits protein synthesis by inactivating an elongation factor 2; this ultimately causes the death of the cell.
2. Necrotizing upper respiratory tract lesions lead to the formation of a tough, gray membrane on the mucous membranes of the throat. This, plus inflammatory swelling in the surrounding tissues, can cause severe respiratory distress.

Pertussis (Whooping Cough)

Pertussis is a prolonged upper respiratory tract infection, characterized by debilitating coughing paroxysms. The paroxysm is followed by a long, high-pitched inspiration, the "whoop," which gives the disease its name. The causative organism is *Bordetella pertussis*, a small, gram-negative coccobacillus. *B. pertussis* causes an extensive tracheobronchitis, with necrosis of the ciliated respiratory epithelium and an acute inflammatory response. The disease has been largely eradicated in the United States through a vaccination program; however, almost 1 million deaths occur worldwide each year, particularly in infants.

Haemophilus influenzae

H. influenzae is an aerobic, pleomorphic gram-negative coccobacillus that exists in both nonencapsulated (type a) and encapsulated (type b) strains. Type b is more virulent and causes more than 95% of invasive bacteremic infections. The capsular polysaccharide of type b organisms allows them to evade phagocytosis, and bacteremic infections are common. The most severe infections occur in children younger than 6 years of age. Epiglottitis, facial cellulites, septic arthritis, and meningitis result from invasive bacteremic infections. Complications can be prevented by inoculating infants with *H. influenzae* type b vaccine.

Neisseria meningitides

N. meningitides, commonly termed meningococcus, appears as paired, bean-shaped, gram-negative cocci. It produces disseminated blood-borne infections, often accompanied by shock and profound disturbances in coagulation. Meningococci spread primarily by respiratory droplets. Between 5% and 15% of the population carries the organism in the nasopharynx as a commensal organism. Although some meningococcal diseases appear as sporadic cases, epidemic disease appears most frequently in young adults in crowded quarters such as among military recruits in barracks.

   N. meningitides attaches to nonciliated epithelium of the upper respiratory tract, and disease occurs if it spreads to the bloodstream before protective immunity can develop. Many of the systemic effects of meningococcal disease are due to the endotoxin of the outer membrane lipopolysaccharide of the bacterium. Endotoxin promotes an increase in TNF production, an activation of the complement and coagulation cascades, disseminated intravascular coagulation, fibrinolysis, and shock.

   In meningococcal meningitis, the leptomeninges and subarachnoid space are infiltrated with neutrophils and the underlying brain parenchyma is swollen and congested. Waterhouse-Friderichsen syndrome, a hemorrhagic necrosis of the adrenals, can occur rarely (3%–4% of all cases).

Sexually Transmitted Bacterial Diseases

Gonorrhea

Neisseria gonorrhoeae is an aerobic, bean-shaped, gram-negative diplococcus also termed gonococcus. It causes gonorrhea, an acute, suppurative infection of the genital tract, which can cause sterility.

Pathogenesis

N. gonorrhoeae have surface pili that form a barrier against phagocytosis by neutrophils. The pili also contain an IgA protease that facilitates attachment of the gonococci to the surface of the mucous membranes of the urethra, endocervix, and fallopian tube.

Clinical Features

- In women, gonococci cause endocervicitis, vaginitis, and salpingitis.
- In men, gonococci cause urethritis, and, sometimes, urethral stricture.
- Neonatal infections derived from the birth canal of an infected mother usually manifest as conjunctivitis. Prophylactic administration of silver nitrate to the eyes of neonates has eliminated this disease in developed countries, but it is still a major cause of blindness in much of Asia and Africa.

Chancroid

Chancroid is an acute, sexually transmitted infection caused by *Haemophilus ducreyi*, a small, gram-negative bacillus that appears in tissue as clusters or chains of parallel bacilli. The disease is characterized by painful genital ulcerations and associated lymphadenopathy.

Granuloma Inguinale

Granuloma inguinale is a sexually transmitted, chronic superficial ulceration of the genitalia and the inguinal and perianal regions. It is caused by *Calymmatobacterium granulomatis*, a small, encapsulated, nonmotile, gram-negative bacillus. The disease is common in tropical and subtropical areas.

Enteropathic Bacterial Infections
Escherichia coli

E. coli, although discussed here as contributing to enteropathic infections, also causes more than 90% of all urinary tract infections. In addition, it is a major opportunistic pathogen, frequently producing pneumonia and sepsis in immunocompromised hosts, and meningitis and sepsis in newborns.

E. coli organisms are a group of antigenically diverse, aerobic (facultatively anaerobic), gram-negative bacteria. Most strains are intestinal commensals, well adapted to growth in the human colon without causing harm. However, *E. coli* can do damage when it gains access to other body sites, such as the urinary tract, meninges, or peritoneum.

E. coli Diarrhea

Strains of *E. coli* that produce diarrhea possess specialized virulence properties, usually plasmid-borne, which confer the capacity to cause intestinal disease. There are four distinct strains of *E. coli* that cause diarrhea, all acquired by ingestion of contaminated food or water:

1. Enterotoxigenic *E. coli* is a major cause of diarrhea in poor tropical areas; it also causes "traveler's diarrhea" among visitors to the region. The strain produces diarrhea by elaborating enterotoxins that cause secretory dysfunction of the small intestine. It produces no macroscopic or microscopic damage to the intestine, although in severe cases, fluid and electrolyte loss can cause extreme dehydration.
2. Enteropathogenic *E. coli* is a major cause of diarrhea in poor tropical areas, especially in infants and young children.
3. Enterohemorrhagic *E. coli* causes a bloody diarrhea. It produces an enterotoxin almost identical to Shiga toxin that destroys the epithelial cells of the colon.
4. Enteroinvasive *E. coli* causes a food-borne dysentery, which is clinically and pathologically indistinguishable from that caused by *Shigella*. It invades and destroys mucosal cells of the distal ileum and colon.

E. coli Urinary Tract Infection

Urinary tract infections with *E. coli* are most common in persons who have structural or functional abnormalities of the urinary tract. These infections are usually caused by fecal contamination of the perineum and periurethral areas. The infection produces an acute inflammatory infiltrate at the site of infection, usually the bladder mucosa. If the infection ascends to the kidney, pyelonephritis ensues, with dilated and congested submucosal blood vessels with a neutrophilic infiltrate.

E. coli Pneumonia

Pneumonias caused by enteric gram-negative bacteria are opportunistic infections occurring in debilitated persons because of decreased gag and cough reflexes, abnormal neutrophil chemotaxis, or injured respiratory epithelium. These pneumonias result from the proliferation of aspirated organisms in the terminal airways. Multifocal areas of consolidation occur, and bronchioles and alveoli are filled with proteinaceous fluid, fibrin, neutrophils, and macrophages.

E. coli Sepsis (Gram-negative Sepsis)

In healthy persons, macrophages and neutrophils usually phagocytose any stray organisms that gain access to the bloodstream.

However, in persons with predisposing conditions, such as neutropenia, pyelonephritis, or cirrhosis, *E. coli* sepsis may develop. The presence of *E. coli* in the bloodstream causes septic shock through the release of TNF, whose release from macrophages is stimulated by bacterial endotoxin.

Neonatal *E. coli* Meningitis and Sepsis

E. coli and group B streptococci are the primary causes of meningitis and sepsis in the first month after birth. Both types of bacteria colonize the vagina, and the newborn acquires the organisms on passage through the birth canal. The pathology of *E. coli* meningitis is identical to that of other bacterial meningitides. Antibiotic treatment is often effective; however, the mortality rate still ranges between 15% and 50%.

Salmonella Enterocolitis and Typhoid Fever

The bacterial genus *Salmonella* comprises over 1,500 antigenically distinct but biochemically and genetically related gram-negative rods, which cause two important human intestinal diseases: *Salmonella* enterocolitis and typhoid fever.

Salmonella enterocolitis is an acute self-limited gastrointestinal illness that is acquired by ingestion of food contaminated with nontyphoidal *Salmonella* strains. The bacteria then proliferate in the small intestine, invade enterocytes in the ileum and colon, and make several toxins that cause dysfunction of the enterocytes. Salmonella food poisoning manifests as a diarrhea beginning 12 to 48 hours after ingestion of contaminated food. This contrasts with staphylococcal food poisoning, which is caused by preformed toxin and begins 1 to 6 hours after ingestion of toxin-contaminated food.

Typhoid fever is an acute systemic illness caused by infection by *Salmonella typhi*. Paratyphoid fever is a clinically similar but milder disease that results from infection with other species of *Salmonella*, including *S. paratyphi*. The term enteric fever includes both typhoid and paratyphoid fever.

Typhoid fever is acquired from convalescing patients or from chronic carriers. Carriers tend to be older women with gallstones or biliary scarring, in whom *S. typhi* colonizes the gallbladder or biliary tree. It is spread through ingestion of contaminated water and food.

S. typhi invade the small bowel where they are engulfed by macrophages; however, they evade them and are not killed. The bacteria multiply within the macrophages, then spread to regional lymph nodes and throughout the body to infect the bone marrow, liver, and spleen. The infection of macrophages stimulates the production of IL-1 and TNF, thereby causing the prolonged fever, malaise, and wasting characteristics of typhoid fever. The intestinal mucosa may become necrotic, producing ulcers that may hemorrhage or perforate into the peritoneal cavity, causing infectious peritonitis.

Treatment of typhoid fever entails antibiotics and supportive care; treatment within 3 days of onset of fever is generally curative.

Shigellosis

Shigellosis is an acute bacterial dysentery characterized by a necrotizing infection of the distal small bowel and colon. It is caused by one of four species of *Shigella*, which are aerobic, gram-negative rods. Of these species, *S. dysenteriae* is the most virulent. *Shigella* organisms are among the most virulent enteropathogens known. Disease is produced by ingestion of as few as 10 to 100 organisms, and there are few asymptomatic carriers. *Shigella* is spread by the fecal–oral route.

Replicating shigellae kill infected enterocytes and spread into the lamina propria. Shigellae produce a potent exotoxin, Shiga toxin, which inhibits protein synthesis. By destroying colonic enterocytes, the toxin causes production of a watery diarrhea by interfering with fluid absorption in the colon.

Treatment with antibiotics is effective, and regeneration and healing of infected colonic epithelium is rapid.

Cholera

Cholera is a severe diarrheal illness caused by the enterotoxin of *Vibrio cholerae*, an aerobic, curved gram-negative rod. The organism proliferates in the lumen of the small intestine and causes profuse, watery diarrhea, rapid dehydration, and (if fluids are not restored) shock and death within 24 hours of the onset of symptoms. Cholera is epidemic enteritis, usually acquired from contaminated water.

V. cholerae organisms themselves do not invade the mucosa of the small intestine, but instead cause diarrhea by the elaboration of the potent cholera toxin. This toxin contains a subunit that catalyzes the chemical modification of a G protein within the enterocyte, causing the continuous activation of adenyl cyclase. The resulting excessive increase in intracellular cAMP results in the massive secretion of electrolytes and water into the intestinal lumen.

Fluid and electrolyte loss can advance to shock and death within hours if fluid volume is not replaced. Replacement of lost salts and water can be accomplished by oral rehydration with preparations of salt, glucose, and water. Cholera subsides in 3 to 6 days, and infection confers long-term immunity.

Campylobacter jejuni

Campylobacter jejuni is a microaerophilic, curved gram-negative rod. The most common cause of bacterial diarrhea in the developed world, it is acquired through contaminated food or water. The bacteria inhabit the gastrointestinal tracts of cows, chickens, sheep, and dogs, which constitute an animal reservoir for infection. Ingested *C. jejuni* multiply in the alkaline environment of the duodenum and produce several toxic proteins, thus causing a superficial enterocolitis of the ileum and colon. The colon crypts often fill with neutrophils, forming so-called crypt abscesses. These pathological changes resolve in 7 to 14 days.

Yersinia Infections

Yersinia enterocolitica and *Yersinia pseudotuberculosis* are gram-negative coccoid or rod-shaped bacteria. These facultative anaerobes are found in the feces of wild and domestic animals, including rodents, sheep, cattle, dogs, cats, and horses. Both organisms have been isolated from drinking water and milk, and tend to localize in lymph nodes and Peyer patches. Fever, painful diarrhea, and abdominal pain may lead to an erroneous diagnosis of appendicitis.

Pulmonary Infections with Gram-negative Bacteria

Klebsiella and *Enterobacter*

Both of these short, encapsulated gram-negative bacilli are responsible for causing hospital-acquired (nosocomial) pneumonia. Debilitated and immunosuppressed patients are especially susceptible. The bacilli are inhaled and multiply within alveoli, causing formation of a mucoid alveolar exudate dominated by macrophages, fibrin, and edema fluid.

Legionnaires Disease (Legionellosis)

Legionella is a genus of gram-negative bacilli that includes the species *L. pneumophila* that causes Legionnaires disease, an acute, sometimes fatal pneumonia. The disease is a noncontagious environmental hazard, caused by the inhalation of aerosols from contaminated cooling towers, water heaters, humidifiers, and evaporative condensers. In the alveoli, *Legionella* are phagocytosed by macrophages but block the fusion of the phagosome with the hydrolytic enzyme-containing lysosome. The bacilli then multiply and are released to infect more macrophages. Affected alveoli and bronchioles become filled with an exudate of fluid, fibrin, neutrophils, and macrophages. Alveolar walls become fibrotic, and some are destroyed. When immunity to the bacilli develops, macrophages are activated and cease to support the intracellular growth of the organisms. With resolution of the pneumonia, the lungs heal with little permanent damage.

Pseudomonas aeruginosa

P. aeruginosa is a ubiquitous aerobic, gram-negative rod found in soil and water. It is a major opportunistic pathogen that can cause disease in the hospital environment, where it is associated with pneumonia, wound infections, and urinary tract disease. Cystic fibrosis, diabetes, and neutropenia are some disorders that predispose to infection with *P. aeruginosa*. Antibiotic use tends to select for *P. aeruginosa* infection, because the organism is resistant to most antibiotics. This is believed to be due to its rapid efflux pumps, which extrude antibiotics.

P. aeruginosa can produce a slime layer that resists phagocytosis. Infection with *P. aeruginosa* is usually accompanied by a "fruity" odor. The bacillus elaborates an array of proteins that allow it to attach to, invade, and destroy host tissues, while avoiding host inflammatory and immune defenses.

P. aeruginosa often invades small vessels, producing vascular thrombosis and hemorrhagic necrosis, mainly in the lungs and skin. Blood vessel invasion predisposes to sepsis and leads to the development of multiple nodular lesions in the lung.

Melioidosis

Melioidosis (Rangoon beggars disease) is an uncommon disease caused by *Pseudomonas pseudomallei*, a small gram-negative bacillus in the soil and surface water of Southeast Asia and other tropical areas. During the conflict in Vietnam, several hundred servicemen acquired melioidosis. The skin is the usual portal of entry. Acute melioidosis is a pulmonary infection ranging from a mild tracheobronchitis to a severe pneumonia.

- Chronic melioidosis is a persistent localized infection causing abscesses in many organs. It may lie dormant for months or years, only to appear suddenly; hence the colloquial name "Vietnamese time bomb."

Clostridial Diseases

Clostridia are gram-positive, spore-forming bacilli that are obligate anaerobes. Anaerobic conditions promote vegetative division, whereas aerobic conditions lead to spore formation. Spores pass in animal feces and contaminate soil. Many Clostridium species produce a variety of toxins; the main species that cause human disease follow:

- *Clostridium perfringens*, which causes food poisoning, necrotizing enteritis, and gas gangrene. Clostridial food poisoning is self-limited. A more serious consequence of *C. perfringens* infection is encountered in children in New Guinea who have eaten contaminated roast pig and develop a necrotizing enteritis. *C. perfringens* may also contaminate wounds, causing gas gangrene. The bacterium elaborates a myotoxin that destroys cell membranes, alters capillary permeability, and causes necrosis of previously healthy skeletal muscle.

- *Clostridium tetani*, which causes tetanus (lockjaw). Spores of *C. tetani* are in soil and enter the site of an accidental wound. Necrotic tissue at the wound site causes spores to vegetate. A potent neurotoxin is produced, which permits unopposed neural stimulation and sustained contraction of skeletal muscle (tetany)
- *Clostridium botulinum*, which causes botulism. *C. botulinum* contaminates improperly canned food and produces a potent neurotoxin. The neurotoxin inhibits the release of acetylcholine, resulting in descending paralysis of cranial nerves, trunk, and limbs, with eventual respiratory paralysis and death.
- *Clostridium difficile*, which can overgrow other bacteria in the gut when antibiotics are given, produces an exotoxin that causes pseudomembranous colitis. The bacterium does not invade the colonic mucosa but rather produces two exotoxins, which cause fluid secretion and destroy enterocytes. An inflammatory exudate called a pseudomembrane often forms over affected areas of the colon.

Bacteria with Animal Reservoirs or Insect Vectors

Brucellosis

Brucellosis is a zootic (disease of animals that can be transmitted to humans). Brucella are small, aerobic, gram-negative rods that in humans mainly infect monocytes/macrophages. Four *Brucella* species cause disease, and each has its own animal reservoir. Almost every type of domesticated animal is affected. Elimination of infected animals and vaccination of herds have reduced the incidence in the United States.

Humans acquire the bacteria by contact with infected tissue, ingestion of contaminated meat or milk, or inhalation of contaminated aerosols. Human brucellosis may be an acute systemic disease or a chronic infection characterized by waxing and waning fevers, sometimes lasting over a period of weeks to months when untreated, which is why it is sometimes called undulant fever. The bacteria multiply in, and cause hyperplasia of, macrophages. Lymphadenopathy and hepatosplenomegaly may ensue.

Plague

Yersinia pestis, a short, gram-negative rod found in animals such as wild rodents, causes plague, an often fatal bacteremic infection. Infected fleas transmit the bacterium to humans.

Spread from rats to people, the plague of the mid-14th century, known as the "Black Death," killed more than one fourth of the European population. Infected patients often develop necrotic, hemorrhagic skin lesions, hence the name "black death." Plague still occurs sporadically in the United States. There are three clinical presentations:

- Bubonic plague: *Y. pestis* replicate intracellularly in macrophages and multiply in regional lymph nodes producing hemorrhagic necrosis in enlarged, painful regional lymph nodes (buboes).
- Septicemic plague: Patients die of overwhelming growth of the bacteria in the bloodstream.
- Pneumonic plague: Pneumonic spread occurs when organisms reach lung alveoli and are expelled by coughing. Affected portions of the lungs show hemorrhagic necrosis.

Tetracycline combined with streptomycin is the recommended therapy.

Tularemia

Tularemia is caused by *Francisella tularensis*, a small, gram-negative coccobacillus. It is an acute, febrile granulomatous disease acquired mainly from contact with infected rabbits or from bites of infected ticks. About 250 cases occur annually in the United States. Lesions occur at the site of inoculation and in the lymph nodes, spleen, liver, bone marrow, lungs, heart, and kidneys. The initial skin lesion is an exudative, pyogenic ulcer. Later, disseminated lesions undergo a granulomatous reaction resembling the lesions of tuberculosis.

Anthrax

Anthrax is a necrotizing disease caused by *Bacillus anthracis*, which is a large, spore-forming, gram-positive rod. It is an infectious disease of domestic animals that can be transmitted to humans. Anthrax spores can survive in the soil for long periods. Humans are infected when spores enter the body through breaks in the skin, by inhalation, or by ingestion. The spores of *B. anthracis* germinate in the human body to yield vegetative bacteria that multiply and release a potent necrotizing toxin.

In most cases of cutaneous anthrax, the infection remains localized, and the organism is eventually eliminated as a result of the host's immunological response. If the infection disseminates, as occurs when the organisms are inhaled or digested, the resulting widespread tissue destruction is usually fatal.

Some nations have experimented with the use of anthrax as an agent of biological warfare. International convention now bans such use.

Listeriosis

Listeriosis is a systemic infection caused by *Listeria monocytogenes*, a small, motile, gram-positive coccobacillus. Listeriosis affects wild and domestic animals, and most human disease results from the ingestion of contaminated dairy products.

L. monocytogenes evades antibacterial defense mechanisms because of its unusual life cycle. After phagocytosis, the organism escapes from the host's phagolysosome into the cytoplasm by disrupting the phagolysosome membrane with listeriolysin O, an exotoxin. It then replicates and usurps the contractile elements of the host cell to form and enter elongated protrusions, which are then engulfed by adjacent cells. In this way, *Listeria* spreads from one cell to another without exposure to the hostile extracellular host environment.

Listeria infections fall into one of two groups:

1. Listeriosis of pregnancy involves maternal infection during pregnancy, leading to abortion, premature delivery, or neonatal infection.
2. Septicemic listeriosis is a severe febrile illness most common in immunodeficient patients. It may lead to shock and disseminated intravascular coagulation.

Cat-scratch Disease

This self-limited granulomatous lymphadenitis is usually caused by *Bartonella henselae*, a small, gram-negative rod. The disease is transmitted by the scratch or bite of a cat and is characterized by a suppurative and granulomatous lymphadenitis. Infections are more common in children than in adults.

Glanders

Glanders, an infection of horses and other equines that is only rarely transmitted to humans, is caused by *Pseudomonas mallei*, a small, gram-negative, nonmotile bacillus. Humans contract the disease by contact with infected animals or by inhalation of contaminated aerosols.

- Acute glanders is characterized by bacteremia and is almost always fatal.
- Chronic glanders features draining skin abscesses, lymphadenopathy, and hepatosplenomegaly. Mortality exceeds 50%.

Bartonellosis

This disease is an infection by *Bartonella bacilliformis*, a small, multiflagellated, gram-negative coccobacillus. It occurs only in Peru, Ecuador, and Colombia, and it is transmitted by the bite of a sandfly. It Bartonellosis causes acute anemia and chronic skin disease.

Infections Caused by Branching Filamentous Organisms

Actinomycosis

Actinomycosis is a slowly progressive, suppurative, fibrosing infection involving the jaw, thorax, or abdomen. The disease is caused by a number of anaerobic and microaerophilic bacteria called *Actinomyces*, the most common being *Actinomyces israelii*. These organisms are branching, filamentous, gram-positive rods that live in the human body as saprophytes, usually without producing disease. Colonies of actinomycoses grow large enough to be visible as hard, yellow grains known as "sulfur granules."

To cause disease, *Actinomyces* must be inoculated into an anaerobic environment. This can occur following dental extraction, aspiration of organisms contaminating dental debris, traumatic or surgical disruption of the bowel, or prolonged use of intrauterine devices. The disease is characterized by abscesses and sinus tracts that burrow across normal tissue into adjacent regions of the body.

Nocardiosis

Nocardiosis is a suppurative infection of the lung that often spreads to the brain and skin. The disease is usually caused by *Nocardia asteroides*. Nocardia are aerobic, gram-positive, filamentous, branching bacteria. They are weakly acid-fast, a characteristic used to distinguish them from the morphologically similar actinomyces. With the Gram stain, they appear as beaded, filamentous, gram-positive rods. They can also be demonstrated by silver impregnation.

Nocardiosis is most common in persons with impaired immunity and debilitating diseases. Nocardia produce pulmonary abscesses that are frequently multiple and confluent. The abscesses are filled with neutrophils, necrotic debris, and scattered organisms.

Spirochetal Infections

Spirochetes are long, spiral bacteria, some too thin to be visible by routine microscopy. Specialized techniques, such as darkfield microscopy, or silver impregnation are needed for their demonstration. Three genera of spirochetes, *Treponema, Borrelia*, and *Leptospira*, cause human disease (Table 9-6).

Syphilis

Syphilis (lues) is a chronic, systemic infection caused by *Treponema pallidum*. It is a worldwide disease transmitted almost exclusively by sexual contact. It can also be passed from an infected mother to her fetus. The organisms reproduce at the site of inoculation, pass to regional lymph nodes, enter the systemic circulation, and are disseminated throughout the body. Chronic infection and inflammation cause tissue destruction, sometimes for decades. The course of syphilis is divided into three stages (Fig. 9-1).

Table 9-6
Spirochete Infections

Disease	Organism	Clinical Manifestations	Distribution	Mode of Transmission
Treponemes				
Syphilis	*Treponema pallidum*	See text	Common worldwide	Sexual contact, congenital
Bejel	*T. endemicum (T. pallidum, subspecies endemicum)*	Mucosal, skin, and bone lesions	Middle East	Mouth-to mouth contact
Yaws	*T. pertenue (T. pallidum, subspecies pertenue)*	Skin and bone	Tropics	Skin-to-skin contact
Pinta	*T. carateum*	Skin lesions	Latin America	Skin-to-skin contact
Borrelia				
Lyme disease	*Borrelia burgdorferi*	See text	North America, Europe, Russia, Asia, Africa, Australia	Tick bite
Relapsing fever	*B. recurrentis* and related species	Relapsing flulike illness	Worldwide	Tick bite, louse bite
Leptospira				
Leptospiro- sis	*Leptospira interrogans*	Flulike illness, meningitis	Worldwide	Contact with animal urine

From Rubin E, Gorstein F, Rubin R, et al. Rubin's Pathology, 4th ed. Philadelphia: Lippincott Williams & Wilkins, 2005, p. 407.

Primary Syphilis

The classic lesion of primary syphilis is the chancre, a painless ulcer, which lasts 3 to 12 weeks. It appears at the site of *T. pallidum* inoculation, usually the penis, vulva, anus, or mouth. Chancres display a characteristic "luetic vasculitis" in which the walls of vessels in the epidermis around the lesion are thickened by lymphocytes and fibrous tissue.

Secondary Syphilis

Secondary syphilis features dissemination of spirochetes. It is characterized by a maculopapular rash, especially of the palms and

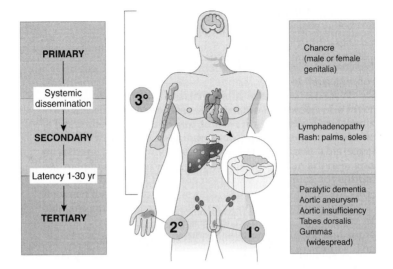

F I G U R E   9-1
Clinical characteristics of the various stages of syphilis. (From Rubin E, Gorstein F, Rubin R, et al. Rubin's Pathology, 4th ed. Philadelphia: Lippincott Williams & Wilkins, 2005, p. 408.)

soles, which may be accompanied by whitish plaques on the vulva or scrotum. Lesions of the mucous membranes, lymph nodes, meninges, stomach, and liver also occur.

Tertiary Syphilis

Tertiary syphilis causes neurological and vascular diseases. An asymptomatic latent period, sometimes lasting for years, is followed by lesions of tertiary syphilis in one third of untreated persons. Focal ischemic necrosis secondary to obliterative endoarteritis is the underlying mechanism for processes associated with tertiary syphilis. Tertiary syphilitic symptoms include the following:

- Syphilitic aortitis with damage to the ascending aorta (*tree-bark appearance* of the intima) and aneurysm formation.
- Neurosyphilis with damage to the meninges (*meningovascular syphilis*), spinal cord (*tabes dorsalis*), and cerebral cortex (*general paresis*).
- Gumma (granulomatous lesions with central necrosis, epithelioid macrophages, and peripheral fibrous tissue) can appear in any organ or tissue and are the hallmark of *benign tertiary syphilis*. They apparently cause no damage.

Congenital Syphilis

Fetal infection acquired in utero from an infected mother, can cause stillbirth or neonatal illness. The lesions of congenital syphilis are identical to those of adult disease.

Nonvenereal Treponematoses

Treponemes indistinguishable from *T. pallidum* cause chronic, non-venereal diseases in tropical and subtropical countries. Like syphilis, they (a) result from inoculation into mucocutaneous surfaces, and (b) pass through defined clinical stages: (a) primary lesion, (b) secondary skin eruptions, (c) a latent period, and (d) a tertiary late stage.

Yaws

Yaws is caused by *T. pertenue*. The primary lesion appears as a "mother yaw," a red papilloma on the skin. The secondary stage brings smaller skin yaws. A latent period is followed by late-stage gummas of the skin.

Bejel

Bejel (also known as "endemic syphilis") is caused by *T. pallidum endemicum*. It is transmitted by nonvenereal routes such as from mouth to mouth or from utensils to mouth. Primary lesions are rare, but secondary lesions appear in the mouth and are identical to mucosal lesions of syphilis.

Pinta

Pinta is caused by *T. carateum* and is characterized by variously colored spots on the skin. Lesions of the three stages of pinta are limited to the skin.

Lyme Disease

Lyme disease is a chronic systemic infection that begins with a characteristic skin lesion and later manifests as cardiac, neurological, or joint disturbances. It is caused by *Borrelia burgdorferi*, a large, microaerophilic spirochete, which is transmitted from its animal reservoir (mainly mice and deer) to humans by the bite of the tiny *Ixodes* tick.

Lyme disease has become the most common tick-borne illness in the United States. It was first described in patients from Lyme, Connecticut, but was later recognized in many other areas. Like other spirochetal diseases, Lyme disease occurs in stages:

- Stage 1: At the site of the tick bite, a "bulls-eye" expanding papule with a red rim and a central clear area develops (called erythema chronicum migrans).

- Stage 2: Migratory musculoskeletal pains develop, along with swollen lymph glands, and cardiac and neurological abnormalities. Meningitis and facial palsy occur in 15% of patients.
- Stage 3: This may begin months to years after the tick bite and is manifested by joint, skin, and neurological abnormalities. Arthritis of the large joints, especially the knee, develops in over half of infected persons. The histopathological changes in the joints are indistinguishable from those of rheumatoid arthritis, with villous hypertrophy and a conspicuous mononuclear infiltrate in the subsynovial lining area.

Leptospirosis

Leptospirosis is an infection with spirochetes of the genus *Leptospira*. It is usually a mild, self-limited febrile disease; however, in persons with more severe infections, hepatic and renal failure may prove fatal. The disease affects animals and humans worldwide, but is most common in the tropics. Between 30 and 100 cases of leptospirosis occur annually in the United States.

Leptospires penetrate the skin following contact with infected rats, contaminated water, or mud. In severe cases, the disease is biphasic:

- *Leptospiremic phase*: The presence of leptospires in the blood and cerebrospinal fluid cause symptoms of fever and myalgias.
- *Immune phase*: IgM antibodies are produced and meningeal irritation becomes apparent. In more severe cases, jaundice, hepatic and renal failure, hemorrhages, and shock may develop. This severe form has been referred to as *Weil disease*.

Relapsing Fever

Relapsing fever is an acute febrile, septicemic illness caused by spirochetes of the genus *Borrelia*. There are two main types:

- *Epidemic relapsing fever* is caused by *B. recurrentis* and is transmitted by the bite of an infected louse. Infection occurs when a feeding infected louse is crushed on the skin, liberating the *Borrelia*. Louse-borne relapsing fever is seen in Ethiopia, Sudan, and the South American Andes.
- *Endemic relapsing fever* is caused by a number of *Borrelia* species and is transmitted from rodents to humans by the bite of an infected tick. Tick-borne relapsing fever occurs sporadically worldwide.

Both types of diseases are characterized by an initial week of fever that ends abruptly, only to begin again a week later; hence the name, relapsing fever. During the afebrile period, spirochetes disappear from the blood and change their antigenic coats. In each relapse, the symptoms are milder. In more severe infections, the spleen exhibits military microabscesses, and the liver exhibits necrotic areas and sinusoids infiltrated with spirochetes.

Chlamydial Infections

Chlamydiae are obligate intracellular parasitic bacteria that must use the metabolic machinery of a host cell to reproduce. Chlamydiae exist in two forms, the infectious *elementary body*, which can survive extracellularly and which attaches to, and is endocytosed by, the host. When inside, the organisms transform into the metabolically active, *reticulate body*, which can now divide repeatedly, forming many daughter elementary bodies. It is the reticulate form that kills the host cell, releasing necrotic inflammatory debris that further damages infected tissue.

Chlamydial infections are widespread in birds and mammals. Three species of chlamydiae cause human infection: (a) *C. trachomatis*, (b) *C. psittaci*, and (c) *C. pneumoniae*.

Chlamydia trachomatis Infections

A variety of strains of *C. trachomatis* cause three distinct types of disease: (a) genital and neonatal, (b) lymphogranuloma venereum, and (c) trachoma.

Genital and Neonatal C. trachomatis Infections

C. trachomatis strains D through K cause a genital epithelial infection that is now the most common sexually transmitted disease in North America. Early disease may be asymptomatic but later may involve the following:

- Men: urethritis, epididymitis, and proctitis. There may be a purulent penile discharge associated with dysuria.
- Women: cervicitis, endometritis, salpingitis, and pelvic inflammatory disease. There may be a mucopurulent drainage from the cervical os.
- Neonates: conjunctivitis and pneumonia caused by perinatal transmission). The conjunctival epithelium often contains characteristic vacuolated cytoplasmic inclusions (inclusion conjunctivitis).

Lymphogranuloma Venereum

Lymphogranuloma venereum is a sexually transmitted disease that begins as a genital ulcer, and progresses to a local necrotizing lymphadenitis. The intense inflammatory process can result in severe scarring. It is caused by *C. trachomatis* strains L1 through L3.

Trachoma

Trachoma is a chronic infection of the conjunctiva that progressively scars the conjunctiva and cornea. Secondary bacterial infections and corneal ulcerations are common. *C. trachomatis* strains A, B, Ba, and C cause the disease. The disease is a major problem in parts of Africa, India, and the Middle East. In endemic areas, infection is acquired early in childhood, becomes chronic, and eventually progresses to blindness.

Psittacosis (Ornithosis)

Psittacosis is a self-limited pneumonia transmitted to humans from infected birds. The causative agent is *C. psittaci*. The disease is known both as psittacosis (association with parrots) or ornithosis (association with birds in general). Fewer than 50 cases of psittacosis are reported annually in the United States.

C. *psittaci* reproduces in alveolar lining cells and destroys them, resulting in an inflammatory response in the lung. Type II pneumocytes appear hyperplastic with cytoplasmic inclusions. In severe disease, *C. psittaci* can spread to produce foci of necrosis in liver and spleen.

Chlamydia pneumoniae

Chlamydia pneumoniae is another member of the Chlamydia family causing pneumonia. The respiratory tract infection is milder than that caused by C. psittaci, and is spread from person to person rather than from birds.

Rickettsial Infections

Rickettsiae are small, gram-negative bacteria that cannot replicate outside a host. They live in animals and are transmitted by bloodsucking arthropods such as fleas, lice and ticks. Humans are accidental hosts for most species of *Rickettsia*; human infections result from insect bites. The human target cell for all rickettsiae is the endothelial cell of capillaries and other small blood vessels. Several species of *Rickettsia* cause different human diseases, which are traditionally divided into the "spotted fever group" and the "typhus group" (Table 9-7).

Rocky Mountain Spotted Fever

Rocky Mountain spotted fever (RMSF) is an acute, potentially fatal, systemic vasculitis. The causative agent, *Rickettsia rickettsii*, is transmitted to humans by tick bites. The name of the disease is misleading, because cases in the Rocky Mountain region are rare; most

Table 9-7

Rickettsial Infections

Disease	Organism	Distribution	Transmission
Spotted fever group			
Rocky Mountain spotted fever	*Rickettsia rickettsii*	Americas	Ticks
Queensland tick fever	*R. australis*	Australia	Ticks
Boutonneuse fever, Kenya tick fever	*R. conorii*	Mediterranean, Africa, India	Ticks
Siberian tick fever	*R. sibirica*	Siberia, Mongolia	Ticks
Rickettsialpox	*R. akari*	United States, Russia, Central Asia, Korea, Africa	Mites
Typhus group			
Louse-borne typhus (epidemic typhus)	*R. prowazekii*	Latin America, Africa, Asia	Lice
Murine typhus (endemic typhus)	*R. typhi*	Worldwide	Fleas
Scrub typhus	*R. tsutsugamushi*	South Pacific, Asia	Mites
Q fever	*Coxiella brunetti*	Worldwide	Inhalation

From Rubin E, Gorstein F, Rubin R, et al. Rubin's Pathology, 4th ed. Philadelphia: Lippincott Williams & Wilkins, 2005, p. 417.

U.S. cases extend from the eastern seaboard westward to Texas, Oklahoma, and Kansas.

In RMSF, inflammatory damage to blood vessels produces a characteristic rash. Necrosis and reactive hyperplasia of vascular endothelium are often associated with thrombosis of smaller vessels. Cutaneous lesions on palms and soles are a distinctive feature of the disease. Extensive damage to vessel walls causes fluid loss, which can lead to shock.

Epidemic (Louse-borne) Typhus

Epidemic typhus is a severe systemic vasculitis, caused by *Rickettsia prowazekii*, an organism that has a human-louse-human life cycle.

A louse taking a blood meal from an infected human becomes infected, and then deposits infected feces on the skin of the next victim. The disease last occurred in the United States. in 1921, although it is widely distributed in some regions of Africa, Asia, and Latin America. The pathological changes are similar to those of RMSF and other rickettsial diseases.

Endemic (Murine) Typhus

Endemic typhus is similar to epidemic typhus but tends to be a milder disease. Humans are infected with *Rickettsia typhi* by interrupting the rat-flea-rat cycle.

Scrub Typhus

Scrub typhus (Tsutsugamushi fever) is an acute, febrile illness of humans caused by *Rickettsia tsutsugamushi*. Rodents are the natural mammalian reservoir. From rats, the organism is passed to trombiculid mites (chiggers). Infected chigger larvae can attach to humans and inoculate the skin. Scrub typhus is found in eastern and southern Asia, Japan, and the South Pacific. Endemic infection does not occur in the western world.

Q Fever

Q fever is a self-limited infection, first reported in Queensland, Australia, in 1935. It is caused by *Coxiella burnetii*, a small, pleomorphic coccobacillus. *Coxiella* is sometimes classified as a rickettsia, so Q fever is listed among the rickettsial diseases. Humans acquire Q fever by exposure to infected animals or by inhalation of contaminated barnyard dust. Lungs and liver are the organs most prominently involved. Lungs show areas of consolidation, and multiple microscopic granulomas appear in the liver. The disease usually resolves in 2 to 14 days.

Mycoplasmal Infections

Mycoplasma are the smallest self-reproducing prokaryotes. They are also called pleuropneumonialike organisms. They lack a true cell wall, and are gram-negative.

Numerous *Mycoplasma* species are known to inhabit the human body, but only three are pathogenic: *M. pneumoniae*, *M. hominis*, and *Ureaplasma urealyticum*. The diseases associated with these organisms are shown in Table 9-8. *M. pneumoniae* causes 15% to 20% of all pneumonias, but the infection is a mild "walking pneumonia," a self-limited lower respiratory tract infection.

Table 9-8

Mycoplasmal Infections

Organism	Disease
Mycoplasma pneumoniae	Tracheobronchitis Pneumonia Pharyngitis Otitis media
Ureaplasma urealyticum	Urethritis Chorioamnionitis Postpartum fever
Mycoplasma hominis	Postpartum fever

From Rubin E, Gorstein F, Rubin R, et al. Rubin's Pathology, 4th ed.
Philadelphia: Lippincott Williams & Wilkins, 2005, p. 420.

Mycobacteria

Mycobacteria are slender rod-shaped aerobic bacteria. The high lipid content of the cell wall make them "acid fast." The two primary mycobacterial pathogens, *Mycobacterium tuberculosis* and *M. leprae*, exclusively infect humans.

Tuberculosis

Tuberculosis is a chronic, communicable disease in which the lungs are the prime target, although any organ may be infected. The disease is caused principally by *M. tuberculosis hominis*. Alternatively, it can be caused by *M. tuberculosis bovis*, which is acquired by the ingestion of infected milk. *M. tuberculosis* is a slender, beaded bacillus that is transmitted from human to human by aerosol droplets.

Tuberculosis is one of the most important bacterial diseases in humans, killing approximately 3 million people each year. In the United States, the annual incidence is 12 per 100,000; the risk of infection is high for HIV-infected persons, malnourished persons, and immigrants from regions in the world where the disease is endemic. Africans, Native Americans, and Eskimos are especially susceptible. Types of tuberculosis include the following:

- *Primary tuberculosis* occurs on first exposure to the organism. Mycobacteria are deposited in lung alveoli and are phagocytosed by alveolar macrophages. The bacilli resist killing by blocking the fusion of the phagosome with the lysosome; they then multiply within the lysosomes of the macrophages.

- ➤ In more than 90% of normal adults, tuberculous infection is self-limited. An immunologically competent host will contain the infection in two ways: (a) sensitized helper T cells secrete γ interferon, which activates the macrophages to kill the mycobacteria, and (b) sensitized killer T cells kill the infected macrophages. If some infected macrophages persist, they are surrounded by fibrous tissue and success-fully contained. When the number of organisms is high, a hypersensitivity reaction produces tissue necrosis with a characteristic caseous consistency.
  - ➤ The lung lesion of primary tuberculous infection is known as the *Ghon focus*—a small area of inflammatory consolida-tion.

- *Progressive primary tuberculosis:* In immunologically incompe-tent hosts, granulomas are poorly formed and infection pro-gresses to regional lymph nodes or disseminates to multiple sites.
- *Miliary tuberculosis:* Infection occurs at disseminated sites.
- *Secondary (cavitary) tuberculosis:* This results from the prolifera-tion of *M. tuberculosis* in a person who has been previously infected.

  - ➤ The source of bacteria is usually from organisms erupting from old granulomas. The ensuing response leads to pro-duction of tuberculous cavities, which contain caseous ma-terial and are teeming with mycobacteria.
  - ➤ The bacteria may remain confined to the lung, or they may spread to other organs. Untreated secondary tuberculosis is a wasting disease that is eventually fatal.

Leprosy

Leprosy (Hansen disease) is a chronic, slowly progressive, destruc-tive process involving peripheral nerves, skin, and mucous mem-branes, caused by *Mycobacterium leprae*. Although leprosy is now rare in developed countries, 15 million people are infected world-wide, primarily in tropical areas. *M. leprae* is a slender, weakly acid-fast rod that cannot be cultured on artificial media or in cell culture. *M. leprae* grows best at temperatures below core body temperature, and lesions tend to occur in the hands and face.

Leprosy is transmitted from person to person, and probably involves inoculation of bacteria carried from nasal secretions into the respiratory tract or into open wounds.

Most people (95%) have a natural protective immunity and are not infected even after prolonged exposure. A small minority (5%) may develop symptoms; those with high resistance develop *tuberculoid leprosy*, whereas those with an inadequate immune re-sponse have low resistance and develop *lepromatous leprosy*. The

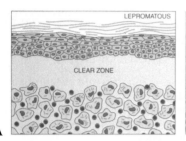
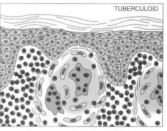

A   B

FIGURE   9-2
The skin lesions of lepromatous leprosy differ from those of tuberculoid leprosy. A: In lepromatous leprosy, the epidermis has flattened (loss of Rete ridges). A characteristic "clear zone" of uninvolved dermis separates the epidermis from tumorlike accumulations of macrophages, each containing numerous lepra bacilli (*Mycobacterium leprae*). B: In tuberculoid leprosy, a macular skin lesion displays a raised, infiltrated margin containing discrete granulomas that extend to the basal layer of the epidermis (without a clear zone). The granulomas are composed of epithelioid cells and Langerhans giant cells, and are associated with lymphocytes and plasma cells. Lepra bacilli are rare. (From Rubin E, Gorstein F, Rubin R, et al. Rubin's Pathology, 4th ed. Philadelphia: Lippincott Williams & Wilkins, 2005, p. 426.)

skin lesions of lepromatous leprosy differ from those of tuberculoid leprosy (Fig. 9-2).

- *Tuberculoid leprosy:* Termed "tuberculoid" because the lesions resemble lesions of tuberculosis, but lack caseous necrosis. Leprosy lesions show circumscribed dermal granulomas, composed of epithelioid macrophages, Langhans giant cells, and lymphocytes. In contrast to lesions of lepromatous leprosy, lesions of the milder tuberculoid leprosy cause minimal disfigurement. Nerve fibers are swollen and infiltrated with lymphocytes. Nerve involvement causes diminished sensation.
- *Lepromatous leprosy:* Exhibits multiple tumorlike lesions of the skin, eyes, testes, nerves, lymph nodes, and spleen. Nodular infiltrates of foamy macrophages teem with bacilli. Dermal infiltrates cause extensive disfigurement of facial regions.

Mycobacterium avium-intracellulare Complex

Mycobacterium avium and *Mycobacterium intracellulare* are similar mycobacterial species, which cause identical diseases and are classed together as *M. avium-intracellulare* (MAI) complex. Prior to the AIDS epidemic, MAI was extremely rare, but today it is the third most common opportunistic infection in AIDS patients in the United States. MAI is found in soil and water, and humans probably acquire it from the environment. The disease is clinically and pathologically similar to tuberculosis but progresses more slowly. Both infections produce pulmonary nodules and cavities, and both show caseating granulomas.

Fungal Infections

Fungi are eukaryotes, and are larger and more complex than bacteria, with nuclei enclosed in nuclear membranes and cytoplasmic organelles such as mitochondria and endoplasmic reticulum.

Fungi grow in soil, air, and the feces of birds and bats. Of the many known fungi, only a few invade and destroy human tissue. Of these, most are opportunists and infect only persons with impaired immune mechanisms. Most fungi are visible on tissue sections stained with H&E. The PAS reaction and Gomori silver stain are commonly used to detect fungal infections in tissues. There are two basic morphological types of fungi: yeasts and molds.

- Yeasts are the unicellular form of fungi. They are round or oval and reproduce by budding.
- Molds are multicellular filamentous fungal colonies that consist of branching tubules called hyphae. The mass of tangled hyphae in the mold form is called a mycelium.

Candida

Members of the genus *Candida* are yeastlike fungi. Many *Candida* species are endogenous human flora. *C. albicans* resides in small numbers in the oropharynx, gastrointestinal tract, and vagina and is the most frequent candidal pathogen; it is responsible for more than 95% of these infections.

Pathogenesis

Normally, resident bacterial flora limit the number of fungal organisms by (a) blocking candidal attachment to epithelial cells (b) competing for nutrients, and (c) preventing conversion of the fungus to its tissue-invasive forms. Antibiotic use results in the suppression of the competing bacterial flora and is the most common precipitating factor for candidiasis. When any of the host defenses are compromised, candidal infections can occur. Table 9-9 lists some of the candidal infections with conditions that predispose to infection.

Clinical Features

Candidal infections may be manifested in several ways:

Table 9-9

Candidal Infections

Disease	Predisposing Conditions
Superficial infections	
Intertrigo (opposed skin surfaces)	Maceration
Paronychia (nail beds)	Maceration
Diaper rash	Maceration
Vulvovaginitis	Alteration in normal flora
Thrush (oral)	Decreased cell-mediated immunity
Esophagitis	Decreased cell-mediated immunity
Deep infections	
Urinary tract infections	Indwelling urinary catheters
Sepsis and disseminated infection	Neutropenia, indwelling vascular catheters, and change in normal flora

From Rubin E, Gorstein F, Rubin R, et al. Rubin's Pathology, 4th ed. Philadelphia: Lippincott Williams & Wilkins, 2005, p. 429.

- Candidal infections of superficial layers of the epidermis or mucous membranes are characterized by thick, white discharge (in vulvovaginitis) or friable white curdlike membranes (in thrush).
- Candidal endocarditis exhibits large vegetations on the valves.
- Candidal sepsis and disseminated candidiasis are rare and often terminal events of an underlying disorder associated with an altered immune system.

Aspergillosis

Aspergillosis species are common environmental fungi that produce opportunistic infections, usually involving the lungs. There are three distinct types of pulmonary aspergillosis.

- **Allergic bronchopulmonary aspergillosis** develops almost exclusively in asthmatics in whom aspergillus antigens initiate an allergic response. The condition is aggravated if spores actually germinate and grow in the airways. In tissues, aspergillus forms branching filaments (hyphae). Lymphocytes, plasma cells, and eosinophils infiltrate airways, which sometimes become impacted with mucus and fungal hyphae.

- **Aspergilloma** occurs in persons with pulmonary cavities or bronchiectasis. An aspergilloma is a dense mass of tangled hyphae within a fibrous cavity.
- **Invasive aspergillosis** afflicts neutropenic patients, commonly those with acute leukemia. Vascular invasion by the fungi may lead to widespread dissemination outside the lungs. Sections of lung may show branching fungal hyphae surrounding blood vessels and invading adjacent parenchyma.

Mucormycosis (Zygomycosis)

Several related environmental fungi are members of the class Zygomycetes, order Mucorales; the infections they produce are called mucormycoses or zygomycoses. The fungi are ubiquitous in the environment and produce spores that can produce lung disease in susceptible persons, particularly in those with severe diabetes. The three predominant forms of mucormycosis follow:

- *Rhinocerebral*: Fungi proliferate in the nasal sinuses but may invade surrounding tissues; extension into the brain leads to a fatal, necrotizing hemorrhagic encephalitis.
- *Pulmonary*: This potentially fatal infection resembles pulmonary aspergillosis with vascular invasion and areas of septic lung infarction.
- *Subcutaneous*: This infection occurs in the tropics; it produces an enlarging inflammatory mass on the shoulder, trunk, or thigh.

Cryptococcosis

Cryptococcosis is a systemic mycosis caused by *Cryptococcus neoformans*, a yeastlike fungus, which primarily affects the lungs and then disseminates to the meninges. The disease occurs in persons with impaired immunity, such as patients with AIDS and patients taking immunosuppressive drugs. More than 95% of cryptococcal infections involve the brain.

Cryptococcus is unique among pathogenic fungi in having a proteoglycan capsule that is essential for its pathogenicity. It stains poorly with H&E; in tissue section it appears as colorless bubbles or holes. The main reservoir for the fungus is pigeon droppings.

Histoplasmosis

Histoplasmosis is a mycosis caused by *Histoplasma capsulatum*, a dimorphic fungus that grows as a mold at ambient temperatures, but as a yeast in the human body. The disease is usually self-limited but may lead to a systemic granulomatous disease. It resembles tuberculosis in that the organisms grow and multiply inside pulmonary macrophages until the host mounts hypersensitivity and cell-mediated immune responses. Disseminated histoplasmosis develops in persons who fail to mount an effective immune response to the organism, and the fungus spreads to organs such as liver, spleen, lymph nodes, and bone marrow.

Coccidioidomycosis

Coccidioidomycosis is a chronic, necrotizing mycotic infection that clinically and pathologically resembles tuberculosis. The disease, caused by *Coccidioides immitis*, is endemic to arid regions of the Americas begins with focal bronchopneumonia, but may spread outside the lungs. With the onset of an immune reaction, a caseous granuloma develops, which will heal leaving a fibrocaseous nodule. In immunocompromised persons, the lung infection may disseminate to the skin, meninges, and bone.

Blastomycosis

Blastomycosis is a chronic granulomatous and suppurative disease of the lungs, which is often disseminated to other body sites, mainly the skin and bone. The disease, caused by *Blastomyces dermatitidis*, is endemic in the Mississippi and Ohio River basins, as well as around the Great Lakes and the St. Lawrence River. The inhaled spores produce yeasts, and a focal bronchopneumonia ensues. The pulmonary disease usually resolves by scarring, but some persons develop progressive miliary lesions or cavities.

Paracoccidioidomycosis (South American Blastomycosis)

Paracoccidioidomycosis is a chronic granulomatous infection that begins with pulmonary involvement and disseminates to involve the skin, oropharynx, adrenals, and the macrophages of the liver, spleen, and lymph nodes. The causal fungus *Paracoccidioides brasiliensis* is endemic in regions of Central and South America. Reactivation of latent infections can occur, even in persons who have moved from the endemic region.

Sporotrichosis

Sporotrichosis is a chronic infection of the skin, subcutaneous tissues, and regional lymph nodes. It is caused by *Sporothrix schenckii*, a dimorphic fungus. It grows in soil and decaying plant matter. The disease is endemic in parts of the Americas and southern Africa, and is acquired by accidental inoculation from thorns or splinters. Cutaneous sporotrichosis is particularly common among rose gardeners. Inoculation induces an inflammatory response that produces ulceronodular lesions.

Chromomycosis

Chromomycosis is a chronic infection of the skin caused by several species of fungi that live as saprophytes in soil and decaying vegetable matter. The infection is common in barefooted agricultural workers in the tropics. The lesions begin as papules and become wartlike with time.

Dermatophyte Infections

Dermatophytes are fungi that cause localized superficial infections of keratinized tissues such as skin, hair, and nails. Most infections are acquired by direct contact with infected persons. The lesions spread centrifugally, giving a ringlike appearance, hence the disease misnomers "ringworm" and "tinea" (from the Latin tinea, "worm").

Dermatophyte infections are named according to the sites of involvement (e.g., scalp, tinea capitis; feet, tinea pedis, "athlete's foot"; nails, tinea unguium; and intertriginous areas of the groin, tinea cruris, "jock itch"). Infections range from asymptomatic disease to chronic, pruritic eruptions. They are treated with topical antifungal agents.

Mycetoma

A mycetoma is a slowly progressive, localized, and often disfiguring infection of the skin, soft tissues, and bone, produced by inoculation of various soil-dwelling fungi and filamentous bacteria. Mycetoma occurs in the tropics, and the foot is the most common site of infection.

Protozoal Infections

The protozoa are single-celled eukaryotes that fall into three general classes:

1. Amebae: Pseudopods provide locomotion. *Entamoeba histolytica* is extracellular and can digest and invade tissues.
2. Flagellates: Threadlike flagella provide locomotion. Trypanosomes are flagellates that damage by causing inflammatory responses.
3. Sporozoites: Are not motile; are produced by multiple fission of a spore. Sporozoites are a stage in the life cycle of the *Plasmodium* organisms that cause malaria.

Protozoa are responsible for extraintestinal as well as intestinal diseases (Table 9-10).

Table 9-10

Protozoal Infections

	Agent	Disease Characteristics	Transmission	Distribution
Intestinal infections				
Amebiasis	*Entamoeba histolytica*	Mild diarrhea to severe dysentery	Fecal contamination of food or water	Tropics
Giardiasis	*Giardia lamblia*	Small intestine, intermittent flatulence to malabsorption	Fecal contamination of food or water	Worldwide
Cryptosporodiasis	*Cryptosporidium*	Diarrheal disease, gastroenteritis	Fecal contamination of food or water	Worldwide
Extraintestinal infections				
Malaria	*Plasmodium* (four species)	Anemia, splenomegaly	Anopheles mosquito	Tropical and subtropical areas
Babesiosis	*Babesia*	Malarialike illness	Deer tick	Europe and North America
African trypanosomiasis	*Trypanosoma brucei*	Generalized lymphadenopathy, often meningoencephalitis	Tsetse fly	West, central, east Africa

American trypanosomiasis (Chagas disease)	*T. cruzi*	Chronic cardiomyopathy, megaesophagus, megacolon	Reduviid bug ("kissing" bug)	North, Central, and South America
Leishmaniasis	*Leishmania* species	Visceral, mucotaneous, or cutaneous disease	Sandfly	Tropical and some temperate areas
Toxoplasmosis	*Toxoplasma gondii*	Lymphadenopathy, to sometimes life-threatening central nervous system disease, chorioretinitis, mental retardation	Cat feces	Worldwide
Primary amebic meningoencephalitis	*Naegleria fowleri*	Fatal suppurative inflammation of meninges	Swimming in ponds and lakes	Very rare; tropical and subtropical regions
Pneumocystis carinii pneumonia	*P. carinii* (transitional between a fungus and a protozoan)	Progressive pneumonia, especially in persons with AIDS	Inhalation	Worldwide

Malaria

Malaria is a mosquito-borne, hemolytic, febrile illness that infects more than 200 million persons and kills more than 1 million yearly. The disease has been eradicated in developed countries but is still prevalent in tropical and subtropical areas.

Pathogenesis

Malaria is a protozoal disease transmitted from person to person by the bite of the female *Anopheles* mosquito. Four species of *Plasmodium* cause malaria: *P. falciparum, P. vivax, P. ovale*, and *P. malariae.* Of the four species, the one that causes the most severe disease the other species and accounts the most deaths is *P. falciparum.*

The following steps occur in the life cycle of malaria:

1. A mosquito bites an infected person, taking blood that contains gametocytes of the malarial parasite.
2. In the mosquito, the parasite produces sporozoites.
3. When the mosquito bites again, it inoculates sporozoites into a naive host.
4. Sporozoites invade and reproduce in host hepatocytes, yielding merozoites.
5. Merozoites exit liver cells and enter red blood cells (RBCs), where they reproduce.
6. Subpopulations of merozoites differentiate into gametocytes.
7. A mosquito, feeding on the infected host ingests gametocytes thereby completing the life cycle of the malarial parasite.

Pathology and Clinical Features

- The rupture of infected RBCs causes anemia and the fever of malaria through the release of pyrogenic material.
- Hepatosplenomegaly reflects the response of liver Kupffer cells and spleen macrophages to the destruction of RBCs. Liver, spleen and lymph nodes are darkened by macrophages filled with breakdown products of RBCs.
- Capillaries become obstructed leading to ischemia of the brain, kidneys, and lungs.
- The brain shows congestion and thrombosis of small blood vessels, which are rimmed with edema and hemorrhage ("ring hemorrhages"). Intravascular hemolysis leads to hemoglobinuric nephrosis (blackwater fever).

Babesiosis

Babesiosis is a malarialike infection caused by protozoa of the genus *Babesia*, which is transmitted by hard-bodies ticks. The causative organisms resemble those of malaria, and they invade and destroy erythrocytes; however, their life cycle differs from that of *Plasmodium*, and they have no exoerythrocytic stage.

Babesiosis is common in animals, mainly cattle, horses, and dogs, but it is rare in humans. In the United States, some human Babesia infections have been reported on islands off the New England coast. Splenectomy and diabetes are predisposing factors. Babesiosis is usually self-limited, but uncontrolled infections can be fatal.

Toxoplasmosis

Toxoplasmosis is a worldwide infectious disease caused by the protozoan *Toxoplasma gondii*. Infections are common, but most are asymptomatic. When they occur in the fetus or in an immunocompromised host, severe necrotizing disease may result.

Toxoplasmosis is acquired by the ingestion of infectious forms of *T. gondii*, which may be present in cat feces, or partly cooked pork, lamb, or venison. Congenital infection is acquired by transplacental transmission from an infected mother to the fetus.

- *Toxoplasma Lymphadenopathy Syndrome*: Affected lymph nodes exhibit numerous epithelioid macrophages surrounding reactive germinal centers. If symptoms appear in an immunocompetent host, they usually manifest as nontender regional lymph node enlargement.
- *Toxoplasmosis in Immunocompromised Hosts:* As with fetal infection, the brain is most commonly affected; infection produces a multifocal necrotizing encephalitis.
- *Congenital Toxoplasma Infections: T. gondii* can travel through the placenta and is more destructive in the fetus than in children or adults. The developing brain and eye are readily infected. Central nervous system infection produces a necrotizing meningoencephalitis; ocular infection causes chorioretinitis.

Pneumocystis carinii (jiroveci) Pneumonia

P. carinii is distributed worldwide; it is one of the most common opportunistic pathogens in persons with AIDS. Although *P. carinii* infection is rapidly contained in immunocompetent persons, it causes progressive, often fatal, pneumonia in persons with severely impaired cell-mediated immunity. Before new protease inhibitors became available for AIDS treatment, 80% of all AIDS patients developed *P. carinii* pneumonia during the course of their illness.

P. carinii reproduces in association with type 1 alveolar lining cells, and active disease is confined to the lungs. Infected alveoli fill with organisms and proteinaceous fluid. Microscopically, alveoli contain a frothy, eosinophilic material, composed of clusters of *P. carinii*, degenerated cells, alveolar macrophages, and cysts. Silver stain shows crescent-shaped organisms, some with a characteristic dark spot in their walls.

Amebiasis

Amebiasis refers to an infection with the pathogenic amoeba, *Entamoeba histolytica*. The infection principally involves the colon and occasionally the liver. The organism reproduces in the human colon and passes in the feces. The disease is usually contracted by ingesting food or water contaminated by amoebic cysts.

- **Intestinal amebiasis** is an ulcerating disease of the colon. Amebae produce flask-shaped ulcers of the mucosa and submucosa, and may invade submucosal venules, thereby disseminating the infection to the liver.
- **Amebic liver abscess** is a major complication of intestinal amebiasis. E. histolytica trophozoites that reach the liver can kill hepatocytes, and produce a necrotic cavity filled with material reported to resemble "anchovy paste." The liver abscess can expand to involve adjacent structures.

Cryptosporidiosis

Cryptosporidiosis refers to an enteric infection with a protozoan of the genus *Cryptosporidium* that causes diarrheal disease in persons with compromised immunity. The disease is acquired by the ingestion of *Cryptosporidium* oocysts, which are shed in the feces of infected humans and animals. Unlike other coccidia, *Cryptosporidium* organisms remain extracellular. They attach to and reproduce on the microvillous surface of the small intestine. The disease is usually self-limited, but in the immunocompromised patient, infections may cause chronic inflammation in the lamina propria and spread to the gallbladder and intrahepatic bile ducts. Diarrhea may persist indefinitely and cause severe fluid loss.

Giardiasis

Giardiasis is an infection of the small intestine caused by the flagellated protozoan *Giardia lamblia*. It causes abdominal cramping and diarrhea. Giardiasis is acquired by the ingestion of infectious cyst forms of the organism, which are shed in the feces of infected humans and animals. Ingested cysts survive the stomach acidity, rupture within the duodenum and jejunum to release trophozoites, which attach to the intestinal epithelium and reproduce. Microscopic examination shows trophozoites on the villi surfaces and within crypts, with minimal mucosal damage.

Leishmaniasis

Leishmaniae are protozoans that are transmitted to humans by the bites of *Phlebotomus* sandflies, which have fed on infected animals. Numerous species of *Leishmania* differ in the type of disease they produce. The protozoans cause clinical syndromes ranging from self-resolving cutaneous ulcers to fatal disseminated disease. Leishmaniasis is endemic in many subtropical and tropical areas.

After inoculation into the skin, leishmaniae are phagocytosed by mononuclear phagocytes, transform into amastigotes, reproduce intracellularly, spread to other phagocytes, and form a cluster of infected phagocytes at the inoculation site. Depending on host susceptibility and species of leishmaniae, three distinct clinical entities may ensue:

1. *Localized cutaneous leishmaniasis*: The overlying epidermis ulcerates, and the lesion becomes granulomatous with epithelioid macrophages, Langerhans giant cells, plasma cells, and lymphocytes. Eventually, the ulcer heals.
2. *Mucocutaneous leishmaniasis*: This late complication of cutaneous leishmaniasis is caused by infection with *Leishmania braziliensis*. Years after the primary lesion has healed, a highly destructive and disfiguring ulcer develops at a mucocutaneous junction such as the larynx, nasal septum, anus or vulva.
3. *Visceral leishmaniasis (kala azar)*: This disseminated leishmaniasis is produced by *Leishmania donovani*. Animal reservoirs of the agent and susceptible age groups vary in different parts of the world. The liver, spleen, and lymph nodes become infected and massively enlarged. Eventually, sheets of parasitized macrophages accumulate in other organs such as the kidney and heart. If untreated, the disease is fatal.

Chagas Disease (American Trypanosomiasis)

Chagas disease causes a systemic infection in humans, with both acute manifestations and long-term sequelae in the heart and gastrointestinal tract. The disease is endemic in Central and South America and is caused by the protozoan parasite *Trypanosoma cruzi*. The parasite is transmitted by "kissing bugs" that infest dwellings of the poor; bugs become infected after biting an animal or person who already has Chagas disease. They then transmit the disease to new hosts.

- *Acute Chagas disease*: *T. cruzi* infects cells at the site of inoculation, reproducing in them to form a localized nodular inflammatory lesion known as a chagoma. The organism then disseminates in the bloodstream, infecting cells throughout the body, including cardiac myocytes. Acute Chagas disease may cause fatal myocarditis. The onset of cell-mediated immunity eliminates the acute manifestations, but chronic tissue damage may continue.
- *Chronic Chagas disease*: Chronic disease may develop years after the acute infection. Chronic myocarditis and massive dilation of the esophagus and colon characterize this phase of the dis-

ease. In congenital Chagas disease, infection in pregnant women leads to infection of the placenta and fetus, with subsequent spontaneous abortion.

African Trypanosomiasis

African trypanosomiasis (sleeping sickness) is an infection with *Trypanosoma brucei* a curved flagellate that produces a life-threatening meningoencephalitis. *T. brucei* is a hemoflagellate protozoan that is transmitted by several species of blood-sucking tsetse flies. The pathogenesis of African trypanosomiasis involves the formation of immune complexes by variable trypanosomal antigens and antibodies. The trypanosome evades immune attack in the human host by periodically altering its glycoprotein antigenic coat.

- Gambian trypanosomiasis is a chronic infection with *Trypanosoma brucei gambiense,* often lasting more than a year. It is endemic in the bush of central and west Africa.
- Rhodesian trypanosomiasis is an infection with *T. brucei rhodesiense* occurs in the woodland savanna of east Africa, is rapidly progressive, and kills the patient in 3 to 6 months.

After the primary inoculation of the trypanosomes, a systemic infection involves enlarged lymph nodes and spleen. Infection eventually localizes to the small blood vessels of the central nervous system, causing a destructive vasculitis, and producing the progressive apathy and somnolence characteristic of sleeping sickness. In the more severe Rhodesian trypanosomiasis, organisms may also localize to the heart, causing a fulminant myocarditis.

Primary Amebic Meningoencephalitis

Amebic meningoencephalitis, caused by *Naegleria fowleri*, is a fatal, suppurative inflammation of the brain and meninges. *N. fowleri* is a free-living soil ameba that inhabits lakes and ponds in tropical and subtropical regions. Primary amebic meningoencephalitis is a rare disease affecting bathers in the waters of these areas. The ameba enters nasal mucosa, invades olfactory nerves and olfactory bulbs, and proliferates in the meninges and brain. The disease is rapidly fatal.

Helminthic Infection

Helminths, or worms, are multicellular animals with differentiated tissues and are among the most common human pathogens. They are the largest and most complex organisms capable of living within the human body. Helminths cause disease in various ways: (a) by competing for nutrients; (b) by blocking vital structures; and (c) by causing inflammation and destructive responses.

Parasitic helminths fall into three broad categories:

1. Roundworms (nematodes) are elongate and cylindrical with tubular digestive tracts; some live in lymphatics, some in the intestines; some may invade muscle
2. Flatworms (trematodes) are dorsoventrally flattened with digestive tracts that end in blind loops; blood-dwelling flukes are examples.
3. Tapeworms (cestodes) are segmented organisms that lack a digestive tract and absorb nutrients through their outer walls; they are parasitic in the intestines.

Filarial Nematodes

Lymphatic Filariasis (Elephantiasis)

Lymphatic filariasis is an inflammatory parasitic infection of lymphatic vessels caused by the filarial roundworms *Wuchereria bancrofti* and *Brugia malayi*. The disease is widespread in southern Asia, the Pacific, Africa, and parts of South America. Infection is acquired from the bites of mosquitoes, which transmit infectious larvae, which mature into adult forms. Adult worms inhabit the lymphatics, where the inflammatory response they induce, causes acute lymphangitis. A chronic inflammatory infiltrate, containing numerous eosinophils, surrounds the worms. In a minority of patients, the worms cause lymphatic obstruction, leading to severe lymphedema. Edematous distortion of body parts is known as elephantiasis.

Onchocerciasis

Onchocerciasis ("river blindness") is a chronic inflammatory disease of the skin, eyes, and lymphatics, caused by the filarial nematode *Onchocerca volvulus*. River blindness is one of the world's major diseases, endemic along rivers and streams in parts of Africa, Mexico, and South and Central America. It afflicts and causes blindness in millions of people.

Blackflies transmit infectious larvae to humans. Adult worms live in the deep dermis and subcutaneous tissues. They become encapsulated by fibrous scars and form onchocercal nodules. Gravid females release microfilariae, which migrate into the skin, eyes, and lymph nodes. Ocular onchocerciasis results from migration of microfilariae into all regions of the eye. Lesions show degenerating microfilariae surrounded by chronic inflammation, which may lead to blindness.

Loiasis

Loiasis is infection by the filarial nematode *Loa loa*, the African "eyeworm." *Loa loa* filariasis is prevalent in the rain forests of central and west Africa. Humans and baboons are the definitive hosts, and infection is transmitted by mango flies.

- Adult worms migrate in the skin and occasionally cross the eye beneath the conjunctiva, hence the local name for the infection: "eyeworm." Migrating worms cause no inflammation but cause a creeping sensation with intense itching.
- Static worms are surrounded by eosinophils, other inflammatory cells, and a foreign body giant cell reaction. In more severe cases, filarial thrombi may cause fatal obstruction of vessels in the brain.

Intestinal Nematodes

The most common chronic intestinal infections in the world are caused by the intestinal nematodes (Table 9-11). Intestinal nema-

Table 9-11
Intestinal Nematodes

Species	Common Name	Site of Adult Worm	Clinical Manifestations
Ascaris lumbricoides	Roundworm	Small bowel	Allergic reactions to lung migration; intestinal obstruction
Ancyclostoma duodenale	Hookworm	Small bowel	Allergic reactions to cutaneous inoculation and lung migration; intestinal blood loss
Necator americanus	Hookworm	Small bowel	Allergic reactions to cutaneous inoculation and lung migration; intestinal blood loss
Trichuris trichiura	Whipworm	Large bowel	Abdominal pain and diarrhea; rectal prolapse (rare)
Strongyloides stercoralis	Threadworm	Small bowel	Abdominal pain and diarrhea; dissemination to extraintestinal sites in immunocompromised persons
Enterobius vermicularis	Pinworm	Cecum, appendix	Perianal and perineal itching

From Rubin E, Gorstein F, Rubin R, et al. Rubin's Pathology, 4th ed. Philadelphia: Lippincott Williams & Wilkins, 2005, p. 459.

todes are endemic in tropical and subtropical environments. Humans are the primary host for all of the intestinal nematodes, and infection spreads from person to person through eggs or larvae. In all intestinal nematode infections, worms live in some part of the intestine and deposit eggs into the feces. Fecal contamination of food and water promotes spread of infection. Diagnosis usually involves identification of the eggs in the feces.

Ascariasis

This, the most common helminth infection, is caused by the large roundworm, *Ascaris lumbricoides*. Infections occur worldwide. The worms live in the small intestine and pass eggs into the host feces. Larvae hatch from eggs ingested by a new host. They may penetrate the intestinal wall, reach the lungs, migrate up the respiratory tract, and are reswallowed; eventually they reach the small intestine, where they mature. Heavy infections may cause intestinal or biliary obstruction and liver abscesses.

Trichuriasis

This disease is caused by the intestinal "whipworm," *Trichuris trichiura*, and is found worldwide; more than 2 million persons in the United States are infected. Adult worms live in the cecum and upper colon and pass eggs into the feces. Their invasion causes small erosions and focal active inflammation.

Hookworms

Hookworms are intestinal nematodes that infect the human small intestine, lacerating the mucosa and causing intestinal blood loss. Both *Ancylostoma duodenale* ("Old World" hookworm) and *Necator americanus* ("American" hookworm) prevail on most continents and have overlapping epidemiological boundaries. Worldwide, more than 700 million persons are infected with hookworms; in the United States, 500,000 people harbor the parasite.

Hookworm larvae penetrate the skin, travel to lung alveoli, migrate up the trachea, are swallowed, lodge in the intestinal mucosa and feed on intestinal villi. With extensive worm infections, blood loss can be considerable. Worldwide, this is the most important cause of chronic anemia.

Strongyloidiasis

The threadworm, *Strongyloidiasis stercoralis*, causes this infection of the small intestine. Infection is most frequent in warm, moist climates. Endemic pockets exist in the Appalachian region of the United States.

Although most cases are asymptomatic, threadworm infection can progress to disseminated disease in immunocompromised persons. In disseminated strongyloidiasis, ulceration of the intestinal wall may lead to sepsis with infection of parenchymal organs. If untreated, this condition is fatal.

Pinworm Infection (Enterobiasis)

Unlike most nematode infections that occur mainly in tropical and subtropical regions, pinworm infection is more frequent in temperate zones. It is caused by *Enterobius vermicularis*, an intestinal nematode, and is most common among young children. It is estimated that 5 million school-age children harbor the worm in the United States.

The adult female worm lives in the cecum and appendix and migrates to the perianal and perineal skin to deposit eggs, which stick to fingers and clothing and which are easily transmitted from person to person. Some infected persons are asymptomatic, but most complain of perineal pruritus caused by migrating worms depositing eggs. Several agents are effective against pinworms.

Tissue Nematodes

Trichinosis

Trichinosis is caused by the roundworm *Trichinella spiralis*. The infection is most common in eastern and central Europe, North America, and South America. Humans acquire trichinosis by eating inadequately cooked pork containing encysted *T. spiralis* larvae. Meat inspection programs and restriction of pig feeding practices have largely eliminated *T. spiralis* from domesticated pigs in many developed countries.

After ingestion, *T. spiralis* larvae emerge from tissue cysts, penetrate the intestinal wall, enter the circulation, and lodge in striated muscle. Early myocyte infection elicits an intense inflammatory infiltrate rich in eosinophils and macrophages. When the larvae encyst, the inflammatory infiltrate subsides. Encysted larvae can remain viable for years. The resulting myositis is especially prominent in the diaphragm, extrinsic ocular muscles, tongue, intercostal muscles, gastrocnemius, and deltoids. Eosinophilia may be a prominent feature. Sometimes the central nervous system or heart is also involved in the inflammatory response, producing a meningoencephalitis or myocarditis.

Visceral Larva Migrans (Toxocariasis)

Visceral larva migrans is an infection of deep organs by *Toxocara* roundworms *T. canis* and *T. cati* that live in the intestines of dogs and cats. Ingestion of their embryonated eggs transmits infection to humans, primarily young children. Larvae invade the intestinal wall and are carried to the liver where a few may be carried to any part of the body via the systemic circulation. Dead larvae stimulate formation of small granulomas, which heal by scarring. Infection is generally self-limited.

Cutaneous Larva Migrans

This infection is caused by the migration of a variety of larval nematodes through the skin. It results in a characteristic pruritic eruption on the skin, with a wavy, raised margin. Dogs and cats infected with hookworms are the major source of the disease.

Dracunculiasis

Dracunculiasis is an infection of the connective and subcutaneous tissues and features long adult guinea worms, *Dracunculus medinensis*, beneath the skin. The disease is common in areas of Africa, the Middle East, India and Pakistan, and is transmitted in drinking water. Worms measuring 120 cm in length may occasionally be extracted from skin papules. Secondary infection of papules is common.

Flukes (Trematodes)

Diseases caused by flukes are summarized in Table 9-12.

Schistosomiasis

Schistosomiasis (bilharziasis, snail fever) is the most important helminthic disease of humans, in which intense inflammatory and immunological responses damage the liver, intestine, or urinary bladder. The disease is caused by infestation with schistosomes through contact with contaminated water. Schistosomiasis affects 10% of the world's population, and ranks second only to malaria as a cause of disabling disease.

Pathogenesis

Three species of *Schistosoma* are responsible for the disease, and inhabit distinct geographical regions: *S. mansoni* (tropical Africa and South America), *S. haematobium* (large regions of Africa), and *S. japonicum* (parts of China, the Philippines, and India).

The schistosomes have complicated life cycles, alternating between asexual generations in the snail and sexual generations in humans. The larvae of the parasite live in snails (the intermediate host), and infect humans who bathe in infested waters. Larvae enter through the skin and migrate through blood vessels to other organs, where they mature into egg-laying worms.

Clinical Features

The basic lesion is a circumscribed granulomas or a cellular infiltrate of eosinophils and neutrophils around an egg. Granulomas that form around eggs obstruct microvasculature, and produce ischemic damage resulting in scarring and dysfunction in the affected organs. The site of involvement is determined by the tropism of the particular schistosome:

Table 9-12

Diseases Caused by Flukes (Trematodes)

Disease	Agent	Affected Organs	Distribution
Liver fluke disease			
Schistosomiasism (bilharziasis)	*Schistosoma mansoni*	Liver, Intestines, Urinary Bladder	Tropical Africa, parts of South America
	S. haematobium		Tropical Africa, Middle East
	S. japonicum		Parts of China, Philippines, Asia, India
Clonorchiasis	*Clonorchis sinensis*	Hepatic biliary system	East Asia
Fascioliasis	Fasciola hepatica	Liver and bile ducts	Wherever sheep are raised
Intestinal fluke disease			
Fasciolopsiasis	Fasciolopsis buski	Small intestine	Much of Asia
Lung fluke disease			
Paragonimiasis	*Paragonimus westermani*	Lung (frequently misdiagnosed as tuberculosis)	Many Asian countries

- *S. mansoni* affects the distal colon and liver.
- *S. haematobium* affects rectum, bladder and pelvic organs.
- *S. japonicum* affects the small intestine, ascending colon, and liver.

Liver disease begins as periportal granulomatous inflammation and progresses to periportal fibrosis (pipestem fibrosis); severe cases may result in portal hypertension. Intestinal disease produces inflammatory polyps and foci of fibrosis. Urogenital disease causes patches of mucosal and mural fibrosis, which can obstruct urine flow, with secondary damage to the bladder, ureters, and kidney. (The bladder disease caused by *S. haematobium* is related to development of squamous cell carcinoma of the bladder.)

Clonorchiasis

Clonorchiasis is an infection of the hepatic biliary system by the Chinese liver fluke, *Clonorchis sinensis*. The disease is endemic in East Asia and is acquired by eating raw, smoked, or undercooked fish containing the *C. sinensis* larvae. In parts of Vietnam, China, and Japan, over 50% of the adult population is infected.

The presence of the fluke in the bile ducts leads to ductal obstruction; masses of eggs may become lodged in the ducts and cause cholangitis. There is an increased incidence of bile duct cancer with long-standing infection. The pancreatic ducts may become dilated, thickened, and lined by metaplastic tissue; pancreatitis may occur.

Paragonimiasis

This is a pulmonary infection by the oriental lung fluke, *Paragonimus westermani*. The infection is common in Asian countries and associated with the ingestion of raw crabs or their juices. The infection is often misdiagnosed as tuberculosis. Eggs in the sputum provide the definitive diagnosis.

Fascioliasis

The sheep liver fluke, Fasciola hepatica, is responsible for this biliary disease. It occurs in areas of Europe, the Middle East, and Asia, where sheep are raised and where humans eat raw vegetables, such as watercress, contaminated with the cysts passed by infected sheep.

Immature flukes gain access to the peritoneal cavity, liver, and bile ducts, where they mature to feed on liver cells and deposit eggs in liver parenchyma and bile ducts. The flukes induce hyperplasia of the bile duct walls, and portal and periductal fibrosis. Symptoms reflect intermittent biliary obstruction and chronic inflammation.

Fasciolopsiasis

Fasciolopsiasis is an infestation of the small intestine caused by *Fasciolopsis buski,* the largest intestinal fluke of humans. The disease prevails in Asia and in the Indian subcontinent, especially in areas where humans raise pigs and consume aquatic vegetables. The fluke attaches to the duodenal or jejunal wall and may cause ulcerations and infections at the point of attachment.

Intestinal Tapeworms (Cestodes)

Taenia saginata, Taenia solium, and *Diphyllobothrium latum* are tapeworms that infect humans. They grow within the intestines but rarely cause damage. They are acquired by eating contaminated undercooked beef (*T. saginata*), pork (*T. solium*), or fish (*D. latum*).

Modern farming practices and meat inspection have largely eliminated beef and pork tapeworms in industrialized countries, but infection is common in developing countries. Fish tapeworm infection occurs in regions where people eat raw or pickled freshwater fish. Tapeworm infections are usually asymptomatic; however, the fish tapeworm competes with its host for vitamin B_{12} and may cause anemia.

Cysticercosis

This is a systemic infection by the eggs of the pork tapeworm *T. solium*. Although infection with the adult pork tapeworm in humans usually is asymptomatic, ingestion of the eggs may lead to more serious infection. Once inside the stomach, the tapeworm egg may hatch and develop into cysticerci, which may infect the brain, causing neurocysticercosis with severe symptoms such as convulsions and possible death.

Echinococcosis (Hydatid Disease)

This disease, which features cysts of the liver and lungs, is caused by *Echinococcus granulosus*. Infection with the tapeworm *E. granulosus* is endemic in sheep, goats, and cattle and their attendant dogs. Hydatid disease is present worldwide among herding populations.

Dogs contaminate their human masters with infectious eggs, and the eggs hatch to release tiny embryos that travel through the blood to lodge in a variety of organs. There, they develop into hydatid cysts. In humans, hydatid cysts occur predominantly in the liver but may also involve the lung, kidney, and brain. The rupture of a cyst into a body cavity may cause severe allergic reactions, and the rupture of a cyst in the lung may cause pneumothorax and empyema.

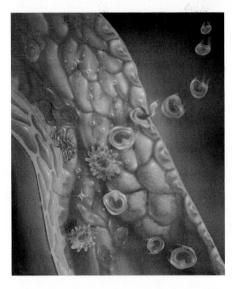

CHAPTER *10*

Blood Vessels

Chapter Outline

Fibromuscular Dysplasia

Vasculitis

    Polyarteritis Nodosa

    Hypersensitivity Angiitis

    Allergic Granulomatosis and Angiitis (Churg-Strauss Syndrome)

    Giant Cell Arteritis (Temporal Arteritis, Granulomatous Arteritis)

    Wegener Granulomatosis

    Takayasu Arteritis

    Kawasaki Disease (Mucocutaneous Lymph Node Syndrome)

    Thromboangiitis Obliterans (Buerger Disease)

    Behçet Disease

    Radiation Vasculitis

    Rickettsial Vasculitis

Aneurysms

    Abdominal Aortic Aneurysms

    Aneurysms of Cerebral Arteries

    Dissecting Aneurysms

    Syphilitic Aneurysms

    Mycotic (Infectious) Aneurysms

Veins

    Varicose Veins of the Leg

    Varicose Veins at Other Sites

    Deep Venous Thrombosis

Lymphatic Vessels

    Lymphangitis

    Lymphatic Obstruction and Lymphedema

Benign Tumors of Blood Vessels

    Hemangiomas

    Glomus Tumors (Glomangiomas)

    Hemangioendotheliomas

Malignant Tumors of Blood Vessels

    Angiosarcoma

    Hemangiopericytoma

    Kaposi Sarcoma

Tumors of the Lymphatic System

    Capillary Lymphangiomas

    Cystic Lymphangiomas

    Lymphangiosarcomas

General Blood Vessel Structure

The walls of all blood vessels in the body, except for the capillaries and postcapillary venules, are composed of three layers called tunics:

- Tunica intima is the innermost layer, facing the lumen. It consists of (a) a single layer of squamous epithelial cells called the endothelium, (b) the basal lamina of the endothelium, and (c) the subendothelial layer containing loose collagenous connective tissue, and occasional smooth muscle cells. A fenestrated elastic sheet, the internal elastic lamina, is part of the subendothelial layer in muscular arteries and arterioles.
- Tunica media is the middle layer and is composed of a layer of circumferentially arranged smooth muscle cells. This layer is relatively thick in arteries and extends from the internal elastic membrane to the thinner external elastic membrane. This external membrane is prominent in larger muscular arteries, and separates the media from the next layer, the tunica adventitia. Between the smooth muscle cells, and made by them, are variable amounts of elastin, collagen fibers, and proteoglycans.
- Tunica adventitia is the outermost connective tissue layer of vessel walls. It consists mainly of collagenous tissue and some elastic fibers. This layer is thicker in veins than in arteries. The adventitia of the larger arteries and veins contains small blood vessels, the vasa vasorum, supplying nutrients to the vascular wall. Small nerves are also present.

The walls of capillaries and venules are made up of a single layer of flattened endothelial cells. Occasional cells called pericytes embrace the outside of capillary walls and may have a contractile function.

Endothelial Cell Function

The endothelium is (a) a macromolecular barrier, (b) a thromboresistant surface, (c) a modulator of vascular smooth muscle cell function, and (d) a highly metabolic cell intimately involved in coagulation, inflammation, and repair. Endothelial cells do not normally proliferate, but after vessel injury, they migrate and proliferate rapidly to reestablish endothelium integrity. Endothelial dysfunction is important in the pathogenesis of vascular disease. For example, accumulation of lipid beneath the endothelium in atherosclerotic lesions reflects the failure of the endothelium to serve as a barrier between tissue and plasma.

Endothelial cells also perform the following:

- Endothelial cells synthesize prostacyclin and nitric oxide, both of which relax smooth muscle and inhibit the aggregation of platelets.
- Endothelial cells make angiotensin-converting enzyme (ACE), which converts angiotensin I to the potent vasoconstrictor, angiotensin II.
- When stimulated, endothelial cells express class II histocompatibility antigens, and so participate in activating lympho-

cytes. Immune responses to endothelial cells are a major part of organ rejection following transplantation.

Table 10-1 lists some additional functions of endothelial cells.

Arteries

Elastic Arteries

Elastic arteries are the largest blood vessels in the body, nearest the heart, and include vessels such as the aorta, pulmonary arteries, common carotid, and subclavian. They are composed of the same three general layers of all arteries and veins previously described; however, they differ in having much thicker tunica intima and tunica media.

- The tunica intima, in addition to the outer endothelium, contains a matrix of collagen, elastin, and proteoglycans. Occa-

Table 10-1
Functions of Endothelial Cells of the Blood Vessels
Permeability barrier
Vasoactive factors: Nitric oxide (EDRF), endothelin
Antithrombotic agent production: Prostacyclin (PGI_2), adenine metabolites
Prothrombotic agent production: Factor VIIIa (von Willebrand factor)
Anticoagulant production: Thrombomodulin, other proteins
Fibrinolytic agent production: Tissue plasminogen activator, urokinaselike factor
Procoagulant production: Tissue factor, plasminogen activator/inhibitor, factor V
Inflammatory mediator production: Interleukin-1, cell adhesion molecules
Receptors for factor IX, factor X, low-density lipoproteins, modified low-density lipoproteins, thrombin
Growth factor production: Blood cell colony-stimulating factors, insulin-like growth factors, fibroblast growth factor, platelet-derived growth factor
Growth inhibitor: Heparin
Replication

From Rubin E, Gorstein F, Rubin R, et al. Rubin's Pathology, 4th ed. Philadelphia: Lippincott Williams & Wilkins, 2005, p. 477.

sional smooth muscle cells, resident lymphocytes, and macrophages are also present.

- The tunica media consists of multiple layers of smooth muscle cells separated by elastic lamellae. The elastic layers minimize energy loss during the pressure changes between systole and diastole. A breakdown of these elastic layers leads to dilation of the wall, called an aneurysm.

Muscular Arteries

The blood conducted by the elastic arteries is distributed to individual organs through large muscular arteries. Smaller muscular arteries play an important role in the regulation of blood flow. The narrow lumen of the smallest of the muscular arteries, the arterioles, produces increased resistance, thereby reducing blood pressure to levels appropriate for the exchange of substances across the thin-walled capillaries. The muscular arteries also maintain systemic pressure by regulating total peripheral resistance.

Capillaries

The capillary endothelium acts as a semipermeable membrane, in which the exchange of plasma solutes with extracellular fluid is controlled by molecular size and charge. Capillary permeability depends on the ultrastructure of the wall of endothelial cells:

- Continuous capillaries, as are found in muscle, lungs, and brain, have occluding tight junctions between endothelial cells.
- Fenestrated capillaries are found in those tissues where there is extensive molecular exchange with the blood; such tissues include the small intestine, endocrine glands, and the kidney. The fenestrations (or windows) act as pores allowing a greater permeability and than that of continuous capillaries.
- Sinusoids are capillaries of wide diameter and irregular shape, found in the liver, spleen, lymph nodes, and bone marrow. Sinusoids allow rapid and intimate exchange of substances between plasma and the surrounding tissue.

Veins

Venules are the first vessels that collect blood from the capillaries. These branch into larger and larger vessels, eventually draining into the large veins returning blood to the heart.

Lymphatics

The lymphatic system drains the lymph from extracellular spaces and returns it to the blood. In the average person, the exchange of fluid across the capillaries throughout the body into the interstitial fluid amounts to about 20 L/day. This moves in both directions, and the majority is returned to the circulation through the walls of the capillaries. However, about 2–4 L/day is returned to the circulation by a circuitous route through the lymphatic system. The composition of this fluid, the lymph, is almost identical to the tissue fluid in the part of the body from which it flows. Lymphatic capillaries are lined by endothelial cells and are highly permeable. Lymphatics pass through regional lymph nodes where foreign material carried by the lymph is filtered.

Hemostasis and Thrombosis

Hemostasis is defined as the arrest of hemorrhage and is a response to vascular injury. The process involves tissue swelling, coagulation, platelet aggregation, and thrombosis. Thrombosis refers to the formation of a blood clot in the circulation. A thrombus is an aggregate of coagulated blood that contains platelets, fibrin, leukocytes, and red blood cells. Its formation involves a "tug of war" between factors that promote thrombosis and those that inhibit it.

Blood Coagulation

Blood coagulation entails the conversion of soluble plasma fibrinogen to an insoluble fibrillar polymer, fibrin, a reaction catalyzed by the proteolytic enzyme, thrombin. This process is called the coagulation cascade (Fig. 10-1) and involves a series of finely tuned steps mediated by a number of coagulation factors, many of which are inhibited by specific inhibitors. This process is carefully controlled, ensuring that clotting will remain restricted and not spread throughout the entire vasculature. Coagulation factors are generally indicated by Roman numerals, with a lowercase *a* appended to indicate an active form.

In blood coagulation, the coagulation cascade is initiated by endothelial injury. This causes the release of tissue factor (TF).

- TF combines with VIIa to form a complex that activates small amounts of X to Xa and IX to IXa.
- The complex of IXa with VIIIa further activates X to Xa.
- The complex of Xa with Va then catalyzes the conversion of prothrombin to thrombin.
- Thrombin functions as a serine protease to convert fibrinogen to fibrin.

Platelet Adhesion and Aggregation

Under normal circumstances circulating platelets are in a nonadherent state. However, injury upregulates platelet adhesiveness, after which platelets interact with each other to form a platelet

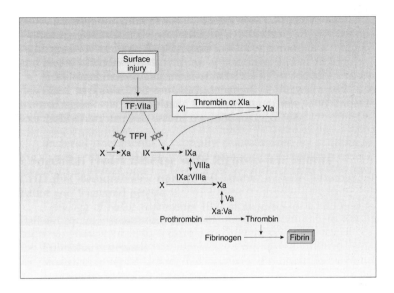

F I G U R E   10-1
The Coagulation Cascade. (From Rubin E, Gorstein F, Rubin R, et al. Rubin's Pathology, 4th ed. Philadelphia: Lippincott Williams & Wilkins, 2005, p. 480.)

thrombus. Platelet aggregates occlude injured small vessels and prevent the leakage of blood. Formation of a platelet thrombus entails a number of steps:

- Platelets adhere and aggregate following vessel wall injury.
- ADP and thromboxane A_2 are released.
- Locally generated thrombin, along with ADP and thromboxane A_2, recruit additional platelets, causing the mass to enlarge.
- Fibrin stabilizes the growing thrombus.
- Leukocytes and red blood cells are also incorporated into the thrombus.
- Endothelial cells release prostacyclin and nitric oxide to control the process by inhibiting platelet aggregation.

Endothelial Factors and Anticoagulant and Procoagulant Processes

For thrombosis to occur, either the endothelial continuity must be disrupted or the endothelial surface must change from an anticoagulant surface to a procoagulant one. The most common denuding injury is the progressive disruption of the endothelium by an atherosclerotic plaque. Endothelium plays a role in clot lysis by synthesizing plasminogen activator, which enhances formation of plasmin and its fibrin-degrading activity. Thus the endothelium plays an active role in control of thrombosis, and can downregulate or upregulate coagulant pathways (Table 10-2).

Atherosclerosis

Atherosclerosis is a disease of large- and medium-sized elastic and muscular arteries and results in the progressive accumulation within the intima of inflammatory cells, smooth muscle cells, lipids, and connective tissue. The fibroinflammatory lipid plaque in the intima, the atheroma, usually develops over several decades. The continued growth of the lesions encroaches on other layers of the arterial wall and narrows the lumen of the vessel wall, leading to reduced or blocked blood flow.

The term arteriosclerosis, which means hardening of the arteries, is sometimes used synonymously with the term atherosclerosis; however, arteriosclerosis is a disease of the walls of smaller arteries and arterioles which become thicker and less elastic, generally as the result of chronic hypertension.

Atherosclerosis as a Disease

Epidemiology

The major complications of atherosclerosis, including heart disease, myocardial infarction, stroke, and gangrene of the extremities account for more than half of the annual mortality in the United States.

Risk Factors

Any factor associated with a doubling in the incidence of ischemic heart disease has been defined as a risk factor.

- Hypertension: An increase in both diastolic and systolic blood pressure is a risk factor for myocardial infarction.
- Blood cholesterol: The amount of cholesterol in the blood is strongly related to the dietary intake of saturated fat. Treatment with cholesterol-lowering drugs (statins) has reduced the incidence of myocardial infarctions.
- Cigarette smoking: Atherosclerosis is more severe and extensive in cigarette smokers than in nonsmokers.
- Diabetes: People with diabetes have a substantially greater risk of occlusive atherosclerotic vascular disease in many organs.
- Increasing age and male sex: Age and sex are strong determinants of the risk for myocardial infarctions, but both are secondary to the accumulated effects of other risk factors.

Table 10-2

Regulation of Coagulation at the Endothelial Cell Surface

Down-regulation
1. Thrombin inactivators
a. Antithrombin III
b. Thrombomodulin
2. Activated protein C pathway
a. Synthesis and expression of thrombomodulin
b. Synthesis and expression of protein S
c. Thrombomodulin-mediated activation of protein C
d. Inactivation of factor V_a and factor VIII_a by APC–protein S complex
3. Tissue factor pathway inhibition
4. Fibrinolysis
a. Synthesis of tissue plasminogen activator, urokinase plasminogen activator, and plasminogen activator inhibitor 1
b. Conversion of GLU-plasminogen to LYS-plasminogen
c. APC-mediated potentiation
5. Synthesis of unsaturated fatty acid metabolites
a. Lipoxygenase metabolites-13-HODE
b. Cyclooxygenase metabolites-PGI_2 and PGE_2
Procoagulant pathways
1. Synthesis and expression of:
a. Tissue factor (thromboplastin)
b. Factor V
c. Platelet activating factor (PAF)
2. Binding of clotting factors IX/IX_a, X (prothrombinase complex)
3. Down-regulation of APC pathway
4. Increased synthesis of plasminogen activator inhibitor
5. Synthesis of 15-HPETE

From Rubin E, Gorstein F, Rubin R, et al. Rubin's Pathology, 4th ed. Philadelphia: Lippincott Williams & Wilkins, 2005, p. 482.

- Physical inactivity and stressful life patterns: These factors have been correlated with increased risk, but their precise relationship to development of atherosclerosis is not established.
- Homocysteine: The increased risk of high levels of plasma homocysteine is comparable to that of smoking or hyperlipidemia. Homocysteine is toxic to endothelial cells and inhibits several anticoagulant mechanisms in endothelial cells.
- C-reactive protein (CRP): CRP is a pentameric protein made in the liver and secreted in increased amounts after an acute inflammatory stimulus. Elevated concentrations of CRP have been linked to increased risk of heart attack and stroke, suggesting that inflammation contributes to atherogenesis.

Pathogenesis

A number of theories explain why and how atherosclerosis develops. Atheromas usually form where arteries branch, possibly because the constant turbulent blood flow in these areas injures the wall of the artery. Injury to the arterial wall may cause the development of an inflammatory response with the release of factors that stimulate cell migration and proliferation.

A hypothetical sequence of events leading to atherosclerotic plaque formation can be formulated (Fig. 10-2):

1. Endothelial dysfunction causes an intimal lesion. Endothelial cells express cell adhesion molecules.
2. Adhesion molecules cause monocytes to move out of the bloodstream into the tunica intima of the artery wall.

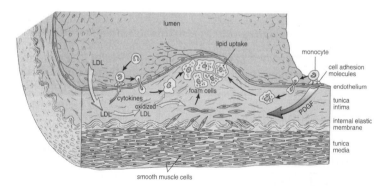

FIGURE 10-2
Schematic diagram of cellular interactions in the formation of an atherosclerotic plaque. (From Ross MH, Kaye G, Pawlina W. Histology, A Text and Atlas, 4th ed. Philadelphia: Lippincott Williams & Wilkins, 2003, p. 333.)

3. Monocytes are transformed into macrophages, which ingest lipids, cholesterol, and other fatty materials to become large foam cells. The lipid is derived from plasma lipoproteins, and low-density lipoprotein (LDL) is the form of lipid most closely associated with accelerated atherosclerosis.

4. Fat-laden foam cells accumulate and release factors, including platelet-derived growth factor (PDGF) that stimulate smooth muscle cells to move from the middle tunica media into the intima.

5. Smooth muscle cells proliferate and also accumulate lipids.

6. Mural thrombosis on the damaged intima stimulates the release of more PDGF, which leads to the secretion of matrix components by the smooth muscle cells.

7. Connective and elastic tissue, cholesterol crystals, and cell debris accumulate to form a patchy plaque. The deeper parts of the thickened intima undergo necrosis.

8. The fibrotic lipid plaque is formed and becomes heterogeneous with respect to inflammatory cell infiltration and matrix organization.

9. As the plaque grows, the lumen of the artery narrows.

10. Complications develop in the plaque, including surface ulceration, fissure formation, calcification, and aneurysm formation.

11. Plaque rupture and ensuing thrombosis and occlusion may precipitate heart attack and stroke.

Pathology

The characteristic lesion of atherosclerosis is the lipid plaque. On gross examination, simple plaques are elevated, pale yellow, smooth-surfaced lesions, irregular in shape. On microscopic examination, plaques are covered by endothelium and involve mainly the intima. The area between the lumen and the necrotic core contains smooth muscle cells, macrophages, lymphocytes, foam cells, and connective tissue components. Cholesterol crystals and foreign body giant cells may be present within the fibrous tissue and the necrotic areas. Plaques may progress with time from a simple fibro-fatty lesion to a complicated plaque with erosion, surface ulceration, plaque hemorrhage, mural thrombosis, calcification, and aneurysm.

Complications

Complications vary with the location and size of the affected vessel (Fig. 10-3). They may include acute occlusion resulting in ischemic necrosis of the tissue supplied by the vessel (e.g., heart attack from occlusion of coronary arteries, stroke from occlusion of brain arteries). Chronic narrowing of the vessel may result in reduced blood flow to the distribution of the artery. An aneurysm may form, weakening the vessel wall, typically in the abdominal aorta. Embo-

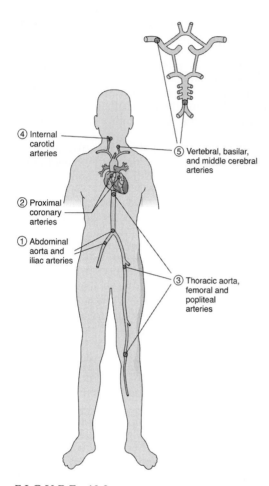

F I G U R E   10-3
Sites of severe atherosclerosis in order of frequency. (From Rubin E, Gorstein F, Rubin R, et al. Rubin's Pathology, 4th ed. Philadelphia: Lippincott Williams & Wilkins, 2005, p. 491)

lization may occur, whereby a thrombus formed over a plaque detaches and lodges in a distant vessel.

Lipid Metabolism and Atherosclerosis

The accumulation of lipid on the wall of an artery is believed to be one of the critical events in the initiation of atherosclerosis. In the body, lipids are important constituents of cell membranes and are stored within cells as a source of fuel.

Because they are insoluble in water, lipids such as cholesterol and triglycerides are transported in the plasma and conjugated to proteins as lipoprotein particles. These consist of a lipid core with associated proteins (apolipoproteins). Lipids have a low density: the higher the lipid content of a particle, the lower the density. High-density lipoprotein (HDL) has a higher ratio of protein to lipid and is therefore the particle with the highest density. The major classes of particles are as follows:

- *Chylomicrons* are formed in intestinal absorptive cells and consist mainly of triglycerides. They transport digested fats to muscle, fat cells and liver.
- *Very-low-density lipoproteins (VLDL)* are formed in the liver and consist mainly of triglycerides and a small percentage of cholesterol. They carry triglycerides from the liver to fat cells.
- *Low-density-lipoproteins (LDL)* are formed from VLDL after delivery of triglycerides to fat cells. More than half of their content is cholesterol, and less than one-tenth triglycerides. They transport cholesterol to different body cells.
- *High-density-lipoproteins (HDL)* are formed in the liver and small intestine. They consist of 25% cholesterol and less than 1% triglycerides. They remove cholesterol from the body tissues and carry it back to the liver. Some of this cholesterol may be excreted in the bile.

Low-density Lipoproteins and Cholesterol Metabolism

Cholesterol is an essential component of cell membranes. Body cells can obtain cholesterol from the diet (exogenous source), or, when dietary sources are low, they can synthesize cholesterol intracellularly (endogenous source). LDL receptors on cell surfaces bind cholesterol-laden LDL, which is taken up via a receptor-mediated pathway. The receptor and lipids are dissociated, and the receptor is returned to the cell surface. The exogenous cholesterol, now in the cytoplasm, causes a reduction in receptor synthesis. At the same time, exogenous cholesterol inhibits the activity of HMG CoA reductase, the key enzyme in the endogenous synthesis of cholesterol. By these two mechanisms exogenous cholesterol inhibits the formation of endogenous cholesterol (Fig.10-4).

High levels of cholesterol in the blood have been associated with atherosclerosis. LDL has been called the "bad cholesterol," because it delivers cholesterol to cells. HDL has been called the "good cholesterol," because it removes cholesterol from body cells and delivers it to the liver for excretion.

LDL has additional "bad" effects. It can be oxidized by the cells that accumulate in the atherosclerotic plaque; oxidized LDL

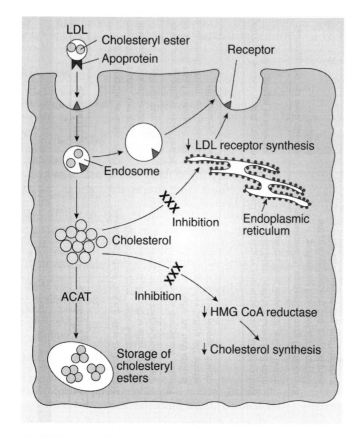

FIGURE   10-4
Low-density lipoprotein and cholesterol metabolism. (From Rubin E, Gorstein F, Rubin R, et al. Rubin's Pathology, 4th ed. Philadelphia Lippincott Williams & Wilkins, 2005, p. 494.)

can activate an inflammatory response. LDL is also toxic to cells in the vascular wall.

Hereditary Disorders of Lipid Metabolism and Atherosclerosis

Familial Hypercholesterolemia

This is an autosomal dominant disease, which results from mutations in the LDL receptor gene. More than 400 mutant alleles for familial hypercholesterolemia have been described. The mutations lead to excessively high levels of plasma cholesterol and cause early onset ischemic heart disease. In addition to the accelerated accumulation of cholesterol in the arteries, LDL cholesterol also deposits in the skin and tendons to form xanthomas.

Apolipoprotein E

In apolipoprotein E, genetic variations in various apoproteins are known to be accompanied by alterations in LDL levels.

Lipoprotein (a)

High levels of the cholesterol-rich lipoprotein (a) are associated with an augmented risk of atherosclerotic disease of the coronary arteries and larger cerebral vessels.

Hypertensive Vascular Disease

Hypertension affects up to 20% of the population in industrial countries and is present in more than half of cases of myocardial infarction, stroke, and chronic renal disease. Most hypertensive persons are described as having "essential" or "primary" hypertension, because the etiology of the disorder remains obscure. Blood pressure varies widely during the course of the day. The World Health Organization has defined hypertension as a systolic pressure greater than 160 mm Hg and a diastolic pressure greater than 90 mm Hg.

Pathogenesis of Hypertension

Blood pressure is simply the product of cardiac output and the systemic vascular resistance to blood flow. Both of these functions are critically influenced by renal function and sodium homeostasis, which interact in the renin-angiotensin system in the following ways:

- A decrease in blood pressure stimulates the kidney juxtaglomerular cells in the wall of the glomerular afferent arteriole to secrete the proteolytic enzyme, renin.
- Renin splits angiotensinogen circulating in the plasma to angiotensin I (an inactive decapeptide).
- Angiotensin I converting enzyme (ACE), located in endothelial cells of the lung and elsewhere, converts angiotensin I to angiotensin II.
- Angiotensin II is a powerful vasoconstrictor, which raises blood pressure. It also stimulates the pituitary to release antidiuretic hormone (ADH), also known as vasopressin. ADH elevates blood pressure by three mechanisms:

  ➤ ADH increases water resorption from the collecting ducts → ⇑ blood volume →⇑ blood pressure

➤ ADH constricts arteriole walls → ⇑ blood pressure
➤ ADH stimulates secretion of aldosterone from the adrenals, which in turn stimulates resorption of NaCl → ⇑ blood volume →⇑ blood pressure

The importance of this system in regulating blood pressure is demonstrated by the therapeutic success in lowering blood pressure by sympathetic antagonists, diuretics, and ACE inhibitors.

Molecular Genetics of Hypertension

The inheritance of essential hypertension is most likely polygenic and not due to single-gene mutations; however, in three hereditary forms of human hypertension, a single gene mutation has been found to cause high blood pressure, and these mutations all result in constitutively increased renal sodium reabsorption. Conversely, mutations that result in sodium wastage are associated with profound hypotension. Thus, these mendelian disorders illustrate the central role for sodium homeostasis in the control of blood pressure.

Acquired Causes of Hypertension

In a small proportion of hypertension, causes are identifiable. These include renal artery stenosis, most forms of chronic renal disease, primary elevation of aldosterone levels, Cushing syndrome, pheochromocytoma, hyperthyroidism, coarctation of the aorta, and renin-secreting tumors. The central lesion in most cases is a decrease in the caliber of the lumen of small muscular arteries and arterioles.

Arteriosclerosis

Chronic hypertension leads to reactive changes in the smaller arteries and arterioles throughout the body, collectively referred to as arteriosclerosis.

- *Benign arteriosclerosis*: This condition reflects mild chronic hypertension, and the major change is a variable increase in the thickness of arterial walls. "Hyaline" refers to the glassy appearance of the vessel walls caused by deposition of plasma proteins.
- *Malignant arteriosclerosis*: Elevated blood pressure results in rapidly progressive vascular disease, with the onset of symptomatic disease in the brain, heart, or kidney. It is ordinarily not evident at pressures less than 160/110 mm Hg. The arterioles exhibit increased amounts of intercellular collagen and glycosaminoglycans, resulting in an "onion-skin" appearance. This restricts the arteriole's capacity to dilate.

Mönckeberg Medial Sclerosis

Mönckeberg medial sclerosis refers to degenerative calcification of the media of large and medium-sized arteries. It occurs principally in older persons, and most often involves the arteries of the upper and lower extremities. This disorder is distinct from atherosclerosis and does not usually lead to any clinical disorder.

On gross examination, the arteries are hard and dilated. Microscopically, the smooth muscle is focally replaced by pale, acellular, hyalinized tissue, with concentric dystrophic calcification.

Raynaud Phenomenon

Raynaud phenomenon refers to intermittent, bilateral attacks of ischemia of the fingers or toes, and sometimes the ears or nose. It is more common in women, and hands are more commonly affected than feet. It is characterized by severe pallor, and is often accompanied by burning, prickling or itching sensations. The symptoms are precipitated by cold or emotional stimuli and relieved by heat.

Raynaud phenomenon may occur as an isolated disorder (Raynaud disease) in young, otherwise healthy women, or as a dominant feature of a number of systemic diseases of connective tissue, such as lupus or scleroderma.

Fibromuscular Dysplasia

This is a rare, noninflammatory thickening of large and medium-sized muscular arteries, which is distinct from atherosclerosis and arteriosclerosis. It is typically a disease of women in their reproductive years. In the renal arteries, the stenosis is an important cause of renovascular hypertension. Fibrous and muscular ridges project into the artery lumen. Smooth muscle is replaced by fibrous tissue. Other than renal hypertension, the major complication of this disorder is dissecting aneurysm of the affected arteries.

Vasculitis

Vasculitis refers to inflammation and necrosis of blood vessels, including arteries, veins, and capillaries. Arteries and veins may be damaged by immune mechanisms, infectious agents, mechanical trauma, radiation, or toxins.

Many vasculitic syndromes are thought to involve immune mechanisms, including (a) the deposition of immune complexes, (b) a direct attack on vessels by circulating antibodies, and (c) various forms of cell-mediated immunity. Inciting agents may be associated with a viral infection. Some vasculitides are associated with antineutrophil cytoplasmic antibodies (ANCA). These can be detected by indirect immunofluorescence assays using the patient's serum and ethanol-fixed neutrophils:

- P-ANCA: a perinuclear immunofluorescence, mainly against myeloperoxidase
- C-ANCA: a more general cytoplasmic immunofluorescence, mainly against proteinase 3

Table 10-3 lists some of the most common properties of various vasculitides. It should be noted that there can be considerable variability in these properties.

Polyarteritis Nodosa

This acute, necrotizing vasculitis affects mainly medium-sized muscular arteries.

Pathology

Lesions are patchy and may not involve the entire circumference of the vessel. The most prominent feature is an area of fibrinoid necrosis in which the media and adventitia are fused into an eosinophilic mass. The inflammatory response involves the entire adventitia (periarteritis). As a result of thrombosis in the artery, infarcts are commonly found in the involved organs. Small aneurysms may form. Healed lesions have a fibrotic media.

Clinical Features

Kidneys, heart, skeletal muscle, skin, and mesentery are most frequently involved. Fever and weight loss are common. Without treatment, polyarteritis nodosa may be fatal, but anti-inflammatory and immunosuppressive therapy can lead to remissions or cures.

Hypersensitivity Angiitis

Hypersensitivity angiitis refers to a broad category of inflammatory vascular lesions representing a reaction to foreign materials such as bacterial products or drugs.

- *Cutaneous vasculitis* may follow the administration of drugs such as aspirin, penicillin, and thiazide diuretics. It may also follow bacterial or viral infections. A palpable purpura of the lower extremities is typical. Microscopically, the superficial cutaneous venules display fibrinoid necrosis and an acute inflammatory reaction. The disease is usually self-limited.
- *Systemic hypersensitivity angiitis* (also referred to as microscopic polyarteritis) may be an isolated entity or a feature of other vascular diseases, and may also exhibit purpuric skin lesions.

Table 10-3
Properties of Vasculitides

Type	Sex Ratio (M:F)	Age Range (years)	Vessel Size	ANCA Association	Distribution
Giant Cell Arteritis (Temporal)	1:3	50–75	Large		Temporal artery
Takayasu's Arteritis	1:9	15–25	Large		Aorta and its branches
Kawasaki Disease	1:5	1–5	Large to medium		Coronary arteries
Polyarteritis nodosa	2:1	40–60	Medium to small	P-ANCA	Kidney, heart, muscle, skin, mesentery
Wegener's Granulomatosis	1:1	30–50	Small	C-ANCA 70% P-ANCA 10%	Respiratory tract, kidney, spleen
Microscopic Polyangiitis			Small	60% P-ANCA 40% C-ANCA	Skin, occasionally renal
Churg-Strauss Syndrome	2:1	40–60	Medium to small	70% exhibit C-ANCA or P-ANCA	Lungs (asthma), kidney, heart, liver, CNS
Buerger Disease	1:9	20–50	Medium to small		Hands and Feet
Behçet Disease	1:1	20–35	Small		Oral, genital, ocular

A feared complication of microscopic polyarteritis is renal involvement, characterized by rapidly progressive glomerulonephritis and renal failure. Microscopic polyarteritis is associated with the presence of ANCA.

Allergic Granulomatosis and Angiitis (Churg-Strauss Syndrome)

This syndrome is a systemic vasculitis that occurs in young people with asthma, and features eosinophilia. Widespread necrotizing vascular lesions of small- and medium-sized arteries are found in multiple organs. There is prominent involvement of the lungs. Two thirds of patients exhibit C-ANCA or P-ANCA.

Giant Cell Arteritis (Temporal Arteritis, Granulomatous Arteritis)

This is the most common vasculitis, with an average age at onset of 70 years. It involves a focal, chronic, granulomatous inflammation, usually of the temporal arteries and their branches.

Pathology

Lesions are characterized by granulomatous inflammation of the media and intima with giant cells at the site of the internal elastic lamina and infiltrates of leukocytes and plasma cells. The internal elastica may be fragmented.

Clinical Features

Patients present with headache and throbbing temporal pain. Visual symptoms occur in almost half the patients. Swelling and tenderness are present in the skin overlying the affected artery.

Wegener Granulomatosis

Wegener granulomatosis is a systemic necrotizing vasculitis characterized by lesions of the nose, sinuses, lungs, and renal glomerular disease. The etiology is unknown. More than 90% of patients have ANCA in their blood; of those, 75% are C-ANCA, which suggests that activated neutrophils are responsible for attack on vessel walls.

Pathology

Lesions of Wegener granulomatosis feature parenchymal necrosis and a granulomatous inflammation composed of neutrophils and other leukocytes. The individual lesions of the lung may be as large as 5 cm across. Vasculitis involves small to medium-sized vessels most frequently in the respiratory tract, kidney, and spleen.

Clinical Features

A persistent bilateral pneumonitis and chronic sinusitis are prominent. Hematuria and proteinuria indicate glomerular involvement. The untreated disease is fatal; immunosuppressive treatment with cyclophosphamide leads to striking improvement.

Takayasu Arteritis

Takayasu arteritis refers to an inflammatory disorder of the aortic arch and its major branches. It affects young women (usually younger than 30 years of age). An autoimmune basis has been proposed.

Pathology

The aorta is thickened and has focal raised plaques. The branches of the aorta display stenosis and occlusion, interfering with blood flow and accounting for the synonym, "pulseless disease."

Clinical Features

Constitutional symptoms (dizziness, visual disturbance, dyspnea) may be noted. Asymmetric differences in blood pressure may develop, and the pulse in one extremity may disappear.

Kawasaki Disease (Mucocutaneous Lymph Node Syndrome)

Kawasaki disease is an acute necrotizing vasculitis of infancy and early childhood characterized by high fever, rash, conjunctival and oral lesions, and lymphadenitis. In 70% of patients, the vasculitis may affect the coronary arteries and cause aneurysms. The disease is usually self-limited. An infectious cause is suspected.

Thromboangiitis Obliterans (Buerger Disease)

This is an occlusive inflammatory disease of medium and small arteries in the distal arms and legs. It is exacerbated by smoking, which plays an etiological role in the disease. An increased prevalence of HLA-A9 and HLA-B5 haplotypes among patients with the disease lends credence to the idea that a genetic hypersensitivity to tobacco is involved in the pathogenesis.

Pathology

Acute inflammation of medium and small arteries, with involvement of the endothelium, may lead to thrombosis and obliteration of the lumen.

Clinical Features

Symptoms usually begin between 25 and 40 years of age with cramping pains in muscles following exercise. Painful ischemic disease can lead to gangrene of the extremity with possible necessity of amputation.

Behçet Disease

Behçet disease is a widespread vasculitis of many organs, characterized by oral and genital ulcers and ocular inflammation, with occasional lesions in the central nervous system, gastrointestinal tract, and cardiovascular system. Large and small vessels are involved; the cause is unknown.

Radiation Vasculitis

This form of vasculitis has an acute phase with injury to the endothelium and a chronic phase with fibrosis of the vessel wall. Radiation damage predisposes to accelerated atherosclerosis.

Rickettsial Vasculitis

Rickettsia are intracellular parasites that produce a characteristic vasculitis. Different rickettsial diseases affect different types of small vessels in extent and severity.

Aneurysms

Arterial aneurysms are localized dilations of blood vessels caused by a congenital or acquired weakness in the media. They are classified by location, configuration, and etiology. The gross morphology of aneurysms reveals different features:

- Fusiform aneurysm: An ovoid swelling parallel to the long axis of the vessel
- Saccular aneurysm: A bubblelike outpouching of the wall
- Dissecting aneurysm: A hematoma in which hemorrhage into the media separates the layers of the vessel wall by a column of blood
- Arteriovenous aneurysm: A direct communication between an artery and a vein

Abdominal Aortic Aneurysms

Abdominal aortic aneurysms are complications of atherosclerosis. They are defined as a dilation of the vessel in which its diameter is increased at least 50%. They are typically found in men older than 50 years of age, and half of the patients are hypertensive.

The aneurysms are usually fusiform and more than 5 to 6 cm in diameter, and the risk of rupture increases with the diameter. Most abdominal aneurysms are lined by raised, ulcerated, and calcified atherosclerotic lesions. The vessel wall is fibrous with a thickened and inflamed adventitia.

Aneurysms of Cerebral Arteries

The most common type of cerebral aneurysm is saccular and is called a "berry aneurysm." It results from a congenital defect in a branch point of the arterial wall.

Dissecting Aneurysms

Dissecting aneurysm refers to the entry of blood into the arterial wall and its extension along the length of the vessel. It usually occurs in the wall of the ascending aorta, and forms a second arterial lumen within the media. It is most common in men in the sixth or seventh decades.

Pathogenesis

Some cases of dissecting aneurysm represent a complication of Marfan syndrome (see Chapter 6). Most cases of dissecting aneurysm show a transverse tear in the intima and internal media. This allows blood from the lumen to enter and dissect the media. Hemorrhage into the extravascular space is a frequent cause of death. Aortic rupture into the pericardial sac can cause fatal cardiac tamponade.

Clinical Features

A severe "tearing" chest pain with acute onset is characteristic of an aortic dissection, which is sometimes diagnosed as myocardial infarction, but electrocardiogram and serum enzymes are normal. Surgical intervention and control of hypertension have reduced the overall mortality to less than 20%.

Syphilitic Aneurysms

Syphilitic (luetic) aneurysms reflect an aortitis and were once the most common form of aortic aneurysm. With better treatment and control of syphilis, its incidence has decreased. The aneurysms affect the ascending aorta with focal necrosis of the vasa vasorum and disruption of the elastic laminae in the media. The scars formed give a "tree bark" appearance to the vessel wall.

Mycotic (Infectious) Aneurysms

These aneurysms result from the weakening of the vessel wall by a microbial infection and have a tendency to rupture and hemorrhage.

Veins

Varicose Veins of the Leg

A varicose vein is an enlarged and tortuous blood vessel. Superficial leg varicosities, usually in the saphenous system, are extremely common.

Pathogenesis

Risk factors for varicose veins include (a) age, with the increase in frequency reflecting degenerative changes in the vein walls, loss of supporting fat and muscle tone, (b) sex; women more affected than men, (c) heredity (familial predisposition), (d) posture, with prolonged standing, and (e) obesity

Pathology and Clinical Features

Varicose veins exhibit variations in wall thickness, patchy calcifications, and deformity of valves. Most require no treatment. Severe varicosities may lead to ulcerations, and may need surgical intervention.

Varicose Veins at Other Sites

- *Hemorrhoids*: Dilations of the veins of the rectum and anal canal may occur inside or outside of the anal sphincter. They are aggravated by constipation and pregnancy, and often bleed.
- *Esophageal Varices*: These are complications of portal hypertension and are caused mainly by liver cirrhosis. High portal pressure leads to distension of the anastomoses between the portal system and the veins at the lower end of the esophagus.
- *Variocele:* This palpable mass in the scrotum is formed by varicosities of the pampiniform plexus.

Deep Venous Thrombosis

This term now refers to conditions that principally affect leg veins, and includes thrombophlebitis (inflammation and thrombosis resulting from an infection), and phlebothrombosis (thrombosis occurring in the absence of an initiating infection). Deep venous thrombosis is associated with prolonged bed rest or reduced cardiac output.

Lymphatic Vessels

Lymphangitis

The thin-walled lymphatic capillaries draining interstitial spaces can pick up foreign material and cellular debris in the area. This can cause an inflammation of the lymphatics (lymphangitis), which can then transport inflammatory products to regional lymph nodes, and cause lymphadenitis. Pathogens such as β-hemolytic streptococci are common offenders. Draining lymph nodes become enlarged and inflamed. These can be accompanied by painful subcutaneous streaks in the region of the inflamed nodes.

Lymphatic Obstruction and Lymphedema

When major lymphatic trunks (especially in the axilla or groin) are obstructed by scar tissue, tumor cells, or parasites, lymphedema can occur. Prolonged obstruction leads to a progressive dilation of lymphatic vessels called lymphangiectasia. The term elephantiasis describes a lymphadematous limb that has become grossly enlarged as the result of filariasis, a tropical infection by a parasitic worm.

Benign Tumors of Blood Vessels

Tumors of the vascular system are common; many are actually hamartomas (masses of disorganized cells and tissues).

Hemangiomas

These are common benign tumors of infancy and are composed of vascular channels, usually in the skin. There are three general types:

- Capillary hemangioma is a lesion composed of capillary-like channels that may be located in the skin, subcutaneous tissues, mucous membranes of the lips and mouth, spleen, kidneys, and liver. They are bright red or blue, depending on the degree of oxygenation of the blood. In the skin, they are known as "birthmarks."
- Juvenile hemangiomas, also called "strawberry hemangiomas," are found on the skin of newborns, grow rapidly in the first few months, and usually regress by 5 years of age. They are composed of packed masses of capillaries separated by connective tissue.
- Cavernous hemangiomas consist of large cavernous channels occurring in the skin where they are called "port wine stains." They may also occur on mucosal surfaces, spleen, liver, and pancreas. Occasionally, they are found in the brain where they may slowly enlarge and cause neurological symptoms. They do not regress spontaneously.

Other hemangiomatous syndromes include the rare von Hippel-Lindau syndrome, characterized by cavernous hemangiomas in the cerebellum and retina, and the Sturge-Weber syndrome, characterized by a developmental disturbance of blood vessels in the brain and skin.

Glomus Tumors (Glomangiomas)

These benign but painful neoplasms of the glomus body (an arteriolar-venous anastomosis) are most frequent in the distal regions of fingers and toes. Histologically, they consist of nests of glomus tumor cells embedded in a fibrovascular stroma.

Hemangioendotheliomas

These vascular tumors are intermediate between benign hemangiomas and malignant angiosarcomas. The epithelioid endothelial cells are eosinophilic with vacuolated cytoplasm. These tumors are usually curative after excision, but one fifth of patients develop metastases.

Malignant Tumors of Blood Vessels

Angiosarcoma

Angiosarcoma is a rare, highly malignant tumor composed of malignant endothelial cells, which most commonly arise in skin, soft tissue, breast, bone, liver, and spleen. It begins as small, sharply demarcated red nodules but enlarges to become a pale fleshy mass without a capsule. It exhibits varying degrees of differentiation, ranging from distinct vessels to few recognizable channels. Liver angiosarcoma has been associated with arsenic (a component of pesticides), vinyl chloride (in plastic production), and the administration of thorium by radiologists.

Hemangiopericytoma

Hemangiopericytoma is a rare malignant neoplasm that arises from pericytes, the contractile cell external to the walls of capillaries. It occurs most frequently in the retroperitoneum and lower extremities.

Kaposi Sarcoma

Kaposi sarcoma is a malignant tumor derived from endothelial cells and is a complication of AIDS. It begins as painful purple or brown nodules in the skin. Histologically, the lesions are quite variable but often contain poorly differentiated, spindle-shaped cells and a vascular lesion filled with red blood cells.

Tumors of the Lymphatic System

Capillary Lymphangiomas

Capillary lymphangiomas (simple lymphangiomas) are benign tumors composed of small grayish pink fleshy nodules. They are subcutaneous and can occur in the skin of the face, lips, chest, genitalia, or extremities. Microscopically, they appear as a network of lymphatics.

Cystic Lymphangiomas

These benign lesions in the neck or axilla are soft, spongy, and pink. They are composed of endothelial-lined spaces filled with a proteinaceous fluid.

Lymphangiosarcomas

These rare malignant tumors may follow lymphedema or radiation. They present as purplish nodules in edematous skin, and may develop in 0.1% to 0.5% of patients with lymphedema of the arm following radical mastectomy.

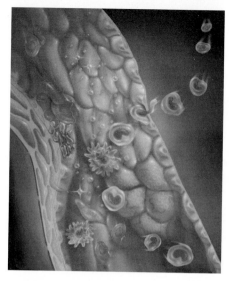

CHAPTER *11*

The Heart

Chapter Outline

Normal Anatomy and Histology

The heart is a fist-sized muscular pump that weighs approximately 240 to 340 grams (Fig. 11-1). The flow of blood out of the heart is influenced by a variety of factors, including the resistance to outflow (systemic venous pressure or pulmonary artery pressure), contractility, heart rate, cardiac fitness, and conduction of electrical impulses. The lower venous pressure and afterload on the right side of the heart is reflected in the thinner wall of the right ventricle (<0.5 cm wall thickness), as compared to the left ventricle (1.3–1.5 cm wall thickness).

The myocardium is a syncytial network of myocytes that are connected by cell-cell mechanical and electrical junctions. Contraction of each myocyte occurs by changes in the sarcomere, which is the basic functional unit of the myocyte. The sarcomere is formed by interdigitated thick and thin filaments. Thick filaments are formed of myosin heavy chains, myosin binding protein C, and myosin light chains. Thin filaments are formed of actin and regulatory components, which include tropomyosin and the troponin complex. The amount of force generated by the cardiac myocyte is reflected in the amount of overlap between thick and thin filaments, with an optimal sarcomere length of 2.0 to 2.2 μm. The Starling law of the heart states that the contractile force of the heart is a function of diastolic fiber length.

Contraction of the heart is regulated by calcium entry into the myocyte, which triggers a conformational change in the regulatory proteins and allows repetitive cycling (by repetitive cross-linking of the actin and myosin within the sarcomere). In general, the force generated by the myocyte is directly proportional to the amount of calcium that enters the cell.

The conduction system of the heart initiates the heartbeat at the sinoatrial node, which then transmits the electrical impulse through the atria, atrioventricular node, bundle of His, and ulti-

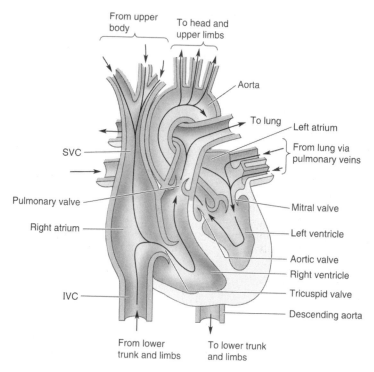

FIGURE   11-1
Diagram of heart demonstrating cardiac chambers and valves. (From Moore KL, Dalley AF. Clinically Oriented Anatomy, 4th ed. Philadelphia: Lippincott Williams & Wilkins, 1999, p. 121.)

mately the right and left branches of the Purkinje system that activate the ventricular muscle. In instances of sinoatrial node dysfunction, the more distal components of the conducting system take over the role of pacemaker and, as a general rule, the more distal the site of electrical impulse, the slower the heart rate.

The coronary arteries supply the cardiac muscle and are composed of the right and left coronary arteries. The left main coronary artery bifurcates early in its course into the left anterior descending artery (LAD) and the left circumflex artery. The "dominance" of the coronary circulation is ascribed to the coronary artery that supplies the posterior descending coronary artery, which is most commonly a right coronary-dominant distribution. Blood flow in the heart typically passes from the coronary artery terminals to the epicardium then endocardium. In cases of myocardial ischemia, the endocardium is generally the most vulnerable site.

Myocardial Hypertrophy and Heart Failure

Cardiac output can be described by the Frank-Starling mechanism, which states that the stroke volume of the heart is a function of the diastolic fiber length and that, within certain limits, the heart will pump whatever volume is brought to it by the venous circulation. Under normal circumstances, the heart typically ejects approximately 60% of the ventricular volume during systole (ejection fraction). In disease states, however, the heart can undergo compensatory changes such as hypertrophy to maintain cardiac output. When compensatory mechanisms begin to fail, patients may develop congestive heart failure. In cases of acute severe impairment, cardiac output cannot be maintained, and patients may experience life-threatening cardiogenic shock.

Myocardial hypertrophy is an adaptive response that increases the contractile strength of the myocyte and develops under conditions of hemodynamic overload, such as chronic hypertension, valvular stenosis, valvular insufficiency, myocardial injury, or other stresses. Hypertrophy is characterized by an increased size of the myocyte and increased amounts of sarcomeric proteins, without an increase in myocyte number. Over time, hypertrophy can lead to ventricular dilation. Multiple factors are involved in the development of cardiac hypertrophy, including the following:

- Angiotensin II: locally secreted factor that promotes hypertrophy and formation of the extracellular matrix
- Endothelin-1: vasoconstrictor and myocyte growth factor produced by the heart
- Insulin-like growth factor-1: locally secreted factor that promotes myocyte growth
- Extracellular matrix: increased collagen synthesis in cardiac overload can lead to impaired oxygen and nutrient diffusion
- β-adrenergic desensitization: decreased cardiac response to catecholamines due to defective coupling of the receptor to adenylyl cyclase
- Calcium homeostasis: decreased numbers of RyR2 channels and decreased calcium uptake by the sarcolemma lead to reduced cytosolic calcium and impaired contractility
- Protooncogene expression: c-jun and c-fos are expressed with acute overload and may promote the expression of fetal genes
- Fetal gene expression: atrial natriuretic factor and brain natriuretic protein are reexpressed in the adult heart following overload and can reduce hemodynamic stress by affecting sodium and water balance. In addition, the failing heart may utilize glucose rather than fatty acids for energy secondary to reexpression of fetal genes.

A variety of disorders may cause heart failure, including ischemic heart disease (80% of cases), cardiomyopathies, and congenital heart disease. The majority of patients with cardiac failure have ventricular hypertrophy. In cases in which the left ventricle hypertrophies and fails, the right ventricle undergoes some level of hypertrophy due to the increased workload. In most cases, ventricular hypertrophy is followed by dilation of the ventricles.

Left-sided heart failure is the most common form of heart failure and often occurs secondary to ischemic heart disease and hypertension. The left atrial and pulmonary venous pressures increase, which results in passive pulmonary congestion, small ruptures of the pulmonary capillaries, and extrusion of fluid from the alveolar capillaries. Patients commonly demonstrate dyspnea on exertion, orthopnea (dyspnea when lying down), paroxysmal nocturnal dyspnea, and often pulmonary edema. The lungs often demonstrate the presence of hemosiderin-laden macrophages ("heart failure cells") due to small capillary rupture. In addition, the inadequate arterial perfusion of end organs results in the retention of sodium and water, leading to volume overloads.

Right-sided heart failure may occur with intrinsic pulmonary disease or pulmonary hypertension or secondary to left-sided heart failure. Patients often demonstrate jugular venous distention, lower extremity edema, and congestion of the liver ("nutmeg liver") and spleen.

Microscopically, the damaged myocytes contain a vacuolated appearance of the cytoplasm due to increased amounts of glycogen and degenerative changes due to loss of myofibrils.

Congenital Heart Disease

Congenital heart disease (CHD) occurs in approximately 1% of all live births and may occur in isolation or in combination with other congenital defects. Table 11-1 lists the defects and the relative inci-

Table 11-1
Relative Incidence of Specific Anomalies in Patients with Congenital Heart Disease

Ventricular septal defects—25% to 30%
Atrial septal defects—10% to 15%
Patent ductus arteriosus—10% to 20%
Tetralogy of Fallot—4% to 9%
Pulmonary stenosis—5% to 7%
Coarctation of the aorta—5% to 7%
Aortic stenosis—4% to 6%
Complete transposition of the great arteries—4% to 10%
Truncus arteriosus—2%
Tricuspid atresia—1%

From Rubin E, Gorstein F, Rubin R, et al. Rubin's Pathology, 4th ed. Philadelphia: Lippincott Williams & Wilkins, p. 530.

dence of each. Both environmental and genetic influences have been implicated in the development of CHD, and risk factors include the use of certain drugs in early pregnancy, maternal diabetes, and maternal infection with rubella virus during the first trimester. Single-gene defects that lead to CHD include Turner syndrome, DiGeorge syndrome, and trisomy 21.

CHD can be categorized by the presence of underlying shunts within the cardiovascular system, as described in Table 11-2. Patients that lack a shunt are typically acyanotic, whereas patients that have a permanent right-to-left shunt or that are in late stages of an initial left-to-right shunt that has reversed the direction of flow (Eisenmenger complex) become cyanotic.

Congenital Heart Disease with Initial Left-to-right Shunts

Initial left-to-right shunts include a broad variety of CHDs, which are described in Table 11-3. Early in the course of disease, patients typically are acyanotic but become cyanotic in later stages when

Table 11-2
Classification of Congenital Heart Disease

Initial left-to-right shunt

Ventricular septal defect
Atrial septal defect
Patent ductus arteriosus
Persistent truncus arteriosus
Anomalous pulmonary venous drainage
Hypoplastic left heart syndrome

Right-to-left shunt

Tetralogy of Fallot
Tricuspid atresia

No shunt

Complete transposition of the great vessels
Coarctation of the aorta
Pulmonary stenosis
Aortic stenosis
Coronary artery origin from pulmonary artery
Ebstein malformation
Complete heart block
Endocardial fibroelastosis

From Rubin E, Gorstein F, Rubin R, et al. Rubin's Pathology, 4th ed. Philadelphia: Lippincott Williams & Wilkins, p. 531.

Table 11-3
Congenital Heart Disease with Initial Left-to-right Shunts

Disease	Description
Ventricular septal defect (VSD)	Most common CHD; often found in the membranous septum below the outflow tract of the pulmonary artery; small VSDs often close spontaneously; large VSDs may lead to heart failure, infective endocarditis, paradoxical emboli, prolapse of an aortic valve cusp, and pulmonary hypertension
Atrial septal defect (ASD)	Normal connection between the atria (foramen ovale, ostium secundum, ostium primum, sinus venosus, atrioventricular canal) is maintained following birth; patients with early disease may show easy fatigability and exertional dyspnea and later show cyanosis and clubbing of the fingers; may be complicated by arrhythmias, pulmonary hypertension, right ventricular hypertrophy, heart failure, paradoxical emboli and bacterial endocarditis
Patent ductus arteriosus (PDA)	Persistence of fetal structure can lead to complications if large, including left ventricular hypertrophy, heart failure, pulmonary hypertension, and bacterial endocarditis; may be corrected by prostaglandin inhibitor application (e.g., indomethacin)
Persistent truncus arteriosus	Common trunk for the aorta, pulmonary arteries, and coronary arteries that always overrides a VSD and receives blood from both ventricles; patients have rapid heart failure, recurrent respiratory tract infections, and early death due to large-volume pulmonary blood flow
Hypoplastic left heart syndrome	Hypoplasia of the left ventricle and ascending aorta and hypoplasia or atresia of the left-sided valves; accompanied by an obligate left-to-right shunt through a patent foramen ovale; systemic blood flow passes from the pulmonary trunk to the aorta via a patent ductus arteriosus
Anomalous pulmonary venous return	Most commonly, total anomalous pulmonary vein drainage demonstrates pulmonary vein drainage into a common pulmonary venous chamber and then through a persistent left superior vena cava; patients can survive only if a patent foramen ovale or atrial septal defect is present

the flow of the shunt reverses to right-to-left, generally secondary to increased pulmonary pressures. In many cases, the initial defect may go unrecognized until late reversal of flow results in cyanosis, left ventricular dilation, and heart failure. In a subset of cases, paradoxical emboli may occur, in which emboli cross from the right side of the heart to the left side (with subsequent systemic embolization) via a septal defect.

The most common form of CHD is a *ventricular septal defect* (*VSD*). The VSD may occur at any point along the muscular or membranous portions of the interventricular septum and can vary tremendously in size. The most common location of a VSD is within the membranous portion of the interventricular septum, which grows downward from the endocardial cushions and is situated below the outflow tract of the pulmonary artery or behind the septal leaflet of the tricuspid valve. Small defects may close spontaneously, whereas larger defects can lead to reversal of flow due to increased pulmonary pressures, left ventricular dilation, and congestive heart failure. Complications of VSDs include infective endocarditis, paradoxical emboli, and prolapse of an aortic valve cusp.

Atrial septal defects (*ASDs*) are also common defects that involve the atrial septum. The development of the atrial septum is complex and includes the formation of a downward growing septum primum that extends to the endocardial cushion, a subsequent defect in this septum primum that allows fetal right-to-left shunting (termed the ostium secundum), and the ultimate development of a second septum (septum secundum) to the right of the septum primum. The ultimate structure formed by these septa is the foramen ovale, which persists until birth and, when sealed, is termed the fossa ovalis. Multiple subtypes of ASDs exist and include the following:

- Patent foramen ovale: as many as 25% of normal adults may harbor an asymptomatic minute opening, which can be identified only by examination with a probe (probe patent foramen ovale), and which may become a true right-to-left shunt with increased right atrial pressure
- Ostium secundum type: is the most common ASD (90% of cases) and is found in the middle portion of the septum; if combined with mitral stenosis is termed *Lutembacher syndrome*
- Ostium primum type: involves the region adjacent to the endocardial cushions
- Sinus venosus defect: is found in the upper portion of the septum near the entry of the superior vena cava
- Atrioventricular canal: may be partial or complete and involves both the atrial and ventricular septum

Figure 11-2 demonstrates the normal development of the atrial and ventricular septa. Early in life, patients with an ASD may describe early fatigability and exertional dyspnea. Later in life, a right-to-left shunt may develop secondary to increased pulmonary pres-

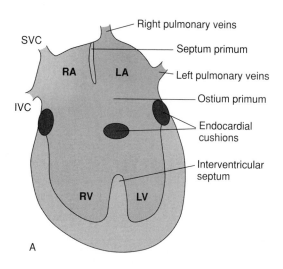

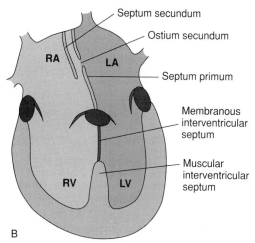

FIGURE 11-2

A. The common atrial chamber is being separated into the right and
left atria (RA and LA) by the septum primum. Because the septum
primum has not yet joined the endocardial cushions, there is an
open ostium primum. The ventricular cavity is being divided by a
muscular interventricular septum into right and left chambers (RV
and LV). SVC, superior vena cava; IVC, inferior vena cava. B. Formation of separate chambers of the heart. (From Rubin E, Gorstein F,
Rubin R, et al. Rubin's Pathology, 4th ed. Philadelphia: Lippincott
Williams & Wilkins, p. 532.)

Table 11-4
Congenital Heart Disease without Shunts

Disease	Description
Transposition of the great arteries	The aorta arises from the right ventricle and the pulmonary artery arises from the left ventricle; survival is only possible in the presence of a communication between the two circulations such as an ASD, VSD, or patent ductus arteriosus
Coarctation of the aorta	Local constriction of the aorta that often occurs below the origin of the left subclavian artery at the site of the ductus arteriosus; may be associated with Turner syndrome or berry aneurysms in the brain; identified clinically by a difference in blood pressure between the upper and lower extremities resulting in left ventricular hypertrophy, dizziness, and headaches; radiologically identified by notching of the inner surfaces of the ribs
Pulmonary stenosis	May involve the pulmonary valves, the right ventricular infundibular muscle with subvalvular stenosis, or peripheral portions of the pulmonary arteries
Congenital aortic stenosis	May be valvular (often with a bicuspid aortic valve), subvalvular (band of fibroelastic tissue or muscular ridge below the valves), or a supravalvular stenosis; over time, may result in a calcified valve with reduced mobility leading to dyspnea and angina pectoris
Coronary artery arising from a pulmonary artery	Region of the myocardium supplied by the aberrant coronary artery may undergo ischemia secondary to the decreased oxygen content of the pulmonary artery
Ebstein malformation	Downward displacement of an abnormal tricuspid valve (often the septal or posterior valve) into an underdeveloped right ventricle; the valves appear elongated and adherent to the ventricular wall; can lead to heart failure, right atrial dilation, arrhythmias, and sudden death
Congenital heart block	Disruption of the conducting system that often complicates other congenital heart defects; can lead to cardiac hypertrophy Arrhythmias, dizziness, and heart failure
Endocardial fibroelastosis	Fibroelastic thickening of the endocardium of the left ventricle that can affect the valves; may be primary or secondary to factors that lead to left ventricular hypertrophy; grossly the heart show gray-white patches
Dextrocardia	A rightward orientation of the base-apex axis of the heart; the heart is functionally normal if dextrocardia occurs in association with situs inversus (inverted position of the visceral organs)

sures, leading to cyanosis and clubbing of the fingers. Complications may include atrial arrhythmias, pulmonary hypertension, right ventricular hypertrophy, heart failure, paradoxical emboli, and bacterial endocarditis.

Additional defects that involve an initial left-to-right shunt are described in Table 11-3 and include a patent ductus arteriosus, truncus arteriosus, hypoplastic left heart syndrome, and anomalous pulmonary venous return.

Congenital Heart Disease with Right-to-left Shunts

CHD that demonstrates right-to-left shunts include tetralogy of Fallot and tricuspid atresia.

Tetralogy of Fallot represents 10% of all cases of CHD and is defined by four anatomical defects:

- Pulmonary stenosis
- Ventricular septal defect that involves the muscular septum and the endocardial cushions
- Dextroposition of the aorta so that it overrides the ventricular septal defect
- Right ventricular hypertrophy

The heart in tetralogy of Fallot undergoes hypertrophy and demonstrates an overall boot shape. In addition, almost half of all patients have additional cardiac anomalies, including ostium secundum ASDs, patent ductus arteriosus, a left superior vena cava, and endocardial cushion defects. If the cardiac defects are not corrected during the first two years of life, patients develop exertional dyspnea, arterial desaturation, and cyanosis. Complications may include heart failure, growth retardation, polycythemia, bacterial endocarditis, and brain abscesses.

Tricuspid atresia is the congenital absence of the tricuspid valve that results in a right-to-left shunt through a patent foramen ovale.

Congenital Heart Disease without Shunts

A variety of CHDs can produce serious symptoms without the presence of a shunt. These conditions are described in Table 11-4.

Ischemic Heart Disease

Ischemic heart disease occurs most commonly in the setting of atherosclerosis, although coronary vasospasm, aortic stenosis, or aortic insufficiency can also induce cardiac ischemia. In general, atherosclerotic heart disease is responsible for the vast majority of

Table 11-5

Risk factors for ischemic heart disease

Systemic hypertension	Obesity
Cigarette smoking	Increasing age
Diabetes mellitus	Male gender
Elevated blood cholesterol: specifically,	Family history
elevated low-density lipoproteins	Sedentary lifestyle
(LDLs) and reduced high-density	Aberrant serum thrombotic or
lipoproteins (HDLs)	thrombolytic factors

deaths related to cardiac disease. Risk factors for ischemic heart disease are listed in Table 11-5.

Any condition that interferes with the blood supply to the heart, oxygenation of the blood, or increased cardiac work may lead to ischemic heart disease (Table 11-6). Blood flow to the heart is only compromised in the setting of extensive luminal narrowing (50% to 75% luminal stenosis); the coronary arteries are small muscular arteries that provide minimal resistance to blood flow and. In many cases, acute myocardial infarction is caused by thrombosis secondary to spontaneous rupture of an atherosclerotic plaque. The distribution of myocardial infarction demonstrates specific locations depending on the coronary artery involved (Fig. 11-3) and different microscopic features based on the age of the infarct.

Myocardial infarcts may be categorized as subendocardial or transmural. Subendocardial infarcts affect the inner third of the left ventricle and often occur as a consequence of hypoperfusion of the heart. In contrast, transmural infarcts involve the full thickness of the ventricular wall and often occur following occlusion of a coronary artery. The infarct can progress over time and the extension of the infarct is related to the volume of arterial collateral flow.

Manifestations of ischemic heart disease include the following:

- *Angina pectoris*: typically, substernal pain that radiates to the left arm, jaw, and epigastric region and may be accompanied by diaphoresis and nausea
- *Stable angina*: angina induced by physical exertion or emotional stress and relieved by rest or sublingual nitroglycerine
- *Unstable angina*: unpredictable onset of angina that may occur during rest or sleep, that is associated with the development of nonocclusive thrombi over atherosclerotic plaques, and that may rapidly progress to myocardial infarction
- *Prinzmetal angina*: atypical form of angina that occurs at rest and is caused by coronary artery spasm

Table 11-6

Causes of Ischemic Heart Disease

Decreased supply of oxygen

Conditions that influence the supply of blood

Atherosclerosis and thrombosis
Thromboemboli
Coronary artery spasm
Collateral blood vessels
Blood pressure, cardiac output, and heart rate
Miscellaneous: arteritis (e.g., periarteritis nodosa), dissecting aneurysm,
    luetic aortitis, anomalous origin of coronary artery, muscular bridging
    of coronary artery

Conditions that influence the availability of oxygen in the blood

Anemia
Shift in the hemoglobin-oxygen dissociation curve
Carbon monoxide
Cyanide

Increased oxygen demand (i.e., increased cardiac work)

Hypertension
Valvular stenosis or insufficiency
Hyperthyroidism
Fever
Thiamine deficiency
Catecholamines

From Rubin E, Gorstein F, Rubin R, et al. Rubin's Pathology, 4th ed.
Philadelphia: Lippincott Williams & Wilkins, p. 543.

- *Myocardial infarction*: discrete focus of infarction that occurs along specific vascular distributions
- *Ischemic cardiomyopathy:* repeated episodes of ischemia results in myocyte damage and left ventricular dysfunction, leading to congestive heart failure
- *Sudden death*: often caused by an acute thrombosis of a coronary artery leading to ventricular fibrillation

During the first 20 to 30 minutes of ischemia, myocyte damage may be reversible. However, ischemia of longer duration results in permanent myocyte damage and grossly identifiable changes. The gross and microscopic findings associated with myocardial infarction vary with time and the major findings are included in Table 11-7.

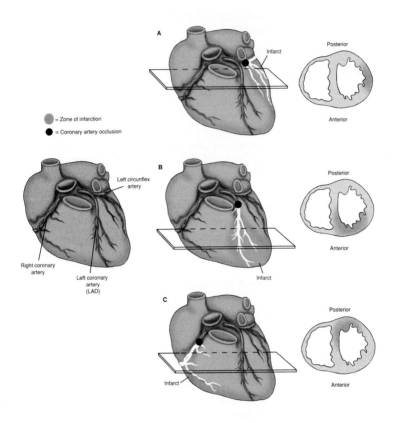

FIGURE 11-3
Position of left ventricular infarcts resulting from occlusion of each of the three main coronary arteries. A. Posterolateral infarct. B. Anterior infarct. C. Posterior infarct. (From Rubin E, Gorstein F, Rubin R, et al. Rubin's Pathology, 4th ed. Philadelphia: Lippincott Williams & Wilkins, p. 524.)

When reperfusion of the ischemic myocytes occurs, the area of infarct appears hemorrhagic, and the myocytes show contraction band necrosis with thick, irregular, eosinophilic in necrotic myocytes.

Myocardial infarcts may present with substernal or precordial crushing pain that may extend into the jaw or down the inside of the left arm. Patients may also experience nausea, vomiting, diaphoresis, and shortness of breath. A subset of myocardial infarc-

Table 11-7

Gross and Microscopic Findings in Cardiac Ischemia

Time Following Onset of Ischemia	Findings
12–18 hours	Infarct becomes visible as gross area of pallor and microscopically contains deeply eosinophilic fibers with coagulation necrosis and formation of "wavy fibers"
24 hours	Infiltration of neutrophils at the periphery of the infarct and myocytes lose nuclei
5–7 days	Grossly the infarct appears mottled and more sharply outlined with a pale necrotic region surrounded by a hyperemic zone and microscopically the neutrophilic response has abated; the periphery shows phagocytosis of the dead muscle by macrophages, fibroblast proliferation, and lymphocyte infiltration
2–3 weeks	Grossly the region is depressed and soft; microscopically, the collagen deposition abates and collagen deposition begins
>1 month	The infarct appears grossly firm and white and microscopically appears as dense fibrous tissue

tions may be silent, especially in diabetic patients. Electrocardiography demonstrates new Q waves and changes in the ST segment. Elevations in cardiac enzymes included cardiac troponins and the MB isoform of CK are present.

Treatment of a myocardial infarction includes restoration of blood flow by thrombolytic enzymes (tissue plasminogen activator or streptokinase) or percutaneous transluminal coronary angioplasty (PTCA). In addition, coronary artery bypass grafting may be used to restore blood flow to a distal segment of an occluded coronary artery.

Complications of myocardial infarctions include the following:

- Arrhythmias
- Left ventricular failure and cardiogenic shock
- Rupture of the free wall of the myocardium
- Rupture of the papillary muscle with resultant mitral regurgitation
- Aneurysms
- Mural thrombosis and embolism

- Pericarditis: *Dressler syndrome* refers to a delayed form of pericarditis that occurs 2 to 10 weeks after infarction that may have an immunologic basis

Hypertensive Heart Disease

Hypertension has been defined as a persistent increase in systemic blood pressure greater than 140 mm Hg systolic or 90 mm Hg diastolic. Chronic systemic hypertension causes pressure overload on the left ventricle that ultimately leads to compensatory changes, including concentric *left ventricular hypertrophy* and septal hypertrophy. On gross examination, the heart is enlarged and heavy, weighing greater than 350 grams. On microscopic examination, the heart demonstrates an increased diameter of the myocytes with enlarged, rectangular ("boxcar") nuclei. In addition, a mild to moderate amount of interstitial fibrosis may be present. Hypertensive heart disease is also associated with a worsening of underlying coronary atherosclerosis.

Persistent chronic hypertension can ultimately overwhelm the compensatory mechanisms of the heart and lead to congestive heart failure. In addition, vascular complications arising from chronic hypertension include intracerebral hemorrhage, myocardial infarction, aortic aneurysm, and renal disease.

Cor Pulmonale

Cor pulmonale is right ventricular hypertrophy and dilation associated with pulmonary hypertension. Increased resistance to flow into the pulmonary arteries or arterioles results in pressure overload on the right ventricle with subsequent compensatory hypertrophy. In addition to increased resistance within the pulmonary vessels, hypoxia, acidosis, and hypercapnia contribute to pulmonary vasoconstriction. Cor pulmonale may occur in the setting of lung parenchymal disease, pulmonary vascular disease, congenital heart disease, or impaired mobility of the thorax (Table 11-8).

Cor pulmonale may be acute or chronic. Acute cor pulmonale is the sudden occurrence of pulmonary hypertension, which most often occurs in the setting of massive pulmonary emboli. Chronic cor pulmonale, in contrast, is much more common and is often associated with chronic obstructive pulmonary disease and pulmonary fibrosis.

Grossly, the right ventricle is hypertrophic with a wall thickness often greater than 1 cm (normal thickness is 0.3–0.5 cm). Often the right ventricle and right atrium appear dilated. Microscopically, the changes are the same as those seen in left ventricular hyperten-

Table 11-8

Causes of Cor Pulmonale

Parenchymal diseases of the lung	*Congenital heart diseases*
Chronic bronchitis and emphysema	*Impaired movement of the thoracic cage*
Pulmonary fibrosis (from any cause)	Kyphoscoliosis
Cystic fibrosis	Pickwickian syndrome
	Pleural fibrosis
	Neuromuscular disorders
Pulmonary Vascular Diseases	Idiopathic hypoventilation
Recurrent pulmonary emboli	
Primary pulmonary hypertension	
Peripheral pulmonary stenosis	
Intravenous drug abuse	
Residence at high altitude	
Schistosomiasis	

From Rubin E, Gorstein F, Rubin R, et al. Rubin's Pathology, 4th ed. Philadelphia: Lippincott Williams & Wilkins, p. 553.

sion, including increased diameter of the myocytes and enlargement of the nuclei.

Acquired Valvular and Endocardial Diseases

Valve disease may occur secondary to inflammation, infection, or degenerative diseases. *Valvular stenosis* occurs when the valves are thickened and fused, which leads to an obstruction of blood flow and hypertrophy of the cardiac muscle proximal to the obstruction because of pressure overload. *Valvular regurgitation* occurs in the setting of valve destruction, which leads to retrograde blood flow, volume overload on the proximal cardiac chamber, and subsequent hypertrophy. In both cases, when the cardiac compensatory mechanisms fail, dilation of the affected chamber with reduced function can occur. A description of acquired valvular diseases is presented in Table 11-9.

Rheumatic Heart Disease

Rheumatic heart disease often begins as an acute rheumatic fever during childhood that often leads to long-term deformities of the cardiac valves. Two types of rheumatic heart disease are summarized in Table 11-9.

Table 11-9
Acquired Valvular Diseases

Disease	Etiology	Pathologic Findings	Complications
Rheumatic heart disease			
Acute rheumatic fever	*Streptococcus pyogenes* (group A β-hemolytic streptococcus)	Myocarditis with Aschoff body formation, "bread-and-butter" pericarditis and endocarditis with nodular fibrin deposition, especially on left-sided valves	Often resolves, although a low mortality rate occurs with persistent myocarditis; chronic rheumatic heart disease may develop
Chronic rheumatic heart disease	Resolution of acute rheumatic fever	Fibrotic, thickened, shrunken, less pliable valve leaflets that are often fused; most commonly affects the mitral valve leading to a "fish mouth" appearance of the valve	Mitral valve regurgitation, mitral stenosis, congestive heart failure, bacterial endocarditis, mural thrombi, adhesive pericarditis
Collagen vascular diseases			
Systemic lupus erythematosus (SLE)	Autoimmune	Endocarditis with verrucous vegetations (Libman-Sacks endocarditis) most common on the mitral valve, fibrinous pericarditis	Coronary artery disease, valvular stenosis or regurgitation
Rheumatoid arthritis	Autoimmune	Rheumatoid granulomatous inflammation with fibrinoid necrosis and palisading lymphocytes and macrophages in the myocardium, pericardium, or valves	Generally does not compromise function
Ankylosing spondylitis	Autoimmune	Dilation of the aortic ring and scarring of the aortic valves leading to aortic regurgitation	Aortic regurgitation

Bacterial endocarditis	Infection of the cardiac valves that may be acute (*Staphylococcus aureus* or *S. pyogenes*) or subacute (*Streptococcus viridans* or *Staphylococcus epidermidis*); occurs in the setting of valve disease, prosthetic valves, bacteremia, IV drug use, or advanced age	Bacterial vegetations often on the left-sided valves (mitral and aortic valves) that are often on the points of closure of the leaflets or cusps; IV drug use may primarily involve the right-sided valves	Destruction of the valve leading to congestive heart failure, septic emboli, glomerulonephritis due to immune-complex deposition in the kidneys
Nonbacterial thrombotic endocarditis	Associated with cancer or wasting diseases	Sterile vegetations on the mitral and aortic valves that do not lead to valve destruction	Embolization of vegetations
Calcific aortic stenosis	Rheumatic aortic valve disease, senile calcific stenosis, or congenital bicuspid aortic stenosis	Dystrophic calcification of the aortic valve that produces nodules on the base and lower half of the aortic cusps that rarely involve the free margins	Concentric left ventricular hypertrophy, congestive heart failure
Calcification of the mitral valve annulus	Elderly patients	Calcific deposits transform the mitral ring into a rigid, curved bar without deformation of the valve leaflets	Often asymptomatic; a murmur may be present
Mitral valve prolapse	Idiopathic, Marfan syndrome, collagen disorders, myotonic muscular dystrophy, hyperthyroidism, among others	Mitral valves are enlarged and redundant and the chordae tendineae are thinned and elongated leading to floppy mitral valves	Most patients are asymptomatic, but may lead to endocarditis

(continues)

301

Table 11-9
(continued)

Disease	Etiology	Pathologic Findings	Complications
Papillary muscle dysfunction	Ischemic heart disease	Scarring of the papillary muscle	Mitral regurgitation
Carcinoid heart disease	Often small intestinal carcinoids that have metastasized to the liver	Plaque-like deposits of dense, pearly gray, fibrous tissue on the tricuspid and pulmonary valves and right ventricular endocardium, associated with deformation of the valves	Pulmonary valve stenosis

Acute Rheumatic Fever

Acute rheumatic fever (ARF) is a multisystem disease of childhood that occurs following an acute streptococcal infection, usually pharyngitis ("strep throat"). Affected children are often between 9 and 11 years of age. The infectious agent is *Streptococcus pyogenes*, which is a member of the group A β-hemolytic *Streptococcus* family. Although the pathogenesis of ARF is unclear, it has been proposed that cross-reacting antibodies against streptococcal antigens may lead to an autoimmune-like reaction within the body.

ARF affects the pericardium, myocardium, endocardium, and valves. Microscopic findings include the following:

- Myocardium: nonspecific myocarditis with lymphocytic and macrophage infiltration, fibrinoid degeneration of collagen, and formation of *Aschoff bodies*, which are granulomatous lesions with a central fibrinoid region surrounded by lymphocytes, plasma cells, macrophages, and giant cells
- Pericardium: shaggy fibrinous deposits on the visceral and parietal surfaces of the pericardium termed "bread-and-butter" pericarditis
- Endocardium and valves: valve leaflets (most commonly left-sided valves) become inflamed and edematous that ultimately leads to the deposition of tiny fibrin nodules along the leaflets termed verrucous endocarditis

The clinical diagnosis of ARF requires the presence of two major or one major and two minor criteria. Major criteria include carditis, polyarthritis, chorea, erythema marginatum, and subcutaneous nodules. Minor criteria include a previous history of rheumatic fever, arthralgia, fever, specific laboratory findings, and electrocardiographic (EKG) changes. Patients often become symptomatic 2 to 3 weeks following infection, and symptoms typically resolve within 3 months. The joints and central nervous system may be involved. Treatment is often symptomatic. ARF may be prevented by prompt treatment of streptococcal pharyngitis with antibiotics.

Chronic Rheumatic Heart Disease

Long-term structural damage often occurs following acute rheumatic fever and is termed chronic rheumatic heart disease. Characteristically, heart valves demonstrate diffuse fibrosis, causing them to be thickened, shrunken, and less pliable. In addition, the valve leaflets or cusps of the affected valves can develop fibrous adhesions, leading to a fusion of the valves and subsequent stenosis. Typically, the most commonly affected valve is the mitral valve, and the second most commonly affected valve is the aortic valve.

The mitral valve may have a "fish mouth" appearance when viewed from the ventricular aspect because of the severity of valve adhesions. Complications of chronic rheumatic heart disease include bacterial endocarditis, mural thrombi, congestive heart failure, and adhesive pericarditis.

Collagen Vascular Diseases

A variety of collagen vascular diseases can lead to valvular disease, including systemic lupus erythematosus and rheumatoid arthritis. Specific collagen vascular diseases are summarized in Table 11-9.

Bacterial Endocarditis

Bacterial endocarditis is an infection of the cardiac valves that most commonly affects the left-sided heart valves. *Acute bacterial endocarditis* often results in rapid destruction of the infected valve and involves colonization of the valves by highly virulent suppurative organisms such as *Staphylococcus aureus* and *S. pyogenes*. Subacute bacterial endocarditis typically affects previously damaged valves and involves infection by less virulent organisms such as *Streptococcus viridans* or *Staphylococcus epidermidis*. Predisposing factors for bacterial endocarditis include the following:

- Congenital heart disease: most common predisposing factor in children
- Mitral valve prolapse
- Rheumatic heart disease
- Intravenous drug use
- Prosthetic valves
- Transient bacteremia: occurs from any procedure that introduces bacteria into the blood, including dental procedures and catheterization
- Advanced age

Grossly, aggregations of bacterial vegetations appear as pink-tan irregular nodules on the valves, often involving the points of closure of the valves or cusps. The underlying valve may appear damaged or eroded. Microscopically, organisms can be identified with the aid of special stains.

Clinically, early bacterial endocarditis manifests with low-grade fever, fatigue, anorexia, and weight loss. Ultimately, patients may develop heart murmurs, splenomegaly, petechiae, and clubbing of the fingers. Treatment involves the administration of an extended course of antibiotics. Complications include the dissemination of infected thromboemboli, focal segmental glomerulosclerosis due to the deposition of immune-complexes in the glomeruli, and congestive heart failure secondary to a damaged valve.

Nonbacterial Thrombotic Endocarditis

Nonbacterial thrombotic endocarditis (NBTE) refers to the presence of sterile vegetations on normal cardiac valves that often occurs in association with an underlying cancer or wasting disease. NBTE appears similar to bacterial endocarditis, except that there is no damage to the underlying valve.

Mitral Valve Prolapse

Mitral valve prolapse is a fairly common condition in which the mitral valve leaflets become enlarged and redundant and the chordae tendineae become thinned and elongated, which leads to prolapse of the mitral valves into the left atrium during systole. Mitral valve prolapse may be primary and can be associated with a strong family history of the disease, or it may occur secondary to several disorders, such as Marfan syndrome, inherited collagen disorders, myotonic muscular dystrophy, hyperthyroidism, congenital heart lesions, and von Willebrand disease.

Grossly, the mitral valves are redundant and deformed and demonstrate a gelatinous appearance. Microscopically, an accumulation of myxomatous connective tissue is present in the center of the valve leaflet.

Most patients with mitral valve prolapse are asymptomatic with an incidental mid-to-late systolic click. If mitral regurgitation is present, a late systolic murmur may be auscultated. Endocarditis may be a complication of this disease. In severe cases of mitral valve prolapse, replacement of the valve is indicated.

Primary Myocardial Diseases

Primary myocardial diseases include myocarditis, metabolic diseases, and cardiomyopathies.

Myocarditis

Myocarditis is an inflammation of the myocardium associated with myocyte necrosis and degeneration that is independent of ischemic heart disease. Myocarditis is most common in children between 1 and 10 years of age, although the disease may occur at any age. In the majority of cases, the etiology has not been absolutely determined, but viral infection has been proposed to be the underlying cause. Etiologic agents of myocarditis are listed in Table 11-10. Complications of myocarditis include acute heart failure, arrhythmias, and sudden death.

Infectious Myocarditis

Viral myocarditis is the most common form of myocarditis and may be caused by a variety of viruses, including coxsackievirus, echovi-

Table 11-10

Causes of Myocarditis

Idiopathic

Infectious

- Viral: Coxsackievirus, echovirus, influenza virus, human immunodeficiency virus, and many others
- Rickettsial: Typhus, Rocky Mountain spotted fever
- Bacterial: Diphtheria, staphylococcal, streptococcal, meningococcal, borrelial (Lyme disease), and leptospiral infection
- Fungi and protozoan parasites: Chagas disease, toxoplasmosis, aspergillosis, cryptococcal, and candidal infection
- Metazoan parasites: *Echinococcus, Trichina*

Noninfectious

- Hypersensitivity and immunologically related diseases: Rheumatic fever, systemic lupus erythematosus, scleroderma, drug reaction (e.g., to penicillin or sulfonamide), and rheumatoid arthritis
- Radiation
- Miscellaneous: Sarcoidosis, uremia

From Rubin E, Gorstein F, Rubin R, et al. Rubin's Pathology, 4th ed. Philadelphia: Lippincott Williams & Wilkins, p. 564.

rus, and influenza virus. Patients with HIV are especially prone to viral myocarditis caused by coxsackie B and adenovirus. Viral myocarditis appears to involve direct viral cytotoxicity or cell-mediated immune reactions. Other infectious causes of myocarditis include bacteria, rickettsia, fungi, toxoplasmosis, and *Trypanosoma cruzi* (Chagas disease).

Grossly, the heart is flabby and shows biventricular dilation, which correlates with the clinical findings of global hypokinesis of the myocardium. Microscopically, a patchy or diffuse interstitial infiltrate of T lymphocytes and macrophages is present. Occasionally, multinucleated giant cells may be seen. Inflammatory cells often surround individual myocytes, which undergo focal myocyte necrosis. As the infection resolves, fibroblast proliferation and interstitial collagen deposition predominate. Viral myocarditis is often associated with a pericarditis.

Hypersensitivity Myocarditis

Hypersensitivity myocarditis occurs in response to drug administration and appears morphologically similar to viral myocarditis, except that eosinophils are commonly present, and myocyte necrosis is rare. Most patients are often asymptomatic, although chest pain and EKG changes may be present. Treatment involves discontinuation of the inciting drug and, occasionally, corticosteroid administration.

Giant Cell Myocarditis

Giant cell myocarditis is a rare, highly aggressive disease characterized by intense inflammation of the heart with extensive areas of myocyte necrosis and the presence of numerous multinucleated giant cells. This disease presents most often during the third to fifth decades and is rapidly fatal. Grossly, the heart appears flabby and dilated with numerous mural thrombi. Microscopically, giant cells, lymphocytes, and macrophages surround serpiginous areas of necrosis. The only treatment for this disease is cardiac transplantation, although the disease recurs in some patients.

Metabolic Diseases of the Heart

A variety of metabolic diseases lead to cardiac manifestations. *Hyperthyroidism* can cause tachycardia and increased cardiac workload that may ultimately lead to angina pectoris and high-output failure. Severe *hypothyroidism* (myxedema) causes decreased cardiac output, reduced heart rate, and impaired myocardial contractility that can result in a flabby and dilated heart with interstitial fibrosis. *Beriberi heart disease* occurs in patients with vitamin B_1 (thiamine) deficiency and results in a dilated heart and high-output failure.

Cardiomyopathy

Cardiomyopathy is a primary disease of the myocardium that includes dilated, hypertrophic, and restrictive forms.

Dilated Cardiomyopathy

Dilated cardiomyopathy (DCM) is the most common form of cardiomyopathy and is characterized by biventricular dilation, impaired contractility, and, eventually, congestive heart failure. The underlying cause of DCM is unknown; however, it has been proposed that genetic factors play a role, and mutations in several genes associated with force generation within the myocyte have been associated with this disease, including dystrophin, desmin, and troponin T.

Secondary dilated cardiomyopathy occurs in conjunction with a variety of conditions including viral myocarditis, ethanol, cobalt, catecholamine overproduction, anthracycline administration, cyclophosphamide, and pregnancy. Cardiomyopathy of pregnancy occurs during the last trimester of pregnancy or during the first 6 months after delivery and is most common in African-American, multiparous women older than 30 years of age.

Cardiac findings are similar regardless of whether the dilated cardiomyopathy is primary or secondary. Grossly, the heart is enlarged with hypertrophy of both ventricles and a weight often exceeding 900 grams. All chambers of the heart are dilated, although the ventricles are often more severely affected than the atria. The myocardium appears flabby and pale, with small subendocardial scars occasionally present. Mural thrombi are often present. Microscopically, the myocardial fibers demonstrate a mixture of atrophy and hypertrophy. Interstitial and perivascular fibrosis is most prominent in the subendocardial zone. Scattered chronic inflammatory cells may be present. By electron microscopy, the myocytes show a loss of sarcomeres and an increase in the number of mitochondria.

Early in the disease, patients experience exercise intolerance that progresses ultimately to congestive heart failure. Patients are at increased risk for ventricular arrhythmias due to abnormalities in intracellular calcium. Ultimately, treatment of severely affected patients includes cardiac transplantation or the use of a ventricular assist device.

Hypertrophic Cardiomyopathy

Hypertrophic cardiomyopathy describes hypertrophic changes of the heart that are out of proportion to the hemodynamic load on the heart. This disease appears to have a strong genetic component, with more than 100 gene mutations associated with the development of this disease. Mutations of the β-myosin heavy chain, myosin-binding protein C, and troponin T genes ultimately affect sarcomeric function and lead to the formation of cardiac hypertrophy.

Grossly, the heart is always enlarged, but the degree of hypertrophy is variable. The left ventricular wall is thick and the cavity of the left ventricle is prominently reduced in size. Many cases show an associated asymmetric hypertrophy of the interventricular septum, which is often thicker than the left ventricular wall. This thickened septum can bulge into the left ventricular outflow tract during ventricular systole, leading to obstruction of the aortic outflow tract. The atria are typically dilated. Microscopically, the myofibers show prominent disarray, which is most extensive in the interventricular septum.

Most patients with hypertrophic cardiomyopathy are asymptomatic but are at increased risk of sudden death during severe exertion. This cardiac abnormality is commonly found at autopsy in young competitive athletes who experience sudden death. Patients may present prior to any severe outcome with dyspnea, angina pectoris, syncope, or notably increased ejection fractions on ultrasound. Pharmacologic treatment includes the administration of β-adrenergic blockers and calcium channel blockers to reduce contractility, decreased outflow-tract obstruction, and improve left ventricular relaxation during diastole. In addition, surgical removal of the affected portion of the interventricular septum has been associated with relief of symptoms but not the risk of sudden death.

Restrictive Cardiomyopathy

Restrictive cardiomyopathy encompasses a group of diseases in which myocardial or endocardial abnormalities limit diastolic filling without interfering with the contractile function of the heart. In the majority of cases, the ultimate result is congestive heart failure. Causes of restrictive cardiomyopathy include the following:

- Amyloid deposition: ventricular walls appear thickened, firm, and rubbery; endocardial surface has a granular appearance and gritty texture.
- Endomyocardial disease: encompasses endomyocardial fibrosis and eosinophilic endomyocardial disease (*Löffler endocarditis*). Löffler endocarditis is associated with hypereosinophilia and a rash, and demonstrates a gray-white layer of thickened endocardium extending from the apex of the left ventricle to the posterior leaflet of the mitral valve.
- Storage diseases: includes type II glycogen storage diseases, mucopolysaccharidoses, sphingolipidoses, and hemochromatosis
- Sarcoidosis: may produce large regions of myocardial necrosis most prominently involving the base of the interventricular septum that may involve the conduction system of the heart

Cardiac Neoplasms and Tumorlike Conditions

The heart may rarely be involved by primary cardiac tumors or by metastatic spread of malignant melanoma or carcinomas of the lung, breast, or gastrointestinal tract.

Cardiac Myxomas

Cardiac myxomas account for up to half of all cardiac tumors. These neoplasms are often sporadic but may be associated with familial autosomal dominant syndromes. The vast majority of myxomas arise in the left atrium. Grossly, they appear as glistening polypoid masses with short stalks that often measure 5 to 6 cm in diameter. Microscopically, polygonal stellate cells are present singly or in small clusters within a loose myxoid stroma. Patients may present with mitral valve dysfunction or with emboli arising from the tumor. Surgical resection of the tumor is curative in most cases.

Rhabdomyoma

Rhabdomyoma is the most common primary cardiac tumor in infants and children and is identified as multiple nodular masses within the myocardium. The origin of rhabdomyomas is controversial, and this entity may represent a hamartoma rather than a neoplastic process. Often, lesions may be associated with tuberous sclerosis. The lesions are multiple and involve both ventricles and often the atria. In half of cases, the mass may project into the cardiac chamber.

Grossly, rhabdomyomas appear as pale masses ranging up to several centimeters in diameter. Microscopically, the lesions are composed of cells with clear cytoplasm and a small central nucleus. The cytoplasm contains small fibrillar processes that contain sarcomere that radiate to the margin of the cells ("spider cells").

Papillary Fibroelastoma

Papillary fibroelastoma is a hamartomatous lesion formed of papillary fronds that measure up to 4 cm in diameter, which often involve the heart valves. Microscopically, these fronds have a central dense core of collagen and elastic fibers surrounded by looser connective tissue and are covered by endothelium. Although this lesion is often asymptomatic by itself, fragments may embolize to other organs.

Pericardial Disorders

Pericardial Effusion

Under normal conditions, the pericardium contains approximately 50 mL of fluid that lubricates the movement of the heart within the pericardial sac. In a pericardial effusion, *excess fluid* accumulates within the pericardial sac. If a pericardial effusion occurs rapidly, even a small increase in volume may lead to a severe, acute compromise of cardiac function. If a pericardial effusion occurs slowly, the pericardium can accommodate up to 2 L of fluid. Subtypes of pericardial effusions include the following:

- Serous pericardial effusion: often occurs with increased extracellular volume in heart failure or the nephrotic syndrome
- Chylous effusion: occurs from a communication of the thoracic duct with the pericardial space secondary to lymphatic obstruction
- Serosanguineous pericardial effusion: may occur after chest trauma or resuscitation
- Hemopericardium: bleeding into the pericardial cavity following cardiac trauma or rupture of the free ventricular wall following infarction

Cardiac tamponade occurs with rapid accumulation of fluid within the pericardial sac. This rapid accumulation can cause the pericardial pressure to exceed the central venous pressure, limiting the return of blood to the heart. Cardiac tamponade is manifested by a decreased blood pressure and pulsus paradoxus (an abnormal decrease in systolic pressure with inspiration). This condition is almost universally fatal if not relieved by pericardiocentesis or surgical intervention.

Acute Pericarditis

Pericarditis is an inflammation of the visceral or parietal pericardium that may occur in the context of viral myocarditis, a serofibrinous or hemorrhagic exudate, or malignant pericardial effusions. *Fibrinous pericarditis* is the most common form of acute pericarditis and is manifested by a dull, granular fibrin-rich exudate on the inflamed pericardial surface. The pericardium contains predominantly a lymphocytic infiltrate. Fibrinous pericarditis can occur in the setting of uremia, viral infection, or myocardial infarction. Other forms of pericarditis include *suppurative pericarditis* or *hemorrhagic pericarditis*.

Patients may present with sudden, severe, substernal chest pain, and a pericardial friction rub. EKG changes reflecting repolarization abnormalities.

Constrictive Pericarditis

Constrictive pericarditis is a chronic fibrosing disease of the pericardium that compresses the heart and restricts inflow. Despite its name, constrictive pericarditis does not demonstrate inflammation, but a progressive obliteration of the pericardial space by fibrous tissue and a fusion of the visceral and parietal pericardium. Risk factors for this condition include mediastinal radiation, cardiac surgery, and tuberculosis infection. Grossly, the heart is small and is surrounded by a rigid pericardium that restricts the diastolic filling of the heart. Treatment preferentially involves total pericardiectomy.

Pathology of Interventional Therapies

Coronary Angioplasty

Coronary angioplasty and stenting are performed to mechanically dilate an artery narrowed by atherosclerosis. In as many as 40% of patients, restenosis of the lumen develops within 6 months because of a fibroproliferative response of intimal smooth muscle cells injured during the procedure.

Coronary Bypass Grafts

Coronary bypass grafts are performed in the setting of proximal coronary artery stenosis and commonly use the internal mammary artery or saphenous vein as a graft. Complications of the grafts most commonly affect saphenous vein grafts and include early thrombosis, intimal hyperplasia, and atherosclerosis of vein grafts.

Prosthetic Valves

Prosthetic valves may be completely mechanical or contain tissue derived from pig or cow valves or pericardium. Tissue valves are subject to tissue degeneration over time, whereas mechanical valves have an increased risk of thrombosis and require long-term anticoagulant therapy.

Heart Transplantation

Allograft rejection is a major complication of heart transplantation and occurs in a variety of forms:

- Hyperacute rejection: occurs with blood-group incompatibility or major histocompatibility differences and involves the presence of preformed antibodies
- Acute humoral rejection: vascular deposition of immunoglobulin and complement
- Acute cellular rejection: most common form of allograft rejection and involves T-cell infiltration and focal acute myocyte necrosis
- Chronic vascular rejection: concentric intimal proliferation that occurs within the first year of transplantation and can lead to significant coronary artery disease and myocardial infarction

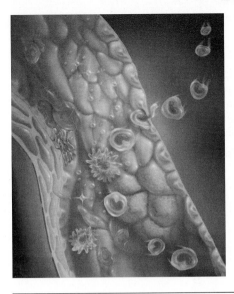

CHAPTER *12*

The Respiratory System

Chapter Outline

Rare Alveolar Diseases
  Alveolar Proteinosis (Lipoproteinosis)
  Diffuse Pulmonary Hemorrhage Syndrome
  Eosinophilic Pneumonia
  Endogenous Lipid Pneumonia
  Exogenous Lipid Pneumonia

Obstructive Pulmonary Diseases
  Chronic Bronchitis
  Emphysema
  Asthma

Pneumoconioses
  Silicosis
  Coal Workers' Pneumoconiosis
  Asbestosis
  Berylliosis
  Talcosis

Interstitial Lung Disease
  Hypersensitivity Pneumonitis (Extrinsic Allergic Alveolitis)
  Sarcoidosis
  Usual Interstitial Pneumonia
  Desquamative Interstitial Pneumonia
  Respiratory Bronchiolitis
  Bronchiolitis Obliterans-organizing Pneumonia
  Lymphoid Interstitial Pneumonia

Langerhans Cell Histiocytosis (Histiocytosis X)

Lymphangioleiomyomatosis

Lung Transplantation

Vasculitis and Granulomatosis
  Wegener Granulomatosis
  Churg-Strauss Syndrome (Allergic Angiitis and Granulomatosis)
  Necrotizing Sarcoid Granulomatosis

Pulmonary Hypertension

Pulmonary Hamartoma

Lung Neoplasms
  Squamous Cell Carcinoma
  Adenocarcinoma
  Bronchioloalveolar Carcinoma
  Small Cell Carcinoma
  Large Cell Carcinoma
  Carcinoid Tumors
  Rare Pulmonary Tumors

The Pleura

Pneumothorax

Pleural Effusion

Pleuritis

Tumors of the Pleura
    Solitary Fibrous Tumor
    Malignant Mesothelioma

THE LUNGS

Normal Histology and Anatomy

The respiratory system is formed by the larynx, trachea, bronchi, bronchioles, alveoli, and pulmonary vasculature. The respiratory system forms progressively during fetal development with the formation of proximal elements occurring first. During the acinar (canalicular) period, which occurs between 17 and 28 weeks of gestation, the framework of the gas-exchanging unit of the lung develops, gas exchange becomes possible, and the fetus becomes viable outside of the uterus. The alveolar period occurs between 34 and 36 weeks of development and encompasses the period of alveolar development, although alveoli can develop through the first 2 years of life.

The trachea measures up to 25 cm in length and divides into the right and left bronchi. The right bronchus diverges at a lesser angle from the trachea than the left; therefore, aspirated material more frequently enters the right bronchus and lung. The bronchi divide into subsequent lobar and segmental bronchi, which supply the 19 segments of lung. Each lung segment can be resected separately because of individual bronchovascular supplies. The tracheobronchial tree contains cartilage and submucosal glands and is lined by pseudostratified, ciliated columnar epithelium. In addition, the tracheobronchial tree contains Clara cells, which detoxify inhaled substances, and Kulchitsky cells, which are neuroendocrine cells that secrete hormonally active products.

The bronchi ultimately branch into bronchioles, which do not contain cartilage or mucous-secreting glands. The last purely conducting bronchiole is termed the terminal bronchiole. Terminal bronchioles divide into the respiratory bronchioles, which merge into the alveolar ducts and alveoli. The acinus, which is the unit of gas exchange, is formed by the respiratory bronchioles, alveolar ducts, and alveoli.

The alveoli are lined by type I and II epithelial cells. Type I cells account for 40% of the alveolar cells, cover 95% of the alveolar surface, and facilitate gas exchange. Type II cells produce surfactant and can reconstitute the alveolar surface after injury. Within the alveolus, the epithelial and endothelial cells are spread very thinly on either side of a basement membrane, which allows the exchange of oxygen and carbon dioxide. Away from the sites of gas exchange, interstitial connective tissue consisting of fibroblasts, myofibroblasts, collagen, elastin, and proteoglycans is present (Fig. 12-1).

The lung has a dual blood supply. The pulmonary arteries accompany the bronchial system within a sheath of connective tissue called the bronchovascular bundle and are elastic arteries proximally and muscular arteries distally. The bronchial arteries arise from the thoracic aorta and supply the lung as far as the respiratory bronchioles. The bronchial arteries are accompanied by veins that ultimately drain into the azygous or hemiazygous veins. There are no lymphatics in the majority of the alveolar walls.

The lung uses a variety of mechanisms to protect itself against infection and particle infiltration. The mechanisms include humidifying the air in the nose and trachea, trapping particles of varying sizes along all levels of the tracheobronchial tree, use of a mucocili-

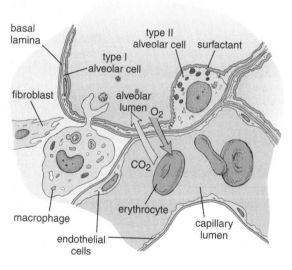

FIGURE   12-1

Diagram of the interalveolar septum. The alveolar septum forms the air-blood barrier and is responsible for most of the gas exchange that occurs in the lung. The arrows indicate the direction of CO_2 and O_2 exchange between the alveolar air space and the blood. (From Ross MH, Kaye G, Pawlina W. Histology: A text and Atlas, 4th ed. Philadelphia: Lippincott Williams & Wilkins, 2003, p. 586.)

ary blanket to push foreign particles back toward the upper airways, and using pulmonary alveolar macrophages to ingest particles that ultimately reach the alveolus.

Congenital Anomalies

Congenital anomalies of the lungs most commonly present within the first 2 years of life and frequently manifest with respiratory distress and cyanosis (Table 12-1). Anomalies that may present later in life include a *bronchogenic cyst* and *intralobar sequestration*. Often, the involved portion of the lung demonstrates signs of recurrent infection and subsequent fibrosis. In certain cases, if the abnormality is localized, the affected lung may be surgically resected to relieve symptoms.

The most common congenital lesion of the lung is *pulmonary hypoplasia*, which often occurs in association with other congenital abnormalities and with trisomy 13, 18, and 21. Pulmonary hypoplasia is the incomplete or defective development of the lung, which results in a lung that is smaller than normal. The major factors that have been implicated in pulmonary hypoplasia include compression of the lung, often by a congenital diaphragmatic hernia, oligohydramnios, and decreased respiration.

Diseases of the Bronchi and Bronchioles

The diseases covered within this section deal with acute conditions and their sequelae. Chronic bronchitis is discussed in the section about chronic obstructive pulmonary disease.

Airway Infections

Many infections that affect the bronchi (*bronchitis*) also often involve the distal (peripheral) airways (*bronchiolitis*). In the majority of infections that affect the bronchi and bronchioles, patients present with cough, chest tightness, and shortness of breath. The most severe cases of bronchitis and bronchiolitis often affect infants and children and are more severe in malnourished children. Certain types of infections can lead to extensive inflammation of the bronchioles, which results in subsequent healing by fibrosis, leading to occlusion or obliteration of the bronchioles, termed *obliterative bronchiolitis*. The most common infectious agents that lead to bronchitis or bronchiolitis include the following:

- Influenza: may result in severe acute inflammation of the respiratory mucosa, which appears fiery red, and occasionally may be fatal
- Adenovirus: may result in obliterative bronchiolitis

Table 12-1

Congenital Anomalies of the Tracheobronchial Tree and Lungs

Congenital Anomaly	Appearance and Pathology of the Lung	Additional Associations/ Findings
Bronchial atresia	Reduced size and development of a bronchus, which often supplies the apical posterior segment of the left upper lobe with resultant overexpansion of the affected segment	May appear as a radiographic mass
Pulmonary hypoplasia	Incomplete/defective lung development resulting in a small lung	Congenital diaphragmatic hernia, oligohydramnios, trisomy 13, 18, or 21
Congenital cystic adenomatoid malformation	Abnormal bronchiolar structures of varying sizes or distribution; usually affects single lobe; multiple cystlike spaces lined by bronchiolar epithelium	Often presents with respiratory distress and cyanosis
Bronchogenic cyst	Discrete, extrapulmonary, fluid-filled mass lined by respiratory epithelium and surrounded by muscle and cartilage, often found in the mediastinum	May compress a major airway or become secondarily infected
Extralobar sequestration	Mass of lung tissue not connected to the bronchial tree, located outside the visceral pleura and supplied by an abnormal artery; contains dilated bronchioles, alveolar ducts, and alveoli, and is covered by pleura	More common in men and associated with other anomalies; manifests with dyspnea, cyanosis, or recurrent infection
Intralobar sequestration	Mass of lung tissue within the visceral pleura, often in the lower lobe, that is isolated from the tracheobronchial tree and is supplied by a systemic artery; cystlike spaces lined by cuboidal or columnar epithelium containing macrophages and eosinophilic material and may show signs of chronic recurrent pneumonia with end-stage honeycomb changes	Often presents in adolescents with cough, sputum production, and recurrent pneumonia

- Respiratory syncytial virus (RSV): self-limited disease that often occurs as epidemics in nurseries and causes peribronchiolar inflammation, disorganization of the epithelium, and overdistention of the lung parenchyma
- Measles: rare in developed countries; may result in obliterative bronchiolitis
- *Bordetella pertussis*: causes *whooping cough*, characterized by fever and severe prolonged bouts of coughing followed by a characteristic deep whooping inspiration
- *Haemophilus influenzae*: may cause exacerbations of chronic bronchitis
- *Streptococcus pneumoniae*: may cause exacerbations of chronic bronchitis
- *Candida albicans*: occurs in cases of trauma, burns, and neutropenia; demonstrates noninvasive growth leading to mucosal ulceration

Irritant Gases

The major irritant gases are oxidants (ozone, oxides of nitrogen) and sulfur dioxide. Oxidants are caused by the action of sunlight on automobile exhaust fumes and bring about respiratory problems in major urban areas. Sulfur dioxide is derived mainly from the burning of fossil fuels. These gases may exacerbate respiratory conditions, such as chronic pulmonary disease and asthma, with exposure. Exposure to high concentrations of these agents may result in bronchiolitis.

Exposure to chlorine and ammonia gases may occur in industrial accidents and can result in the development of extensive bronchial and bronchiolar mucosal injury. Secondary inflammation can result in extensive *bronchiectasis* (irreversible dilation of bronchioles).

Bronchocentric Granulomatosis

Bronchocentric granulomatosis refers to nonspecific granulomatous inflammation centered on bronchi or bronchioles.

Patients with asthma who develop bronchocentric granulomatosis typically have allergic bronchopulmonary aspergillosis and also may demonstrate bronchial mucous plugs, bronchiectasis and bronchiolectasis, and eosinophilic pneumonia. *Aspergillus* hyphae may be found in the mucous plugs.

Patients without asthma who develop bronchocentric granulomatosis commonly have an infection, especially tuberculosis or histoplasmosis. In other cases, patients may have rheumatoid arthritis, ankylosing spondylitis, or Wegener granulomatosis. In idiopathic cases, patients may respond well to corticosteroid therapy.

Obliterative (Constrictive) Bronchiolitis

Obliterative bronchiolitis is an uncommon disorder in which an initial inflammatory bronchiolitis is followed by bronchiolar scarring and fibrosis, resulting in constrictive narrowing and eventually complete obliteration of the airway lumen. Patients may have dyspnea and wheezing secondary to severe obstruction. The chest radiograph or computed tomography (CT) scan may be normal or show overinflation caused by air trapping distal to the obliterated bronchioles. Obliterative bronchiolitis may occur in the following conditions:

- Graft-versus-host disease
- Chronic rejection in lung transplantation
- Collagen vascular disease
- Postinfectious viral disorders
- Inhalation of toxins
- Use of certain drugs, such as penicillamine

Microscopically, the bronchioles show chronic mural inflammation and varying amounts of submucosal fibrosis. These lesions are often focal, and an elastic stain may help identify scarred bronchioles. Adjacent airways may show bronchiolectasis and mucous plugs. The surrounding lung is normal.

In many patients, obliterative bronchiolitis has a progressive course. There is no known effective therapy, although many patients are treated with corticosteroids.

Bronchial Obstruction

Bronchial obstruction may occur secondary to endobronchial extension of tumors or mucous plugs from aspirated material. In partial obstruction, the trapped air may lead to overdistention of the distal segment of lung. In complete obstruction, the distal lung develops atelectasis and is susceptible to pneumonia, pulmonary abscess, or bronchiectasis.

Atelectasis

Atelectasis refers to the collapse of expanded lung tissue and may occur with bronchial obstruction, direct compression of the lung (i.e., pneumothorax), or as a postoperative complication. If atelectasis is severe, hypoxemia may occur. In cases of long-standing atelectasis, the collapsed lung becomes fibrotic and the bronchi dilate. Permanent bronchial dilation may result, which is termed *bronchiectasis*.

Right middle lobe syndrome refers to atelectasis caused by obstruction of the bronchus to the right middle lobe, which often is caused by external compression by enlarged hilar lymph nodes.

The affected right middle lobe may demonstrate bronchiectasis, chronic bronchitis and bronchiolitis, lymphoid hyperplasia, abscess formation, and dense fibrosis.

Bronchiectasis

Bronchiectasis is the irreversible dilation of bronchi caused by the destruction of the muscular and elastic elements of the bronchial walls. Bronchiectasis is obstructive or nonobstructive in nature, as described in the following:

- *Obstructive bronchiectasis* is localized to a segment of lung distal to a mechanical obstruction of a central bronchus by any cause, including tumor, mucous plugs, or foreign bodies.
- Nonobstructive bronchiectasis often occurs secondary to respiratory infections or defects in the mucociliary defense mechanism, including cilia disorders. Nonobstructive bronchiectasis may be localized or generalized.
- Localized nonobstructive bronchiectasis often occurs after childhood respiratory infections.
- Generalized nonobstructive bronchiectasis occurs secondary to acquired disorders or the inherited impairment of the host defense mechanisms that allows the introduction of infectious organisms into the airways. Acquired disorders that lead to generalized nonobstructive bronchiectasis include neurologic disorders, incompetence of the lower esophageal sphincter, nasogastric intubation, and chronic bronchitis. Inherited conditions include cystic fibrosis, hypogammaglobulinemias, IgG subclass deficiency, and dyskinetic ciliary syndromes. Generalized bronchiectasis is usually bilateral and is most common in the lower lobes.

Kartagener syndrome is an immotile cilia syndrome that includes the triad of dextrocardia, bronchiectasis, and sinusitis. This syndrome is caused by an absence of inner or outer dynein arms of the cilia that result in cilia immotility. Sterility in men and women is common in this syndrome because of impaired ciliary motility in the reproductive tract.

Grossly, bronchial dilation is classified as saccular (severe dilation with dilated blind-ended sacs), varicose (irregular dilations and constrictions), and cylindrical (uniform, moderate dilation). The bronchi appear dilated and have white or yellow thickened walls. The bronchial lumen often contains thick, mucopurulent secretions.

Microscopically, the bronchi and bronchioles show severe inflammation with destruction of all components of the bronchial wall. After collapse of the distal lung, the damaged bronchi dilate. There is an increased number of goblet cells and squamous metaplasia of the central airways and lymphoid follicles often are seen in the bronchial walls. The distal bronchi and bronchioles are scarred and often obliterated.

Patients with bronchiectasis present with a chronic productive cough, often producing several hundred milliliters of mucopurulent sputum per day. Often, hemoptysis, dyspnea, and wheezing are present. Patients often experience pneumonia as a complication and ultimately may develop chronic hypoxia and pulmonary hypertension. A definitive diagnosis often is made by CT scan, in which the bronchi appear dilated with thickened walls. Occasionally, an acute, reversible dilation of bronchi may occur after bacterial or viral bronchopulmonary infection, although the bronchi do not return to normal size for several months after resolution of the infection.

Pulmonary Infections

Pulmonary infections may be caused by bacteria, fungi, or viruses and the etiologic agent often varies with exposure, immune status, and age. In addition, the type of etiologic agent may demonstrate different radiographic and pathologic findings.

Bacterial Pneumonia
General Considerations

Pneumonia is a generic term that refers to inflammation and consolidation (solidification) of the pulmonary parenchyma and often is caused by bacteria. Pneumonia often occurs in three settings:

- Community-acquired pneumonia: occurs in persons with no primary disorder of the immune system
- Nosocomial pneumonia: caused by organisms spread in a hospital environment to susceptible persons
- Opportunistic pneumonia: affects immunocompromised persons

The majority of bacteria that cause pneumonia are normal inhabitants of the oropharynx. Bacteria can reach the alveoli by aspiration of secretions, inhalation of microorganisms, hematogenous spread, or direct spread. Risk factors for bacterial pneumonia include cigarette smoking, chronic bronchitis, alcoholism, severe malnutrition, wasting diseases, and poorly controlled diabetes. The more common forms of bacterial pneumonia are described in Table 12-2.

Pneumonia is subdivided into *lobar pneumonia* (consolidation of an entire lobe) or *bronchopneumonia* (scattered foci in one or several lobes). Lobar pneumonia is most commonly caused by pneumococcus or klebsiella infection and demonstrates a well-described series of pathologic findings that include the following:

Table 12-2
Bacterial Pneumonia

Organism	Demographics	Lung Findings	Complications
Streptococcus pneumoniae (streptococcus)	Young to middle-aged adults	Often follows a viral infection; early stage has protein-rich edema in the alveoli; neutrophils and hemorrhage; later stage has neutrophil lysis and macrophage infiltrate; firm lung; often lobar pneumonia	Pleuritis, effusion, pyothorax, empyema, bacteremia, pulmonary fibrosis, lung abscess
Klebsiella pneumoniae	Middle-aged men, alcoholics, diabetics, patients with COPD	Neutrophils, congestion, and hemorrhage; may produce a mucoid appearance of the cut lung surface owing to the bacterial capsule; increased size of affected lobe; often lobar pneumonia	Tissue necrosis, abscess formation, bronchopleural fistula
Staphylococcus aureus	Cystic fibrosis after viral infection	Bronchopneumonia with the formation of many small abscesses; rupture of an abscess into a bronchiole may lead to the formation of a pneumatocele (thin-walled cyst lined by respiratory epithelium)	Cavitation, pleural effusions
Streptococcus pyogenes (group A streptococcus)	After viral infection, debilitated persons	Heavy lungs with bloody edema; alveoli filled with fibrin-containing fluid and rare neutrophils; often bronchopneumonia	Alveolar necrosis, empyema
Streptococcus agalactiae (group B strep)	Infants after exposure in the birth canal	Similar to previous	Respiratory distress syndrome, toxemia

(continues)

Table 12-2
(continued)

Organism	Demographics	Lung Findings	Complications
Legionella pneumophila	Caused by contaminated air-conditioning systems, often elderly and immunocom-promised persons	Multiple lobes have bronchopneumonia with large confluent areas; alveoli contain fibrin, neutrophils, and macrophages; may have extensive necrosis of inflammatory cells; fibrous organization over time	Empyema
Gram-negative bacteria (*Escherichia coli*, *Pseudomonas*)	Immunosuppressed persons	*E. coli* presents as bronchopneumonia; *Pseudomonas* may have an infectious vasculitis and infarction	
Anaerobic bacteria (e.g., *Bacteroides*)	Patients with swallowing disorders or seizures, alcoholics	Necrotizing bronchopneumonia	Lung abscess
Chlamydia psittaci (psittacosis)	Inhalation of contaminated bird excreta	Minimal lung findings; may have irregular consolidation and interstitial findings	
Bacillus anthracis (anthrax)	Direct contact with spores	Hemorrhagic pneumonia, hemorrhagic bronchitis, hemorrhagic mediastinitis	
Yersinia pestis (plague)	Inhalation of spores or person-to-person spread	Extensive hemorrhagic bronchopneumonia, pleuritis, enlargement of mediastinal lymph nodes	

- Multiplication of organisms, edema, and congestion
- Red hepatization: development of an alveolar exudate containing neutrophils and red blood cells that causes the lung to become firm and red, with an appearance similar to liver
- Gray hepatization: ingestion of debris by macrophages and a fibrin suppurative exudate that makes the lung firm and appear gray
- Resolution: degradation of consolidated exudate

Bacterial pneumonia is typically characterized by a filling of the alveoli with polymorphonuclear leukocytes and often is associated with an abrupt onset of fever, malaise, and a productive cough

Pneumococcal Pneumonia

Pneumococcal pneumonia is one of the more common forms of bacterial pneumonia and is caused by *Streptococcus pneumoniae*. Infection with this organism commonly occurs after a viral infection of the upper respiratory tract. The capsule of pneumococcus prevents phagocytosis by alveolar macrophages; therefore, the bacteria first must be opsonized before they can be ingested and killed. Pneumococcal pneumonia most commonly results in a lobar pneumonia, which progresses through the previously described stages of congestion, hepatization, and resolution. Pneumococcal pneumonia has an abrupt onset with fever, chills, and chest pain. Patients often describe "rusty" sputum caused by degraded red blood cells in the alveoli. This disease responds rapidly to antibiotics, although the radiographic abnormalities may only resolve after several days.

Complications related to pneumococcal pneumonia include the following:

- Pleuritis: painful inflammation of the pleura
- Pleural effusion: serous exudate in the pleural cavity
- Pyothorax: purulent exudate in the pleural cavity that may heal by fibrosis
- Empyema: localized collection of pus with fibrous walls in the pleural cavity
- Lung abscess
- Bacteremia
- Pulmonary fibrosis: intraalveolar exudates becomes organized and forms intraalveolar plugs of granulation tissue, also termed *organizing pneumonia*

Mycoplasma Pneumonia

Mycoplasma infection causes an atypical pneumonia with an insidious onset, minimal leukocytosis, and a prolonged course. Radiographs show a patchy intraalveolar pneumonia or an interstitial infiltrate. The infection commonly causes bronchiolitis with neutro-philic intraluminal exudates and an intense lymphoplasmacytic in-filtrate in the bronchiolar wall. The diagnosis is often established by serology to detect *M. pneumoniae* antibodies or cold agglutinins. Erythromycin is an effective antibiotic against this organism.

Tuberculosis

Mycobacterium tuberculosis often is acquired via inhalation of aero-sols and has demonstrated a recent resurgence, especially in pa-tients with AIDS. Tuberculosis is divided into primary and second-ary (reactivation) tuberculosis.

Primary Tuberculosis

Primary tuberculosis occurs after initial exposure to *M. tuberculosis*. After inhalation of the organism, the organism replicates in the alveolus and ultimately leads to the formation of a Ghon focus. The Ghon focus consists of a peripheral parenchymal granuloma, often in the upper lobes, which is well circumscribed, often 1 to 2 cm in diameter, and contains central necrosis. If this lesion is associ-ated with enlarged mediastinal lymph nodes, it is termed a Ghon focus. Resolution of the Ghon focus results in a calcified lesion. The majority of primary tuberculosis infections are asymptomatic.

Secondary Tuberculosis

Secondary tuberculosis represents either reactivation of primary tuberculosis or reinfection in a previously sensitized host. Second-ary tuberculosis is characterized by multiple granulomas and ex-tensive tissue necrosis that is most common in the upper lobes, but which may affect any part of the lung. These lesions may heal and calcify or may erode into an adjacent bronchus and cause a tuberculous cavity. The wall of this cavity is composed of an inner, thin, gray membrane encompassing soft necrotic nodules, a middle zone of granulation tissue, and an outer collagenous border. The caseous material contains macrophages filled with the acid-fast ba-cilli. If the cavity is in communication with a bronchus, the infec-tious material disseminates into the airways and within the lung.

Complications of secondary tuberculosis include the fol-lowing:

- Miliary tuberculosis: multiple, minute granulomas in many or-gans
- Hemoptysis: caused by the erosion of small pulmonary arteries
- Bronchopleural fistula: occurs when a subpleural cavity rup-tures into the pleural space
- Tuberculous laryngitis

- Intestinal tuberculosis: may follow swallowing of infectious material
- Aspergilloma: fungal mass caused by superinfection by *Aspergillus*

Fungal Infections

Fungal infections are caused by a variety of organisms and occur most commonly in immunocompromised patients or persons in certain geographic areas who are exposed to the organisms. The more common respiratory infections caused by fungal organisms are described in Table 12-3.

Viral Pneumonia

Viral infections of the pulmonary parenchyma produce diffuse alveolar damage and interstitial (rather than alveolar) pneumonia. Infection of the lung by viruses first affects the alveolar epithelium and causes a mononuclear infiltrate in the interstitium. Necrosis of type I epithelial cells and the formation of hyaline membranes cause a morphologic appearance identical to diffuse alveolar damage. The most common viruses to cause viral pneumonia include cytomegalovirus, measles, varicella, herpes simplex influenza, and adenovirus. Typically, viral inclusions are identified within the epithelial cells, and occasionally multinucleation may occur.

Lung Abscess

A lung abscess is a localized accumulation of pus accompanied by the destruction of the pulmonary parenchyma, including alveoli, airways, and blood vessels. The most common cause of lung abscess is aspiration, often in the setting of depressed consciousness. The infections are often polymicrobial and contain anaerobic organisms derived from the oral cavity. Other causes of lung abscess include bronchial obstruction, necrotizing pneumonia, penetrating trauma, and infected pulmonary emboli. Lung abscess occurs more commonly on the right side because of the bronchial architecture and often is multiloculated. The abscess is filled with polymorphonuclear leukocytes, macrophages, and debris and is surrounded by hemorrhage, fibrin, and inflammatory cells. Over time, a fibrous wall forms around the abscess and it may become lined by squamous epithelium. Patients often present with cough, fever, and the production of foul-smelling sputum. Complications of lung abscess include rupture into the pleural space or drainage into a bronchus with subsequent dissemination to other parts of the lung.

Table 12-3
Fungal Infections of the Lung

Organism	Distribution	Pulmonary Findings
Histoplasma capsulatum (histoplasmosis)	Midwest and southeast United States (Ohio and Mississippi valleys), in bird droppings	Most are asymptomatic and cause a Ghon-like complex; granulomas often calcify in a concentric laminar pattern; can involve lymph nodes draining the infectious site; may reactivate
Coccidioides immitis (coccidiomycosis)	Southwest United States	Similar to tuberculosis and histoplasmosis, but without lymph node involvement
Cryptococcus neoformans (cryptococcosis)	Often found in pigeon droppings; often affects immunocompromised persons	Range from small parenchymal granulomas to several large granulomas, pneumonic consolidation, and cavitation
Blastomyces dermatitidis (North American blastomycoses)	Canada, basins of the Missouri, Mississippi, and Ohio rivers	Most cause a Ghon-like complex or progressive pneumonitis
Aspergillus species (aspergillosis)	Ubiquitous	May cause invasive aspergillosis resulting in vessel invasion and pulmonary infarction in immunocompromised persons, aspergilloma creating a fungal ball in preexisting cavities of tuberculosis or bronchiectasis, or allergic bronchopulmonary aspergillosis is asthmatic persons with bronchocentric granulomas and eosinophilic pneumonia
Pneumocystis carinii pneumonia (PCP)	Ubiquitous	Often affects immunocompromised persons and causes an interstitial infiltrate of plasma cells and lymphocytes, diffuse alveolar damage, and a foamy alveolar exudates with the organisms appearing as tiny bubbles

Diffuse Alveolar Damage (Acute Respiratory Distress Syndrome)

Diffuse alveolar damage (DAD) is a nonspecific pattern of injury of the alveolar epithelial and endothelial cells that results from a variety of acute insults that are listed in Table 12-4. The clinical counterpart of DAD is *acute respiratory distress syndrome* (ARDS), in which patients with previously normal pulmonary function experience pulmonary damage that leads to rapidly progressive respiratory failure. The counterpart of ARDS in newborns is termed *respiratory distress syndrome* (RDS) *of the newborn* and, when associated with DAD, is termed *hyaline membrane disease*. RDS may occur secondary to bronchopulmonary dysplasia, decreased alveolarization, or surfactant deficiency in newborns.

In general, microscopic examination of the lung does not reveal the cause of DAD, except in instances in which a specific infectious agent is identified or in which bizarre, atypical, hyperchromatic nuclei in type II cells point to chemotherapeutic injury. It has been proposed that activation of the complement system with subsequent recruitment and activation of neutrophils may play a role.

DAD can be divided into two stages, an exudative phase and an organizing phase, as follows:

- Exudative phase: develops during the first week after pulmonary injury. Injury to the endothelial cells results in leakage of

Table 12-4
Important Causes of Adult Respiratory Distress Syndrome

Nonthoracic trauma	*Drugs and therapeutic agents*
Shock due to any cause	Heroin
Fat embolism	Oxygen (high concentrations
	Radiation
Infection	Paraquat
Gram-negative septicemia	Cytotoxic drugs (e.g., bleomycin,
Other bacterial infections	methotrexate)
Viral infections	
Aspiration	
Near-drowning	
Aspiration of gastric contents	

From Rubin E, Gorstein F, Rubin R, et al. Rubin's Pathology, 4th ed. Philadelphia: Lippincott Williams & Wilkins, 2005, p. 606.

protein-rich fluid from the alveolar capillaries into the interstitial space. Damage to and loss of type I pneumocytes allows the passage of fluid into the alveolar spaces, in which the deposition of plasma proteins causes the formation of eosinophilic, glassy, fibrin-containing precipitates termed hyaline membranes. Plasma cells, lymphocytes, and macrophages accumulate in the interstitial space in response to injury. By the end of the first week, cuboidal type II pneumocytes line the denuded alveolar septa. The alveolar capillaries and pulmonary arterioles may show fibrin thrombi.

- Organizing phase: begins approximately 1 week after pulmonary injury and features the proliferation of fibroblasts within the alveolar walls. Hyaline membranes are no longer formed at this stage.

Clinically, patients exposed to pulmonary injury typically do not begin to demonstrate symptoms for several hours, after which tachypnea and dyspnea become prominent. Blood gases show arterial hypoxemia and decreased PCO_2. The arterial hypoxemia cannot be reversed by increasing the oxygen tension of the inspired air and patients require mechanical ventilation. Radiographically, extensive bilateral opacities are present in both lungs, which is termed "whiteout."

In patients who recover from DAD, the fibrosis resolves and the extra collagen and hyaline membranes are resorbed. Pulmonary function can return to normal in these instances. However, in patients who progress, severe fibrosis leads to restructuring of the pulmonary parenchyma with the development of honeycombing and end-stage lung. In patients who do not recover, the lungs appear heavy, edematous, and virtually without air at autopsy.

Rare Alveolar Diseases

Alveolar Proteinosis (Lipoproteinosis)

Alveolar proteinosis is a condition in which the alveoli are filled with a granular eosinophilic material, which is periodic acid-Schiff (PAS)–positive, diastase resistant, and rich in lipids. This disease occurs in patients who have compromised immunity, in patients with leukemia and lymphoma in conjunction with respiratory infections, and in patients with exposure to environmental inorganic dusts. Although no etiologic agent has been identified, it has been proposed that impaired alveolar macrophage activity and increased surfactant production by type II pneumocytes underlie the pathophysiology.

Grossly, the lungs are very heavy, viscid, and demonstrate yellow fluid leaking from the cut surface. Scattered, firm, yellow-white nodules are present. Microscopically, granular material is noted in the alveoli, alveolar ducts, and respiratory bronchioles. This material stains with antibodies against surfactant apoprotein and by electron microscopy demonstrates lamellar bodies similar to those found within type II pneumocytes. The interstitial structure of the lung is intact and little inflammation is present.

This disease most commonly occurs in adults and presents with fever, productive cough, and dyspnea. Patients often experience repeated respiratory tract infections, often with fungi or *Nocardia*. Radiographically, diffuse, bilateral, symmetric, alveolar infiltrates, which may radiate from the hilar regions, are identified. Treatment involves repeated bronchoalveolar lavage to remove the material.

Diffuse Pulmonary Hemorrhage Syndrome

Diffuse alveolar hemorrhage can occur in a variety of settings and is characterized by acute hemorrhage, with numerous intraalveolar red blood cells, or chronic hemorrhage, with hemosiderin-laden macrophages within the alveoli. Often, a neutrophilic infiltrate is present in the alveolar wall and involves the capillaries, termed neutrophilic capillaritis. Diffuse pulmonary hemorrhage syndromes can be classified into associated antibody patterns demonstrated by immunofluorescence into linear, granular, or pauciimmune/negative. A list of conditions associated with diffuse pulmonary hemorrhage is presented in Table 12-5.

Goodpasture Syndrome

Goodpasture syndrome is a triad of diffuse alveolar hemorrhage, glomerulonephritis, and a circulating cytotoxic autoantibody to a component of the basement membranes of the glomerulus and alveolus. This disease typically affects young men who often present with hemoptysis, dyspnea, weakness, and mild anemia. Pulmonary disease may precede renal disease by several months. Patients with Goodpasture syndrome experience extensive intraalveolar hemorrhage, resulting in heavy, dark red or rusty-colored lungs. Microscopically, red blood cells and hemosiderin-laden macrophages fill the alveoli and the alveolar septa are mildly thickened by interstitial fibrosis and hyperplasia of type II pneumocytes. Immunofluorescence shows a linear deposition of IgG and complement on the basement membrane. Radiographically, diffuse, bilateral alveolar infiltrates are present that may resolve within days after red blood cell breakdown. The diagnosis is established by renal or pulmonary biopsy. Treatment involves corticosteroids, cytotoxic drugs, and plasmapheresis.

Idiopathic Pulmonary Hemorrhage

Idiopathic pulmonary hemorrhage often affects children and is distinguished from Goodpasture syndrome by the absence of renal

Table 12-5

Conditions Resulting in Pulmonary Hemorrhage

Disease	Immunologic Mechanism	Immunofluorescence Pattern
Goodpasture syndrome	Antibasement membrane antibody	Linear
Systemic lupus erythematosus	Immune complexes	Granular
Mixed cryoglobulinemia		
Henoch-Schönlein purpura		
IgA disease		
Wegener granulomatosis	Antineutrophil cytoplasmic antibody (ANCA)	Negative or pauciimmune
Idiopathic glomerulonephritis		
Idiopathic pulmonary hemorrhage	No immunological marker	

From Rubin E, Gorstein F, Rubin R, et al. Rubin's Pathology, 4th ed. Philadelphia: Lippincott Williams & Wilkins, 2005, p. 610.

involvement or circulating autoantibodies. Microscopically, this disease is identical to Goodpasture syndrome. Patients present with cough, dyspnea, substernal chest pain, fatigue, iron deficiency anemia, and occasionally hemoptysis. Pulmonary hemorrhages are recurrent. The course is more protracted. Treatment involves corticosteroid administration, but the response is variable. One fourth of patients die of massive pulmonary hemorrhage, whereas many other patients develop progressive fibrosis and, ultimately, cor pulmonale.

Eosinophilic Pneumonia

Eosinophilic pneumonia refers to the accumulation of eosinophils in the alveolar spaces and may be idiopathic or secondary to a variety of conditions listed in Table 12-6. Idiopathic eosinophilic

Table 12-6
Types of Eosinophilic Pneumonia

Idiopathic	*Drug-induced*
Chronic eosinophilic pneumonia	Antibiotics
Acute eosinophilic pneumonia	Cytotoxic drugs
Simple eosinophilic pneumonia	Antiinflammatory agents
(Löffler syndrome)	Antihypertensive drugs
	L-Tryptophan (eosinophilic fasciitis)
Secondary eosinophilic pneumonia	*Immunologic or systemic diseases*
Infection	
Parasitic	Allergic bronchopulmonary as-
Tropical eosinophilic pneumonia	pergillosis
Ascaris lumbricoides, Toxara	Churg-Strauss syndrome
canis, filaria	Hypereosinophilic syndrome
Dirofilaria	
Fungal	
Aspergillus	

From Rubin E, Gorstein F, Rubin R, et al. Rubin's Pathology, 4th ed. Philadelphia: Lippincott Williams & Wilkins, 2005, p. 606.

pneumonia may be subdivided into three categories based on the severity of findings and the presence of symptoms.

- Simple eosinophilic pneumonia (Löffler syndrome): mild condition with transient pulmonary infiltrates that are often asymptomatic
- Acute eosinophilic pneumonia: symptoms of fever, hypoxemia, and diffuse interstitial and alveolar infiltrates on chest radiograph that occur within a week; may be accompanied by DAD. Patients respond well to corticosteroids, and the disease does not recur.
- Chronic eosinophilic pneumonia: symptoms of fever, night sweats, weight loss, cough productive of eosinophils, and dyspnea often in a background of asthma; alveoli are filled with eosinophils, macrophages, and a proteinaceous exudate; radiographs show peripheral alveolar infiltrates with sparing of the hilum. Patients respond dramatically to corticosteroids.

In industrialized countries, secondary eosinophilic pneumonia most commonly is caused by drug hypersensitivity, especially antibiotics, antiinflammatory agents, and cytotoxic drugs. In temperate climates, infectious agents such as *Ascaris lumbricoides* and *Aspergillus* may induce an eosinophilic pneumonia.

Endogenous Lipid Pneumonia

Endogenous lipid pneumonia (golden pneumonia) is localized distal to an obstructed airway and is characterized by lipid-laden macrophages in the alveolar spaces. Grossly, the lungs appear golden-yellow. Microscopically, the alveoli are filled with foamy macrophages that contain needle-shaped cholesterol clefts. The alveolar walls maintain their structure, and a mild chronic inflammation and fibrosis may be present.

Exogenous Lipid Pneumonia

Exogenous lipid pneumonia is caused by aspirated mineral, vegetable, or animal oil. Grossly, the lung demonstrates a poorly demarcated, gray, greasy lesion. Microscopically, foamy macrophages are present in the alveoli and interstitium. Large oil droplets are surrounded by a foreign-body giant cell reaction. Patients often are asymptomatic, and the lesion is detected commonly as an incidental radiographic finding.

Obstructive Pulmonary Diseases

Chronic obstructive pulmonary disease (COPD) is a general term that describes patients who demonstrate a decrease in forced expiratory volume, as determined by spirometric pulmonary function tests (PFTs). COPD encompasses a variety of diseases, including chronic bronchitis, asthma, and emphysema. COPD is characterized by decreased air flow, either by an increased resistance within the airways (narrowed airways in chronic bronchitis or asthma) or a reduction in the outflow pressure (loss of elastic recoil in emphysema).

Chronic Bronchitis

Chronic bronchitis is defined clinically as the presence of a chronic productive cough without discernible cause for more than half the time over a period of 2 years. This disease is caused by cigarette smoking primarily, with more than 90% of cases occurring in smokers. The frequency and severity of acute respiratory tract infections is increased in patients with chronic bronchitis. Often, chronic bronchitis is accompanied by emphysema, with both diseases contributing to the clinical presentation.

Initially, cough and sputum production are more severe in the winter months, but over time these symptoms occur throughout the year. Patients have an increased risk of acute respiratory failure precipitated by infections or air pollution. In addition, patients have an increased risk of infections by *H. influenzae* and *S. pneumoniae* caused by retained mucous secretions. As the disease progresses, exertional dyspnea, cyanosis, and cor pulmonale may develop, and patients are described as "blue bloaters."

Microscopically, chronic bronchitis is characterized by hyperplasia and hypertrophy of the mucous cells and an increased proportion of mucous to serous cells. Additional microscopic findings include the following:

- Excess mucus in the central and peripheral airways
- Pits in the bronchial epithelium that represent dilated bronchial gland ducts
- Thickening of the bronchial wall caused by mucous gland enlargement and edema
- Increased numbers of goblet cells (hyperplasia)
- Increased amounts of bronchial smooth muscle
- Squamous metaplasia of the bronchial epithelium caused by tobacco smoke

Emphysema

Emphysema is a chronic lung disease characterized by enlargement of the airspaces distal to the terminal bronchioles with destruction the bronchiole wall. Compared to patients with chronic bronchitis, patients with emphysema are at lower risk for recurrent pulmonary infections and are less likely to develop cor pulmonale.

The major cause of emphysema is cigarette smoking, and moderate to severe emphysema is uncommon in nonsmokers. It has been proposed that emphysema results from an imbalance in elastin synthesis in the lung and breakdown of elastic tissue, leading to an overall loss of elastin and damage to the alveolar wall. Smoking both increases the number of neutrophils in the alveoli (which contain elastase) and reduces α_1-antitrypsin activity (which normally blocks elastase activity).

Another cause of emphysema is a hereditary deficiency in α_1-antitrypsin. This form of emphysema typically affects younger persons and most often is associated with the *PiZ* allele. In addition to emphysema, these patients also develop cirrhosis of the liver.

Emphysema is classified according to the portion of the alveolus involved (Fig. 12-2), although the disease may demonstrate various admixtures of these types:

- Centrilobular emphysema: most common and is associated with cigarette smoking and clinical symptoms; destruction of the cluster of terminal bronchioles near the end of the bronchiolar tree; most severe in the upper zones of the lung

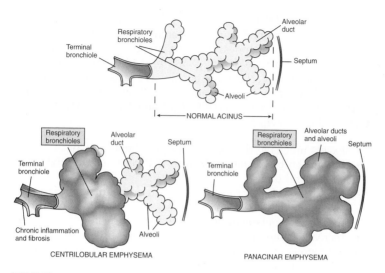

F I G U R E   12-2
Types of emphysema. The acinus is the gas-exchanging structure of
the lung situated distal to the terminal bronchiole. In centrilobular
(proximal acinar) emphysema, the respiratory bronchioles are predominantly involved. In panacinar (distal acinar) emphysema, the
acinus is uniformly damaged. (From Rubin E, Gorstein F, Rubin R,
et al. Rubin's Pathology, 4th ed. Philadelphia: Lippincott Williams &
Wilkins, 2005, p. 618.)

- Panacinar emphysema: acinus is uniformly affected, with destruction of the alveolar septa from the center to the periphery
  of the acinus; may result in a lacy network of supporting tissue;
  occurs in α_1-antitrypsin deficiency and smokers; tends to occur
  in the lower zones of the lung
- Localized emphysema: destruction of alveoli and emphysema
  in only one or a few locations; often at the apex of an upper
  lobe; can result in bullae

Patients with emphysema often present after the 60 years of
age with a prolonged history of exertional dyspnea and minimal,
nonproductive cough. These patients often require the use of accessory muscles to breathe, are tachypneic, and have a prolonged expiratory phase. Because they have a higher respiratory rate and an
increased minute volume, they can maintain arterial hemoglobin
saturation at near-normal levels and are referred to as "pink puf-
fers." Radiologically, there is overinflation of the lung, demon-

strated by enlarged lungs, depressed diaphragms, and an increased posteroanterior diameter (barrel chest). Fibrosis generally is not a characteristic of emphysema. The disease progresses over time, and no treatment is essentially effective.

Asthma

Asthma is a chronic lung disease caused by increased responsiveness of the airways to a variety of stimuli. Asthma affects up to 10% of children and 5% of adults in the United States, and the prevalence appears to be increasing. Previously, asthma had been subclassified into extrinsic (allergic) asthma and intrinsic (idiosyncratic) asthma, although this terminology is no longer used.

The underlying pathophysiology of asthma is proposed to be a bronchial hyperresponsiveness to an inflammatory reaction to diverse stimuli. Following exposure to an inciting factor, the inhaled allergen interacts with T_H2 cells and IgE antibody bound to the surface of mast cells. Activated macrophages, mast cells, eosinophils, and basophils then release inflammatory mediators, which result in bronchoconstriction, increased vascular permeability, and mucous secretions. These inflammatory mediators include histamine, bradykinin, leukotrienes, prostaglandins, thromboxane A_2, platelet-activating factor, and interleukins.

A variety of triggering factors can induce asthma, including the following:

- Allergy: most common trigger and often found in children
- Infection: RSV in children younger than 2 years of age and often rhinovirus, influenza, and parainfluenza in older patients
- Exercise: related to increased heat or water loss from the airway epithelium
- Occupational exposure
- Drug exposure: often aspirin and other nonsteroidal antiinflammatory agents
- Air pollution
- Emotional factors

Grossly, the lungs from patients who die during status asthmaticus are distended with air and the airways are filled with thick, tenacious, adherent mucous plugs. Microscopically, the mucous plugs contain epithelium, eosinophils, and Charcot-Leyden crystals, which are derived from phospholipids of the eosinophil cell membrane. Occasionally, the mucoid exudates form a cast of the airways, termed a Curschmann spiral. Compact clusters of epithelial cells, termed Creola bodies, also can be seen in the sputum. The submucosa is edematous and contains a mixed inflammatory infiltrate. Squamous metaplasia, goblet cell hyperplasia, and a thickened basement membrane may be present.

Patients often present with paroxysms of wheezing, dyspnea, and cough, and acute episodes may be superimposed on a background of chronic airway obstruction. When acute asthma is severe and unresponsive to therapy, it is termed status asthmaticus and often requires hospitalization. Treatment for asthma classically includes the administration of β-adrenergic agonists, inhaled corticosteroids, cromolyn sodium, methylxanthines, and anticholinergic agents. Systemic corticosteroids are reserved for status asthmaticus or resistant chronic asthma.

Pneumoconioses

Pneumoconioses are diseases caused by inhalation of inorganic dusts, and includes silicosis, coal dust pneumoconiosis, asbestosis, and berylliosis. Generally, the lung lesions produced by these dusts reflects the dose and size of the particle inhaled, and the symptoms are often a result of the amount of fibrosis produced secondary to these factors. Often, the most severe disease is that produced by particles that reach the more peripheral regions of the lung.

Silicosis

Silicosis is caused by inhalation of silicon dioxide (silica) and may affect persons involved in sandblasting, mining, ceramic manufacturing, and metal polishing, among others. Silicosis is most caused by the crystalline form of silica (quartz). A pro-fibrogenic cycle is formed that involves such processes as the ingestion of silica particles by macrophages, death of macrophages with release of silica and fibrogenic factors, and reingestion of silica by new macrophages. The following are the forms of silicosis that occur:

- Simple nodular silicosis: nodules smaller than 1 cm in diameter, composed of concentrically arranged collagen, around which lymphocytes and fibroblasts coalesce; often asymptomatic
- Progressive massive fibrosis: nodules larger than 2 cm in diameter, leading to cavitation and fibrosis; may present with exertional dyspnea or dyspnea at rest
- Acute silicosis: diffuse fibrosis without nodules; rapidly progressive dyspnea

Coal Workers' Pneumoconiosis

Coal workers' pneumoconiosis (CWP) can occur in mine workers and is caused by inhalation of coal dust, which contains silica, carbon, and other molecules. Simple CWP demonstrates nonpalpable black nodules that are smaller than 1 cm in diameter, which are composed of carbon-laden macrophages associated with mild dilation of the respiratory bronchioles and occasionally a fibrotic stroma. Complicated CWP demonstrates lesions larger than 2 cm in diameter, progressive fibrosis, and often significant respiratory impairment.

Asbestosis

Asbestosis occurs with inhalation of long, thin fibrous silicate minerals, which are found in older insulation, construction material, and brake linings, and form deposits at the bifurcations of alveolar ducts. Some particles are ingested by macrophages, whereas others penetrate the interstitium and activate inflammatory and fibrogenic cascades. Asbestosis is characterized by bilateral, diffuse interstitial fibrosis, and the presence of asbestos bodies (ferruginous bodies), which appear as a thin golden-brown fibers surrounded by a beaded iron-protein coat with terminal rounded protrusions (dumbbell shaped). These molecules stain with Prussian blue iron stain. A variety of complications may result from asbestos exposure and include the following:

- Benign pleural effusion
- Pleural plaques: pearly white with a smooth or nodular surface formed of acellular, dense, hyalinized fibrous tissue with numerous slitlike spaces
- Diffuse pleural fibrosis: fibrosis restricted to the pleura
- Rounded atelectasis: caused by pleural fibrosis and adhesions associated with atelectasis
- Honeycomb lung
- Mesothelioma: discussed later

Berylliosis

Berylliosis can occur with inhalation of beryllium, which is used in aerospace industries, industrial ceramic manufacturing, and atomic reactors. Acute berylliosis occurs within hours or days of exposure and is reflected pathologically as diffuse alveolar damage. Chronic berylliosis is reflected pathologically by the presence of numerous noncaseating granulomas situated along the pleura, septa, and bronchovascular bundles. Patients may progress to end-stage fibrosis and honeycomb lung.

Talcosis

Talcosis occurs with prolonged and heavy exposure to talc dust or by intravenous drug use when talc is used as a carrier material. Microscopically, foreign-body granulomas are associated with birefringent platelike talc particles in a background of fibrotic nodules and interstitial fibrosis.

Interstitial Lung Disease

A variety of diseases are categorized as interstitial lung diseases and present with restrictive pulmonary function, interstitial inflammatory infiltrates, and similar clinical and radiologic patterns. Pulmonary tests often reveal decreased lung volume and decreased oxygen-diffusion capacity. A summary of interstitial lung diseases is presented in the following.

Hypersensitivity Pneumonitis (Extrinsic Allergic Alveolitis)

Hypersensitivity pneumonitis may be induced by a wide variety of antigens, including moldy hay (farmer's lung), fungi in stagnant water sources, and long-term exposure to bird feathers and excrement (bird fancier's lung). Hypersensitivity pneumonitis may be acute or chronic. Acute hypersensitivity pneumonitis is characterized by neutrophils in the alveoli and respiratory bronchioles.

- Chronic hypersensitivity pneumonitis is characterized by bronchiolocentric cellular interstitial lymphocytes, plasma cells and macrophages, noncaseating granuloma formation, and organizing pneumonia. End-stage hypersensitivity pneumonitis may result in pulmonary fibrosis.

Patients often present initially with dyspnea, cough, and mild fever 4 to 6 hours after allergen exposure. The symptoms remit within a day, but reemerge on reexposure and may become chronic, resulting in cor pulmonale if severe. Pulmonary function tests demonstrate a restrictive pattern with reduced compliance, reduced diffusion capacity, and hypoxemia. Removal of the offending environmental agent is the only effective treatment, although steroids may help a subset of patients.

Sarcoidosis

Sarcoidosis most commonly affects the lungs but also may involve the skin, lymph nodes, and eyes. In North America, the prevalence of sarcoidosis is highest in African Americans, but may affect persons of any background or gender and often occurs in younger persons. Although the underlying etiology of sarcoidosis is unclear, a possible exaggerated helper T-cell response may underlie the pathogenesis of this disease.

Pulmonary sarcoidosis affects the lung and hilar lymph nodes and results in the formation of multiple noncaseating granulomas in the interstitium, pleura, and around the bronchovascular bundles. This cellular granulomatous phase may be followed by a fibrotic phase in which the granulomas become fibrotic beginning at the periphery and may demonstrate an onion skin appearance. Asteroid-bodies (star-shaped crystals) and Schaumann bodies (small lamellar calcifications) may be present in the granulomas. Radiographically, sarcoidosis demonstrates diffuse reticulonodular infiltrates are present.

Acute sarcoidosis has an abrupt onset and often demonstrates a spontaneous remission within 2 years. Chronic sarcoidosis has an insidious onset and is often progressive. Patients often present with cough and dyspnea. The prognosis is favorable for these patients and the active stages can be treated with corticosteroids.

Usual Interstitial Pneumonia

Usual interstitial pneumonia (UIP) is often idiopathic (termed idiopathic pulmonary fibrosis), but may be secondary to collagen vascular disease, drug toxicity, and asbestosis, among other causes. The etiology may be immunologic, viral, or genetic, although the exact cause remains to be determined.

The lungs in UIP are small and fibrosis tends to be worse in the lower lobes, subpleural regions and interlobular septa, which leads to a retraction of the lungs along the scars, giving the lung a hobnail appearance. Pathologically, chronic interstitial inflammation and interstitial fibrosis is patchy, with focal areas of scarring and honeycomb cystic change. The fibrosis tends to be worse under the pleura and foci of fibrosis are found adjacent to regions of normal lung. The fibroblastic foci demonstrate temporal heterogeneity, with foci of different ages present within the lung. Fibroblastic foci are best demonstrated by a Movat stain.

UIP begins insidiously, with the gradual onset of exertional dyspnea and dry cough over a period of 5 to 10 years that ultimately leads to severe restrictive lung disease. The radiographs show diffuse bilateral reticular infiltrates that are most prominent in the lower lobes. Physical examination reveals fine rales at the lung bases and late inspiratory crackles. Over time, tachypnea at rest, cyanosis, and cor pulmonale may develop. Patients may be treated with corticosteroids and cyclophosphamide, but lung transplantation is often the only option for a cure. The mean survival for these patients is 4 to 6 years.

Desquamative Interstitial Pneumonia

Desquamative interstitial pneumonia (DIP) is a chronic, fibrosing, interstitial pneumonitis of unknown etiology that often occurs in cigarette smokers in the fourth or fifth decades. DIP is distinguished from UIP by the preservation of normal alveolar architecture and the lack of patchy scarring and honeycomb change. The alveoli are filled with macrophages that contain a fine, granular golden-brown pigment and the interstitium demonstrates mild chronic inflammation and fibrosis. DIP has been proposed to represent a spectrum with respiratory bronchiolitis (see below).

Radiographs show bilateral ground glass infiltrates, predominantly in the lower lobes. Patients respond well to corticosteroids and smoking cessation.

Respiratory Bronchiolitis

Respiratory bronchiolitis (RB) occurs in cigarette smokers and may be an incidental finding or may cause interstitial lung disease. Microscopically, a prominent accumulation of pigmented macrophages is present in the airways, especially centered on the bronchioles. The process is patchy and there may be focal interstitial fibrosis centered around the bronchioles. Patients generally have only mild respiratory dysfunction. Radiographs show a thickening of the peripheral bronchioles most prominently in the upper lobes. Symptoms often resolve after smoking.

Bronchiolitis Obliterans-organizing Pneumonia

Bronchiolitis obliterans-organizing pneumonia (BOOP), is characterized by polypoid plugs of tissue that fill the bronchiolar lumen and adjacent airways. BOOP may occur in a variety of conditions, including inhalation of toxic materials, drug administration, and respiratory tract infections. Microscopically, plugs of loose organizing fibrosis and chronic inflammatory cells occlude bronchioles (bronchiolitis obliterans), alveolar ducts, and alveoli (organizing pneumonia), but the architecture of the lung is preserved. The alveolar septa are only slightly thickened and contain chronic inflammation.

Organizing pneumonia demonstrates a mean onset of 55 years and presents with acute onset of fever, cough, and dyspnea approximately 4 to 6 weeks after a flulike illness. Radiographs demonstrate localized opacities or bilateral interstitial infiltrates, which migrate over time. Corticosteroid therapy is effective and many patients within weeks to months even without therapy.

Lymphoid Interstitial Pneumonia

Lymphoid interstitial pneumonia (LIP) is a rare disease that most commonly affects adults and may be idiopathic or associated with a variety of conditions (Table 12-7).

LIP is characterized by a diffuse infiltration of alveolar septa and peribronchiolar spaces by lymphocytes, plasma cells, and macrophages and noncaseating granulomas may be present. The

Table 12-7

Interstitial Lung Disease

Disease	Etiology	Pathologic Findings	Radiologic Findings
Hypersensitivity pneumonitis	Inhaled allergens	Acute form has neutrophils in alveoli Chronic form has bronchiolocentric interstitial inflammation with plasma cells, lymphocytes, and noncaseating granulomas	
Sarcoidosis	Probable exaggerated T-cell response	Multiple noncaseating granulomas in the interstitium and pleura that may fibrose; Schaumann bodies; asteroid bodies	Diffuse reticulonodular infiltrate
Usual interstitial pneumonia (UIP)	Often idiopathic, many secondary causes	Small lungs; fibrosis worse in lower lobes; patchy chronic inflammation and interstitial fibrosis worse under the pleura; foci of normal lung present; fibroblast foci of varying ages	Diffuse bilateral reticular infiltrates worse in the lower lobes
Desquamative interstitial pneumonia (DIP)	Unknown, but related to smoking	Preserved alveolar architecture without scarring; mildly thickened alveolar walls with chronic inflammation and interstitial fibrosis; macrophages with golden-brown pigment	Bilateral ground-glass infiltrates, more predominant in the lower lobes
Respiratory bronchiolitis	Smoking	Patchy accumulation of pigmented macrophages in the air spaces, centered on the bronchioles; mild peribronchiolar fibrosis and chronic inflammation	Thickened peripheral bronchioles in the upper lobes

(continues)

Table 12-7
(continued)

Disease	Etiology	Pathologic Findings	Radiologic Findings
Bronchiolitis obliterans-organizing pneumonia (BOOP)	Drugs, toxins, inflammation, viral	Patchy areas of loose organizing fibrosis and chronic inflammation in the distal airways (bronchiolitis obliterans) and alveoli (organizing pneumonia) adjacent to normal lung; plugs of interstitial organizing fibrosis in the airways; architecture preserved	Localized opacities or bilateral infiltrates that migrate over time
Lymphoid interstitial pneumonia (LIP)	Idiopathic Dysproteinemia Collagen vascular disease Immunodeficiency Infection Iatrogenic	Diffuse infiltration of alveolar septa and peribronchiolar spaces by lymphocytes, plasma cells and macrophages; lung architecture preserved	

alveolar architecture is preserved without evidence of scarring. The alveolar spaces often contain proteinaceous exudates.

Patients often present with cough and progressive dyspnea, which may progress in some instances to end-stage lung. Corticosteroids and cytotoxic drugs may prove of some benefit.

Langerhans Cell Histiocytosis (Histiocytosis X)

Langerhans cell histiocytosis (LCH) encompasses a several conditions, including eosinophilic granuloma, Hand-Schüller-Christian disease, and Letterer-Siwe disease. In adults, LCH is often an isolated disease termed pulmonary eosinophilic granuloma, and is almost always associated with cigarette smoking. Pulmonary LCH often affects patients in the third or fourth decades of life Children are often affected by Hand-Schüller-Christian disease or Letterer-Siwe disease (see Chapter 20).

Microscopically, pulmonary LCH demonstrates scattered nodular infiltrates with stellate borders that are centered on the bronchioles or in a subpleural location and frequently extend into the interstitium. The lesions demonstrate Langerhans cells admixed with lymphocytes, eosinophils, and macrophages. Langerhans cells are characterized by prominently grooved nuclei, small nucleoli, cytoplasmic Birbeck granules demonstrated by electron microscopy, and CD1a and S-100 expression. The disease can progress to end-stage fibrosis and honeycomb lung.

Presenting symptoms of pulmonary LCH may be a nonproductive cough, dyspnea on exertion, and spontaneous pneumothorax. Radiographs show diffuse bilateral reticulonodular lesions in the upper lobes that may undergo cavitation. Cessation of smoking is beneficial early in the disease.

Lymphangioleiomyomatosis

Lymphangioleiomyomatosis (LAM) occurs in women of childbearing age and is characterized by the widespread, abnormal proliferation of smooth muscle in the lung, mediastinal and retroperitoneal lymph nodes, and the major lymphatic ducts. This proliferation appears to be under hormonal control and may occur in association with tuberous sclerosis.

Grossly, the lungs are enlarged and show extensive cystic changes. Microscopically, the cystic spaces are lined by nodules or bundles of rounded or spindle-shaped smooth muscle cells that lack normal parallel organization. The smooth muscle cells follow a lymphatic distribution within the interlobular septa, along the pleura, and around blood vessels and bronchioles. These cells immunolabel for HMB45 and occasionally for estrogen and progesterone receptors.

Patients present with shortness of breath, hemoptysis, cough, spontaneous pneumothorax or chylous effusions. As the disease progresses, the radiographs demonstrate a diffuse interstitial reticular or cystic pattern. Although some patients have an indolent course, many die from progressive respiratory failure. Hormonal ablation therapy may be of benefit in some patients.

Lung Transplantation

Patients undergo lung transplantation for a variety of disease, and the major complications of lung transplant include acute and chronic rejection and infection.

Acute rejection demonstrates perivascular infiltrates of lymphocytes, macrophages, and eosinophils. Chronic rejection shows bronchiolitis obliterans, with late formation of bronchiectasis. Numerous opportunistic infections may occur in these patients, including infection with cytomegalovirus, *Candida*, and *Aspergillus*. Lymphoproliferative disorders can occur in 3% to 8% of cases and often are associated with Epstein-Barr virus (EBV) infection.

Vasculitis and Granulomatosis

Wegener Granulomatosis

Wegener granulomatosis (WG) is a disease of unknown etiology that is characterized by aseptic, necrotizing, granulomatous inflammation, and vasculitis that most commonly affects the head and neck, followed by the lung, kidney, and eye. In most cases, the lung nodules are multiple and bilateral and have a tan-brown or hemorrhagic cut surface, often with cavitation. Microscopically, these nodules demonstrate tissue necrosis, granulomatous inflammation, and fibrosis. Vasculitis may affects arteries, capillaries, or veins and may consist of acute, chronic, or granulomatous inflammation that destroys the internal and external elastic lamina. The lungs may show acute or chronic hemorrhage. Neutrophilic infiltration of the alveolar walls, termed neutrophilic capillaritis, is often present.

Patients may present with cough, hemoptysis, or pleuritis, and may demonstrate systemic symptoms including arthralgias, skin lesions, fever, weight loss, peripheral neuropathy, central nervous system disorders, and pericarditis. Diffuse pulmonary hemorrhage, resulting in severe respiratory failure and renal failure, may be fatal. Radiographs show multiple bilateral intrapulmonary nodules.

Serum studies indicate elevated levels of classical and perinuclear antineutrophil cytoplasm antibody (C-ANCA and P-ANCA, respectively). Most patients are treated effectively with corticosteroids and cyclophosphamide.

Churg-Strauss Syndrome (Allergic Angiitis and Granulomatosis)

Churg-Strauss syndrome is a disease of unknown etiology that is characterized by vasculitis composed of varying types of inflammatory cells including eosinophils, lymphocytes, plasma cells, macrophages, giant cells, and neutrophils. In addition, the lungs show changes of asthmatic bronchitis or bronchiolitis, eosinophilic pneumonia, and parenchymal necrosis. Three clinical phases occur, including the following:

- Prodrome: allergic rhinitis, asthma, peripheral eosinophilia, eosinophilic pneumonia or eosinophilic enteritis
- Systemic vasculitic phase: extrapulmonary manifestations, including cutaneous leukocytoclastic vasculitis or peripheral neuropathy
- Postvasculitic phase: often characterized by persistent asthma and allergic rhinitis, sometimes with cardiovascular manifestations of pericarditis, hypertension, and cardiac failure

Patients are often positive for P-ANCA during the vasculitic phase. Most patients respond to corticosteroids, but severe cases may require cyclophosphamide.

Necrotizing Sarcoid Granulomatosis

This disease consists of nodular confluent sarcoid granulomas and a pulmonary-specific vasculitis containing giant cells, necrotizing granulomas, and chronic inflammation. Radiographs show multiple well-circumscribed pulmonary nodules. Most patients are asymptomatic, and corticosteroids are used in patients with multiple pulmonary nodules.

Pulmonary Hypertension

The mature lung is a high-volume, low-pressure system in adults, with increased pulmonary pressure defined as a mean pressure exceeding 25 mm Hg at rest. Pulmonary hypertension can occur in instances of increased flow or increased vascular resistance and may be conceptualized as precapillary or postcapillary, with the source of abnormality localized proximal or distal to the capillary bed.

Causes of precapillary pulmonary hypertension include the following:

- Left-to-right cardiac shunts
- Primary pulmonary hypertension (see below)
- Thromboembolic pulmonary hypertension
- Hypertension secondary to fibrotic lung disease and hypoxia

Causes of postcapillary pulmonary hypertension include the following:

- Pulmonary venoocclusive disease
- Hypertension secondary to left-sided cardiac disorders such as mitral stenosis and aortic coarctation

In general, pulmonary atherosclerosis is present in the largest pulmonary arteries. Pulmonary hypertension can be graded from 1 through 6, with grades 1 to 3 being reversible and grades 4 to 6 being irreversible. The grades include the following:

- Grade 1: medial hypertrophy of the muscular pulmonary arteries and the appearance of smooth muscle in the pulmonary arterioles
- Grade 2: intimal proliferation with increasing medial hypertrophy
- Grade 3: intimal fibrosis of muscular pulmonary arteries and arterioles, which may be occlusive
- Grade 4: formation of plexiform lesions together with dilation and thinning of the pulmonary arteries
- Grade 5: plexiform lesions in combination with dilation or angiomatoid lesions
- Grade 6: fibrinoid necrosis of the arteries and arterioles

Over time, pulmonary hypertension from any cause can result in right ventricle hypertrophy and cor pulmonale.

Primary pulmonary hypertension is a rare disease caused by increased tone in the pulmonary arteries and is most common in women in their 20s and 30s. Patients manifest an insidious onset of dyspnea, and radiographs may be normal in the early stages of the disease. Medical treatment is ineffective for primary pulmonary hypertension, and a heart-lung transplant is the only effective means of treatment.

Pulmonary venoocclusive disease is characterized by extensive occlusion of small pulmonary veins and venules by loose, sparsely cellular, intimal fibrosis. This cause of pulmonary hypertension has a more fulminant course than other causes of pulmonary hypertension and the radiographs show scattered pulmonary infiltrates.

Pulmonary Hamartoma

Pulmonary hamartomas most commonly occur during the sixth decade and often are discovered incidentally. These lesions are benign neoplasms that often present in the peripheral lung and occasionally cause bronchial obstruction if located within the bronchiole. Grossly, these lesions are solitary, circumscribed, lobulated masses that average 2 cm in diameter and have a white or gray, cartilaginous cut surface. The tumor contains elements that normally are present within the lung, including cartilage, fibromyxoid connective tissue, fat, bone, smooth muscle, and clefts lined by respiratory epithelium. Radiographically, these lesions demonstrate a characteristic "popcorn" pattern of calcification.

Lung Neoplasms

The lung may be affected by metastatic disease, in which lesions are often well-demarcated and multiple, and primary lung cancer. Lung cancer is the most common cause of cancer death worldwide. The main distinction is between small cell and non-small cell carcinoma; small-cell carcinoma may respond to chemotherapy and is generally not amenable to surgical resection. Lung carcinoma often presents between 60 to 70 years of age and has a male predominance, although the number of affected women is increasing.

Lung cancer is the most common cause of cancer death worldwide and is caused by cigarette smoking in the vast majority of cases. In addition, a variety of genetic alterations have been implicated in the development of lung cancer, including the following:

- *K-ras* oncogene mutations: occur in 25% of adenocarcinomas, 20% of large cell carcinomas, and 5% of squamous cell carcinomas; rare in small cell carcinoma
- *Myc* oncogene overexpression: occurs in 10% to 40% of small cell carcinomas, but is rare in other types
- *P53* mutations: occur in 80% of small cell carcinomas and 50% of non-small cell carcinoma
- *Rb* mutations: occur in 80% of small cell carcinomas and 25% of non-small cell carcinoma
- *Bcl-2* protooncogene expression: occurs in 25% of squamous cell carcinomas and 5% of adenocarcinomas

All subtypes of lung cancer share many common features, including the following:

- Pulmonary effects: cough, dyspnea, hemoptysis, chest pain, obstructive pneumonia, and pleural effusion
- Pancoast syndrome: involvement of the lung apex by tumor may involve the eighth cervical and first and second thoracic nerves, which results in shoulder pain radiating in an ulnar distribution down the arm
- Horner syndrome: a Pancoast tumor that paralyzes the cervical sympathetic nerves leading to depression of the eyeball (enophthalmos), ptosis of the upper eyelid, constriction of the pupil (miosis), and absence of sweating on the affected side of the face (anhidrosis)
- Superior vena cava syndrome: mediastinal tumor growth may obstruct the superior vena cava

- Metastases: regional lymph nodes and distal spread to the brain, bone, liver, and adrenal glands
- Paraneoplastic syndromes: acanthosis nigricans, dermatomyositis/polymyositis, myasthenic syndromes, Cushing syndrome, syndrome of inappropriate antidiuretic hormone secretion (SIADH), hypercalcemia

Overall, the 5-year survival for patients with lung cancer is 15%, although the cancer subtype specific survival varies from 42% for bronchoalveolar carcinoma to 5% for small cell carcinoma.

Squamous Cell Carcinoma
Squamous cell carcinoma accounts for approximately 30% of lung carcinomas in the United States. These cancers often arise in the central portion of the lung from the major or segmental bronchi and appear grossly as firm, gray-white lesions that may ulcerate the bronchial wall and invade the pulmonary parenchyma. Central cavitation may be present. Well-differentiated squamous cell carcinomas demonstrate keratin pearls and often individual cell keratinization, whereas poorly differentiated carcinomas may be difficult to distinguish from other subtypes.

Adenocarcinoma
Adenocarcinoma accounts for approximately 30% of lung carcinomas in the United States. These cancers most commonly arise in the periphery of the lung and grossly appear as irregular gray-white lesions that may cause puckering of the overlying pleura. Adenocarcinomas may be subdivided into acinar, papillary, solid with mucus formation, and bronchoalveolar carcinoma (see next paragraph), and generally there is at least focal gland formation and intracytoplasmic mucin as demonstrated by PAS stain. Adenocarcinomas demonstrate surrounding parenchymal invasion and occasionally involvement of the pleura.

Bronchioloalveolar Carcinoma
Bronchioloalveolar carcinoma (BAC) is a rare subtype of adenocarcinoma (1%–5%) that grows along preexisting alveolar walls without invasion of the underlying pulmonary parenchyma. The cells in BAC appear as atypical cuboidal to low columnar cells with occasional mucinous features. Invasive tumor growth arising from a BAC often defines the tumor as an adenocarcinoma. BAC is a form of lung carcinoma that is not strictly linked to cigarette smoking.

Small Cell Carcinoma
Small cell carcinoma ("oat cell carcinoma") accounts for approximately 20% of all lung carcinomas in the United States. Small cell

carcinoma often appears as a perihilar mass with rapid growth and frequent lymph node metastases. As many as 70% of patients present at an advanced stage. Grossly, small cell carcinoma appears soft and white with extensive hemorrhage and necrosis on cut section. Microscopically, the cells appear round or oval with hyperchromatic nuclei, scant cytoplasm, absent or inconspicuous nucleoli, and nuclear molding (nuclei appear to embrace one another). Although termed "small cell," the cells are actually significantly larger than surrounding lymphocytes. Necrosis is common and the mitotic index is extremely high in these tumors. Often, small cell carcinoma may present with paraneoplastic syndromes, especially diabetes insipidus and Cushing syndrome. Small cell carcinoma must be distinguished from other subtypes of lung carcinoma because of the different treatment options.

Large Cell Carcinoma

Large cell carcinoma is typically a diagnosis of exclusion when the lesion does not morphologically fit into the classification of squamous cell carcinoma, adenocarcinoma, or small cell carcinoma. Generally, the neoplastic cells are large with ample cytoplasm. This subtype accounts for approximately 10% of all lung carcinomas.

Carcinoid Tumors

Carcinoid tumors are neuroendocrine tumors that are derived from the pluripotential basal layer of the respiratory epithelium and account for 2% of all lung carcinomas. These tumors may be situated in any part of the lung and appear grossly as fleshy, smooth, polypoid masses that protrude into the bronchial lumen. Microscopically, these tumors show an organoid, trabecular, or rosette-like growth pattern with uniform cells containing finely granular ("salt and pepper") nuclei. Carcinoids are classified as atypical if they have increased mitotic activity (2–10 mitotic figures per 10 high-power fields), necrosis, disorganization of the architecture, and nuclear pleomorphism. Carcinoid tumors often are indolent lesions and symptoms, when present, include hemoptysis, postobstructive pneumonitis, and dyspnea, as well as occasional endocrinopathies such as Cushing syndrome. These lesions may occur at any age, but account for the most common form of primary lung carcinoma presenting in childhood. The prognosis for these patients is excellent, with a 90% 5-year survival for typical carcinoids and a 60% 5-year survival for atypical carcinoids.

Rare Pulmonary Tumors

A variety of uncommon tumors occur in the lungs, including the following:

- Inflammatory pseudotumor: circumscribed nodular masses of inflammatory cells and fibroblasts that occur often before 40 years of age and contain a mixture of inflammatory cells
- Pulmonary epithelioid hemangioendothelioma: low-grade vascular neoplasms that often occur in young adult women who present with multiple oval-shaped nodules with a central, sclerotic hypocellular zone and a peripheral cellular zone
- Carcinosarcoma: mixture of epithelioid and spindled cells that may represent a dedifferentiation of a lung carcinoma
- Pulmonary blastoma: malignant tumor that resembles embryonal lung with a glandular component of poorly differentiated columnar cells in tubules and spindled intervening cells that occurs in adults
- Mucoepidermoid carcinoma and adenoid cystic carcinoma: identical to the lesions that occur in the salivary glands and arise within the tracheobronchial mucous glands
- Pulmonary artery sarcoma: mesenchymal tumor that may represent lesions such as fibrosarcoma, leiomyosarcoma, or angiosarcoma that grows in an intraluminal fashion with proximal arteries and extends in a wormlike fashion into branching arterioles
- Lymphomatoid granulomatosis: lymphoproliferative disorder of EBV-infected B cells characterized by a pulmonary nodular lymphoid infiltrate with central necrosis and vascular permeation that occurs in middle-aged persons

THE PLEURA

Pneumothorax

A pneumothorax refers to air within the pleural cavity that may occur secondary to traumatic perforation of the pleura or that may be spontaneous. Spontaneous pneumothorax most commonly occurs in young adults and is often caused by the rupture of an emphysematous bleb. A tension pneumothorax is a life-threatening pneumothorax large enough to shift the mediastinum to the opposite side that may result in compression of the opposite lung.

Pleural Effusion

A pleural effusion is a collection of excess fluid within the pleural cavity that may be caused by a variety of benign or malignant inciting factors. Pleural effusions may be differentially labeled based on the content of the effusion:

- Hydrothorax: watery effusion that occurs secondary to increased hydrostatic pressure in the capillaries in patients with heart failure, pulmonary edema, or systemic edema
- Pyothorax: effusion containing large amounts of neutrophils that occurs with infections of the pleura or as a complication of bacterial pneumonia
- Empyema: variant of pyothorax in which thick pus accumulates within the pleural cavity, often accompanied by loculation and fibrosis
- Hemothorax: bloody effusion that occurs following trauma or a ruptured vessel
- Chylothorax: milky, lipid-rich effusion caused by lymphatic obstruction

Pleuritis

Inflammation of the pleura (pleuritis) can result from the extension of a pulmonary infection to the pleura, bacterial infections within the pleural cavity, viral infections, collagen vascular disease, or pulmonary infarction. Patients generally describe a sharp, stabbing chest pain on inspiration.

Tumors of the Pleura

Solitary Fibrous Tumor

Solitary fibrous tumor is a localized neoplasm that may occur at many sites, including the visceral and parietal pleura. These lesions occasionally are pedunculated and may be very large in size. Grossly, these lesions demonstrate a nodular, whorled, or lobulated gray-white cut surface with occasional cyst formation. The tumor cells are spindle-to-oval shaped and commonly form a "patternless pattern," which describes a random or disorderly appearance. Interspersed ropy collagen is often a defning feature. A subset of these lesions is malignant and demonstrates increased cellularity, pleomorphism, necrosis and more than 4 mitoses per 10 high power fields. Solitary fibrous tumor presents at an average age of 55 years and patients may have chest pain, shortness of breath, cough, hypoglycemia, weight loss, hemoptysis, fever, or night sweats. Patients have a good prognosis if the lesions are completely excised.

Malignant Mesothelioma

Malignant mesothelioma arises from mesothelial cells and may occur in the pleura, peritoneum, pericardium, and the tunica vaginalis. The average age of onset is 60 years and the majority of patients describe a prior exposure to asbestos. Grossly, pleural mesothelioma appears to encase and compress the lung, extending into fissures and interlobar septa. Often, only superficial invasion into the periphery of the lung is present. Microscopically, malignant mesothelioma has a biphasic appearance, with epithelial and sarcomatous patterns. The epithelial component resembles adenocarcinoma with gland formation. The sarcomatous component demonstrates spindled cells. Mesotheliomas are positive for cytokeratin and WT-1. In contrast to adenocarcinomas of the lung, mesotheliomas are negative for CEA, Leu-M1, B72.3, and BER-EP4. Patients with malignant mesothelioma may present with pleural effusions, a pleural mass, chest pain, and generalized nonspecific symptoms. Metastases may occur to the lung parenchyma or mediastinal lymph nodes, as well as more distant sites such as liver, bone, and adrenals. There is no effective treatment.

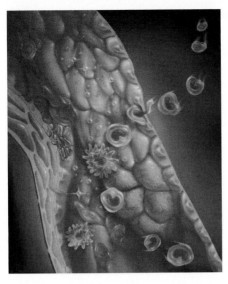

CHAPTER *13*

The Gastrointestinal Tract

Chapter Outline

THE ESOPHAGUS

Normal Anatomy and Histology

The esophagus resides in the thoracic cavity, dorsal to the trachea, and functions as a 25-cm-long food conduit. Esophageal motility is mediated by a combination of striated and smooth muscle in the upper portion and only smooth muscle in the lower portion. The histologic layers of the esophagus follow:

- Mucosa: nonkeratinized stratified squamous epithelium
- Submucosa: mucous glands and lymphatics
- Muscularis propria: circular and longitudinal smooth muscle with or without striated muscle
- Adventitia: surrounding fat and larger vessels without serosal lining

Congenital Disorders

A variety of congenital disorders affects the esophagus (Table 13-1). The most common anomaly is a *tracheoesophageal fistula*, which involves a connection between the trachea and esophagus and often the formation of a blind esophageal pouch (esophageal atresia).

The vast majority (90%) of tracheoesophageal fistulas involves a connection between the trachea and lower portion of the esophagus with a concomitant blind pouch corresponding to the upper portion of the esophagus (Fig. 13-1). In these cases, the upper pouch fills with swallowed mucus, which may be regurgitated and then aspirated. Tracheoesophageal fistulas may be associated with the *Vater syndrome* (*v*ertebral defects, *a*nal atresia, *t*racheoesophageal fistula, *r*enal dysplasia, and often esophageal atresia).

Motor Disorders

Motor function mediates the muscular activity of the esophagus, and disorders in motor function commonly result in difficulties in swallowing (dysphagia). Motor disorders may be caused by the following:

- Dysfunction of the striated muscle of the upper esophagus
- Systemic skeletal muscle disorders (myasthenia gravis)
- Neurologic diseases
- Peripheral neuropathy (diabetes, alcoholism)

Achalasia reflects a lack of esophageal motility combined with an inability of the lower esophageal sphincter to relax with swallowing. Symptoms include pain on swallowing (odynophagia) and dysphagia. Achalasia is caused by a loss or absence of ganglion cells in the myenteric plexus of the esophagus, as may occur by infection with *Trypanosoma cruzi* (*Chagas disease*). The esophagus ultimately becomes dilated and may develop squamous carcinoma.

Scleroderma is a systemic sclerosing disease that results in fibrosis of the inner circular muscle layer of the esophagus, especially adjacent to the lower esophageal sphincter. Dysphagia and heartburn are frequent symptoms.

Hiatal Hernia

Hiatal hernias are caused by a herniation of the stomach through the esophageal hiatus in the diaphragm. Hiatal hernias may be sliding or paraesophageal (Fig. 13-2). Sliding hernias are common

Table 13-1

Congenital and Acquired Disorders of the Esophagus

Disorder	Description	Associations(s)	Clinical Presentation
Tracheoesophageal fistula	Connection between trachea and esophagus	Congenital heart disease	Aspiration pneumonia
Congenital esophageal stenosis	Narrowing of esophagus	None	Dysphagia
Bronchopulmonary foregut malformation	Abnormal lung tissue that connects with esophagus	None	Repeated pulmonary infections
Esophageal webs	Mucosal webs in esophagus lumen	None	Dysphagia
Plummer-Vinson syndrome	Cervical esophageal web, mucosal lesions, iron-deficiency anemia	Adenocarcinoma	Dysphagia, aspiration
Schatzki ring	Narrowing of lower esophagus	None	Mostly asymptomatic
Zenker diverticulum	Upper esophageal diverticulum	Cricopharyngeal muscle disorder	Regurgitation of food eaten in previous days
Traction diverticulum	Midesophageal diverticulum	Motor dysfunction	Asymptomatic
Epiphrenic diverticulum	Lower esophageal diverticulum	Motor dysfunction; reflux esophagitis	Nocturnal regurgitation of large amounts of fluid
Intramural pseudodiverticulosis	Numerous small diverticula	None	Dysphagia

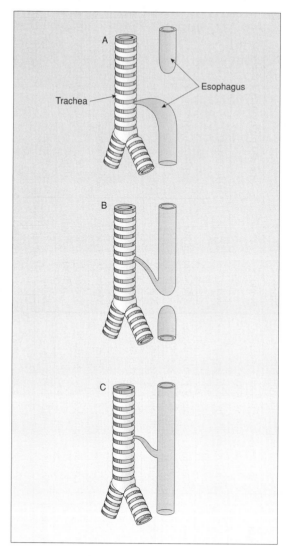

FIGURE   13-1

Congenital tracheoesophageal fistulas. A: The most common type is a communication between the trachea and lower portion of the esophagus. The upper segment of the esophagus ends in a blind sac. B: In a few cases, the proximal esophagus communicates with the trachea. C: The least common anomaly, the H type, is a fistula between a continuous esophagus and the trachea. (From Rubin E, Gorstein F, Rubin R, et al. Rubin's Pathology, 4th ed. Philadelphia: Lippincott Williams & Wilkins, 2005, p. 664.)

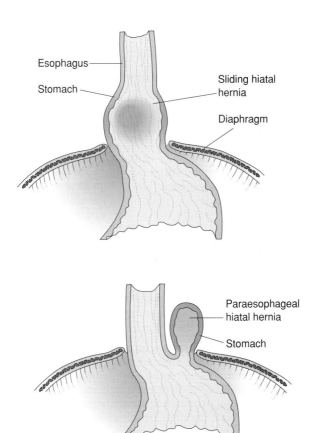

FIGURE 13-2
Comparison of sliding and paraesophageal hiatal hernias. (From Rubin E, Gorstein F, Rubin R, et al. Rubin's Pathology, 4th ed. Philadelphia: Lippincott Williams & Wilkins, 2005, p. 666.)

and occur when a portion of the proximal gastric mucosa slides above the diaphragm. Paraesophageal hernias occur when a portion of the gastric fundus protrudes through a defect in the diaphragmatic connective tissue membrane and is situated alongside the esophagus, thereby having an increased risk of incarceration.

Symptoms include heartburn and regurgitation. Treatment of hiatal hernias includes medical therapy and Nissen fundoplication in which the fundus is wrapped around the esophagus.

Esophagitis

Esophagitis refers to inflammation of the esophagus and may have a variety of causes, including reflux, infection, drugs, systemic illness, and physical agents.

Reflux Esophagitis

- This is the most common type of esophagitis and is caused by reflux of gastric contents into the esophagus (*gastroesophageal reflux disease*), often resulting from a hiatal hernia or decreased lower esophageal sphincter tone. Decreased tone may be caused by alcohol, chocolate, or cigarette use, as well as pregnancy, central nervous system (CNS) depressants, and the presence of a nasogastric tube. The esophagus may demonstrate a reddened appearance (hyperemia) or a thickened, white appearance (leukoplakia). The squamous mucosa undergoes specific morphologic changes with reflux esophagitis, including elongated vascular papillae (>two thirds of the thickness of the epithelium), a thickened basal cell layer (often greater than three cell layers thick), and infiltration by eosinophils, neutrophils, and lymphocytes.

  With continued injury, the esophagus may undergo gastric metaplasia. When goblet cell-containing columnar (intestinal-type) epithelium is present within the metaplastic epithelium, the lesion is termed Barrett esophagus of the distinctive type and may represent a precursor lesion for esophageal adenocarcinoma. Distinctive type Barrett esophagus may undergo progression to low-grade dysplasia, high-grade dysplasia, and ultimately adenocarcinoma in some instances. These patients often are monitored by endoscopy and biopsy. In addition to the preceding changes, reflux esophagitis may lead to the development of erosions, ulcerations, and esophageal strictures. Patients often describe the presence of heartburn and dysphagia.

Infective Esophagitis

Infective esophagitis often occurs in a setting of functional immunosuppression. *Candida esophagitis* may occur with chemotherapy, AIDS, diabetes, or antibiotics, and is manifested by dysphagia and odynophagia. White plaques surrounded by hyperemic mucosa are present on the esophagus and hyphae and yeast forms are identified microscopically. *Herpetic esophagitis* is caused by herpesvirus type 1 and presents with severe odynophagia. Vesicles and erosions are seen on the mucosa, and multinucleated epithelial cells with nuclear inclusions are identified microscopically. *Cytomegalovirus* (CMV) infection manifests as ulceration, and enlarged endothelial or fibroblast cells containing nuclear and cytoplasmic inclusions are identified microscopically. Immunostains for CMV and herpes are available to aid in the microscopic diagnoses of these entities.

Drug-induced Esophagitis

A variety of drugs can induce esophagitis ("pill esophagitis"), including iron tablets and bisphosphonates. Pill esophagitis is often localized.

Chemical Esophagitis

Chemical esophagitis is caused by the ingestion of alkaline (lye) or acidic (hydrochloric acid) solutions. Alkali injury causes liquefactive necrosis with inflammation and saponification of the entire esophageal wall. Acidic injury causes immediate coagulation necrosis limited to the epithelium of the esophagus.

Esophagitis Related to Systemic illness

This type of esophagitis may be caused by such conditions as graft-versus-host disease and pemphigus. Graft versus host disease occurs in the setting of a prior transplant and can present with infiltrations of cytotoxic T lymphocytes into the esophageal mucosa with subsequent epithelial injury and submucosal fibrosis.

Esophagitis Produced by Physical Agents

Physical agents that damage the esophagus include external radiation and nasogastric tube placement.

Esophageal Varices

The veins of the lower third of the esophagus drain into the portal vein via gastroesophageal anastomoses. Resistance to portal blood flow from prehepatic, posthepatic, or intrahepatic causes results in portal hypertension and can lead to dilation of the esophageal veins below the mucosa. These veins are prone to rupture, resulting in life-threatening hemorrhage. Upper gastrointestinal (GI) bleeding, such as from esophageal varices, classically presents as "coffee-ground" emesis and, occasionally, tarry stools.

Lacerations and Perforations

Lacerations of the esophagus may be caused by blunt trauma, instrumentation, or severe vomiting. *Mallory-Weiss syndrome* occurs in the setting of severe vomiting in alcoholic or bulimic patients and results in mucosal lacerations with subsequent emesis of bright red blood. Rupture of the esophagus after vomiting is referred to as *Boerhaave syndrome*. Perforation of the esophagus may occur from trauma or vomiting and can allow the escape of esophageal contents into the mediastinum, resulting in severe infection and tissue destruction.

Neoplasms

Benign Esophageal Neoplasms

Leiomyomas make up the vast majority of benign esophageal neoplasms. These lesions arise from smooth muscle cells and appear as firm, white submucosal lesions made up of monotonous spindled cells. Additional benign lesions that can occur in the esophagus and involve the mucosa include fibrovascular polyps, inflammatory fibroid polyps, and squamous papillomas.

Malignant Neoplasms

Squamous Cell Carcinoma

Squamous cell carcinoma (SCC) is the most common esophageal cancer worldwide. Males are more frequently affected. SCC may be asymptomatic in early stages but ultimately can present with dysphagia and odynophagia at later stages. Only 20% of patients survive 5 years. Risk factors for SCC include the following:

- Alcohol use
- Cigarette smoking
- Nitrosamines
- Lack of fresh fruit, vegetables, and animal protein
- Plummer-Vinson syndrome, celiac sprue, achalasia
- Chemical injury with esophageal stricture
- Webs, rings, and diverticula
- Chronic esophagitis

Most squamous cell carcinomas are formed in the lower third of the esophagus and may appear grossly as polypoid, ulcerating, or infiltrating lesions. Microscopically, the tumors are made up of squamous cells with keratin "pearl" formation, when the tumor is well differentiated. Metastatic spread occurs through the submucosal lymphatic plexus of the esophagus, resulting in lymph node, lung, or liver metastases.

Adenocarcinoma

Adenocarcinoma of the esophagus is the most common esophageal cancer in the United States. As with SCC, men are more frequently affected. Adenocarcinoma most often arises in a background of Barrett esophagus, and the degree of dysplasia and length of esophagus involved in Barrett esophagus appears to correlate with risk of adenocarcinoma development. Additional risk factors include smoking, chronic reflux, and hiatal hernia. Grossly, adenocarcinoma may appear as an ulcerated or polypoid mucosal growth that most commonly occurs in the distal portion of the esophagus.

Microscopically, infiltrating glands are present in the esophageal wall. Adenocarcinoma can metastasize via the lymphatic plexus located in the submucosa.

THE STOMACH

Normal Anatomy and Histology

The stomach is situated just below the diaphragm, between the esophagus and duodenum The stomach is shaped by the lesser curvature and the greater curvature, from which the greater omentum extends. Branches of the celiac, hepatic, and splenic arteries supply the stomach. Venous drainage is directed into the portal system or the splenic and superior mesenteric veins. The stomach receives both sympathetic and parasympathetic innervation. The lining of the stomach contains gastric rugae, or folds. The wall of the stomach is composed of the following:

- Mucosa: contains mucus-secreting, columnar epithelium that extends into pits containing region-specific glands, including cardiac, body/fundic, and pyloric glands
- Submucosa: contains lymphatics and vascular drainage
- Muscularis propria: contains circular, longitudinal, and oblique layers
- Serosa: single-layer epithelial lining

The five regions of the stomach with glands and specific cell types follow (Fig. 13-3).

Congenital Disorders

Pyloric stenosis, which involves a concentric hypertrophy of the circular muscle of the pylorus with subsequent obstruction of the gastric outlet, is one of the more common congenital anomalies of the stomach. Patients present within the first few months of life with projectile vomiting. Frequently, a palpable pyloric mass (enlarged sphincter) and hypochloremic alkalosis may be present. This anomaly is more common in boys than girls and firstborn children. This disorder can be cured by pyloric muscle incision.

Additional congenital anomalies that may involve the stomach include diaphragmatic hernias, duplication cysts, diverticula, situs inversus, presence of ectopic pancreatic tissue, partial atresia, and congenital pyloric and antral membranes.

Defects that may involve the abdominal wall with extrusion of abdominal contents include omphalocele and gastroschisis. *Omphaloceles* are saclike protrusions of all or a portion of the abdominal

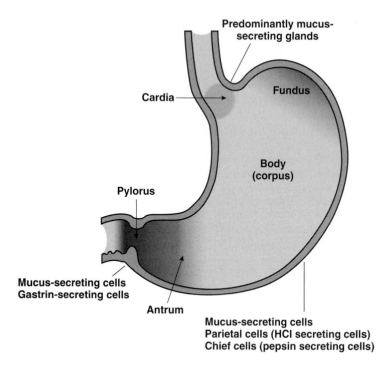

FIGURE 13-3
Anatomical regions of the stomach containing distinctive cell populations. (From Rubin E, Gorstein F, Rubin R, et al. Rubin's Pathology, 4th ed. Philadelphia: Lippincott Williams & Wilkins, 2005, p. 672.)

contents that are covered by amnion and peritoneum and often are associated with other congenital anomalies. *Gastroschisis* is a protrusion of the bowel through an abdominal wall defect without the protection of an overlying membranous covering. Gastroschisis may be associated with nonrotation and intestinal atresia, although other types of congenital anomalies rarely are associated with this condition.

Gastritis

Gastritis refers to an inflammation of the stomach that may be caused by a variety of mechanisms, including pharmaceutical drug use, stress, autoimmune conditions, infection with *Helicobacter pylori*, and bile reflux. Gastritis is subdivided into acute and chronic forms, with several types in each category.

Acute Gastritis

Acute gastritis commonly presents with epigastric pain, nausea, or vomiting. A variety of etiologic factors may lead to acute gastritis, including the following:

- Nonsteroidal antiinflammatory drugs (NSAIDs) or aspirin
- Alcohol
- Ischemic injury
- Extensive burns leading to stress ulcers (Curling ulcer)
- CNS trauma (Cushing ulcer)
- Shock, sepsis
- Gastric acid hypersecretion

Microscopically, the gastric mucosa demonstrates edema, neutrophilic infiltrates, mucosal erosions, and, if severe, ulceration. *Acute hemorrhagic gastritis* is a form of acute gastritis in which extensive necrosis of the gastric mucosa may be associated with life-threatening hemorrhage.

Chronic Gastritis

Chronic gastritis refers to chronic inflammation of the gastric mucosa associated with either environmental or autoimmune conditions (Table 13-2). Patients may be asymptomatic or present with dyspepsia and epigastric pain. The most common cause of chronic gastritis is infection with *Helicobacter pylori*. These organisms appears as small, curved (seagull-like), gram-negative rods with polar flagella that attach to the surface epithelium but do not invade the mucosa. *H. pylori* are associated with a mucosal lymphoplasmacytic infiltrate that is accompanied by involvement of the gastric epithelium and glands by neutrophils. *H. pylori* gastritis has been proposed to represent a risk factor for the development of mucosa-associated lymphoid tissue (MALT) lymphoma. Diagnosis of *H. pylori* infection may be established by gastric biopsy or serologic tests. Treatment in most cases of *H. pylori* infection consists of a combination of agents that reduce acid secretion, increase mucosal protection, and eliminate infectious organisms. Antibiotic administration often includes the triad of bismuth, metronidazole, and tetracycline.

Atrophic gastritis (autoimmune atrophic gastritis, multifocal atrophic gastritis) describes the presence of inflammation of the mucosa accompanied by loss of oxyntic cells and associated neuroendocrine cell hyperplasia. On occasion, the inflammation in atrophic gastritis may be severe enough to be confused with lymphoma. Intestinal metaplasia may occur in atrophic gastritis (as evidenced by the presence of goblet cells) and may represent a risk factor for the development of adenocarcinoma tumors of the stomach.

Additional forms of gastritis include reactive gastropathy, idiopathic granulomatous gastritis, and eosinophilic gastritis.

Table 13-2

Chronic Gastritis

Form	Stomach Region	Etiology	Association(s)
Helicobacter pylori gastritis	Antrum, body	*Helicobacter pylori, Helicobacter heilmannii*	Peptic ulcer disease; MALT lymphoma
Multifocal atrophic gastritis	Antrum, body	*Helicobacter pylori* infection, diet	Gastric cancer
Autoimmune atrophic gastritis	Body, fundus	Autoantibodies to parietal cells (H+/K+ ATPase proton pump) and intrinsic factor	Pernicious anemia; autoimmune disease; gastric cancer
Reactive (chemical) gastropathy	Antrum, body	Reflux of bile and duodenal contents, NSAIDs, alcohol, stress	None
Idiopathic granulomatous gastritis	Diffuse	Unknown; unrelated to infection	Atrophic gastritis
Eosinophilic gastritis	Antrum, pylorus	Unknown	Food allergy, peripheral eosinophilia

MALT, mucosa-associated lymphoid tissue; NSAIDs, nonsteroidal antiinflammatory drugs.

Menetrier Disease

Menetrier disease (hyperplastic hypersecretory gastropathy) is characterized by massively enlarged rugae and an increased stomach weight. This disease is more common in men and presents as postprandial pain relieved by antacids. The oxyntic (parietal) mucosa demonstrates elongated, corkscrew glands lined by mucus-secreting epithelium. The altered epithelium leads to loss of plasma proteins from the epithelium, resulting in weight loss and peripheral edema. Menetrier disease may be related to CMV infection in childhood and tumor necrosis factor-α overexpression in adulthood. Although the childhood form is self-limited, the adult form is considered preneoplastic and requires frequent endoscopic surveillance.

Peptic Ulcer Disease

Peptic ulcer disease (PUD) is an ulceration of the distal stomach or proximal duodenum caused by a variety of factors (Fig. 13-4), and often related to *H. pylori* infection. Peptic ulcers classically present with epigastric pain experienced 1 to 3 hours after a meal or pain that awakens the patient at night. The symptoms are often relieved by alkali substances (milk) and food.

Gastric ulcers appear as punched out lesions on the lesser curvature (chronic gastritis–associated) or greater curvature (NSAID-

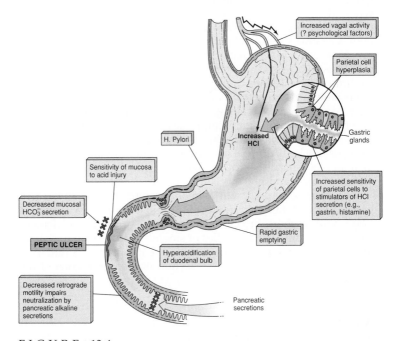

F I G U R E   13-4
Gastric and duodenal factors in the pathogenesis of duodenal peptic ulcers. (From Rubin E, Gorstein F, Rubin R, et al. Rubin's Pathology, 4th ed. Philadelphia: Lippincott Williams & Wilkins, 2005, p. 682.)

associated). These lesions are usually single and less than 2 cm in diameter. Care must be taken to distinguish ulcers from ulcerating carcinomas by histologic examination. *Duodenal ulcers* are also usually solitary and are located on the anterior or posterior wall of the proximal duodenum.

Microscopically, peptic ulcers demonstrate necrotic tissue throughout the thickness of the epithelium, filled in by granulation tissue and containing a fibrotic base with chronic inflammation. A superficial fibrinopurulent exudate is present.

Complications related to PUD include hemorrhage, perforation, pyloric obstruction, and rarely malignant transformation.

Neoplasms

Benign Lesions

The majority of *gastrointestinal stromal tumors* (GISTs) located in the stomach are benign lesions. GISTs are derived from the interstitial (pacemaker) cells of Cajal and appear as submucosal white, whorled lesions made up of spindled cells with vacuolated cytoplasm embedded in a collagenous stroma. GISTs stain with antibodies against CD117 (c-kit).

Hyperplastic polyps make up the majority of gastric polyps and may be variably sized and either sessile (flat) or pedunculated (protruding). These lesions are present in the body and fundus and often arise in a background of chronic atrophic gastritis. They appear microscopically as elongated, branched crypts lined by foveolar epithelium with underlying pyloric or gastric glands.

Fundic gland polyps arise in a background of familial adenomatous polyposis (FAP) or use of proton pump inhibitors. They appear microscopically as dilated oxyntic glands lined by parietal and chief cells, and mucous cell metaplasia often is present.

Peutz-Jeghers polyps are hamartomatous polyps that often present in childhood or adolescence and appear as a lobulated polyp with a short, broad stalk. The stalk of the polyp demonstrates finely branching bundles of smooth muscle that are characteristic of this polyp and the mucosa often appears disorganized. This is discussed further in the section on benign lesions of the small intestine.

Adenomas

Adenomas (*adenomatous polyps*) occur most commonly in the antrum and have an average size of 4 cm. The majority of these polyps are single, sessile lesions made up of tubular or tubulovillous structures. The glands of these polyps demonstrate dysplasia (classified as low- or high-grade) and have a malignant potential that is related to the size of the lesion.

Malignant Lesions

Adenocarcinoma

More than 95% of malignant gastric tumors are gastric adenocarcinomas, which primarily affect the distal stomach. The highest incidence of gastric cancer is in Japan and Chile. Although gastric cancer was a common cause of cancer death within the United States in the mid-1920s, the incidence has dramatically declined, most likely because of changes in environmental exposures. Risk factors for gastric cancer include the following:

- Diet: starch, smoked fish and meat, pickled vegetables
- Nitrosamines: soil, water, processed meats and vegetables
- Genetic factors: blood type A, hereditary nonpolyposis colorectal cancer (HNPCC)
- Age older than 50 years
- Male gender
- *Helicobacter pylori* infection
- Low socioeconomic environment
- Atrophic gastritis, pernicious anemia, subtotal gastrectomy, gastric adenomatous polyps

Gastric cancer may present in early or late (advanced) stages, as categorized by depth of invasion. Both early and advanced gastric adenocarcinoma may appear as protruding, polypoid masses, flat lesions, or ulcerated, irregular lesions. Early gastric cancer, or *superficial spreading carcinoma*, accounts for approximately 5% to 30% of gastric adenocarcinomas. These lesions are confined to the mucosa or submucosa of the stomach, although up to 20% may demonstrate metastases at the time of diagnosis. Advanced gastric cancer, which penetrates through the submucosa, also may appear grossly as a diffusely thickened gastric wall without a mucosal lesion, called *linitis plastica*. Early and advanced gastric adenocarcinoma most likely represents separate lesions, although clinical and pathologic features overlap.

Adenocarcinoma may range in microscopic appearance from well-differentiated lesions with gland formation to poorly differentiated lesions with single, mucin-filled, signet ring cells. Gastric adenocarcinoma metastasizes primarily through lymphatic channels, although hematogenous spread also occurs. A *Virchow node* represents a gastric cancer metastasis to an enlarged supraclavicular node, and a *Krukenberg tumor* represents metastases of signet-ring gastric cancer to an ovary with a prominent desmoplastic reaction.

Patients with gastric cancer often present with weight loss, anorexia and nausea. Epigastric or back pain, relieved by antacids or H_2-antagonists, is common. Occasionally, gastric outlet obstruction or chronic bleeding may be evident.

Carcinoid (Neuroendocrine) Tumors

Carcinoid tumors arise from neuroendocrine cells within the GI tract and harbor potential for recurrence and metastatic spread. The majority of gastric carcinoids are hormonally inactive, although a subset does produce serotonin, which results in the carcinoid syndrome.

Gastric Lymphoma

Gastric lymphomas often present in a similar manner to gastric adenocarcinoma and typically affect patients between 40 and 65 years of age. The majority of these lesions are low-grade B-cell lymphomas (*MALT lymphomas*) arising in a background of *H. pylori* gastritis.

Malignant Gastrointestinal Stromal Tumor

These lesions share many similarities with their benign counterparts, although they are typically larger, and the cells demonstrate an increased number of mitoses. Often, the presence of metastases is necessary to identify the malignant nature of a GIST.

Mechanical Disorders

Mechanical disorders of the stomach include the following:

- *Rupture* after blunt trauma
- *Perforation* with overdistention or severe vomiting
- *Volvulus* with a gastric tumor or nasogastric decompression
- *Diverticulum* formation from congenital weakness or prolonged stress

Bezoars

Bezoars are foreign bodies composed of plant material (phytobezoar) or hair (trichobezoar) that has been altered by the digestive process. Phytobezoars occur in persons who eat an excess of persimmons, swallow unchewed bubble gum, or have delayed gastric emptying. Cellulase may be used for treatment. Trichobezoars occur typically in young women who eat their own hair as a nervous habit.

THE SMALL INTESTINE

Normal Anatomy and Histology

The small intestine extends from the pylorus to the ileocecal valve and may measure 3.5 to 6.5 m in length. The small intestine is divided into three parts, including the following:

- Duodenum: Primarily retroperitoneal, ends at the ligament of Treitz; supplied by the pancreaticoduodenal branch of the hepatic artery
- Jejunum: Contains plicae circularis giving the mucosa a folded appearance; supplied by the superior mesenteric artery
- Ileum: Contains Peyer patches (submucosal lymphoid aggregates); supplied by the superior mesenteric artery

Venous drainage from the intestine passes through the portal venous system. The small intestine is innervated by both sympathetic (celiac plexus) and parasympathetic (vagus nerve) innervation. Four histologic layers make up the wall of the small intestine:

- Mucosa: villi composed of columnar epithelium (enterocytes) resting on a basement membrane, lamina propria, and muscularis mucosae
- Submucosa: vasculature, lymphatic channels, Brunner glands in the duodenum, Meissner nerve plexus
- Muscularis propria: outer longitudinal and inner circular layers with intervening myenteric nerve plexus of Auerbach
- Serosa: loose connective tissue with a single outer layer of mesothelium

Congenital Disorders

Intestinal Atresia and Stenosis

Intestinal atresia is a complete occlusion of the intestinal lumen, and *intestinal stenosis* is an incomplete stricture of the intestine that does not entirely occlude the lumen. Newborns with these conditions often demonstrate persistent vomiting of bile-containing fluid, lack of meconium passage, and a dilated intestine proximal to the stenosis or obstruction.

Intestinal Duplications (Enteric Cysts)

Duplications are formed of gastrointestinal mucosa, often gastric mucosa, and a smooth muscle wall. They may communicate with the lumen of the gastrointestinal tract or be present as an adjacent cyst. Duplications appear grossly as round or tubular structures and occur most commonly in the ileum.

Meckel Diverticulum

Meckel diverticulum is the most common congenital anomaly of the small intestine and is caused by a persistent vitelline duct. A Meckel diverticulum is a true diverticulum that contains all layers of the gastrointestinal tract, including the muscularis propria. It appears grossly as an outpouching of the gastrointestinal wall along the antimesenteric border of the ileum, often 60 to 100 cm from the ileocecal junction. Complications are often related to the presence of ectopic mucosa and include the following:

- Hemorrhage: caused by ectopic gastric mucosa; accounts for half of all instances of lower gastrointestinal bleeding in children
- Intestinal obstruction: Meckel diverticulum may be a leading point for intussusception of the small intestine (telescoping of the bowel inside itself)
- Diverticulitis: inflammation of Meckel diverticulum
- Perforation
- Fistula

Malrotation

Malrotation predisposes to volvulus and ischemia of the small and large bowel because of improper intestinal rotation in development.

Meconium Ileus

Thickened meconium leads to an obstruction of the small intestine, often the ileum, in this condition. *Meconium ileus* is caused by cystic fibrosis, in which deficiency in pancreatic enzyme secretion leads to thickened intestinal mucus. Complications include volvulus, perforation, and intestinal atresia. Treatment involves a hypertonic enema with detergent or surgery.

Infections

The small intestine is susceptible to bacterial, viral, and parasitic infections, which contribute significantly to mortality worldwide.

Bacterial Infections (Infectious Enterocolitis)

Infectious enterocolitis may occur as a result of the following:

- Ingestion of preformed toxins
- Colonization by bacteria with subsequent enterotoxin production
- Invasion of the bacterium into the wall of the intestine with subsequent intracellular growth and cell-to-cell spread

In contrast to the colon, which contains a large number of aerobic and anaerobic microorganisms, the small intestine is relatively sterile, with $<10^4$/mL of primarily aerobic microorganisms.

"Food poisoning" refers to enterocolitis produced by eating food containing preformed bacteria-produced toxins (*S. aureus, B. cereus*); symptoms often occur within hours of eating contaminated food.

Toxigenic bacteria include *Vibrio cholerae* and certain *Escherichia coli* strains (ETEC, EHEC), which bind to enterocytes, establish colonization of the intestine, and secrete enterotoxins. These toxins bind to the enterocytes and stimulate secretion of electrolytes into the intestinal lumen, causing a watery diarrhea that can lead to dehydration. In general, the intestinal mucosa is not extensively damaged in these infections.

Invasive bacteria include *Shigella, Salmonella, Yersinia, Campylobacter*, and certain *E. coli* strains (EIEC), which often affect the distal ileum and colon. These organisms directly damage the intestinal mucosa by entering and proliferating within intestinal cells. Invasion by these bacteria also increases prostaglandin production, which potentiates fluid secretion.

Bacterial diarrhea often presents with abdominal pain, fever, vomiting, watery diarrhea, or bloody diarrhea (*dysentery*). Increased intestinal secretion, stimulated by bacterial toxins and enteric hormones, plays a major role in the diarrheal process. A summary of bacterial enterocolitis, with major pathologic findings, is presented in Table 13-3.

Viral Infections

A variety of viruses affect the small intestine, including *echovirus, coxsackievirus, adenovirus,* and *coronavirus. Rotavirus* is a common cause of infantile diarrhea and causes duodenal mucosal injury and impaired intestinal absorption lasting up to 2 months. *Norwalk virus* causes patchy mucosal lesions and malabsorption leading to vomiting and diarrhea; symptoms often resolve within 2 days.

Intestinal Tuberculosis

Intestinal tuberculosis is an uncommon disease that is caused by *Mycobacterium bovis* or *Mycobacterium tuberculosis*. Infection occurs by ingestion of contaminated food or swallowing of infectious sputum. The organism invades the bowel wall at the lymphoid-rich tissue of the ileocecal region. Infection results in granuloma formation, as well as ulcers and full-thickness inflammation in certain

Table 13-3

Bacterial Infections of the Small Intestine

Organism	Mechanism	Source	Gastrointestinal Presentation	Pathology
Shigella (shigellosis)	Invasion	Humans	Diarrhea, dysentery	Superficial ulceration and hemorrhage of the terminal ileum and colon; purulent exudate
Salmonella typhi (typhoid fever)	Invasion	Contaminated food or water	Hemorrhagic, perforation	Necrosis of lymphoid tissue in terminal ileum with scattered ulcers; large macrophages with bacilli
Nontyphus salmonella	Invasion	Milk, eggs, beef, poultry	Diarrhea, dysentery	Mild mucosal ulceration, edema, neutrophil infiltration; villous blunting; potential for hematogenous spread; osteomyelitis in patients with sickle cell anemia
Escherichia coli (ETEC, EHEC)	Enterotoxin	Water, beef	Diarrhea	Mild mucosal ulceration, edema, neutrophil infiltration; termed "traveler's diarrhea"; may cause hemorrhagic colitis or hemolytic uremic syndrome

				See previous
E. coli (EIEC)	Invasion	Humans, water	Dysentery	See previous
Yersinia enterocolitica, pseudotuberculosis	Invasion	Milk, pork	Diarrhea, cramps	Peyer patch hyperplasia, mucosal ulceration with fibropurulent exudate; epithelioid granulomas with central necrosis; mesenteric lymphadenitis; rarely, pharyngitis, pericarditis
Campylobacter jejuni	Invasion, enterotoxin	Humans, milk, poultry	Diarrhea, dysentery	Villous blunting, mild mucosal ulceration
Staphylococcus aureus	Preformed toxin	Nonrefrigerated food	Severe vomiting, cramps	Mild mucosal edema; minimal changes
Clostridium perfringens	Enterotoxin	Poultry, meat, fish	Vomiting, diarrhea	Mild mucosal edema; minimal changes
Clostridium botulinum	Preformed toxin	Canned foods	Diarrhea	Minimal intestinal changes; neurotoxin may cause respiratory failure
Vibrio cholerae	Enterotoxin	Shellfish, humans, water	Diarrhea, cholera	Mild mucosal edema, minimal changes

cases. Patients present with chronic abdominal pain, malnutrition, weight loss, fever, weakness, and frequently a palpable right lower quadrant mass.

Intestinal Fungal Infections

Fungal infections of the small intestine occur primarily in immuno-compromised patients. Common organisms include *Candida*, *Histoplasma*, and *Mucor*. In general, fungal forms invade the intestinal mucosa and produce mucosal erosion. Progression to ulceration, hemorrhage, and necrosis may occur. Certain fungi, such as *Mucor*, also may demonstrate invasion of blood vessels. Blood-borne dissemination and perforation are rare complications.

Intestinal Parasites

The majority of small intestine parasites are transmitted by fecal-oral spread or undercooked meat products. Categories of parasites include the following:

- Protozoon: *Giardia Entamoeba*
- Roundworms (nematodes): *Ascaris, Strongyloides*, hookworm, *Trichuris*
- Tapeworms (cestodes)
- Fluke (trematode)

Vascular Diseases

Acute Intestinal Ischemia

Decreased blood flow to the small intestine may result from systemic decreases in blood pressure (severe hypotension) or occlusion of mesenteric blood vessels, such as the superior mesenteric artery, by a thrombus or embolus. Rapid occlusion of a large artery may lead to either segmental or diffuse small bowel infarction, whereas severe hypotension produces primarily diffuse infarction.

Thrombosis of the mesenteric veins in patients with hypercoagulable states, stasis, or venous inflammation also may lead to acute intestinal ischemia. The most commonly affected vein is the superior mesenteric vein; however, collateral drainage often prevents infarction of the small intestine.

Infarcted bowel appears purple and edematous and is malodorous. If the infarction is segmental, sharp delineations between normal and affected bowel are present. In cases of arterial occlusion, sloughing of the mucosa and hemorrhage of the mucosa and submucosa occur. The wall of the small intestine becomes thin and may demonstrate intramural gas bubbles (pneumatosis). In cases of nonocclusive intestinal ischemia, only the mucosa may demonstrate changes, which range from dilated capillaries to extensive necrosis.

Patients with acute intestinal ischemia present with the abrupt onset of severe abdominal pain and frequently bloody diarrhea, hematemesis, or shock. The majority of patients require surgical resection of the infarcted bowel.

Chronic Intestinal Ischemia

Atherosclerosis of the major splanchnic arteries may lead to intermittent abdominal pain, termed *intestinal angina*. Pain often begins within 30 minutes of eating and lasts for a few hours. Chronic ischemia results in intestinal fibrosis, which may lead to stricture formation, obstruction, malabsorption, and occasionally acute intestinal ischemia and infarction.

Malabsorption

Malabsorption refers to any clinical condition in which nutrients are not properly processed and absorbed. The majority of absorption occurs in the proximal small intestine, although the distal small intestine is important in the absorption of bile salts and vitamin B_{12}.

Absorption may be described via luminal and intestinal phases (Fig. 13-5). Luminal absorption describes processes that occur in the intestinal lumen that subsequently allow nutrients to be absorbed. Conditions that cause luminal-phase malabsorption include the following:

- Interruption of the continuity of the stomach and duodenum after surgery
- Pancreatic dysfunction: cystic fibrosis, chronic pancreatitis, cancer
- Deficient or ineffective bile salts: impaired bile excretion, bacterial overgrowth, and ileal bypass

Intestinal-phase malabsorption is caused by abnormalities in the intestinal wall and enterocyte transport mechanisms, which include the following:

- Microvillus abnormalities: sprue, primary disaccharidase deficiency
- Decreased absorptive area: resection, gastrocolic fistula, mucosal damage from celiac disease, Whipple disease
- Altered metabolic function of the enterocytes: abetalipoproteinemia
- Decreased enterocyte transport: Whipple disease, intestinal lymphoma

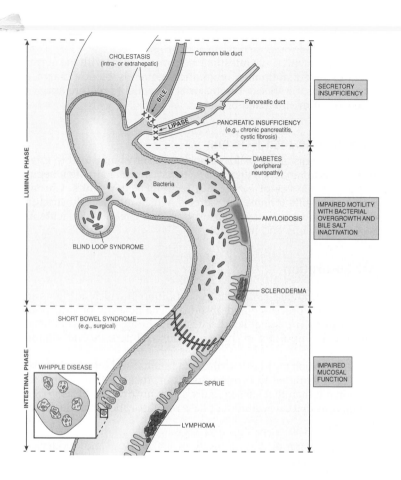

F I G U R E   13-5
Causes of malabsorption. (From Rubin E, Gorstein F, Rubin R, et
al. Rubin's Pathology, 4th ed. Philadelphia: Lippincott Williams &
Wilkins, 2005, p. 698.)

Malabsorption may be specific (isolated) or generalized. *Specific malabsorption* is an identifiable molecular defect that causes malabsorption of a single nutrient; for example, *pernicious anemia* occurs with malabsorption of vitamin B_{12}. *Generalized malabsorption* describes malabsorption of several or all major nutrient classes. Generalized malabsorption leads to malnutrition, presenting as weight loss or failure to thrive in children. A summary of clinical and pathologic findings in malabsorption is presented in Tables 13-4 and 13-5.

Diarrhea may be a secondary symptom in malabsorption, as residual, nonprocessed nutrients in the intestinal lumen may stimulate bacterial fermentation or increased colonic secretion.

Laboratory tests have been developed that examine generalized absorption, as well as the absorption of specific nutrients. General tests include the following:

- D-Xylose absorption: intestinal phase of absorption
- $^{14}CO_2$-cholyl-glycine breath test: bacterial overgrowth or ileal absorptive function

Specific tests include the following:

- Lactose-tolerance test: measurement of blood sugar after disaccharide administration
- Schilling test: vitamin B_{12} absorption

Mechanical Obstruction

Mechanical obstruction may be caused by a luminal mass, intrinsic bowel wall lesion, or extrinsic compression. *Intussusception*, in which a portion of the bowel telescopes into an adjacent portion of the bowel, may be caused by a Meckel diverticulum or inflamed Peyer's patch. *Volvulus* describes a twisting of the bowel on its mesentery, which may obstruct the bowel and interrupt the blood supply. *Adhesions* are fibrous bands caused by prior surgery and may externally obstruct the intestine. Finally, *hernias* may become incarcerated and may potentially develop a compromised blood supply.

Neoplasms

Benign Lesions

Peutz-Jeghers Syndrome and Hamartomatous Polyps

Peutz-Jeghers syndrome is an autosomal dominant disorder characterized by intestinal hamartomatous polyps and mucocutaneous melanin pigmentation on the face, buccal mucosa, hands, feet, and perianal and genital areas. The disease is caused by inactivating mutations of the *LKB1* gene, which encodes a protein kinase.

In Peutz-Jeghers syndrome, hamartomatous polyps often occur in the stomach, proximal small intestine, and colon. These polyps appear grossly as flat or pedunculated lesions that vary greatly in size. Microscopically, the key feature of these polyps is a prominently branching pattern of smooth muscle fibers that is

Table 13-4

Pathologic Manifestations of Intestinal Malabsorption

Disease	Pathology
Specific malabsorption	
Lactose intolerance	Normal to mildly blunted villi
Abetalipoproteinemia	Normal villous morphology ; lipid vacuoles in epithelial cells (enterocytes)
Tropical sprue	Normal to severely blunted villi; inflammation of the lamina propria
Generalized malabsorption	
Celiac disease (celiac sprue)	Normal bowel wall thickness; blunting or absence of villi., numerous intraepithelial lymphocytes, increased plasma cells in the lamina propria
Whipple disease	Thickened, edematous bowel wall; flat, thickened villi; extensive infiltration of the lamina propria by large foamy macrophages containing PAS-positive glycoprotein granules in the cytoplasm; dilated mucosal and submucosal lymphatics; electron-microscopy reveals small bacilli in the macrophage cytoplasm and free within the lamina propria
Hypogammaglobul inemia-associated (acquired)	Normal to blunted villous architecture; paucity or lack of plasma cells in the lamina propria and nodular lymphoid hyperplasia; *Giardia* organisms
Congenital lymphangiectasia	Normal to blunted villous architecture; grossly identifiable white spots on the intestinal mucosa; dilated lymphatics (lacteals) in the lamina propria
Radiation enteritis	Mucosal ulceration, selling and detachment of the endothelial cells of the small arterioles, fibrin plugs in the arteriolar lumens, and large foam cells (macrophages) in the vessel intima

Table 13-5

Clinical Manifestations of Intestinal Malabsorption

Disease	Process	Genetic Association	Symptoms	Treatment
Specific malabsorption				
Lactose intolerance	Lactase (disaccharidase) deficiency	Rare	Abdominal distention, flatulence, diarrhea with dairy ingestion	Lactase administration
Abetalipoproteinemia	Failure of apoprotein B synthesis	Autosomal recessive	Loss of deep tendon reflexes, ataxia, erythrocytic acanthocytosis	Ingestion of medium-chain triglycerides
Tropical sprue	Long-standing bowel contamination with bacteria	None	Steatorrhea, anemia, weight loss, folic acid and vitamin B_{12} deficiency, hypoalbuminemia	Tetracycline and folic acid
Generalized malabsorption				
Celiac disease (celiac sprue, gluten-sensitive enteropathy)	Epithelial damage, ?adenovirus, ?antigliadin antiendomysial antibodies	HLA-B8, DR8, DQ2	Generalized malabsorption with wheat, barley, rye ingestion (gliadin exposure); dermatitis herpetiformis	Gluten-free diet
Whipple disease	*Tropheryma whippelii*	None	Generalized malabsorption; systemic findings	Antibiotics
Hypogammaglobulinemia-associated (acquired)	Immune dysfunction, with associated *Giardia*	None	Generalized malabsorption	Metronidazole
Lymphangiectasia	Lacteal dilation	None	Steatorrhea, protein-losing enteropathy, lymphopenia, chylous ascites	Treat underlying conditions (pancreatitis, sarcoidosis), surgery
Radiation enteritis	Irradiation	None	Anorexia, cramps, diarrhea	Symptomatic

continuous with the muscularis mucosa. The glands that are present within the polyp demonstrate normal components for the location of the polyp (i.e., intestinal type epithelium in intestinal polyps). Although these polyps do not undergo malignant transformation in many cases, instances of adenocarcinoma arising from these lesions have been reported. Patients with Peutz-Jeghers syndrome also are at increased risk of cancer of the breast, pancreas, gastrointestinal tract, testis, and ovary.

Gastrointestinal Stromal Tumors

GISTs are intramural lesions made up of interstitial cells of Cajal that are covered by normal intestinal mucosa (see section on gastric neoplasms).

Lipomas

Lipomas are benign tumors of mature adipose tissue that occur often in the distal ileum. Complications include intussusception, ulceration, and mucosal bleeding.

Adenomas

Adenomas are classified by morphology as tubular, villous, or tubulovillous. Low-grade dysplasia is a defining characteristic of all adenomas. Although many adenomas behave in a benign manner, a subset of lesions may develop high-grade dysplasia and invasive adenocarcinoma. Complications include bleeding and intussusception.

Malignant Neoplasms

Adenocarcinoma

Adenocarcinoma accounts for half of all malignant small bowel neoplasms, although the frequency of this entity is generally rare. The majority of small intestine adenocarcinomas occur in middle-aged persons, primarily in the duodenum and jejunum. Patients with Crohn disease, FAP, HNPCC syndrome, and celiac disease are at increased risk. Affected patients often present with progressive intestinal obstruction, intussusception, or occult bleeding. Overall 5-year survival is less than 20%.

Grossly, adenocarcinoma may appear ulcerated or polypoid and occasionally demonstrate a circumferential growth pattern. Microscopically, atypical glands are identified infiltrating the wall of the intestine.

Primary Intestinal Lymphoma

Lymphoma is the second most common malignancy of the small intestine and it originates in the MALT present in the mucosa and submucosa. Chronic stimulation of intestinal lymphocytes has been proposed to induce the development of intestinal lymphoma. Primary intestinal lymphoma has been subclassified as Western-type intestinal lymphoma and Mediterranean lymphoma.

Western-type intestinal lymphoma affects adults older than 40 years of age and children younger than 10 years of age. The disease affects the ileum and presents as a fungating mass, elevated ulcerated lesion, diffuse segmental thickening of the bowel wall, or plaquelike mucosal nodule. Complications include obstruction, intussusception, perforation, and bleeding. Patients often present with chronic abdominal pain, diarrhea, and clubbing of the fingers.

Mediterranean lymphoma occurs in developing countries, often in young men, and may have an environmental cause. Mediterranean lymphoma is associated with intestinal B lymphocyte dysfunction in which heavy chains of immunoglobulin A are secreted without associated light chains. The duodenum and proximal jejunum are involved primarily. The lesion appears as a diffusely thickened bowel wall that leads to mucosal atrophy and severe malabsorption.

Sprye-associated lymphoma is a T-cell lymphoma that occurs in association with long-standing celiac disease.

Carcinoid (Neuroendocrine) Tumor

Approximately 20% of small bowel malignancies are *carcinoid tumors*, which most frequently present in the appendix or ileum. Two percent of carcinoid tumors are associated with Meckel diverticulum. Carcinoids are often multifocal and may be associated with multiple endocrine neoplasia (MEN) I. The malignant potential of a carcinoid parallels lesion size.

Carcinoids may be functional and secrete peptides and amines, most commonly serotonin. Carcinoids appear often as submucosal nodules with intact, overlying mucosa. Microscopically, nests, cords, rosettes, and trabeculae, made up of uniform small cells with fine granular chromatin, are present within a highly vascular stroma. Mitoses are rare. Lymph node and liver metastases can occur in a subset of patients.

Carcinoid syndrome is caused by excess serotonin and presents with diarrhea, episodic flushing, bronchospasm, cyanosis, telangiectasia, and skin lesions. Occasionally, right-sided cardiac valvular disease may occur. The serotonin metabolic product 5-hydroxyindoleacetic acid is detectable in the urine in carcinoid syndrome.

Malignant Gastrointestinal Stromal Tumors

Malignant GISTs also may occur in the small intestine.

Metastatic Tumors

The most common malignant tumors affecting the small bowel are metastatic lesions from sites such as the pancreas, lung, and ovary, as well as metastatic melanoma.

Pneumatosis Cystoides Intestinalis

This disease describes gas pockets found within the wall of the gastrointestinal tract anywhere along its length. Most cases are discovered incidentally, although symptoms such as episodic diarrhea may occur. The outcome of pneumatosis cystoids intestinalis is dependent on the underlying cause of disease, which includes the following:

- Intestinal obstruction
- Peptic ulcer
- Crohn disease
- Mesenteric ischemia
- Volvulus
- Neonatal necrotizing enterocolitis

Microscopically, cysts ranging up to several centimeters in diameter are present below the serosa or in the submucosa. These cysts often are lined by macrophages and giant cells.

THE LARGE INTESTINE

Normal Anatomy and Histology

The large intestine consists of the colon and rectum and measures 0.9 to 1.25 m in length. The colon is subdivided into the cecum, ascending colon, transverse colon, descending colon, and sigmoid colon. The superior mesenteric artery supplies the proximal half of the large intestine, and the inferior mesenteric artery supplies the distal half. The regular outpouchings of the colon are termed haustra.

Microscopically, the colonic wall is made up of the following:

- Mucosa: flat with regularly spaced pits, termed crypts of Lieberkühn; columnar epithelium with interspersed goblet cells; the lamina propria contains chronic inflammatory cells and occasional eosinophils
- Submucosa: lymphatic channels, blood vessels, and Meissner nerve plexus
- Muscularis propria: inner circular and outer longitudinal layer; the longitudinal layer is separated into three bundles called taeniae coli; Auerbach nerve plexus
- Serosa

Congenital Disorders

Congenital Megacolon (Hirschsprung Disease)

Hirschsprung disease is the most common cause of congenital intestinal obstruction. It results from a lack of ganglion cells, predominantly in the rectum. Patients often present early in life with constipation. The rectum, in the absence of neural signals that allow relaxation, becomes constricted and spastic. The bowel is prominently dilated proximal to this region. A rectal biopsy demonstrating lack of ganglion cells confirms the diagnosis.

Although most cases are sporadic, 10% are familial and may occur with *RET* mutations (MEN II syndrome) or mutations of the endothelin-B receptor and ligand. An increased association of Hirschsprung disease occurs with Down syndrome. Treatment requires surgical resection of the affected portion of bowel.

Acquired megacolon occurs secondary to agents that decrease colonic motility, including diabetic neuropathy, scleroderma, inflammatory bowel disease, infection, amyloidosis, and hypothyroidism, as well as psychogenic causes. Acquired megacolon most frequently occurs in adults.

Anorectal Malformations

These developmental defects result from arrested development of the caudal region of the gut during the first 6 months of development. Malformations range from relatively minor to severe and include the following:

- Anorectal agenesis: failure of anal and rectal development
- Rectal atresia
- Imperforate anus: anus covered by a cutaneous membrane
- Fistula

Infections

Pseudomembranous Colitis

Pseudomembranous colitis is an inflammatory condition of the colon most often associated with antibiotic use and colonization by *Clostridium difficile*. The bacterium elaborates toxins that cause necrosis of the colonic epithelium and neutrophilic crypt inflammation. The exudate formed by the necrotic epithelium, mucus, fibrin, and neutrophils forms an overlying "pseudomembrane." Gross examination of the colon reveals irregularly shaped yellow-gray plaques that most often affect the rectosigmoid region. Patients have diarrhea, fever, leukocytosis, and abdominal cramps. Treatment involves antibiotics and supportive therapy.

Neonatal Necrotizing Enterocolitis

Neonatal necrotizing enterocolitis (NEC) represents one of the most common surgical emergencies of newborns and occurs most commonly in premature infants. The etiology of NEC most likely reflects an ischemic event leading to secondary bacterial colonization. Patients may present with ileus, bilious vomiting, and bloody stools and progress. With progression of the disease, lethargy and signs of shock become apparent. The large intestine may demonstrate a variable appearance, from pseudomembrane formation to frank gangrene.

Inflammatory Bowel Disease

Inflammatory bowel disease (IBD) encompasses two chronic inflammatory diseases of the intestinal tract: *Crohn disease* and *ulcerative colitis*. Both diseases generally are intermittently active disease processes that are classically distinguished on the basis of location and gross and microscopic examination of the bowel (Table 13-6).

Despite these defining features, the distinction between Crohn disease and ulcerative colitis may be unclear in specific patients because of nonspecific findings on biopsy specimens and evolution of the disease process, which leads to a diagnosis of "indeterminate colitis."

Microscopic Colitis

Collagenous Colitis

Collagenous colitis is characterized by chronic watery diarrhea. Examination of specimens from affected patients reveals a grossly normal bowel mucosa. Microscopically, a thickened band of collagen containing blood vessels is present below the surface epithelium, which measures up to 10 times the normal thickness. The epithelium contains an increased number of intraepithelial lymphocytes, and the lamina propria contains increased numbers of chronic inflammatory cells.

Lymphocytic Colitis

Lymphocytic colitis is also characterized by chronic watery diarrhea. Patients with this disease have an increased incidence of HLA-A1 and a decreased incidence of HLA-A3. Lymphocytic colitis is also common in patients with celiac disease. Grossly, the colonic mucosa appears normal. On microscopic examination, a marked increase in the number of lymphocytes (>10 lymphocytes/100 epithelial cells) is in the colonic epithelium.

Radiation Enterocolitis

Pelvic or abdominal radiation can lead to radiation colitis up to a year after treatment. This entity may range from mucosal ulceration to progressive ischemia. Fistula formation, hemorrhage, perforation, and strictures may complicate this disease.

Table 13-6
Comparison of Crohn Disease and Ulcerative Colitis

Features	Crohn Disease	Ulcerative Colitis
Clinical manifestations		
Onset	Late teens/early adult	Early adult
Location	Skip lesions throughout gastrointestinal tract	Continuous lesions of colon, rectum
Rectal involvement	Uncommon	Common
Symptoms	Abdominal pain, fever, diarrhea, colonic bleeding	Diarrhea, rectal bleeding, cramps
Systemic conditions	Sclerosing cholangitis, cholelithiasis, amyloidosis	Arthritis, uveitis, erythema nodosum, pyoderma gangrenosum, sclerosing cholangitis
Association with smoking	Increased risk	?Protective
Genetic loci	Chromosome 16	Unknown
Bacterial association	?*Pseudomonas,* mycobacteria	?Enterobacter
ANCA formation	Uncommon	Common
Risk of colon cancer	Slightly increased	Greatly increased
Treatment	Corticosteroids, cyclosporine, anti-TNF antibodies	Corticosteroids, azathioprine
Macroscopic features		
"Skip" lesions	Common	Absent
Thickened wall	Common	Uncommon
Strictures	Common	Uncommon
Right colon predominance	Common	Absent
Fistulas	Common	Absent

(continues)

Table 13-6
(continued)

Features	Crohn Disease	Ulcerative Colitis
Circumscribed ulcers	Common	Absent
Confluent linear ulcers	Common	Absent
Pseudopolyps	Absent	Common
Microscopic features		
Transmural inflammation	Common	Uncommon
Submucosal fibrosis	Common	Absent
Fissures	Common	Uncommon
Granulomas	Common	Absent
Crypt abscess	Uncommon	Common

Modified from Rubin E, Gorstein F, Rubin R, et al. Rubin's Pathology, 4th ed. Philadelphia: Lippincott Williams & Wilkins, 2005, p. 719.

Diverticular Disease

Diverticulosis describes an acquired condition in which the mucosa and submucosa herniate through the muscularis propria of the large intestine. The herniated tissue does not include all layers of the intestinal wall; thus, these lesions are considered pseudodiverticula. Examination of the mucosa containing a diverticulum reveals a round opening, which may contain stool. The muscular wall of the intestine surrounding the diverticula appears thickened. Microscopically, diverticula appear as flask-like structures that originate at the intestinal lumen and extend through the muscularis propria.

Diverticulosis primarily affects the sigmoid colon (95% of cases) but may involve additional portions of the large intestine. This disease is more common in elderly persons and those residing in Western countries. Primary etiologic factors that may promote diverticulum formation include the following:

- Low dietary fiber, leading to sustained bowel contractions and increased intraluminal pressure
- Decreased resilience of the intestinal connective tissue

More than 80% of persons with diverticulosis are asymptomatic. Occasionally, patients may experience episodic colicky pain, flatulence, diarrhea, or constipation. A potentially serious complication of diverticulosis is sudden, painless, severe bleeding. Lower GI bleeding often occurs as bright red blood per rectum or as black tarry stools.

Diverticulitis is an inflammation of a diverticulum, often occurring secondary to fecalith impaction. It may result in perforation, abscess formation, peritonitis, fibrosis, or fistula formation. Patients with diverticulitis present with persistent left lower quadrant abdominal pain, fever, changes in bowel habits, and leukocytosis. The majority of patients respond to antibiotics, although surgery is required in 20% of patients.

Vascular Diseases

Ischemic Colitis

Ischemic colitis often occurs in elderly patients who have atherosclerosis of the mesenteric blood vessels. The most common pattern of ischemic colitis is chronic segmental disease that affects watershed areas of the bowel such as the splenic flexure and rectosigmoid area. The rectum is frequently spared. Patients present with abdominal pain, rectal bleeding, and a change in bowel habits. This clinical presentation may also be seen in patients with IBD and infective colitis.

The mucosa in ischemic colitis may demonstrate mucosal ulcers, hemorrhagic nodular lesions, or a pseudomembrane on endoscopy and gross examination. Microscopically, mucosal ulcerations, crypt abscesses, edema, and hemorrhage are identified.

Based on the extent and severity of disease, patients are treated with supportive measures or surgery. Long-term complications include colonic stricture and obstruction.

Angiodysplasia (Vascular Ectasia)

Angiodysplasia occurs in elderly patients, often secondary to localized arteriovenous malformations. This disease may be associated with aortic valve disease. Patients present with multiple episodes of lower GI bleeding of unknown etiology. On pathologic examination, the large intestine demonstrates multiple hemangiomatous lesions smaller than 0.5 cm diameter, which consist of tortuous, thin-walled, dilated veins and capillaries in the submucosa. The cecum and ascending colon are affected most commonly.

Hemorrhoids

Hemorrhoids are dilated, thick-walled venous channels that occur frequently in the elderly population and during pregnancy. *Internal hemorrhoids* arise from the superior hemorrhoidal plexus above the pectinate line and *external hemorrhoids* originate from the inferior hemorrhoidal plexus below the pectinate line. Patients may present with rectal bleeding or iron-deficiency anemia. Painful thrombosis of hemorrhoids may occur.

Solitary Rectal Ulcer Syndrome

Internal mucosal prolapse of the rectum may lead to mucosal irritation and ulceration, demonstrated microscopically as smooth muscle proliferation from the muscularis mucosa into the lamina propria. Ulceration may or may not be present.

Colorectal Polyps

Polyps are raised lesions present on the GI mucosa. These lesions may be precancerous (adenomas) or nonneoplastic (hyperplastic, juvenile, inflammatory, and lymphoid polyps). Polyps are defined macroscopically as sessile (flat) or pedunculated (containing a stalk).

Nonneoplastic Polyps

Hyperplastic Polyps (Metaplastic Polyps)

Hyperplastic polyps are small, sessile mucosal projections that are nonneoplastic and are often multiple. The most common form of colonic polyp, hyperplastic polyps occur in more than 75% of elderly patients. Microscopically, these lesions demonstrate elongated, branched, starfishlike glands that are dilated and lined by goblet cells. It is proposed that hyperplastic polyps develop from slowed migration of epithelial cells from the base of the crypts.

Juvenile Polyps (Retention Polyps)

Described as hamartomatous proliferations of the colonic mucosa, *juvenile polyps* occur most commonly in children younger than 10 years of age. Juvenile polyps generally are single, pedunculated, nonneoplastic lesions. Microscopically, these lesions demonstrate dilated and cystic epithelial crypts filled with mucus and a fibrovascular lamina propria.

Inflammatory Polyps

These nonneoplastic polyps are nodular mucosal structures caused by inflamed and regenerating epithelium.

Lymphoid Polyps

These nonneoplastic polyps are caused by submucosal lymphoid follicles that produce an overlying projection of the mucosa. *Nodu-*

lar lymphoid hyperplasia describes an excess of lymphoid tissue within the colon, often leading to the appearance of multiple polyps.

Adenomas

Adenomatous polyps are neoplastic growths of the colonic epithelium that demonstrate at least low-grade dysplasia. Approximately half of all adenomas occur in the rectosigmoid region and frequently are asymptomatic.

Adenomas are separated into tubular, villous, and tubulovillous forms based on histologic appearance. Tubular adenomas demonstrate a flat surface, whereas villous adenomas demonstrate fingerlike villous projections. Tubular adenomas are the most common form of adenoma encountered. Patients with larger tubular adenomas, as well as all villous adenomas, are at increased risk for malignant transformation to adenocarcinoma. Figure 13-6 illustrates general morphologic features of tubular versus villous adenomas.

Adenomas arise from an increase in epithelial proliferation relative to apoptosis. All adenomas contain at least low-grade dysplasia, which appears as stratified nuclei in the colonic epithelium with a decrease in the number of goblet cells. High-grade dysplasia demonstrates loss of nuclear polarity, cribriform architecture, and frequent mitoses.

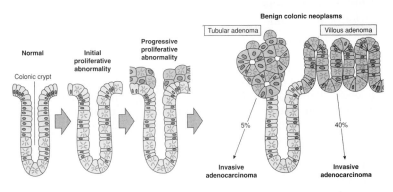

FIGURE 13-6
The histogenesis of adenomatous polyps of the colon. The initial proliferative abnormality of the colonic mucosa, the extension of the mitotic zone in the crypts, leads to the accumulation of mucosal cells. The formation of adenomas may reflect epithelial-mesenchymal interactions. (From Rubin E, Gorstein F, Rubin R, et al. Rubin's Pathology, 4th ed. Philadelphia: Lippincott Williams & Wilkins, 2005, p. 724.)

Serrated adenomas are a special type of adenoma that demonstrates a starfishlike branching of the glands, as seen in hyperplastic polyps, but demonstrates epithelial dysplasia. These lesions may be precancerous.

Familial adenomatous polyposis (FAP), also termed *adenomatous polyposis coli* (APC), is a rare, autosomal dominant condition that accounts for a minor (1%) subset of colorectal carcinomas. The disease is caused by mutations in the APC gene on chromosome 5. Subtypes of FAP include the following:

- Attenuated FAP: less than 100 adenomas of the colon
- Gardner syndrome: extracolonic lesions including osteomas, epidermoid cysts, desmoid tumors, congenital hypertrophy of the retinal pigment epithelium
- Turcot syndrome: malignant CNS tumor, such as medulloblastoma

Patients with FAP develop hundreds to thousands of adenomas during the course of the disease, which often has an onset during childhood or adolescence. The majority of adenomas are of the tubular variety, although tubulovillous and villous adenomas occur. Patients have an increased risk of colorectal cancer, with a mean age of onset of 40 years. Total colectomy before the onset of cancer is curative, although a subset of patients may develop precancerous adenomas in other sites of the GI tract.

Malignant Tumors
Adenocarcinoma

Colorectal carcinoma is a frequent cause of cancer death in Western society, with approximately 5% of Americans developing this cancer during their lifetime. Although classified as a single disease entity, cancer of the colon and cancer of the rectum appear to demonstrate slightly different demographics, suggesting an underlying difference in disease biology. The majority of colorectal cancers arise in adenomatous polyps. Risk factors for colorectal cancer include the following:

- Increased age (>40 years)
- Prior colorectal cancer
- Ulcerative colitis or Crohn disease
- FAP
- HNPCC
- Family history of colorectal cancer
- Diet low in indigestible fiber
- Diet high in animal fat
- Increased intestinal content of anaerobic bacteria

Protective factors include a high selenium content of the soil and plants, exogenous antioxidants, and diets rich in cruciferous vegetables (e.g., cauliflower).

In the early stages, colorectal cancer is often silent. With progression of the disease, symptoms may become apparent. These symptoms include occult or bright red fecal blood, iron-deficiency anemia, fistulas, perforation, or malignant ascites. Cancers arising in the left colon, which contains a smaller-caliber lumen, may present with obstruction accompanied by abdominal pain and change in bowel habits. The only effective treatment for colorectal cancer is surgical resection, often accompanied by chemotherapy and radiation therapy.

The pathogenesis of colorectal carcinoma is complex, with multiple genetic alterations affecting the progression of this disease, including changes in oncogenes (*RAS*) and tumor suppressor genes (*APC, DCC, p53*) expression, alterations in DNA methylation, and deficiencies in DNA mismatch repair (*MLH1*). Figure 13-7 summarizes the basic pathophysiology of colorectal carcinoma progression.

HNPCC syndrome is an autosomal dominant disease that accounts for 3% to 5% of colorectal cancers. HNPCC is caused by a germline mutation in one of the DNA mismatch repair genes, such as *hMSH2* or *hMLH1*, accompanied by a second "hit" or genetic defect in the accompanying allele. Defects in DNA mismatch repair prevent the correction of spontaneous replication errors of DNA, leading to genetic mutations. Over time, replication defects give rise to genomic instability, especially in areas of repetitive sequences (microsatellites) that are prone to DNA replication errors. HNPCC is defined by a number of criteria, including the following:

- Onset of colorectal cancer at a young age (<50 years)
- Few adenomas
- High frequency of carcinomas proximal to the splenic flexure
- Multiple synchronous or metachronous colorectal cancers
- Extracolonic cancers: endometrial, ovarian, gastric, small intestine, hepatobiliary, or urothelial

When developed, the pathologic appearance of colorectal carcinoma is similar regardless of etiology. The gross appearance may be polypoid, ulcerating, or annular and constricting. Colorectal cancer invades the wall of the intestine and may spread by direct extension, lymphatic invasion, or hematogenous (blood-borne) spread. Extension through the intestinal wall is correlated with patient prognosis, as described by the Dukes and TNM systems of pathologic staging (Table 13-7).

Carcinoid (Neuroendocrine) Tumors

These tumors are similar in appearance and behavior to carcinoid tumors of the small intestine (see previous section). Approximately 50% of these tumors have metastasized at the time of discovery.

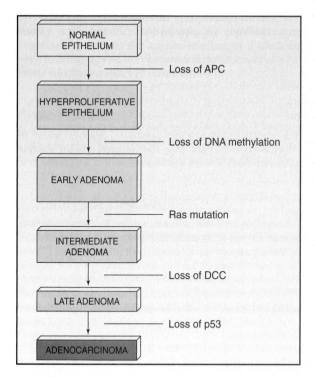

FIGURE   13-7
Model of some of the genetic alterations involved in colonic carcino-genesis. (From Rubin E, Gorstein F, Rubin R, et al. Rubin's Pathol-ogy, 4th ed. Philadelphia: Lippincott Williams & Wilkins, 2005, p. 728.)

Large Bowel Lymphoma

These are uncommon lesions of the large intestine that may present as a segmental thickening, polypoid lesion, or mass extending through the bowel wall. The majority of these lesions are derived from B cells.

Epidermoid Carcinoma of the Anal Canal

Anal cancers constitute 2% of large bowel cancers and may present with bleeding, pain, or an anal mass. Risk factors include infections with *human papillomavirus* (HPV), chronic inflammation, fissures, and trauma. Anal cancers often penetrate directly through the rec-tal wall into adjacent tissues. These cancers may demonstrate squa-

Table 13-7

Classification of Colorectal Cancer

Dukes System

Stage A: tumor confined to the mucosa
Stage B_1: tumor invading into, but not through, the muscularis propria
Stage B_2: tumor invading to the serosa without lymph node metastases
Stage C_1: B_1 tumors with regional lymph node metastases
Stage C_2: B_2 tumors with regional lymph node metastases
Stage D: distant metastases (liver, lung)

Tumor-node-metastasis (TNM) classification

T1: tumor invades the submucosa
T2: tumor invades into, but not through, the muscularis propria
T3: tumor invade the subserosal tissue
T4: tumor penetrates the serosa or adjacent organs

mous, basaloid, or mucoepidermoid appearances and are generally classified as "epidermoid."

Miscellaneous Disorders

Additional disorders that may affect the large intestine include endometriosis, melanosis coli secondary to laxative use, fecal impaction with associated stercoral ulcers, and infectious diseases associated with AIDS (e.g., CMV, *Candida, Cryptosporidium*).

THE APPENDIX

Normal Anatomy and Histology

The appendix measures 8 to 10 cm in length and is attached to the cecum at the level of the ileocecal junction. The appendix contains a mucosa, submucosa, muscularis propria, and serosa. The appendiceal submucosa contains prominent lymphoid tissue.

Appendicitis

Acute appendicitis is the most common disease of the appendix and may occur at any age, although the incidence peaks in the second to third decades. Appendicitis may be caused by luminal obstruction from a fecalith or lymphoid hyperplasia; however, in 50% of all patients, no obstruction is identified. Ultimately, acute appendicitis causes increased intraluminal pressure; venous stasis; ischemia; transmural inflammation; and occasionally, perforation and peritonitis.

Patients with acute appendicitis present with perigastric or right lower quadrant abdominal pain, nausea, vomiting, low-grade fever, and leukocytosis. Complications arising from acute appendicitis include the following:

- Perforation
- Periappendiceal abscess
- Fistula
- Pylephlebitis (thrombophlebitis of the intrahepatic portal vein radicals)
- Diffuse peritonitis and septicemia

On gross examination, the appendix appears congested, tense, and covered with a fibrinous exudate. The lumen contains hemorrhagic or purulent material. Microscopically, neutrophils involve the mucosal surface and may extend through the appendiceal wall to involve the serosa.

Mucocele

A *mucocele* refers to a mucus-filled appendix caused by non-neoplastic (chronic obstruction) or neoplastic (*mucinous cystadenocarcinoma*) conditions. Rupture of a mucinous cystadenocarcinoma may result in extensive seeding of the peritoneum and filling of the abdominal cavity with mucin, termed *pseudomyxoma peritonei*.

Neoplasms

Carcinoids of the appendix are common, generally arise in the distal portion of the organ, and rarely metastasize.

THE PERITONEUM AND PERITONITIS

The peritoneum is the mesothelial lining that covers the abdominal cavity and organs. The visceral peritoneum invests the abdominal organs, whereas the parietal peritoneum covers the abdominal wall and retroperitoneum.

Peritonitis is an inflammation of the peritoneum caused by bacterial infection or chemical irritation. Bacterial sources occur in the context of abdominal viscus perforation, peritoneal dialysis, cirrhosis accompanied by portal hypertension and ascites, the nephrotic syndrome, and disseminated tuberculosis. Chemical sources include bile, hemorrhage, hydrochloric acid from a perforated stomach, pancreatic enzymes from acute pancreatitis, urine, and foreign bodies. Patients present with severe abdominal pain and tenderness, nausea, vomiting, and high fever.

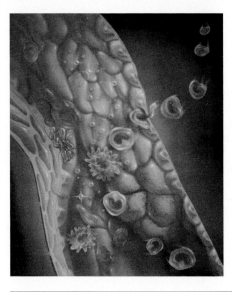

CHAPTER 14

The Liver and Gallbladder

Chapter Outline

THE LIVER

Normal Anatomy and Histology

The liver is composed predominantly of the large right and left lobes, with lesser segments of the right lobe that include the caudate and quadrate lobes. The gallbladder rests in a fossa of the right hepatic lobe. The liver receives a dual blood supply from the hepatic artery, which arises from the celiac axis, and the portal vein, which is formed by the convergence of the splenic and superior mesenteric veins. Venous outflow from the liver proceeds via the hepatic veins, which drain into the inferior vena cava. Bile synthesized in the liver is transported through bile canaliculi to the right and left hepatic ducts, which lead to the common hepatic duct, which in turn is joined by the cystic duct to form the common bile duct. The common bile duct joins with the pancreatic duct to empty at the ampulla of Vater.

The liver lobule is classically represented as a hexagonal structure, with the central vein located in the middle of the hexagon and portal triads (tracts) situated at each point of the hexagon (Fig. 14-1). The portal triads are formed by the bile ducts and branches of the hepatic artery and portal vein. Surrounding the portal tracts is a layer of hepatocytes called the limiting plate. Radiating out from the portal tracts are one-cell-layer thick hepatocyte plates. Between these plates are the hepatic sinusoids, which are lined by fenestrated endothelial cells, phagocytic Kupffer cells, and specialized storage cells called satellite cells (or cells of Ito). Blood that arrives at the portal tract passes through the sinusoids to the central vein, which ultimately empties into the hepatic veins. In contrast, bile formed by the hepatocytes travels in the opposite direction by contraction of the pericanalicular cytoskeleton of the hepatocytes.

The liver acinus, in which the central veins actually form the periphery, is used to describe the microscopic liver. The regions of the liver acinus reflect physiologic differences within the liver and include the highly oxygenated zone surrounding the portal tracts (zone 1), the intermediate zone (zone 2), and the most poorly oxygenated region and region most sensitive to drug injury (zone 3).

Hepatocytes make up approximately 90% of the volume of the liver and each hepatocyte has three specialized surfaces, including the sinusoidal (adjacent to regions of blood flow), lateral (between hepatocytes), and canalicular (adjacent to bile flow). The sinusoidal surface is separated from the endothelial cells by the space of Disse. Hepatocytes contain a centrally placed, spherical nucleus with one or more nucleoli; the nuclei can vary in size significantly.

The liver has several functions, including the following:

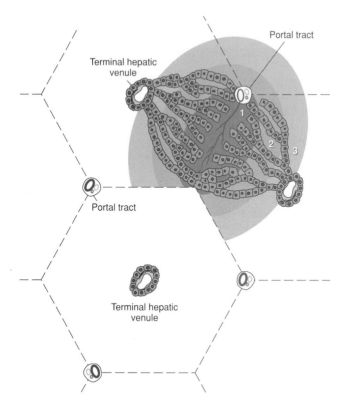

Portal tract

Terminal hepatic
venule

1

2

3

Portal tract

Terminal hepatic
venule

FIGURE 14-1
Morphologic and functional concepts of the liver lobule. In the morphologic liver lobule, the periphery of the hexagonal lobule is anchored in the portal tracts, and the central vein is in the center. The functional liver lobule is derived from the gradients of oxygen and nutrients in the sinusoidal blood. In this scheme, the portal tract, with the richest content of oxygen and nutrients, is in the center (zone 1). (From Rubin E, Gorstein F, Rubin R, et al. Rubin's Pathology, 4th ed. Philadelphia: Lippincott Williams & Wilkins, 2005, p. 744.)

- Metabolism: gluconeogenesis from amino acids, lactate, and glycerol and glycogenolysis
- Synthesis: formation of serum proteins including albumin, clotting factors, complement, and serum-binding proteins
- Storage: storage site of glycogen, triglycerides, iron, copper, and lipid-soluble vitamins
- Catabolism: breakdown of hormones, serum proteins, and site of detoxification of foreign compounds

- Excretion: excretion of bile, which contains a mixture of conjugated bilirubin, bile acids, phospholipids, cholesterol, and electrolytes

The liver is unusual in that it can regenerate after injury to assume its original size.

Bilirubin Metabolism

Bilirubin Formation and Metabolism

Bilirubin is a breakdown product of heme, and the majority of bilirubin in the blood arises from the breakdown of senescent erythrocytes by the mononuclear phagocytic system of the spleen, bone marrow, and liver. Bilirubin is released from phagocytes into the circulation, where it is bound to albumin for transport to the liver. Free bilirubin (i.e., not bound to carrier molecules) may cause irreversible brain injury in newborns if it is present in high concentrations, a condition termed *kernicterus*. Bilirubin is ultimately excreted into the bile by the liver in a four-step process that includes the following:

- Uptake of bilirubin by the liver: most likely carrier-mediated transport process
- Binding of bilirubin to cytosolic proteins termed glutathione S-transferases
- Conjugation of bilirubin to glucuronic acid by the enzyme uridine diphosphate-glucuronyl transferase to form a water-soluble compound
- Excretion of conjugated bilirubin into the bile

When conjugated bilirubin is excreted, it remains intact until it reaches the distal small bowel and colon, where it is hydrolyzed by bacterial flora to free bilirubin that is subsequently reduced to urobilinogen and excreted in the feces. A small amount of urobilinogen and the majority of the bile acids are reabsorbed in the distal ileum and colon and returned to the liver, a process called enterohepatic circulation of bile.

Abnormalities of Bilirubin Metabolism

Abnormalities of bilirubin metabolism may occur at any step in the processing of bilirubin (Fig. 14-2). Terms that are used to describe bilirubin abnormalities include the following:

- Hyperbilirubinemia: increased concentration of bilirubin in the blood (>1.0 mg/dL)
- Jaundice and icterus: yellow skin and sclerae, respectively, that occur when bilirubin concentrations are greater than 2.0 to 2.5 mg/dL

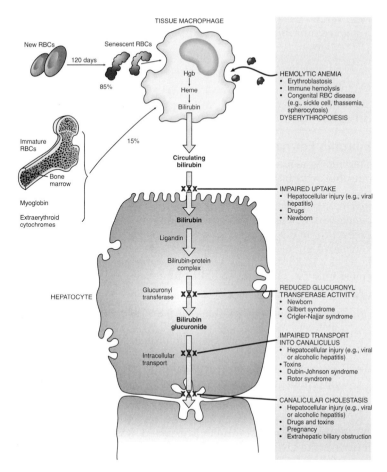

TISSUE MACROPHAGE

New RBCs

Senescent RBCs

120 days

85%

Hgb

Heme

Bilirubin

Immature RBCs

15%

Bone marrow

Myoglobin

Extraerythroid cytochromes

Circulating bilirubin

HEPATOCYTE

Bilirubin

Ligandin

Bilirubin-protein complex

Glucuronyl transferase

Bilirubin glucuronide

Intracellular transport

HEMOLYTIC ANEMIA
• Erythroblastosis
• Immune hemolysis
• Congenital RBC disease (e.g., sickle cell, thassemia, spherocytosis)
DYSERYTHROPOIESIS

IMPAIRED UPTAKE
• Hepatocellular injury (e.g., viral hepatitis)
• Drugs
• Newborn

REDUCED GLUCURONYL TRANSFERASE ACTIVITY
• Newborn
• Gilbert syndrome
• Crigler-Najjar syndrome

IMPAIRED TRANSPORT INTO CANALICULUS
• Hepatocellular injury (e.g., viral or alcoholic hepatitis)
• Toxins
• Dubin-Johnson syndrome
• Rotor syndrome

CANALICULAR CHOLESTASIS
• Hepatocellular injury (e.g., viral or alcoholic hepatitis)
• Drugs and toxins
• Pregnancy
• Extrahepatic biliary obstruction

FIGURE 14-2
Mechanisms of jaundice at the level of the hepatocyte. (From Rubin E, Gorstein F, Rubin R, et al. Rubin's Pathology, 4th ed. Philadelphia: Lippincott Williams & Wilkins, 2005, p. 748.)

- Cholestasis: microscopic plugs of inspissated bile in dilated bile canaliculi and visible bile pigment in hepatocytes
- Cholestatic jaundice: hyperbilirubinemia accompanied by microscopic cholestasis

Diseases that involve abnormalities of bilirubin metabolism are listed in Table 14-1. Categories of bilirubin metabolic abnormalities include the following:

Table 14-1
Abnormalities of Bilirubin Metabolism

Disease	Description
Overproduction of bilirubin	
Hemolytic anemia	Increased destruction of erythrocytes in many diseases including erythroblastosis, immune hemolysis, sickle cell disease, thalassemia, and spherocytosis
Dyserythropoiesis	Ineffective production of red blood cells leading to increased erythrocyte breakdown
Decreased hepatic uptake of bilirubin	
Generalized hepatocellular injury	Causes include certain drug toxicities (rifampin and probenecid), viral hepatitis, and in the newborn; demonstrates increased levels of unconjugated bilirubin
Decreased bilirubin conjugation	
Crigler-Najjar syndrome type I	Recessively inherited disease that results in a severe, unconjugated hyperbilirubinemia due to an absence in UGT activity in the liver; the bile is colorless and the liver is histologically normal; treated by liver transplantation
Crigler-Najjar syndrome type II	Less severe than type I disease and demonstrates only a partial reduction in UGT activity; treatment with phenobarbital can decrease unconjugated bilirubin levels
Gilbert syndrome	Inherited mild chronic unconjugated hyperbilirubinemia caused by impaired clearance of bilirubin in the absence of any detectable functional or structural liver disease; may be caused by mutations of the UGT promoter; common disease that is often recognized after puberty and demonstrates minimal symptoms
Neonatal (physiologic) jaundice	Occurs in 70% of newborns; a transient condition caused by reduced activity of hepatic UGT in the newborn that slowly increases after birth; more pronounced in premature infants; caused by increased levels of unconjugated bilirubin; treated by phototherapy

(*continues*)

Table 14-1

(continued)

Disease	Description
Decreased transport of conjugated bilirubin	
Dubin-Johnson syndrome	Benign autosomal recessive disease caused by complete absence of MRP2 protein in hepatocytes and characterized by chronic conjugated hyperbilirubinemia and coarse, iron-free brown-black pigment deposition in the liver with a grossly black liver; patients experience mild intermittent jaundice; also characterized by urinary coproporphyrin excretion of 80% of the isomer I form
Rotor syndrome	Clinically similar to Dubin-Johnson syndrome except without pigmentation of the liver; patients have few symptoms
Canalicular cholestasis	
Benign recurrent intrahepatic cholestasis	Self-limited, periodic episodes or intrahepatic cholestasis preceded by malaise and itching with approximately three to five episodes in a lifetime; liver shows centrilobular cholestasis and few mononuclear inflammatory cells in the portal tracts; no permanent sequelae
Intrahepatic cholestasis of pregnancy	Pruritus and cholestatic jaundice that usually occurs in the last trimester of each pregnancy and disappears after delivery; does not affect maternal health but may cause fetal distress, stillbirth, and premature delivery
Familial intrahepatic cholestasis (Byler syndrome)	Uncommon, inherited autosomal recessive disorders of infancy or early childhood in which intrahepatic cholestasis progresses relentlessly to cirrhosis; linked to mutations in hepatocellular bile transport systems, including MRP proteins; high association with retinitis pigmentosa; most children die by age 2 years

MRP, multidrug resistance protein; UGT, uridine diphosphate-glucuronyl transferase.

- Overproduction of bilirubin: may result from increased destruction of erythrocytes (hemolytic anemia) or ineffective erythropoiesis (dyserythropoiesis); primarily causes an increase in unconjugated bilirubin. In the presence of underlying hepatic parenchymal damage (e.g., hepatitis), an accompanying conjugated hyperbilirubinemia may be present as well.
- Decreased hepatic uptake: may occur in cases of generalized liver injury, such as viral hepatitis or drug toxicity, or in newborns; reflected by increased unconjugated bilirubin
- Decreased bilirubin conjugation in the liver: occurs in a number of hereditary syndromes, including Crigler-Najjar syndrome and Gilbert syndrome, as well as physiologically in newborns
- Decreased transport of conjugated bilirubin into the canaliculi: often involves mutations in the multidrug resistance protein family and includes Dubin-Johnson syndrome, Rotor syndrome, toxic drug injury, and general hepatocellular injury
- Canalicular cholestasis: hepatocellular injury; toxic drug injury; pregnancy; extrahepatic biliary obstruction

Cholestasis

Cholestasis reflects impaired canalicular bile flow that may be caused by intrahepatic (owing to intrinsic liver disease) or extrahepatic (large bile duct) biliary obstruction and is characterized by the accumulation of bilirubin, cholesterol, and bile acids in the blood (Fig. 14-3). A variety of mechanisms may cause cholestasis, including the following:

- Abnormalities of the canalicular microvilli
- Damage to the canalicular plasma membrane resulting in decreased secretion of bile by the Na^+/K^+-ATPase: chlorpromazine, ethinyl estradiol
- Alterations of the contractile properties of the canaliculus: cytochalasin, phalloidin
- Alterations in the permeability of the canalicular membrane: possibly estrogens and taurolithocholate

Microscopically, cholestasis more commonly affects the centrilobular region of the liver and is characterized by brownish canalicular bile plugs within dilated canaliculi and in hepatocytes. In cases of long-standing cholestasis, scattered necrosis of hepatocytes can occur because of the toxic effects of bile, as well as the formation of extracellular collections of pigment and debris termed a "bile lake." Chronic cholestasis is reflected by the presence of peripheral bile plugs in addition to those present in the centrilobular region.

An additional cause of severe conjugated hyperbilirubinemia is sepsis, especially sepsis caused by gram-negative bacteria. In

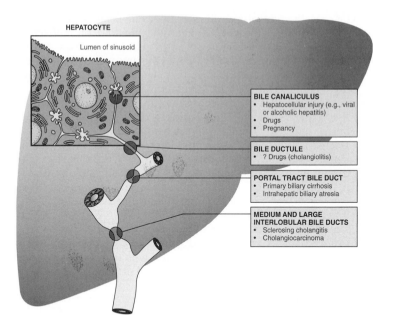

F I G U R E   14-3
Sites of cholestasis. (From Rubin E, Gorstein F, Rubin R, et al. Rubin's Pathology, 4th ed. Philadelphia: Lippincott Williams & Wilkins, 2005, p. 753.)

cases of sepsis, the serum alkaline phosphatase activity and cholesterol levels usually are low, suggesting an isolated defect in the excretion of conjugated bilirubin. Microscopically, the liver demonstrates mild canalicular cholestasis and slight fat accumulation.

Cirrhosis

Cirrhosis occurs as the end-stage of chronic liver disease and reflects irreversible injury to the liver. The majority of cases are caused by chronic viral hepatitis or alcoholism, although up to 15% of cases have an unknown etiology and are termed *cryptogenic cirrhosis*. The normal architecture of the liver is replaced by nodules of regenerating hepatocytes surrounded by bands of fibrosis. At this late stage of liver injury, the inciting cause of liver damage often is difficult to determine, and many different disease processes can lead to this final outcome (Table 14-2).

Grossly, the liver demonstrates a misshapen surface with irregular nodules and fibrous bands of varying widths on cut surface.

Table 14-2	
Causes of Cirrhosis	
Alcoholic liver disease	α_1-Antitrypsin deficiency
Chronic viral hepatitis	Glycogen storage disease, types II and IV
Primary biliary cirrhosis	Galactosemia
Autoimmune hepatitis	Hereditary fructose intolerance
Extrahepatic biliary obstruction	Hereditary fructose intolerance
Sclerosing cholangitis	Hereditary storage diseases:
Hemochromatosis	Gaucher, Niemann-Pick, Wolman,
Wilson disease	mucopolysaccharidoses
Cystic fibrosis	

From Rubin E, Gorstein F, Rubin R, et al. Rubin's Pathology, 4th ed. Philadelphia: Lippincott Williams & Wilkins, 2005, p. 754.

Microscopically, persistent liver cell necrosis, bile duct proliferation, and infiltration of the portal tracts by mononuclear inflammatory cells are present. Commonly, two patterns of cirrhosis are present:

- Micronodular cirrhosis: nodules are usually less than 3 mm in diameter surrounded by thin fibrous septae, often early in the course of cirrhosis and commonly seen in alcoholic cirrhosis
- Macronodular cirrhosis: large nodules separated by broad fibrous bands and often associated with chronic hepatitis or continued regeneration of micronodular cirrhosis

Micronodular and macronodular cirrhosis often present as a spectrum of disease.

Hepatic Failure

Hepatic failure is a clinical syndrome that occurs when liver function is inadequate to sustain metabolic, detoxifying, and synthetic activities. Hepatic failure may develop acutely (e.g., after viral hepatitis or toxic liver injury) or in the context of chronic liver injury (e.g., chronic viral hepatitis or cirrhosis). A variety of complications may result from hepatic failure, including the following:

- Jaundice: caused by inadequate clearance of bilirubin by the injured liver

  ➤ Hepatic encephalopathy: progresses in stages that include sleep disturbance, irritability, and personality changes

(stage I), lethargy and disorientation (stage II), deep somnolence (stage III), and coma (stage IV)

- Coagulation defects and bleeding: reduced hepatic synthesis of
  coagulation factors leading to coagulopathy and occasionally
  disseminated intravascular coagulation
- Hypoalbuminemia: decreased hepatic synthesis of albumin
  that contributes to generalized edema
- Hepatorenal syndrome: oliguria, azotemia, and increased
  plasma creatinine levels that is caused by decreased renal
  blood flow, leading to renal vasoconstriction and often related
  to a poor prognosis
- Decreased arterial oxygen saturation that may be severe
  enough to result in cyanosis
- Endocrine complications: gynecomastia, female body habitus,
  testicular atrophy, loss of libido, palmar erythema, spider angi-
  omas of the upper trunk and face, gonadal failure, amenorrhea

Hepatic encephalopathy is one of the most severe complications of hepatic failure and may be related to toxic compounds
absorbed from the intestine, elevated ammonia levels, or increased
levels of benzodiazepine-like molecules. Hepatic encephalopathy
may be associated with *asterixis* (flapping hand tremor) or fetor
hepaticus, which is associated with the colonic breakdown of sulfur-containing amino acids leads to this characteristic breath odor.
Central nervous system findings include cerebral edema, laminar
necrosis and spongiform change of the deep layers of the cerebral
cortex and subcortical white matter, and astrocytic swelling, nuclear enlargement, and nuclear inclusions.

Portal Hypertension

Portal hypertension is a sustained increase in portal venous pressure caused by obstruction to blood flow at any point in the portal
circuit, and may be characterized as prehepatic, intrahepatic, and
posthepatic (Table 14-3; Fig. 14-4). The portal vein delivers two
thirds of the hepatic blood flow and normally maintains a pressure
of 5 to 10 mm Hg (7 to 14 cm H_2O). Increased portal vein pressure
exceeding 30 cm H_2O leads to portal hypertension.
    Complications of portal hypertension include the following:

- Esophageal varices: arise from the opening of portal-systemic
  collaterals as an adaptation to decompress the portal venous
  system and are often located in the submucosa of the esophagus and upper stomach

  ➤ Exsanguinating hemorrhage may result from rupture of
    these arteries, with a mortality rate as high as 40%
  ➤ May be treated by direct balloon tamponade, injection of

Table 14-3

Causes of Portal Hypertension

Disease	Description
Prehepatic	
Portal vein thrombosis	May occur in the setting of cirrhosis, tumors, infections, hypercoagulability states, pancreatitis, or surgical trauma
Increased splenic flow	Myeloid metaplasia
Intrahepatic	
Cirrhosis	Regenerative nodules in the liver impinge on the hepatic veins leading to obstruction distally; also central vein sclerosis and sinusoidal fibrosis contribute to the disease in alcoholic liver disease
Schistosomiasis	Ova released from intestinal veins lodge in the intrahepatic portal venules, which results in a granulomatous inflammation that heals by scarring
Primary biliary cirrhosis	Granulomatous inflammation that surrounds and destroys small and medium-sized bile ducts that often affects middle-aged women
Congenital hepatic fibrosis	
Toxins	Arsenic
Posthepatic	
Vena cava obstruction	May result from various causes, including hypercoagulable states and emboli
Budd-Chiari syndrome	Thrombosis of hepatic veins that occurs in association with polycythemia vera, hypercoagulable states, oral contraceptives, pregnancy, bacterial infections, tumors, and paroxysmal nocturnal hematuria; often larger veins are affected; appears as centrilobular necrosis and hemorrhage
Alcoholic central sclerosis	Fibrosis around the central vein
Venoocclusive disease	Variant of Budd-Chiari syndrome with occlusion of the central venules and small branches of the hepatic veins that occurs in association with pyrrolizidine alkaloid ingestion, chemotherapy, hepatic irradiation, or graft-versus-host-disease

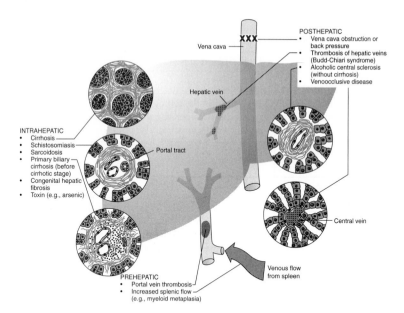

FIGURE 14-4
Causes of portal hypertension. (From Rubin E, Gorstein F, Rubin R, et al. Rubin's Pathology, 4th ed. Philadelphia: Lippincott Williams & Wilkins, 2005, p. 757.)

> sclerosing agents, endoscopic variceal ligation, or intravenous vasopressin
> ➤ Repeated episodes may be treated with construction of portasystemic shunts

- Caput medusae: collateral veins radiating about the umbilicus
- Anorectal varices
- Splenomegaly: Enlarged spleen with inapparent white pulp on cut surface, dilated splenic sinusoids lined by thickened walls containing fibrous tissue and hyperplastic splenic parenchyma. Gamma-Gandy bodies may form following focal hemorrhage and appear as fibrotic, iron-laden nodules.
- Ascites: accumulation of fluid in the peritoneal cavity that occurs as a result of sodium and water retention, decreased oncotic pressure owing to hypoalbuminemia in cirrhosis, and increased hydrostatic pressure in cirrhosis
- Spontaneous bacterial peritonitis: occurs in patients with both cirrhosis and ascites when the ascitic fluid is seeded by bacteria from the blood or by transit through the bowel wall

Viral Hepatitis

A variety of infectious agents can produce hepatitis, including viruses and parasites. Viral hepatitis is caused by hepatotropic viruses, named from A to G, that infect hepatocytes and produce inflammation and necrosis of the liver.

Forms of Viral Hepatitis

Table 14-4 presents a comparison among the more common viral hepatitides.

Hepatitis A

Hepatitis A virus (HAV) is a small, RNA-containing enterovirus of the picornavirus group that infects hepatocytes as well as gastrointestinal epithelial cells. HAV is transmitted from person to person by the fecal-oral route and may occur in crowded and unsanitary conditions. Other modes of transmission involve traveling internationally or ingesting contaminated shellfish. HAV most commonly affects children in day care centers. The incubation period is 3 to 6 weeks, and infected persons develop nonspecific symptoms, including fever, malaise, and anorexia. HAV is not directly cytopathic, and liver injury is postulated to occur from immune reaction to the infected hepatocyte. Although a resulting increase is serum aminotransferases (AST, ALT) and jaundice may occur, many patients remain anicteric. The virus is shed in the feces between 4 and 8 weeks after infection. Serum IgM anti-HAV is elevated and is followed by persistent increases in IgG anti-HAV (Fig. 14-5). HAV does not pursue a chronic course, no carrier state occurs, and infection provides lifelong immunity.

Hepatitis B

Hepatitis B virus (HBV) is a member of the hepatotropic DNA virus family of hepadnaviruses. Humans are the only significant reservoir of HBV. Transmission of the virus occurs by transfer of blood products by contaminated needles or by intimate contact, because the virus is contained within blood, saliva, and semen. Routine screening of blood products for HBsAg has virtually eliminated the transmission of virus by transfusion. A carrier state occurs in approximately 0.3% of infected persons in the United States and in as many as 20% in infected persons in Southeast Asia and Africa. Synthetic vaccines against HBsAg confer lifelong immunity.

The genome of HBV is a partial DNA duplex that contains four long open-reading frames that include the following:

- Core (C) coding region: encodes the core antigen (HBcAg) and the e antigen (HBeAg)

Table 14-4
Viral Hepatitides

	Hepatitis A	Hepatitis B	Hepatitis C	Hepatitis D	Hepatitis E
Genome	ssRNA, unenveloped	ds DNA, enveloped	ssRNA, enveloped	ssRNA, enveloped	ssRNA, unenveloped
Incubation Period	3–6 weeks	4 weeks to 6 months	7–8 weeks	Requires HBV	35–40 days
Transmission	Fecal-oral	Parenteral, intimate contact	Parenteral, intimate contact	Parenteral, intimate contact	Water-borne
Fulminant necrosis	Very rare	Yes	Rare	Unknown	No
Chronic hepatitis	No	10%	80%	Yes (HBV)	No
Carrier state	No	Yes	Yes	Yes	Unknown
Liver cancer	No	Yes	Yes	Same as HBV	Unknown

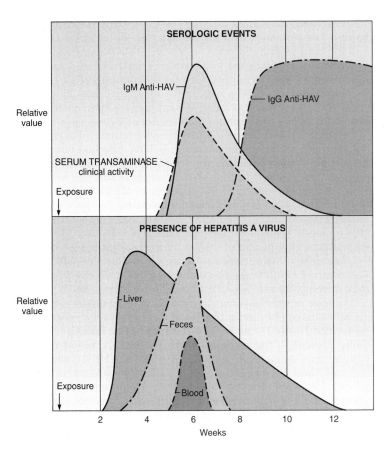

F I G U R E   14-5
Typical serological events associated with hepatitis A (HAV) infection. (From Rubin E, Gorstein F, Rubin R, et al. Rubin's Pathology, 4th ed. Philadelphia: Lippincott Williams & Wilkins, 2005, p. 763.)

- Surface coding region: encodes the noninfective hepatitis B surface antigen (HBsAg) that is present in the coat that encompasses the HBV core (i.e., envelope glycoprotein); used as antigen in synthetic vaccine
- DNA polymerase (P) coding region: encodes enzyme that replicates viral DNA and has reverse transcriptase activity
- X coding region: small protein that activates viral transcription and may function in hepatocellular carcinogenesis in chronic infection

HBV binds to surface receptors on the hepatocyte and is internalized and transported to the nucleus, where the DNA is closed and the viral replication cycle begins. Viral RNA is transported to the cytoplasm, where the viral proteins are translated and viral particles are either enveloped for release from the cell or recycled to the cell nucleus. HBV is not directly cytopathic, and liver injury occurs from cytotoxic (CD8[+]) T lymphocytes that are directed against multiple HBV epitopes within hepatocytes.

Acute or primary hepatitis B may be symptomatic or asymptomatic. The majority of patients with acute HBV infection have a self-limited hepatitis with subsequent clearance of the virus, complete recovery, and lifelong immunity. The serum of patients with acute HBV infection demonstrate the appearance of HBsAg 1 week to 2 months after exposure, which is followed by the appearance of anti-HBcAg antibody, circulating HBeAg, and, importantly, anti-HBs antibody (Fig. 14-6). The persistence of HBeAg in the serum correlates with a period of intense viral replication and therefore maximal infectivity of patients. In cases in which acute HBV infection does not result in clearance of the virus and recovery, patients may develop chronic hepatitis B or fulminant hepatitis B.

Chronic hepatitis B occurs in patients who do not have detectable anti-HBs antibodies in the blood for more than 6 months and consequently are unable to clear the HBV virus. HBsAg is persistently present in the serum of these patients. A subset of these patients may demonstrate active hepatitis when HBV continues to replicate, and is evidenced by persistent elevations in serum HBeAg. Liver inflammation and necrosis are present, and patients are symptomatic with persistent elevation of serum aminotransferase levels. Some of these patients may produce anti-HBs antibodies, but these antibodies are bound to antigen and form circulating immune complexes that may cause a serum sickness–like syn-

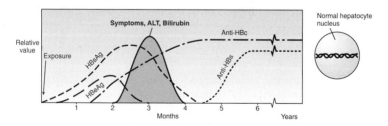

FIGURE   14-6

Acute hepatitis B (HBV) infection with subsequent resolution and recovery. (From Rubin E, Gorstein F, Rubin R, et al. Rubin's Pathology, 4th ed. Philadelphia: Lippincott Williams & Wilkins, 2005, p. 765.)

drome. Patients with chronic infection and active disease are likely to develop cirrhosis and are at increased risk for hepatocellular carcinoma. A *chronic carrier* state may occur in other patients when persistent HBV infection results in subclinical disease, with normal liver functions and minimal alteration of liver histology.

Fulminant hepatitis B occurs rarely and is characterized by massive liver cell necrosis, hepatic failure, and a high mortality rate.

Hepatitis C

Hepatitis C virus (HCV) is a member of the flavivirus family and is an enveloped, single-stranded RNA virus. The prevalence of HCV infection ranges from 1.8% in the United States to greater than 20% in Egypt. Viral spread occurs by parenteral exposure or intimate contact and risk factors for disease include intravenous drug use and high-risk sexual behavior. Screening of blood products has greatly reduced the risk of transmission by transfusion. The HCV genome contains a single open reading frame, which encodes a polyprotein that is subsequently cleaved into three structural proteins (one core and two envelope proteins) and four nonstructural proteins. The incubation period for HCV ranges from weeks to months, and elevated serum aminotransferase levels usually are present within 1 to 3 months of exposure. HCV RNA is detected in the blood within approximately 1 month after infection and is followed by the appearance of anti-HCV antibodies (Fig. 14-7). Similar to HBV, HCV is not directly cytopathic, and liver injury most likely occurs from cytotoxic (CD8$^+$) T lymphocytes that are directed against infected hepatocytes.

Approximately 20% of patients who are infected with HCV develop an acute, self-limited infection that resolves in a few months. The remainder of patients develop chronic disease, and as many as 20% develop cirrhosis and an increased risk for hepatocellular carcinoma. Chronic HCV infection also is associated with essential mixed cryoglobulinemia, membranoproliferative glomerulonephritis, porphyria cutanea tarda, sicca syndrome, and lymphoma.

Hepatitis D

Hepatitis D virus (HDV) is a defective RNA virus that requires the synthesis of HBsAg for assembly. HDV infection may occur simultaneously with HBV (co-infection) or after HBV infection (superinfection). Typically, superinfection of an HBV carrier with HDV increases the severity of an existing chronic hepatitis.

Hepatitis E

Hepatitis E virus (HEV) is an enteric undeveloped, single-stranded RNA virus that spreads by the fecal-oral route. HEV often occurs as large outbreaks and often affects young to middle-aged persons.

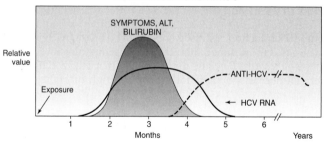

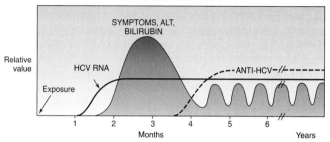

FIGURE 14-7
Clinical course of hepatitis C (HCV) infection. (From Rubin E, Gorstein F, Rubin R, et al. Rubin's Pathology, 4th ed. Philadelphia: Lippincott Williams & Wilkins, 2005, p. 768.)

The virus causes a self-limited, acute, icteric disease with associated hepatomegaly, fever, and arthralgias. The disease is especially dangerous in pregnant women. No chronic disease or carrier state has been identified.

Acute Hepatitis

Acute viral hepatitis is morphologically similar among all forms of viral hepatitis and demonstrates scattered necrosis of single cells or clusters of hepatocytes. Some apoptotic liver cells appear small and deeply eosinophilic and are termed Councilman bodies. Hepatocytes may appear swollen and lobular disarray may be present because of scattered foci of regenerating liver cells. Chronic inflammatory cells, especially lymphocytes, diffusely infiltrate the lobule, surround individual necrotic liver cells, and accumulate in areas of focal necrosis. Often, lymphocytes are present between the wall of the central vein and the liver plates, which is termed central phlebitis. In addition, lymphocytes accumulate within the portal tracts and may form follicles, especially in hepatitis C. Cholestasis is common. With recovery, the normal architecture of the liver is restored.

Confluent hepatic necrosis is a severe form of acute viral hepatitis in which extensive hepatocyte cell death leads to geographic regions of necrosis. This condition occurs most commonly in patients with HBV infection and is subdivided into varying degrees of severity:

- Bridging necrosis: bands of necrosis that stretch between portal tracts, central veins, and between portal tracts and central veins
- Submassive confluent necrosis: necrosis of entire lobules or groups of adjacent lobules with clinically severe hepatitis
- Massive hepatic necrosis: necrosis of virtually all hepatocytes with the appearance of a shrunken, soft, flabby liver with a wrinkled capsule associated with a high mortality rate

Chronic Hepatitis

Chronic hepatitis occurs as a complication of HBV and HCV infection and may demonstrate varying degrees of inflammation and necrosis:

- Piecemeal necrosis: periportal lesion with destruction of the limiting plate of hepatocytes with a periportal chronic inflammatory infiltrate between the portal tracts and the lobular parenchyma
- Portal tract lesions: variable infiltration of the portal tracts by lymphocytes, plasma cells, and macrophages with a mild-to-severe proliferation of bile ducts
- Intralobular lesions: focal necrosis and inflammation within the parenchyma; HBV infection may produce ground-glass hepatocytes with large granular cytoplasm
- Periportal fibrosis: deposition of collagen caused by the piecemeal necrosis of hepatocytes that may ultimately bridge between portal tracts

Autoimmune Hepatitis

Autoimmune hepatitis is a severe chronic hepatitis of unknown cause that commonly affects young women and is associated with circulating autoantibodies and high levels of serum immunoglobulins. Many patients demonstrate other forms of autoimmune disease in addition to autoimmune hepatitis.

Type I autoimmune hepatitis is the most common form of this disease and predominantly affects young women. This disease is associated with antinuclear and anti-smooth muscle antibodies. The asialoglycoprotein receptor on hepatocytes may be the most likely target of circulating antibodies. The disease may be asymptomatic for long periods and present with cirrhosis in as many as 25% of patients. Susceptibility is associated with the *DRB1* gene.

Type II autoimmune hepatitis occurs in children between 2 and 14 years of age and demonstrates circulating antibodies to liver and kidney microsomes (anti-LKM). The target antigen is a P450-type drug-metabolizing enzyme (CYP 2D6).

Microscopically, the liver appears similar to that of chronic viral hepatitis. A subset of patients may progress to cirrhosis. Therapy includes corticosteroids, immunosuppressive drugs, and liver transplantation.

Alcoholic Liver Disease

Alcoholic liver disease can occur with excessive intake of any form of ethanol. A dose-dependent relationship exists between the lifetime dose of alcohol (duration and daily amount) and the appearance of cirrhosis. Approximately 15% of chronic alcoholics develop cirrhosis, often after 10 years of alcohol abuse, and many of these persons die from hepatic failure or other complications of cirrhosis. A complicating factor in the pathogenesis of alcoholic liver disease and cirrhosis is the finding that chronic alcoholics have an apparently higher incidence of HBV and HCV infection, although the underlying cause of this is unknown.

After ingestion, ethanol is rapidly absorbed from the stomach and distributed in the body water space. Ethanol is oxidized in the liver by cytosolic alcohol dehydrogenase (ADH) to form acetaldehyde and acetate, although a minor microsomal ethanol-oxidizing pathway also is present in the endoplasmic smooth reticulum. The clearance of ethanol is linear (fixed amount per unit of time), although chronic alcoholics metabolize alcohol at a higher rate.

A variety of lesions occur in the liver after excessive alcohol consumption that may occur sequentially or coexist:

- Fatty liver (steatosis): Reversible deposition of fat droplets within hepatocytes that is manifested by an enlarged, yellow liver and is caused by increased hepatic fatty acid synthesis, decreased mitochondrial oxidation of fatty acids, increased triglyceride production, and impaired release of lipoproteins from the liver
- Alcoholic hepatitis: acute necrotizing lesion characterized by central zone hepatocyte necrosis, cytoplasmic eosinophilic hyaline inclusions of intermediate filaments in hepatocytes (Mallory hyaline), neutrophilic inflammatory response, and

perivenular fibrosis that may suddenly develop after many years of drinking

- Severe fibrosis often is present around the central vein and leads to perivenular sinusoidal obliteration and is termed *central hyaline sclerosis*. Patients present with malaise, anorexia, fever, right upper quadrant pain, jaundice, mild leukocytosis, elevated transaminases, and elevated alkaline phosphatase.
- Alcoholic cirrhosis: occurs in 15% of alcoholics; many patients progress to end-stage liver disease

Chronic alcohol ingestion can result in increased activity of the cytochrome P450–dependent mixed-function oxidases, which can augment the metabolism of hepatic toxins, including carbon tetrachloride and acetaminophen.

Nonalcoholic Fatty Liver Disease

Nonalcoholic fatty liver disease (NAFLD) appears morphologically similar to alcoholic liver disease but is caused by a variety of factors, including obesity, type 2 diabetes mellitus, and hyperlipidemia. Histologic features occur along a spectrum and include steatosis, lobular and portal inflammation, hepatocyte necrosis, Mallory hyaline, and fibrosis that is often centrilobular. Steatosis in association with hepatitis in this population is termed *nonalcoholic steatohepatitis* (NASH). Weight loss may improve NAFLD, although some patients may progress to cirrhosis.

Primary Biliary Cirrhosis

Primary biliary cirrhosis (PBC) is a chronic progressive cholestatic liver disease characterized by the destruction of the intrahepatic bile ducts (nonsuppurative destructive cholangitis). This disease predominantly affects middle-aged women between 30 and 65 years of age, and the majority of cases are sporadic. Immunologic abnormalities are associated with this disease, including the presence of circulating antimitochondrial antibodies and infiltrating CD8[+] T cells, and many patients demonstrate other coexistent autoimmune diseases. The pathology of PBC occurs in three stages:

- Stage I, ductal lesions: Chronic destructive cholangitis affects the intrahepatic small- and medium-sized bile ducts and is predominantly mediated by lymphocytes, although plasma cells and macrophages are present; may be accompanied by lymphoid follicles and epithelioid granulomas in the portal tracts. The bile duct epithelium is irregular and hyperplastic with nuclear stratification and occasional papillary ingrowths.

- Stage II, scarring: Small bile ducts virtually disappear, medium-sized bile ducts are scarred, bile duct proliferation within the portal tracts is florid, and collagenous septa extend from the portal tracts into the lobular parenchyma.
- Stage III, cirrhosis: Dark green, bile-stained liver that exhibits fine nodularity with rare small bile ducts and no inflammation

Patients often present with severe pruritus (caused by bile acid deposition in the skin) and progressive increases in serum bilirubin levels. Serum aminotransferase levels are only moderately increased. Cholesterol-laden macrophages accumulate in the subcutaneous tissues in lesions termed xanthomas. Because of impaired bile secretion and subsequent fat and fat-soluble vitamin malabsorption, steatorrhea, osteomalacia, and osteoporosis may occur. Many patients develop gallstones.

Some patients progress to cirrhosis and often die of complications, including hepatic failure and portal hypertension. In other patients, PBC may pursue an indolent course for 20 to 30 years, and end-stage PBC may be treated by liver transplantation.

Primary Sclerosing Cholangitis

Primary sclerosing cholangitis (PSC) commonly affects men younger than 40 years of age, many of who have ulcerative colitis. PSC is characterized by inflammation and fibrosis of the intrahepatic and extrahepatic bile ducts, which may eventually lead to progressive biliary obstruction, persistent obstructive jaundice, and secondary biliary cirrhosis. Although the cause of PSC is unknown, the disease is associated with haplotypes HLA B8 and DR3, and circulating antineutrophil cytoplasmic antibodies (pANCAs) are common.

The disease is commonly segmental, may affect the gallbladder, and can be subdivided into three stages:

- Stage I: periductal inflammation and fibrosis in the portal tracts
- Stage II: obliteration of bile ducts and extension of fibrous septa into the parenchyma
- Stage III: secondary biliary cirrhosis

Inflammation of intrahepatic and extrahepatic ducts of all sizes can occur and, because of the segmental nature of the lesion, appears as a beading of intrahepatic biliary tree by imaging. PSC has a poor prognosis, with a mean survival after symptoms of only 6 years. Patients have a markedly increased risk of cholangiocarcinoma. Liver transplantation may be curative, although PSC may recur.

Extrahepatic Biliary Obstruction

The extrahepatic biliary tree may be obstructed by a variety of lesions, including carcinoma of the biliary tract, pancreas or ampulla, gallstones, external compression by enlarged lymph nodes, strictures, or congenital biliary atresia.

Early in the course of obstruction, the liver is swollen and bile stained, with centrilobular cholestasis and edema of the portal tracts. With increasing severity of obstruction, the portal tracts demonstrate a mononuclear infiltrate, bile duct proliferation, distended bile ducts, and occasional rupture of bile ducts leading to the formation of bile lakes, which appear as focal, golden-yellow deposits surrounded by degenerating hepatocytes. Foamy, lipid-laden macrophages accumulate in the portal tracts and may lead to granuloma formation. Damaged hepatocytes with large amounts of intracellular bile undergo feathery degeneration, with a characteristic reticulated cytoplasm. A superimposed suppurative cholangitis may be present. Over time, the portal tracts become enlarged and may demonstrate onion skin fibrosis.

If untreated, extrahepatic biliary obstruction may progress to micronodular cirrhosis.

Iron Overload Syndromes

The excess accumulation of iron in the body (siderosis) may occur in a variety of circumstances (Table 14-5), including hereditary hemochromatosis (HH) and secondary iron overload syndromes. The body contains 3 to 4 grams of iron, approximately two thirds of which is present in hemoglobin, myoglobin, and iron-containing enzymes. The remainder is present in stored iron, which exists as soluble ferritin and insoluble hemosiderin. Ferritin is present in the cytoplasm of all cells and in small amounts in the circulation. Hemosiderin is a product of ferritin degradation that is present as golden-yellow granules that stain with the Prussian blue stain. The liver and bone marrow are the major sites of iron storage in the ·

Table 14-5

Causes of Iron Overload

Increased iron absorption	Parenteral iron overload
Hereditary hemochromatosis	Multiple blood transfusions
Chronic liver disease	Injectable medicinal iron
Iron-loading anemias	
Porphyria cutanea tarda	Focal iron overload
Congenital disease (e.g., atransferrinemia)	Idiopathic pulmonary
Dietary iron overload (Bantu siderosis)	hemosiderosis
Excess medicinal iron	Renal hemosiderosis

From Rubin E, Gorstein F, Rubin R, et al. Rubin's Pathology, 4th ed. Philadelphia: Lippincott Williams & Wilkins, 2005, p. 785.

body. Iron is absorbed in the gastrointestinal tract and this absorption is dependent on dietary ascorbate.

Hereditary Hemochromatosis

HH is inherited as an autosomal recessive disorder and most commonly affects men between 40 and 60 years of age. The gene involved in HH is *Hfe*, which is located on chromosome 6 and encodes a transmembrane protein similar to MHC class-1 molecules. The mutant Hfe protein, which is present on many cells including duodenal enterocytes, cannot promote iron intake into the cytoplasm. As a result, duodenal crypt cells sense a general iron deficiency and therefore upregulate DMT-1 expression that then increases absorption of dietary iron. Iron levels may increase within the body as high as 20 to 40 grams.

HH is characterized by excessive iron absorption and toxic accumulation of iron in parenchymal cells, especially the liver, heart, and pancreas. The clinical hallmarks of advanced HH are cirrhosis, diabetes, skin pigmentation, and cardiac failure. A number of organs are affected in HH, including the following:

- Liver: enlarged, reddish brown liver with micronodular cirrhosis and iron granules within hepatocytes and bile duct epithelium
- Skin: increased pigmentation
- Pancreas: rust-colored, fibrotic pancreas with increased iron in exocrine and endocrine cells and resulting in glucose intolerance and diabetes
- Heart: iron pigment is present within myocardial fibers and is associated with myocyte necrosis, fibrosis, and congestive heart failure
- Endocrine system: pituitary, adrenal, thyroid, and parathyroid abnormalities can occur, including the development of testicular atrophy from pituitary damage
- Joints: severe arthropathy in the fingers and hands may occur

Iron levels may increase within the body as high as 20 to 40 grams. The normal laboratory value for plasma iron is 80 to 100 g/dL, and transferrin is usually one third saturated.

In patients with HH, the serum iron concentration is more than doubled and transferrin is completely saturated. The liver disease in HH is indolent but may develop into cirrhosis with or without associated hepatocellular carcinoma. Repeated phlebotomy may be effective. Life expectancy in patients who have not yet developed cirrhosis or diabetes is identical to that of the general population.

Secondary Iron Overload

Secondary iron overload often occurs in the setting of a hemolytic anemia, such as sickle cell anemia or thalassemia major, in which ineffective erythropoiesis prevents the use of iron that is obtained from the diet or from transfused blood. Liver findings generally are less severe than those in patients with HH, and include iron deposition in the periphery of the lobules and initial deposition within Kupffer cells that eventually spill over into the hepatocytes.

Heritable Disorders Associated with Cirrhosis

Wilson Disease (Hepatolenticular Degeneration)

Wilson disease (WD) is an autosomal recessive disease that occurs in 1 in 50,000 live births and is characterized by the deposition of excess copper in the brain and liver. Copper intake from the diet generally exceeds required amounts, and excess copper is cleared by the liver by both excretion into the bile and secretion into the blood by conjugation with ceruloplasmin.

WD is caused by mutations in *ATP7B*, which encodes an ATP-dependent transmembrane cation channel that transports copper within the hepatocyte. *ATP7B* mutations render copper transport ineffective and both biliary excretion of copper and incorporation into ceruloplasmin are deficient. As a result, copper accumulates in the liver, where it ultimately leads to hepatocyte death, release of copper into the blood, and deposition of copper in extrahepatic tissues.

Liver injury in WD progresses from mild to severe chronic hepatitis, and cirrhosis may develop even during childhood. In addition, Mallory hyaline may be contained within periportal hepatocytes and cholestasis may be present. With persistent injury, chronic hepatitis and cirrhosis may result in jaundice, portal hypertension, and hepatic failure. WD is not associated with an increased risk of hepatocellular carcinoma.

The brain is also strikingly affected by WD and demonstrates a reddish brown discoloration of the corpus striatum and subthalamic nuclei. In addition, the central white matter of the cerebral or cerebellar hemispheres may show spongy softening or cavitation, with atrophy of the overlying cortex. Incoordination, tremors, dysarthria, dysphagia, dystonia, spasticity, and psychiatric disorders may be present.

Other organs affected in WD include the following:

- Eye: development of Kayser-Fleischer rings (golden-brown, bilateral, discoloration of the cornea that encircles the periphery of the iris) caused by copper deposition in Descemet membrane
- Bones: osteomalacia, osteoporosis, spontaneous fractures, and various arthropathies
- Kidney: renal glomerular and tubular dysfunction, including proteinuria, lowered glomerular filtration, aminoaciduria, and phosphaturia
- Blood: transient acute hemolytic episodes

Half of all patients with WD present during adolescence, primarily with hepatic, neurologic, or psychiatric manifestations. Treatment involves the administration of D-penicillamine, a copper-chelating agent that promotes excretion of copper in the urine. Liver transplantation is curative.

Cystic Fibrosis

In cystic fibrosis, tenacious mucous plugs accumulate in the intrahepatic biliary tree, which may lead to hepatic failure during the first weeks of life or secondary biliary cirrhosis later in life.

α_1-Antitrypsin Deficiency

This autosomal recessive disease can lead to hepatic or pulmonary disease because of defective section of the mutant protein by the liver. The PiZ isoform of the α_1-antitrypsin protein undergoes abnormal folding and forms insoluble aggregates within the lumen of the endoplasmic reticulum of the hepatocyte. Microscopically, the hepatocytes demonstrate faintly eosinophilic, PAS-positive cytoplasmic droplets. Micronodular cirrhosis develops in many patients by 2 to 3 years of age and may become macronodular over time. The cirrhosis is complicated by a high incidence of hepatocellular carcinoma.

Inborn Errors of Carbohydrate Metabolism

A variety of disorders of carbohydrate metabolism can lead to cirrhosis, including the following:

- Glycogen storage diseases: Glycogenosis type IV (brancher deficiency, Andersen disease) leads to severe hepatomegaly and cirrhosis by 4 years of age.

  ➤ Sharply circumscribed, PAS-positive inclusions of abnormal glycogen are present in enlarged hepatocytes.
  ➤ Deposition also may occur in the heart, skeletal muscle, and brain.

- Galactosemia: autosomal recessive deficiency of galactose-1-phosphate uridylyl transferase, which converts galactose to glucose, leading to an accumulation of galactose in the liver and other organs

  ➤ Infants who are fed milk rapidly develop hepatosplenomegaly, jaundice, and hypoglycemia.
  ➤ Cataracts and mental retardation are common.

> Within 2 weeks of birth, the liver shows extensive fat accumulation, bile duct proliferation, cholestasis, and fibrosis shortly thereafter.
> Cirrhosis occurs within 6 months.

- Hereditary fructose intolerance: autosomal recessive disease caused by a deficiency of fructose-1-phosphate aldolase, which prevents fructose breakdown. After ingestion of fructose, infants develop hepatomegaly, jaundice, and ascites.
- Tyrosinemia: autosomal recessive disease characterized by a deficiency of fumarylacetoacetate hydrolase that converts tyrosine to fumarate and acetoacetate

> Acute tyrosinemia occurs within weeks of birth and is characterized by hepatosplenomegaly and is associated with liver failure and death.
> Chronic tyrosinemia begins in the first year of life and is characterized by growth retardation, renal disease, and hepatic failure. The disease is associated hepatocellular carcinoma and death before 10 years of age.

Indian Childhood Cirrhosis

Indian childhood cirrhosis primarily affects preschool boys on the Indian subcontinent and is frequently fatal. The liver demonstrates micronodular cirrhosis and abundant Mallory bodies.

Toxic Liver Injury

Acute, chemically induced hepatic injury demonstrates a broad spectrum of liver disease, ranging from transient cholestasis to fulminant hepatitis. Chronic injury may result in a range of manifestation from mild chronic hepatitis to active cirrhosis. Certain hepatotoxic chemicals, such as acetaminophen, carbon tetrachloride, phalloidin, and yellow phosphorus produce a predictable, dose-dependent liver cell necrosis that is characteristically zonal and occurs shortly after administration of the drug. These compounds are metabolized by the mixed-function oxidase system of the liver, which produces activated oxygen species and reactive metabolites. In contrast, other drugs may produce an idiosyncratic reaction, which is independent of the dose of the drug administered.

The hepatic necrosis that occurs in conjunction with toxic drug injury is most commonly centrilobular and is most likely caused by greater activity of drug-metabolizing enzymes in the central zones. Within this region, hepatocytes show coagulative necrosis, hydropic swelling, and variable amounts of fat but only sparse inflammation. Fatty liver, with accumulation of triglycerides within the hepatocytes often occurs in a predictable fashion and may be macrovesicular or microvesicular.

- Macrovesicular steatosis: often occurs in association with chronic ethanol ingestion, carbon tetrachloride, phalloidin, corticosteroids, and methotrexate; a form that resembles alcoholic hepatitis is termed steatohepatitis
- Microvesicular steatosis: characterized by small fat vacuoles dispersed throughout the cytoplasm of the hepatocyte that retains a central location of the nucleus; often associated with severe liver disease and may occur in pregnancy, phospholipidosis, and Reye syndrome. Reye syndrome, which occurs after administration of aspirin in children following the onset of a febrile illness, results in microvesicular steatosis, hepatic failure, and encephalopathy.

Additional abnormalities of the liver that occur in association with toxic drug injury include the following:

- Acute intrahepatic cholestasis: often manifests with mild jaundice, pruritus, and elevated serum alkaline phosphatase levels
- Lesions that resemble viral hepatitis
- Chronic hepatitis: may occur with persistent use of hepatotoxic drugs
- Granulomatous hepatitis: noncaseating granulomas in the portal tracts and the lobular parenchyma
- Vascular lesions: occlusion of the hepatic veins (Budd-Chiari syndrome) may occur with administration of oral contraceptives, and peliosis hepatis (cystic, blood-filled cavities not lined by endothelial cells) may occur with administration of anabolic sex steroids, contraceptive steroids, and tamoxifen
- Hepatic adenomas: can occur following oral contraceptive or anabolic steroid use (see below)
- Hemangiosarcoma: may occur many years after the intravenous administration of thorium dioxide (Thorotrast)

Porphyrias

The porphyrias are inherited and acquired deficiencies in the heme biosynthesis pathway that are characterized by the accumulation of porphyrin intermediates. The site of abnormal heme metabolism and porphyrin accumulation classifies porphyria as hepatic or erythropoietic. The inherited porphyrias are autosomal dominant traits that may be precipitated by administration of drugs, sex hormones, starvation, hepatitis C, HIV, and alcohol. The liver in hepatic porphyrias displays steatosis, hemosiderosis, fibrosis, and cirrhosis. Among the various types of porphyria are the following:

- Acute intermittent porphyria: most common genetic porphyria and affects young adults; results from deficient porphobilinogen deaminase activity in the liver; presents with colicky abdominal pain and neuropsychiatric symptoms
- Porphyria cutanea tarda: may be inherited or acquired and affects middle-aged to elderly persons; results from deficient uroporphyrinogen decarboxylase activity, causes cutaneous photosensitivity and liver disease

Vascular Lesions

Congestion of the liver may occur in a variety of acute and chronic conditions. *Acute passive congestion* often occurs during the agonal period, resulting in a liver with diffuse red speckles that represent dilated and congested sinusoids and central veins in the centrilobular zone.

Chronic passive congestion occurs with persistent congestive heart failure, when venous outflow from the liver is reduced secondary to increased peripheral venous resistance. Grossly, the liver is often reduced in size and demonstrates a mottled light and dark pattern on cut section, which is termed nutmeg liver. Microscopically, the centrilobular central veins and adjacent sinusoids are dilated, and the surrounding liver cell plates are thinned by pressure atrophy. Severe, long-standing, right-sided heart failure also can result in varying degrees of hepatic fibrosis that radiate from the central vein.

In cases of shock, the centrilobular hepatocytes may undergo ischemic necrosis, as they are located most distally from the blood supply arriving at the portal tracts. *Infarction* of the liver is uncommon because of the dual blood supply and overlapping vascular distribution; however, acute occlusion of the hepatic artery (or its branches) may occur after emboli, polyarteritis nodosa, or accidental ligation during surgery. Acute occlusion of the intrahepatic branches of the portal vein may occur with elevated hepatic venous pressure and produces a triangular dark-red infarction with the base of the triangle located on the surface of the liver (Zahn infarct).

Liver Infections

Bacterial Infections

Bacterial infections of the liver are uncommon in industrialized countries and may occur as a complication of a systemic disease. Various forms of abscesses include the following:

- Pyogenic liver abscesses: caused by staphylococci, streptococci, and gram-negative enterobacteria; may reach the liver by the blood or biliary tract

- Pylephlebitic abscess: results from intraabdominal infection that spreads to the liver in the portal blood
- Cholangitic abscess: results from obstruction of the biliary tree with a secondary retrograde infections, often because of *Escherichia coli*, and most commonly affects the right lobe

Patients with a hepatic abscess present often with high fever, rapid weight loss, right upper quadrant abdominal pain, hepatomegaly, and occasionally jaundice. Serum alkaline phosphatase levels often are elevated. Treatment involves surgical drainage and antibiotics, but the mortality from this condition ranges from 40% to 80%.

Parasitic Infections

Parasitic infections of the liver are uncommon in industrialized countries, but may include protozoal and helminthic infections, among others.

Protozoal infections include the following:

- Amebiasis (*Entamoeba histolytica*): Well-circumscribed, 8- to 12 cm diameter cysts that contain thick, dark material that appears similar to anchovy paste or chocolate; trophozoites are present in the periphery of the necrotic debris
- Malaria: hepatomegaly that arises from Kupffer cell hypertrophy and hyperplasia caused by phagocytosis of cellular debris
- Visceral leishmaniasis (*kala azar*): hepatomegaly that arises from Kupffer cell hyperplasia that ingest the parasitic organisms to form cytoplasmic Donovan bodies

Helminthic infections include the following:

- Schistosomiasis: See Chapter 9 and the discussion of portal hypertension.
- Ascariasis (*Ascaris lumbricoides*): This results in a severe, suppurative cholangitis when the worms lodge in the intrahepatic biliary tracts and subsequently disintegrate, leading to the release of eggs.
- Liver flukes (*Clonorchis sinensis* and *Fasciola hepatica*): Organisms lodge in the intrahepatic biliary tree, where they produce a hyperplasia of the biliary epithelium and may promote the development of cholangiocarcinoma.
- Echinococcosis (cystic hydatid disease; *Echinococcus granulosus*): Tapeworms form slowly enlarging cysts within the liver and may result in toxic or allergic reactions to the contents.

Leptospira spirochetes may produce *Weil syndrome*, which demonstrates prolonged fever, jaundice, and occasionally azotemia, hemorrhage, and altered consciousness.

Lesions of *syphilis* may occur in the context of congenital syphilis, with neonatal hepatitis resulting in fibrosis of the portal tracts and around hepatocytes, or tertiary syphilis, which is characterized by hepatic gummas.

Cholestatic Syndromes of Infancy

Prolonged cholestasis and jaundice in infants may occur with hepatocyte disease or obstruction of the biliary tract. Neonatal hepatitis may be idiopathic or occur as a result of α_1-antitrypsin deficiency, viral hepatitis B, and TORCH infections (toxoplasmosis, rubella, cytomegalovirus, and herpes simplex). The multiple causes of neonatal hepatitis are described in Table 14-6. Microscopically, the hepatocytes undergo giant cell transformation, with up to 40 nuclei per cell and distended cytoplasm. In addition, cholestasis, extramedullary hematopoiesis, chronic inflammation around the portal tracts and in the lobular parenchyma, and fibrous tissue septa extending from the portal tracts are identified.

Biliary Atresia

Biliary atresia is a disease of neonates in which the biliary tree does not demonstrate a lumen. The disease may be categorized as extrahepatic or intrahepatic. *Extrahepatic biliary atresia* is a cholestatic disease characterized by obliteration of the lumen of all or part of the biliary tree external to the liver. The microscopic spectrum of disease can vary from acute and chronic periluminal inflammation with epithelial necrosis to fibrosis of the original lumen with mature connective tissue with minimal inflammation. Cholestasis and bile duct proliferation are notable. Occasionally, giant multinucleated hepatocytes may be identified. A subset of these lesions is associated with other congenital anomalies, including heart, intestine, and splenic abnormalities.

Intrahepatic biliary atresia is a paucity of bile ducts within the liver, which also demonstrates cholestasis and bile duct proliferation. Intrahepatic biliary atresia may be idiopathic, associated with known causes of neonatal hepatitis (e.g., α_1-antitrypsin deficiency), or with *Alagille syndrome*, which is an autosomal dominant disorder of Notch signaling characterized by bile duct paucity, and heart, eye, skeleton, kidney, and abnormalities of the central nervous system.

Benign Tumors and Tumorlike Lesions

Hepatic Adenoma

Hepatic adenomas are benign tumors that occur in young to middle-aged women, most commonly in association with the use of

Table 14-6
Causes of Neonatal Hepatitis

Idiopathic
  Idiopathic neonatal hepatitis
  Prolonged intrahepatic cholestasis
  Arteriohepatic dysplasia
    (Alagille syndrome)
  Paucity of intrahepatic bile ducts not
    associated with specific syndromes
  Zellweger syndrome (cerebrohe-
    patorenal syndrome)
  Byler disease

Mechanical obstruction of the intra-
    hepatic bile ducts
  Congenital hepatic fibrosis
  Caroli disease (cystic dilation of
    intrahepatic ducts)

Metabolic disorders
  Defects of carbohydrate metabolism
    Galactosemia
    Hereditary fructose intolerance
    Glycogenesis type IV
  Defects of lipid metabolism
    Gaucher disease
    Niemann-Pick disease
    Wolman disease
    Tyrosemia (defect of amino acid
    metabolism)
    α_1-Antitrypsin deficiency
    Cystic fibrosis
      Parenteral nutrition

Hepatitis
  Hepatitis B
  TORCH agents
  Varicella
  Syphilis
  ECHO viruses
  Neonatal sepsis

Chromosomal abnormalities
  Down syndrome
  Trisomy 18
Extrahepatic biliary atresia

From Rubin E, Gorstein F, Rubin R, et al. Rubin's Pathology, 4th ed. Philadelphia: Lippincott Williams & Wilkins, 2005, p. 795.

oral contraceptives. Grossly, these lesions appear as solitary, sharply demarcated, encapsulated masses up to 40 cm in diameter. The lesions have a risk of intraabdominal bleeding in certain instances. Microscopically, the neoplastic hepatocytes appear similar to normal hepatocytes, but with loss of lobular architecture and an absence of portal tracts and central veins. Occasionally the cells are large and eosinophilic or clear because of increased amounts of cytoplasmic glycogen. Often, large, thick-walled arteries are present in the capsule.

Focal Nodular Hyperplasia

Focal nodular hyperplasia (FNH) is a benign, nodular lesion that may range up to 15 cm in diameter and demonstrates a characteristic central scar on cut section. This lesion most commonly affects young women, although both sexes may be affected. Hepatocytic nodules are surrounded by fibrous septa that contain bile ducts, large arteries and veins, and mononuclear inflammatory cells. Lobular architecture is absent.

Nodular Regenerative Hyperplasia

Nodular regenerative hyperplasia can occur in association with oral contraceptives, anabolic steroids, extrahepatic infections, neoplasms, chronic inflammation, and autoimmune disease and is characterized by small, hyperplastic nodules without fibrosis in an otherwise normal liver. The lesion may be localized or diffuse, and often the nodules form thickened liver cell plates that compress the surrounding parenchyma. In many cases, nodular regenerative hyperplasia may be associated with portal hypertension.

Hepatic Hemangioma

A hemangioma in the liver is commonly benign, and it is often small and asymptomatic. Grossly, the lesion is less than 5 cm in diameter and appears solitary, although it may be multiple. Microscopically, the lesion is morphologically consistent with a cavernous hemangioma, with large vascular spaces lined by endothelium. A rare form of hemangioma is the *infantile hemangioendothelioma*, which appears during the first 2 years of life and contains arteriovenous shunts large enough to cause congestive heart failure.

Cystic Disease of the Liver

A variety of benign diseases can form cystic lesions within the liver, including the following:

- Bile duct hamartomas (von Meyenburg complexes): a collection of anomalous small, cystic bile ducts embedded in a fibrous stroma and are often multiple and appear as gray-white foci; these lesions are lined by bile duct epithelium and may contain inspissated bile
- Solitary and multiple simple cysts: unilocular cysts lined by cuboidal to columnar epithelium
- Congenital hepatic fibrosis: recessively inherited disorder that manifests in children and adolescents characterized by enlarged portal tracts that exhibit extensive fibrosis and numerous bile ducts; may result in severe portal hypertension with recurrent bleeding from esophageal varices

Malignant Tumors of the Liver

Metastatic Cancer

Metastatic cancer is the most common malignancy of the liver and can occur with virtually any form of cancer, although melanoma and gastrointestinal, breast, lung, and pancreatic primaries are the most common primary lesions. The liver may show single or multiple lesions that are commonly firm and white, but may contain regions of hemorrhage and necrosis. Complications may include weight loss, portal hypertension, and gastrointestinal bleeding.

Hepatocellular Carcinoma

Hepatocellular carcinoma (HCC) is a malignant tumor that derives from hepatocytes. Risk factors for the development of HCC include the following:

- Hepatitis B infection
- Hepatitis C infection
- Alcoholic cirrhosis
- Hemochromatosis
- α_1-Antitrypsin deficiency
- Aflatoxin B_1 ingestion: fungal contaminant of many foods, especially in less developed countries

Grossly, HCC appears as a soft tan mass in the liver with occasional hemorrhage. Multiple lesions may be present. Microscopically, well-differentiated lesions may be difficult to distinguish from normal liver, although there is an absence of normal portal tract structures associated with these nodules. Trabecular, pseudoglandular, and solid patterns may be present. A subset of tumors may display a more poorly differentiated or anaplastic appearance.

HCC typically may be asymptomatic or present as an enlarging mass in the liver. Paraneoplastic syndromes may be present, and patients may demonstrate polycythemia, hypoglycemia, and hypercalcemia. α-Fetoprotein levels are often elevated in serum of patients with HCC.

Fibrolamellar HCC is a variant of HCC that occurs in adolescents and young adults and demonstrates a characteristic appearance of large, eosinophilic hepatocytes arranged in clusters and surrounded by delicate collagen fibers. The prognosis of fibrolamellar HCC is more favorable than that of typical HCC.

Cholangiocarcinoma

Cholangiocarcinoma originates at any location within the biliary tract, often affects elderly persons with an average age of 60 years, and is more frequent in Asia. Cholangiocarcinomas are commonly composed of small cuboidal cells in a ductal or glandular configuration with surrounding desmoplasia. Cholangiocarcinomas that arise at the confluence of the right and left hepatic ducts are termed *Klatskin tumors*, or *hilar cholangiocarcinomas*. Klatskin tumors can result in obstruction of the hepatic ducts and infiltration through the wall of the bile ducts and into surrounding structures. Cholangiocarcinomas can metastasize to many extrahepatic sites.

Hepatoblastoma

Hepatoblastoma is a rare malignant tumor of children that is often diagnosed before 3 years of age. Grossly, these lesions may range up to 25 cm in diameter, are circumscribed, and may appear necrotic or hemorrhagic in appearance. Microscopically, cells of epithelial and mesenchymal appearance are present, although mesenchymal cells occasionally are absent. The epithelial component resembles embryonal cells, which are small, fusiform, and arranged in ribbons or rosettes, and fetal cells, which closely resemble hepatocytes but containing glycogen and fat. The mesenchymal elements may demonstrate connective tissue, cartilage, or osteoid differentiation.

Children with hepatoblastoma may present with abdominal enlargement, vomiting, and failure to thrive. Associated congenital anomalies of the heart and kidney may be present. Serum α-fetoprotein levels are elevated and occasional ectopic gonadotropin secretion can lead to sexual precocity. Treatment options include surgical resection or liver transplantation.

Hemangiosarcoma

Hemangiosarcoma is a malignant vascular tumor that arises after exposure to thorium dioxide, vinyl chloride, or inorganic arsenic. Patients often present with hepatomegaly, jaundice, or ascites, and hemolytic anemia and pancytopenia may be present. Grossly, the liver demonstrates multiple foci of hemorrhagic tumor. Microscopically, the tumor cells are spindle-shaped endothelial cells that line the sinusoids and compress the liver cell plates. Occasionally, cavernous spaces or solid masses of cells may be present. Often, widespread metastases are present. These tumors are at increased risk of rupture and may cause extensive bleeding into the abdominal cavity.

Liver Transplantation

Liver transplantation is used to treat a variety of conditions from cirrhosis to certain tumors, and success of transplant generally is related to recurrence of the underlying disease or the level of transplant rejection.

Acute rejection is characterized by portal inflammation, with lymphocytes adhering to the endothelium of terminal venules and small branches of the portal veins, with or without subendothelial inflammation (*endothelialitis*). In addition, bile duct atypia may be present.

Chronic rejection is characterized by damage to interlobular bile ducts, resulting in destruction of small bile ducts and cholestasis *(vanishing bile duct syndrome)*. Subintimal foam cells, intimal sclerosis, and myointimal hyperplasia may result in narrowed or occluded arteries.

THE GALLBLADDER

Normal Anatomy and Histology

The gallbladder is a saclike structure that measures approximately 8 cm in length and that contains approximately 50 mL of bile. The gallbladder stores, concentrates, and excretes bile into the cystic duct, which ultimately empties into the common bile duct. The wall of the gallbladder is composed of a mucosa, muscularis, and adventitia. The mucosa is thrown into irregular folds, which can extend into the wall of the gallbladder as *Rokitansky-Aschoff sinuses*.

Congenital Anomalies

The most common congenital anomalies of the gallbladder are gallbladder duplication and accessory bile ducts. In addition, cystic dilations of the bile duct can occur and are termed choledochal cyst, choledochal diverticulum, and choledochocele (Fig. 14-8). Multiple cysts may appear as segmental dilations of the biliary tree, either extrahepatically or intrahepatically (termed Caroli disease).

Cholelithiasis

Biliary stones (cholelithiasis) may affect the gallbladder or any portion of the extrahepatic biliary tree. In industrialized countries, the majority of stones are cholesterol gallstones, and the remainder are made up of calcium bilirubinate or other calcium salts (pigment stones). In contrast, pigment stones are more common in the tropics and Asia. The majority of gallstones are not radiopaque; they can be visualized by ultrasonography.

Cholesterol stones are the most common form of gallstone and appear round or faceted, yellow-tan, and may range from 1 to 4 cm in diameter. Greater than 50% of the stone is composed of cholesterol, with flthe remainder of the stone formed by calcium salts

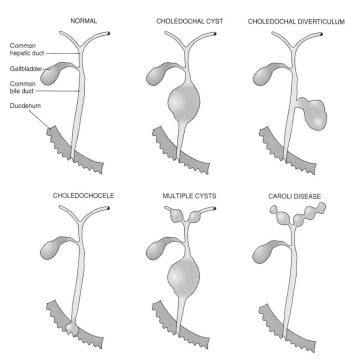

NORMAL

CHOLEDOCHAL CYST

CHOLEDOCHAL DIVERTICULUM

Common hepatic duct

Gallbladder

Common bile duct

Duodenum

CHOLEDOCHOCELE

MULTIPLE CYSTS

CAROLI DISEASE

F I G U R E   14-8
Congenital dilations of the bile ducts. (From Rubin E, Gorstein F, Rubin R, et al. Rubin's Pathology, 4th ed. Philadelphia: Lippincott Williams & Wilkins, 2005, p. 803.)

and mucin. The most common risk factors for the development of cholesterol gallstones are female gender, reproductive age, and obesity (female, fat, forty, and fertile or "the four Fs"). In addition, familial predisposition, certain ethnicities, and increased serum cholesterol levels can increase the risk of developing gallstones. The pathogenesis of cholesterol gallstones involves increased levels of cholesterol in the bile, increased precipitation of bile in the gallbladder by pronucleating biliary proteins and mucus, and impaired gallbladder motility.

Pigment stones are subdivided into black and brown pigment stones.

- Black pigment stones: Irregular, measure less than 1 cm in greatest dimension, and appear glassy; composed of calcium bilirubinate, bilirubin polymers, calcium salts, and mucin. Risk factors include increased age, malnourishment, cirrhosis, and

hemolytic anemia. Increased amounts of secreted, unconjugated bilirubin precipitate as calcium bilirubinate.
- Brown pigment stones: Spongy, laminated, and composed of calcium bilirubinate mixed with cholesterol and calcium soaps of fatty acids; found more frequently in the intrahepatic and extrahepatic bile ducts rather than in the gallbladder. Brown stones are almost always associated with bacterial cholangitis, especially *E. coli*–induced infection. In addition, patients with mechanical obstruction to bile flow may demonstrate the formation of brown stones.

Patients with gallstones may be asymptomatic, but they may have biliary colic if the gallstones are lodged within the cystic or common bile duct. Treatment of gallstones includes the oral administration of bile acids and extracorporeal lithotripsy. Complications of cholelithiasis include obstruction of the cystic duct or common bile duct, acute and chronic cholecystitis, obstructive jaundice, cholangitis, and pancreatitis.

Cholecystitis

Acute Cholecystitis

Acute cholecystitis is a diffuse inflammation of the gallbladder, often secondary to obstruction of the gallbladder outlet, most commonly by gallstones. Grossly, the external surface of the gallbladder is congested and layered with fibrinous exudates. The wall demonstrates edema and the gallbladder mucosa is red to purple in color. Gallstones often are present within the gallbladder. Microscopically, acute and chronic inflammation involves the mucosa and the wall of the gallbladder demonstrates edema and hemorrhage. Focal ulceration or widespread necrosis of the gallbladder mucosa may occur.

Patients often present with right upper quadrant pain that often follows repeated bouts of biliary colic. Mild jaundice may be present. Often, acute cholecystitis resolves within a week, with fibrosis of the gallbladder wall. In a subset of cases, progression is heralded by persistent pain, fever, leukocytosis, and shaking chills. Complications include secondary bacterial infection and perforation.

Chronic Cholecystitis

Chronic cholecystitis is the most common disease of the gallbladder and reflects a persistent inflammation of the gallbladder wall that is almost always associated with gallstones. In addition, chronic cholecystitis can occur after repeated bouts of acute cholecystitis. Grossly, the gallbladder wall appears thickened and firm, and fibrous adhesions may be present on the serosal surface. Gallstones often are present. Microscopically, the wall is fibrotic and often is penetrated by Rokitansky-Aschoff sinuses. Chronic inflammation may involve the mucosa and the wall of the gallbladder, and on occasion, the gallbladder wall may become calcified and is termed *porcelain gallbladder*. Patients often describe nonspecific abdominal symptoms.

Cholesterolosis

Cholesterolosis is defined as the accumulation of cholesterol-laden macrophages in the submucosa of the gallbladder that appears grossly as small, yellow, punctate mucosal lesions (*strawberry gallbladder*). Patients generally are asymptomatic.

Benign Tumors of the Gallbladder

Benign tumors of the gallbladder and extrahepatic ducts are rare, and may include papillomas, adenomyomas, fibromas, lipomas, leiomyomas, and myxomas.

Adenocarcinoma

Adenocarcinoma is the most common malignant tumor of the gallbladder and often is associated with cholelithiasis and chronic cholecystitis; therefore, it is more common in women. Gallbladder carcinoma is most common in the fundus of the gland and demonstrates infiltrating, often well-differentiated glands in a desmoplastic stroma. The tumor can readily metastasize or locally invade. The prognosis is poor in patients with biliary adenocarcinoma.

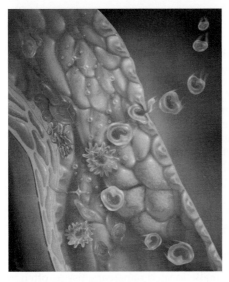

The Pancreas

Chapter Outline

Normal Anatomy and Histology

The pancreas is a mixed endocrine-exocrine organ that resides in the retroperitoneum, situated between the duodenum and the hilum of the spleen. The pancreas is divided into a head, body, and tail.

The exocrine portion of the pancreas is composed of acinar units, which appear microscopically as a rounded single layer of pyramidal cells containing acidophilic zymogen granules that opens onto a central lumen. Acini produce up to 20 digestive enzymes (e.g., trypsin, chymotrypsin, lipase), which empty into a progressively enlarging duct system that ultimately opens at the ampulla of Vater. The digestive enzymes are produced as inactive proenzymes that are activated in the lumen of the intestine. Approximately 80%–85% of the pancreas is exocrine tissue.

The endocrine portion of the pancreas is formed by diffusely distributed islets of Langerhans, which account for approximately 2% of the pancreatic mass. Islets of Langerhans are made up of cells that produce a variety of hormones that are secreted directly into the blood (Table 15-1). Production and secretion of insulin and glucagon, which regulate blood glucose levels, occur in the islets of Langerhans.

Congenital Anomalies

These occur rarely and include the following:

- *Ectopic pancreas*: abnormally located pancreatic tissue, often in the duodenum, stomach, and jejenum
- *Annular pancreas*: head of pancreas encircles the duodenum; may be associated with partial or complete duodenal obstruction in Down's syndrome
- *Pancreas divisum*: failure of pancreatic fusion resulting in two separate glands
- *Cysts*: secondary to faulty pancreatic duct development

Pancreatitis

Pancreatitis is an inflammation of the pancreas caused by injury to acinar cells, resulting in leakage and activation of digestive enzymes within the pancreatic parenchyma (autodigestion). Under normal conditions, protection against pancreatic enzyme activation is accomplished via isolation of enzymatic granules within the cytoplasm, storage of enzymes in an inactive, proenzyme form, and enzymatic inhibitors (α_1-antitrypsin, α_2-macroglobulin, C_1 esterase inhibitor, and pancreatic secretory trypsin inhibitor). Pancreatitis may present as an acute or chronic process, with a wide spectrum of clinical presentations.

Acute Pancreatitis

Acute pancreatitis is a medical emergency that classically presents as severe epigastric pain radiating to the back, associated with nausea and vomiting. Epigastric tenderness, fever, tachycardia, left flank ecchymosis (Grey-Turner's sign), and periumbilical ecchymosis (Cullen's sign) may be present. Diagnosis is based on the clinical impression in conjunction with radiographic and laboratory findings, including elevated serum amylase and lipase. Patients may progress to shock within hours unless treatment is initiated. The

Table 15-1

Cell Types and Neoplasms (Islet Cell Tumors) of the Endocrine Pancreas

Cell Type	Product	Physiological Effect	Tumor	Clinical Manifestations
Alpha	Glucagon	Glycogenolysis, gluconeogenesis (elevation of blood glucose)	Glucagonoma	Mild diabetes, necrotizing rash, anemia, venous thrombosis, severe infections
Beta	Insulin	Reduction of blood glucose; glycogenesis, lipogenesis	Insulinoma	Sweating, nervousness, hunger; hypoglycemia
Delta (D)	Somatostatin	Inhibits pituitary growth hormone release; regulates α, β, δ_1 cells	Somatostatinoma	Mild diabetes, gallstones, steatorrhea, hypochlorhydria
Delta (D_1)	VIP	Same as glucagon; regulates GI motility; $\uparrow$ intestinal cell cAMP	VIPoma	Verner-Morrison syndrome: explosive watery diarrhea, hypokalemia, hypochlorhydria
PP	Pancreatic polypeptide	$\uparrow$ Gastric secretions; $\downarrow$ intestinal motility and bile secretion		Asymptomatic
Enterochromaffin	Serotonin; motilin	Vasodilation; $\uparrow$ vascular permeability; $\uparrow$ gastric motility; $\downarrow$ tone lower esophageal sphincter		Atypical carcinoid syndrome: facial flush, hypotension, periorbital edema, lacrimation
Possible primitive cell of origin	Gastrin	$\uparrow$ Gastric acid secretion	Gastrinoma	Zollinger-Ellison syndrome

GI, gastrointestinal; PP, pancreatic polypeptide; VIP, vasoactive intestinal peptide.

severity and prognosis of acute pancreatitis may be judged using Ranson's criteria, which encompass a variety of clinical and laboratory parameters. Acute pancreatitis has a variety of causes, including the following:

- Cholelithiasis (gallstones): 25-fold increased risk of pancreatitis
- Chronic alcohol use
- Viral infection: mumps, coxsackievirus, and cytomegalovirus
- Drugs: sulfonamides, diuretics, azathioprine, and others
- Blunt trauma
- Acute ischemia
- Metabolic: hyperlipidemia, hypercalcemia
- Familial
- Idiopathic

Initiation of acute pancreatitis may occur following duct obstruction, such as in cholelithiasis; however, the physiology underlying acute pancreatitis in many instances is unclear. Figure 15-1 illustrates known mechanisms of pancreatitis. In its most severe form, acute pancreatitis presents as *acute hemorrhagic pancreatitis*, with widespread hemorrhagic necrosis of the pancreas.

Grossly, the pancreas may appear normal, edematous, hyperemic (red, inflamed), or friable and hemorrhagic. Often, yellow-white, chalklike, areas of fat necrosis may occur in the pancreas and surrounding mesentery. This process of saponification is characterized by calcium and magnesium soap deposition caused by fat necrosis. Microscopically, acinar cell necrosis, intense acute inflammation, and necrotic fat cells are identified.

Acute pancreatitis is generally managed with supportive measures, including intravenous fluids, nasogastric suction to prevent pancreatic enzyme secretion, analgesia, and monitoring. Complications resulting from acute pancreatitis include the following:

- Acute respiratory distress syndrome
- Acute renal failure
- Sepsis
- Pancreatic pseudocyst: cystlike space lined by connective tissue (not epithelium), filled with debris, blood, and pancreatic enzymes
- Fistula formation

Chronic Pancreatitis

Chronic pancreatitis involves the progressive destruction of the pancreas with associated fibrosis and exocrine and endocrine insufficiency. Chronic pancreatitis may occur following repeated episodes of acute pancreatitis. Clinically, chronic pancreatitis presents with recurrent or persistent epigastric pain and weight loss; occasionally, it is silent. Secondary manifestations of pancreatic damage

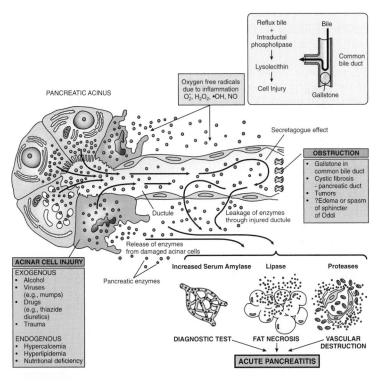

The pathogenesis of acute pancreatitis. Injury to the ductules or the
acinar cells leads to the release of pancreatic enzymes. Lipase and
proteases destroy tissue, thereby causing acute pancreatitis. The release of amylase is the basis of a test for acute pancreatitis. (From
Rubin E, Gorstein F, Rubin R, et al. Rubin's Pathology, 4th ed. Philadelphia: Lippincott Williams & Wilkins, 2005, p. 1003.)

occur with loss of acinar and islet cells, and include steatorrhea,
malabsorption, and insulin-dependent diabetes mellitus. Causes of
chronic pancreatitis include the following:

- Chronic alcohol use (cause of two thirds of cases)
- Chronic acinar cell injury: hemochromatosis
- Chronic renal failure
- Autoimmune chronic pancreatitis
- Cystic fibrosis
- Familial hereditary pancreatitis: rare autosomal dominant dis-
  ease; 15% develop pancreatic ductal adenocarcinoma
- Idiopathic chronic pancreatitis: *CFTR* gene mutations in 30%
  of patients

Grossly, the pancreas appears firm and fibrotic; occasionally, calcifications are present. The pancreatic duct may be dilated secondary to intraductal proteinaceous plugs, stones, or strictures. True cysts (lined by epithelium) and pseudocysts may be present. Microscopically, the pancreatic parenchyma is fibrotic with loss of the exocrine and endocrine elements. A chronic inflammatory component (plasma cells, lymphocytes, and macrophages) may be identified. Variably sized calcified proteinaceous material may be identified in the pancreatic ducts.

Diagnosis of chronic pancreatitis is primarily based on clinical impression; radiographic findings may include pancreatic calcification and ductal dilation. Treatment involves alcohol abstinence, pain management and treatment of secondary disorders related to pancreatic insufficiency. Surgery is indicated in instances of obstruction, fistula, or pseudocyst formation.

Neoplasms

Pancreatic Cystadenoma

Pancreatic cystadenomas are large, multiloculated, cystic lesions that often occur in the pancreatic body or tail and frequently affect women between 50 and 70 years of age. Cystadenomas arise from the pancreatic ductal system. Serous cystadenomas are lined by cuboidal epithelium with clear, glycogen-rich cytoplasm. Mucinous cystadenomas are lined by tall, mucin-producing columnar epithelium and have the potential to develop into a cystadenocarcinoma, a malignant form of this lesion.

Pancreatic Cancer

Pancreatic Ductal Adenocarcinoma

Ductal adenocarcinoma accounts for approximately 90% of all pancreatic cancers. Pancreatic cancer is the fourth most common cause of cancer death in men and the fifth most common cause in women, with a mortality rate approaching 100%. The majority of pancreatic cancers occur in patients older than 60 years of age. Causative factors include:

- Smoking: two- to three-fold increased risk
- Chemical carcinogens: polycyclic hydrocarbons, nitrosamines
- Dietary factors: high intake of meat and fat
- Diabetes mellitus
- Chronic pancreatitis
- Genetic mutations: *K-ras, DPC-4*

Pancreatic cancer occurs most frequently in the head of the gland (60%), followed by the body (10%) and the tail (5%). In the remaining cases, the gland is diffusely involved.

Patients often present late in the disease process with abdominal pain, weight loss, and anorexia. If the cancer is located in the head of the pancreas, biliary obstruction and jaundice may be present; Courvoisier sign refers to a painless dilation of the gallbladder accompanied by jaundice. Ten percent of patients have migratory thrombophlebitis, also termed *Trousseau syndrome*, due to a hypercoagulable state.

Grossly, pancreatic cancer appears as a firm, white, irregular mass invading the pancreas and often the surrounding tissues. Microscopically, irregular, angulated glands are seen invading the pancreatic parenchyma and surrounding nerves. A prominent deposition of collagen is seen surrounding the invading glands (desmoplastic reaction). The majority of pancreatic ductal adenocarcinomas have metastasized to lymph nodes by the time of diagnosis.

Acinar Cell Carcinoma

Acinar cell carcinomas are uncommon pancreatic cancers that appear grossly as large, lobulated, sometimes cystic lesions that frequently present in the head of the pancreas. The majority are metastatic on presentation. Acinar cell carcinoma has a male predominance and often affects elderly patients. Microscopically, these cancers may demonstrate solid, trabecular, acinar, or glandular patterns. The cells have basally situated nuclei and granular, eosinophilic cytoplasm. Some patients develop a syndrome of subcutaneous and bone marrow fat necrosis and polyarthralgia due to release of digestive enzymes from the tumor.

Neoplasms of the Endocrine Pancreas (Islet Cell Tumors)

The endocrine portion of the pancreas is composed of islets of Langerhans scattered throughout the organ; these islets are made up of a variety of cell types, with the majority of islet mass consisting of beta (60%–70%) and alpha (15%–20%) cells. A major function of the pancreatic islets is to regulate blood glucose levels. Elevation of blood glucose results in the release of insulin from beta cells with resultant glycogenesis, lipogenesis, protein synthesis, and decrease in blood glucose. Conversely, low blood glucose stimulates release of the catabolic hormone glucagon with glycogenolysis.

Islet cell tumors make up less than 10% of pancreatic neoplasms. Islet cell tumors may be functional (hormone secretion associated with a clinical syndrome) or nonfunctional. Often functional islet cell tumors may be associated with the multiple endocrine neoplasia syndrome type I (MEN I); MEN I is characterized by multiple adenomas of the pituitary, parathyroids, and endocrine pancreas.

Islet cell tumors are often solitary, circumscribed lesions amenable to surgical resection. Microscopically, these lesions appear solid or trabecular. Tumor cells appear as nests often surrounded by amyloid and numerous small blood vessels. Only the presence

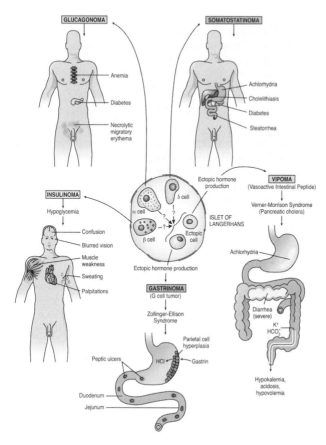

FIGURE 15-2
Syndromes associated with islet cell tumors of the pancreas. (From Rubin E, Gorstein F, Rubin R, et al. Rubin's Pathology, 4th ed. Philadelphia: Lippincott Williams & Wilkins, 2005, p. 1003.)

of metastases determines whether an islet cell tumor is malignant. Islet cell tumors that frequently metastasize include gastrinomas, glucagonomas, somatostatinomas, and VIPomas.

The most common type of islet cell tumor is an insulinoma, followed by gastrinoma. Gastrin-producing cells are normally not present within the pancreas, and the cell of origin of gastrinomas is unknown. Gastrinomas produce the Zollinger-Ellison syndrome, with gastric acid hypersecretion, resulting in severe peptic ulceration, and elevated serum gastrin levels. Figure 15-2 and Table 15-1 summarize the effects of islet cell tumors of the pancreas.

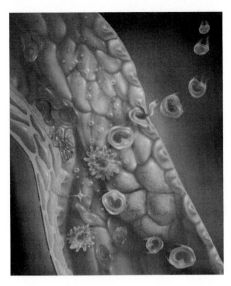

CHAPTER *16*

The Kidney

Chapter Outline

Normal Anatomy and Histology

The kidneys are situated in the retroperitoneal space and maintain electrolyte, acid-base, and water balance; filter toxic molecules; and regulate blood pressure via the renin-angiotensin-aldosterone system. The kidney is surrounded by a fibrous capsule and cushioned by perirenal fat. The outer portion of the kidney is the cortex, which contains the glomeruli and associated tubules (Fig. 16-1). The inner portion of the kidney, or medulla, consists of approximately 12 pyramidal structures containing tubules and collecting ducts. The main architectural unit of the kidney is the nephron, which includes the glomerulus and its associated tubule (Figs. 16-2 and 16-3).

The kidney has four primary elements:

- Blood vessels: abdominal aorta → renal artery → interlobar arteries → arcuate arteries → interlobular arteries → intralobular arteries → glomerular afferent arteriole → glomerular capillary loops → efferent arteriole (gives rise to vasa recta and peritubular capillary network)
- Tubular system: renal corpuscle → proximal convoluted tubule → straight proximal tubule (descending) → descending thin loop of Henle → ascending thin loop of Henle → ascending thick limb of Henle → distal convoluted tubule → collecting duct → papillary ducts that pierce the papilla
- Interstitium: composed of fibroblast-like cells and matrix; secretes erythropoietin and prostaglandins
- Glomerulus: situated in Bowman's capsule; capillary loops with fenestrated endothelium; podocytes; mesangial cells that support the glomerular structure; glomerular basement membrane containing type IV collagen; the filtration barrier (endo-

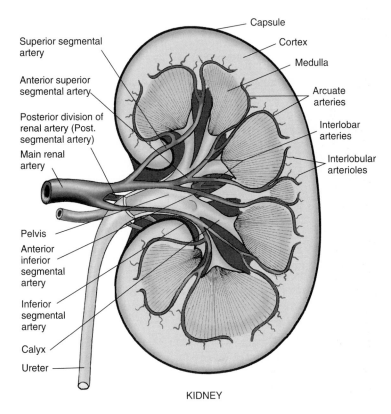

Superior segmental
artery

Anterior superior
segmental artery

Posterior division of
renal artery (Post.
segmental artery)

Main renal
artery

Pelvis

Anterior
inferior
segmental
artery

Inferior
segmental
artery

Calyx

Ureter

Capsule

Cortex

Medulla

Arcuate
arteries

Interlobar
arteries

Interlobular
arterioles

KIDNEY

FIGURE 16-1
Structure of the kidney. (From Rubin E, Gorstein F, Rubin R, et al. Rubin's Pathology, 4th ed. Philadelphia: Lippincott Williams & Wilkins, 2005, p. 826.)

thelium, basement membrane, and podocytes) filters molecules by size and charge

The juxtaglomerular (JG) apparatus is situated at the vascular pole of the glomerulus and includes the macula densa, extraglomerular mesangial cells, terminal afferent arteriole, and proximal efferent arteriole. The JG apparatus regulates blood pressure and glomerular filtration rate via secretion of renin, which promotes the conversion of angiotensinogen to angiotensin I. Angiotensin I is converted by angiotensin-converting enzyme (ACE) to angio-

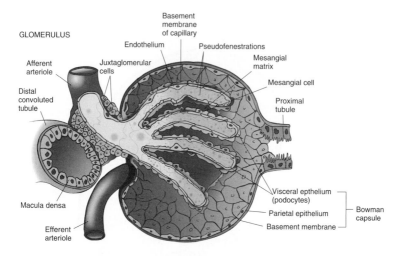

FIGURE   16-2
Glomerular structure. (From Rubin E, Gorstein F, Rubin R, et al.
Rubin's Pathology, 4th ed. Philadelphia: Lippincott Williams & Wil-
kins, 2005, p. 826.)

tensin II, which increases sodium reabsorption, increases vascular
resistance, and induces the release of aldosterone from the adrenal
gland.

Congenital Abnormalities

Congenital abnormalities may be *inherited* or *acquired*. Changes in
the fetal environment may lead to acquired abnormalities. For example, *Potter sequence* occurs after decreased urine production by
the fetus, which causes oligohydramnios (decreased level of amniotic fluid), compression of the fetus against the uterus, and resulting physical deformities. Inherited abnormalities include *autosomal
dominant polycystic kidney disease (ADPKD)* and *autosomal recessive
polycystic disease (ARPKD)*. Additional anomalies are listed in Table
16-1.

Autosomal Dominant Polycystic Kidney Disease

Autosomal dominant polycystic kidney disease (ADPKD) is the
most common inherited abnormality of the kidney, affecting 1 in
200 to 1 in 1,000 persons in the United States. ADPKD is an adult-

RENAL LOBE

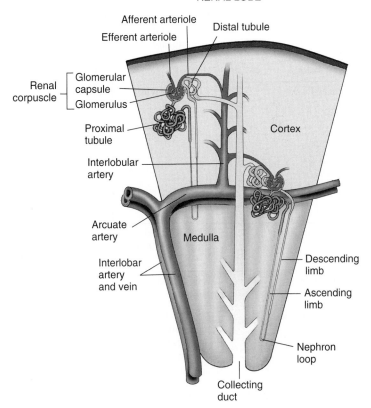

FIGURE 16-3
Structure of the nephron with glomerulus and associated tubule. (From Rubin E, Gorstein F, Rubin R, et al. Rubin's Pathology, 4th ed. Philadelphia: Lippincott Williams & Wilkins, 2005, p. 826.)

onset disease, and 50% of all patients progress to end-stage renal disease (ESRD). The vast majority of ADPKD (85%) is caused by *PKD1* mutations, and the remainder is caused by mutations in the *PKD2* and *PKD3* genes.

Grossly, the kidneys are enlarged, weighing as much as 4,500 grams each (normal is 150 g). Numerous cysts filled with straw-colored fluid are present throughout the kidney; expansion of these cysts occurs secondary to a defective basement membrane. Microscopically, the cysts are lined by cuboidal to columnar epithelium; normal, compressed renal parenchyma is present between cysts.

Table 16-1

Additional Congenital Anomalies of the Kidneys

Disease	Etiology	Manifestation
Potter sequence	Reduced amniotic fluid/fetal urine production	Fetal compression with deformities (e.g., beaklike nose), pulmonary hypoplasia
Renal agenesis	$\downarrow$ Renal growth	Absence of renal parenchyma: $\pm$ Potter sequence Bilateral renal agenesis: Stillborn infant (Potter sequence) Unilateral agenesis: Increased risk of glomerular sclerosis
Renal hypoplasia	$\downarrow$ Renal growth, Down syndrome	Six or fewer normal renal lobes (normal kidney has 12)
Ectopic kidney	Failure of kidney migration	Abnormal pelvic location of kidney
Horseshoe kidney	Abnormal kidney migration Genetic and somatic causes	Fusion of both kidneys, usually at lower poles; increased risk of obstruction and pyelonephritis
Renal dysplasia	Abnormal metanephric differentiation	Undifferentiated tubular structures surrounded by primitive mesenchyme. $\pm$ cartilage $\pm$ cysts associated with urinary outflow obstruction; may be unilateral or bilateral; aplastic, multicystic, diffuse cystic, and obstructive variants; palpable flank mass may be present in newborns

(continues)

Table 16-1

(continued)

Disease	Etiology	Manifestation
Glomerulocystic disease	Genetic and somatic causes *HNF-1 ?* mutation	Numerous small round cysts (<1 cm diameter); small or large kidneys; dilation of Bowman's capsule in many glomeruli
Nephronophthisis–medullary cystic disease complex	Autosomal recessive and dominant variants	Small kidneys with cysts at the corticomedullary junction (up to 1 cm diameter); 10%–25% of renal failure in childhood
Medullary sponge kidney		Multiple small cysts in the renal papillae (<5 mm diameter); symptomatic in adulthood with dysuria, hematuria, flank pain, and "gravel" in the urine
Simple renal cysts	Acquired	Found in one half of all persons older than age 50; incidental, cysts in outer cortex
Acquired cystic disease	Acquired (dialysis-associated)	Multiple cortical and medullary cysts; occur in 75% of patients on dialysis after 5 years

Approximately 30% of patients have hepatic cysts lined by biliary-type epithelium, 10% have splenic cysts, and 5% have pancreatic cysts. Twenty percent of patients with ADPKD develop a berry aneurysm of the Circle of Willis in the brain, which causes death in 15% of patients with ADPKD.

Autosomal Recessive Polycystic Kidney Disease

Autosomal recessive polycystic kidney disease (ARPKD) occurs in 1 in 10,000 to 1 in 50,000 live births, and patients become symptomatic during infancy. Approximately 75% of patients die in the perinatal period, often secondary to pulmonary hypoplasia from Potter sequence. *PKHD1* mutation results in a defective fibrocystic protein, which contributes to the cystic transformation of collecting ducts.

On gross examination, the external surface of the kidney appears smooth. Numerous internal cysts are identified on cut section, which often are radially oriented.

Glomerular Diseases

Analysis of glomerular disease requires detailed examination of the glomerulus by light microscopy, immunofluorescence (IF), and electron microscopy (EM), as well as close correlation with clinical information (Table 16-2).

Common Clinical Terminology of Glomerular Disease

- Asymptomatic proteinuria: protein in the urine without associated symptoms
- Asymptomatic hematuria: blood in the urine without associated symptoms
- Azotemia: elevated blood urea nitrogen (BUN) and creatinine; evident in many renal diseases
- Uremia: clinical syndrome of azotemia with endocrine, gastrointestinal, hematologic, or neuromuscular dysfunction
- Nephrotic syndrome: greater than 3.5 g of urine protein/24 h, hypoalbuminemia (decreased albumin in the blood), edema, hyperlipidemia (elevated lipid levels in the blood), and lipiduria (lipids in the urine); often in noninflammatory glomerulonephropathy
- Nephritic syndrome: hematuria, proteinuria less than 3.5 g of urine protein/24 h, decreased glomerular filtration rate, increased BUN and serum creatinine, oliguria (decreased levels of urine), salt and water retention, edema, and hypertension.

Table 16-2

Microscopic Manifestations of Glomerular Disease

Disease	Histology	Immunofluorescence Immunostain	Appearance on Electron Micrography
Primarily nephrotic syndrome			
Minimal change disease	Normal	6 weak mesangial IgM, C3	Effacement of podocyte foot processes
FSGS	Partial sclerosis of a subset of glomeruli	IgM, C3 trapping in sclerotic areas	Effacement of podocyte foot processes
HIV-associated nephropathy (subtype of FSGS above)	Collapsing pattern of focal sclerosis		Tubuloreticular inclusions in endothelial cells
Membranous glomerulopathy	Normocellular glomeruli, "spikes" (silver stain), thickened capillary walls	Diffuse granular capillary loop IgG, C3	Subepithelial electron-dense deposits
Diabetic glomerulosclerosis	Diffuse GBM thickening, 6 nodular sclerosis	Linear GBM IgG, albumin, fibrinogen	GBM widening, increased mesangial matrix
Amyloidosis-associated renal disease	Eosinophilic deposits in mesangial loops	Congo red apple green birefringence	Nonbranching fibrils in glomerulus
Light-heavy chain deposition diseases	Thickened GBM, 6 nodular mesangial increases	Linear monoclonal Ig chains on GBM*	Finely granular dense material on inner aspect of GBM

(continues)

Table 16-2

(continued)

Disease	Histology	Immunofluorescence Immunostain	Appearance on Electron Micrography
Primarily nephrotic syndrome			
Hereditary nephritis/Alport syndrome	Hypercellularity to sclerosis; tubular atrophy	Absent alpha chains of collagen	Irregularly thickened GBM with splitting
Thin GBM nephropathy	Normal	No specific findings	Reduced GBM thickness by 1/2 to 1/3
Acute postinfectious glomerulonephritis	Neutrophils, hypercellular glomeruli	Granular Ig G and C3 in capillary walls, mesangium	Subepithelial "humps" typical
Type I membranoproliferative glomerulonephritis	Enlarged hypercellular glomeruli, lobular segmentation of glomeruli, 20% crescents	Granular C3in mesangium and capillaries; 6 immunoglobulins	Subendothelial deposits and duplication of GBM
Dense deposit disease (type II membranoproliferative glomerulonephritis)	Hypercellular glomeruli; capillary wall thickening; occasional crescents	Bands of capillary wall C3 staining, granular mesangial staining	Dense deposits in GBM, GBM thickening

Lupus glomerulonephritis	Variable patterns of hypercellularity; capillary wall thickening	Variable mesangial, subendothelial, subepithelial granular deposits; may have "full-house" immunostaining	Dense deposits in various locations; endothelial tubuloreticular inclusions
IgA nephropathy (Berger disease)	Mesangial hypercellularity	Mesangial IgA stain $\geq$IgG or IgM	Mesangial and variable capillary loop dense deposits
Anti-GBM	Fibrinoid necrosis, then crescents	Linear IgG staining of GBM*	Focal GBM breaks
ANCA glomerulonephritis	Focal glomerular necrosis, then crescents	Absence of Ig staining	No dense deposits identified

* Linear IgG staining of GBM is seen in anti-GBM glomerulonephritis and diabetic glomerulonephritis.

ANCA, antineutrophil cytoplasmic autoantibody; FSGS, focal segmental glomerulosclerosis; GBM, glomerular basement membrane.

Red cell casts in the urine are common, often in inflammatory glomerulonephropathy.

- Rapidly progressive glomerulonephritis: rapid progression to renal failure unless aggressive treatment is instituted
- Chronic nephritic syndrome: persistent or intermittent nephritic syndrome with slow progression to renal failure
- Crescent formation: increase in the number of parietal epithelial cells in Bowman's space; frequently associated with a rapid decrease in renal function
- Acute renal failure: rapid onset of decreased glomerular filtration; may be associated with alterations in urine production (polyuria, oliguria, and anuria) over a period of hours to days and may be associated with azotemia. Acute renal failure may result from prerenal, intrinsic, or postrenal disease.
- Chronic renal failure: occurs after long-standing renal disease of many causes and is characterized by uremia and frequently hypertension
- ESRD: kidneys are globally damaged, scarred, and reduced in size
- Dysuria: pain on urination

Mechanisms of Glomerular Injury in Disease

Glomerular disease may occur in a variety of disease processes, including inflammatory and noninflammatory conditions. The pathogenesis of glomerular disease generally may be categorized as follows:

- Damage to the podocyte is identified by effacement of the foot processes, often with vacuolization and microvillous change by EM, and includes minimal change disease (MCD), focal segmental glomerulosclerosis (FSGS), and HIV nephropathy
- Disorders of the glomerular basement membrane are identified by a thin, thickened, or otherwise defective glomerular basement membrane (GBM) and includes thin basement membrane disease, diabetic nephropathy, and Alport's disease
- In situ immune complex deposition occurs with binding of antibodies to an intrinsic glomerular antigen or a foreign antigen deposited within the glomerulus and includes anti-GBM nephritis and some cases of membranous nephropathy
- Deposition of circulating immune complexes in the glomerulus occurs when antigens in the blood are trapped within the glomerulus, which then leads to secondary inflammation; these diseases include post-infectious glomerulonephritis, membranoproliferative glomerulonephritis, cryoglobulinemic glomerulonephritis, IgA nephropathy, and lupus nephritis. Antineu-

trophil cytoplasmic autoantibodies (ANCAs) are associated with neutrophil activation and adhesion to the endothelium and includes pauci-immune crescentic glomerulonephritis, microscopic polyarteritis, and Wegener's granulomatosis

In certain diseases, overlap of pathogenetic mechanisms occurs (e.g., thickening of the GBM secondary to immune complex deposition). Each disease should therefore be considered as a unique entity with potential for overlap of pathologic features shared with other glomerular diseases.

Glomerular Diseases Presenting with Nephrotic Syndrome

Multiple diseases present with the nephrotic syndrome. Diseases in this category generally demonstrate a normal cellularity of the glomerulus and lack of immune deposits. Figure 16-4 is a diagram of the pathophysiology of nephrotic syndrome. A summary of glomerular diseases presenting with the nephrotic syndrome is presented in Figure 16-5.

Minimal Change Glomerulopathy (Lipoid Nephrosis)

Minimal change glomerulopathy (lipoid nephrosis) is responsible for 90% of the nephrotic syndrome in children and may be idiopathic or associated with either allergic disease or a lymphoid neoplasm. The proteinuria in MCD is selective (albumin > globulin). Light microscopy demonstrates a normal glomerulus; an effacement of podocyte foot processes is identified by EM. Patients often respond well to corticosteroids, although they may have intermittent relapses for up to 10 years after steroid withdrawal. Life span is usually normal in this disease.

Focal Segmental Glomerulosclerosis

Focal segmental glomerulosclerosis is common in children and adults. The hallmark of *FSGS* is *focal* (some glomeruli) and *segmental* (portion of single glomerulus) scarring or sclerosis of the glomeruli, which appears microscopically as a replacement of normal glomerular structure with increased matrix and adhesions to Bowman's capsule. Hyalinosis and foam cells may be seen in these areas. EM demonstrates effacement of the epithelial foot processes and vacuolization of the epithelial cells. FSGS may be primary (idiopathic) or secondary to obesity, reduced renal mass, sickle cell nephropathy, cyanotic congenital heart disease, HIV, pamidronate, or intravenous drug abuse. Glomerular sclerosis has been proposed to result from hyperfiltration and hypertrophy in secondary forms.

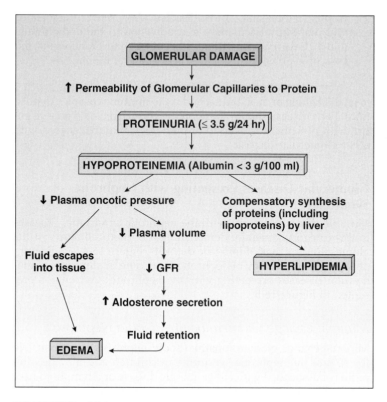

FIGURE 16-4
Pathophysiology of nephrotic syndrome. (From Rubin E, Gorstein F, Rubin R, et al. Rubin's Pathology, 4th ed. Philadelphia: Lippincott Williams & Wilkins, 2005, p. 836.)

Sclerosis limited to the area of the capillary tuft near the tubular take-off is categorized as "tip lesion," a potentially more benign variant of FSGS. HIV-associated nephropathy is a "collapsing" variant of FSGS that demonstrates rapid progression to ESRD and a poor prognosis. Involution of capillary loops, podocyte hypertrophy and hyperplasia, and tubuloreticular inclusions in endothelial cells are seen by EM in this variant. Collapsing FSGS also may occur in HIV-negative patients.

Corticosteroid treatment may yield a mild to moderate response. ACE-inhibitors are additionally used in obese patients or those with reduced renal mass.

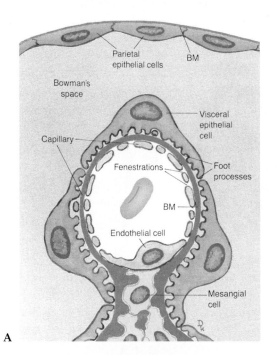

A

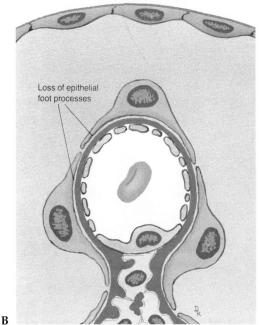

B

FIGURE 16-5
Normal glomerulus (A), minimal change disease (B), (*continues*)

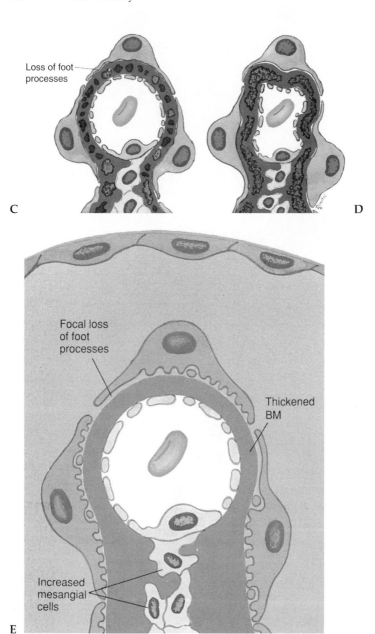

Loss of foot
processes

C

D

Focal loss
of foot
processes

Thickened
BM

Increased
mesangial
cells

E

F I G U R E   16-5 (*continued*)
membranous glomerulonephropathy (C,D), diabetic glomeruloscle-
rosis (E), and (*continues*)

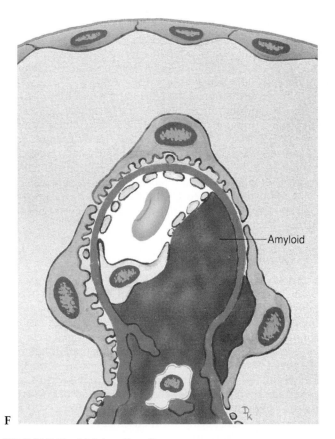

F

FIGURE   16-5 *(continued)*
amyloid nephropathy (F). (From Rubin E, Gorstein F, Rubin R, et al. Rubin's Pathology, 4th ed. Philadelphia: Lippincott Williams & Wilkins, 2005, part A, p. 829; part B, p. 839; parts C and D, p. 844; part E, p. 845; part F, p. 847.)

FSGS may be incorrectly diagnosed as MCD owing to sampling error if the focal region of affected glomeruli is missed on biopsy. A diagnosis of MCD with development of azotemia or nonresponse to steroid therapy suggests reevaluation for FSGS.

Membranous Glomerulopathy

Membranous glomerulopathy is the most common cause of the nephrotic syndrome in white and Asian adults in the United States.

This disease may be idiopathic or secondary to autoimmune disease, infectious disease, therapeutic agents, or neoplasms. Membranous glomerulopathy occurs after the accumulation of immune complexes in the subepithelial zone of the glomerular capillaries with resultant capillary wall thickening.

Light microscopy demonstrates spikes along the GBM by silver staining, which represent projections of the basement membrane around deposited immune complexes. IF reveals confluent granular deposits of IgG and C3 along the capillary loops. Membranous glomerulopathy is described as stage I (subepithelial depositions only) through stage IV (rarefaction of deposits within the GBM).

Membranous glomerulopathy has a variable prognosis, with 25% of patients progressing to ESRD. Patients with progressive renal failure are treated with corticosteroids and cyclophosphamide.

Diabetic Glomerulosclerosis

Diabetes is a systemic disease that produces vascular sclerosis of small vessels throughout the body. Half of all diabetic patients develop diabetic glomerulosclerosis, which results in diffuse global thickening of the GBM and diffuse mesangial matrix expansion.

By light microscopy, acellular nodular mesangial sclerosis (*Kimmelstiel-Wilson* nodules), "hyaline" accumulations in glomeruli and between Bowman's capsule and the parietal epithelium (*capsular drops*), GBM thickening, capillary microaneurysms, and hyaline arteriolosclerosis may be seen. The material deposited in within the mesangium is strongly periodic acid-Schiff (PAS) and silver stain positive. Nonspecific linear basement membrane staining for IgG and albumin is present.

One third of all patients with diabetic glomerulosclerosis develop chronic renal failure. Diabetic glomerulosclerosis is the most common cause of ESRD in the United States. Regulation of blood glucose, dietary protein, and blood pressure is used to control disease progression.

Amyloidosis-associated Renal Disease (Amyloid Nephropathy)

Amyloid deposits involve the glomerulus, arteries, and interstitial areas. Specifically, AA amyloid is derived from serum amyloid A protein during chronic inflammatory conditions and AL amyloid is derived from neoplastic B cells or plasma cells. Other amyloidogenic proteins are rarely implicated.

Light microscopy reveals acellular, eosinophilic deposits irregularly involving the mesangium, capillary wall, arterial wall, or interstitial areas. In contrast to diabetic glomerulonephropathy, these deposits are weakly PAS positive and silver negative. AA and AL amyloid are distinguished by immunohistochemistry; amyloid stains with Congo red and is apple-green and birefringent under polarized light. By EM, fine, nonbranching, randomly oriented fibrils are identified.

Treatment includes chemotherapy for AL amyloidosis and colchicine for AA amyloidosis.

Light Chain and Heavy Chain Deposition Diseases

In these disorders, deposition of monoclonal light or heavy chains occurs within the GBM, mesangial matrix, and tubular basement membranes. Light and heavy chain deposition diseases are caused by an underlying B-cell neoplasm. The deposits stimulate mesangial matrix production, which may mimic diabetic glomerulosclerosis by light microscopy. However, light and heavy chain deposition disease is distinguished by immunostaining for light and heavy chains of immunoglobulin, and demonstration of finely granular deposits along the internal GBM on EM. Resolution of light and heavy chain deposition disease is dependent on treatment of the underlying B-cell neoplasm.

Glomerular Diseases Presenting Solely with Hematuria

Hereditary Nephritis (Alport Syndrome)

Alport syndrome is a basement membrane nephropathy caused by a defect in type IV collagen, which leads to a progressively sclerosing glomerular disease. The most common molecular alteration in Alport syndrome is a mutation of the $\alpha 5$ chain of type IV collagen (*COL4A5* gene), which is inherited in an X-linked fashion. Males generally develop ESRD by age 40 to 50 years, whereas females only develop hematuria. Additional findings in Alport syndrome include ocular and ear defects. The most common somatic mutation is an autosomal recessive form owing to defects in the $\alpha 3$ domain of collagen.

Light microscopic findings in Alport syndrome include nonspecific accumulation of interstitial foamy macrophages, reflecting chronic proteinuria and progressive sclerosing changes in glomeruli. IF using antibodies to the $\alpha 3$ and $\alpha 5$ chains of type IV collagen can reveal a lack of staining for the alpha chain encoded by the mutant gene. EM is essential for the diagnosis of Alport syndrome, revealing variable thinning and thickening of the GBM, with lamination and a basket weave pattern developing in later stages.

Management of Alport's syndrome involves treatment of symptoms.

Thin Glomerular Basement Membrane Nephropathy (Benign Familial Hematuria)

Thin GBM nephropathy is another hereditary GBM disorder that manifests with asymptomatic microscopic hematuria and occasional gross hematuria. Various mutations in collagen genes cause this disease. The diagnosis is confirmed by the finding of extremely thin GBMs by EM analysis.

Thin GBM nephropathy generally is a benign disorder.

Glomerular Diseases Presenting with Nephritic Syndrome

Acute Postinfectious Glomerulonephritis

Acute postinfectious glomerulonephritis is primarily a childhood disease caused by infection with group A (β-hemolytic) streptococci, other bacteria, and occasionally other infections. This disease represents one of the most common renal diseases affecting children. Patients often demonstrate pharyngeal or skin infections before the onset of renal symptoms. Immune complex deposition in the kidney may result from entrapment of circulating preformed complexes or an antibody reaction to bacterial antigens trapped in the glomerulus.

Light microscopy reveals a lesion that varies with stage of the disease. Early in the disease there are hypercellular glomeruli with increased mesangial matrix and an influx of neutrophils. Late in the disease, microscopy may only reveal mildly hypercellular glomeruli. IF reveals a "lumpy-bumpy" pattern of deposits of IgG and C3 along the capillaries and in the mesangium. EM reveals characteristic subepithelial "humps."

Management of postinfectious glomerulonephropathy involves treatment of symptoms, and the majority of patients return to baseline within months.

Type I Membranoproliferative Glomerulonephritis

Type I membranoproliferative glomerulonephritis (MPGN) primarily affects older children and young adults and may be primary (idiopathic) or secondary to an underlying infection, such as bacterial endocarditis or osteomyelitis. Patients may present with a mixed nephritic-nephrotic syndrome. Pathogenic mechanisms include immune complex formation against foreign antigens that subsequently localize to the mesangium and subendothelial region of the glomerulus.

Light microscopy reveals a hypercellular, hyperlobulated glomerulus. PAS and silver stains may reveal a segmental double contour of the GBM ("tram-tracks") that represent a duplication of the GBM around interposed mesangium. Electron-dense deposits are identified in the subendothelial space as well as the mesangium by EM.

Twenty percent of patients develop crescentic disease. The remainder of patients exhibit persistent disease, with up to 50% of patients developing ESRD after 10 years.

Management involves treatment of symptoms, and therapy may be targeted against the underlying disease process, if known.

Dense Deposit Disease (Type II Membranoproliferative Glomerulonephritis)

Dense deposit disease (DDD) is caused by the extensive localization of complement in the GBM and complement activation. The etiology of this disease is proposed to be to prolonged C3 cleaving activity induced by a circulating IgG autoantibody, the "C3 nephritic factor." Immunoglobulin deposition is not identified in the glomerulus.

Light microscopy reveals hypercellular and hyperlobulated glomeruli. A duplication of the GBM is not as evident as that identified in dense deposit disease. EM reveals dense deposits within the GBM that appear "sausagelike."

Unlike MGPN type I, dense deposit disease is a persistent disease with an overall worse prognosis. Management primarily involves treatment of symptoms.

Lupus Nephritis

Systemic lupus erythematosus (SLE) is an autoimmune disease with broad systemic manifestations. Dysregulation of B-cell function and production of autoantibodies against DNA, RNA, nucleoproteins, and phospholipids underlie this disorder. Nephritis is a common finding in patients with SLE. The classification of lupus nephropathy falls into six classes:

- Class I: glomeruli appear normal and do not contain deposits
- Class II: subendothelial immune complexes; mesangial hypercellularity and matrix expansion
- Class III: focal proliferative glomerulonephritis; overt glomerular, mesangial, and intracapillary hypercellularity; involvement of <50% of glomeruli; mesangial and subendothelial deposits
- Class IV: diffuse proliferative glomerulonephritis; overt glomerular involvement of >50% of glomeruli; mesangial and subendothelial deposits
- Class V: subepithelial immune complexes; membranous glomerulopathy
- Class VI: advanced chronic sclerosing disease

Patients with lupus nephropathy demonstrate a variable outcome, with <25% of overall patients progressing to ESRD within

5 years. Class IV lupus nephritis represents the most common type of lupus nephritis, but affected patients also have the worst prognosis. In general, patients may shift between classes of nephritis with disease progression.

A characteristic lesion of class III and IV lupus nephritis that may be seen by light microscopy is the "wire-loop" appearance of the glomerular capillaries, caused by subendothelial immune complex deposition. IF often reveals positive staining for all antibodies tested, including IgG, IgA, IgM, C3, and C1q (a "full-house" pattern). By EM, tubuloreticular inclusions may be identified in endothelial cells.

Treatment of lupus nephritis involves high-dose corticosteroids for class III and IV disease, which typically demonstrate poorer outcomes.

IgA Nephropathy (Berger Disease)

IgA nephropathy (IgAN) is caused by the deposition of IgA immune complexes within the glomerulus, which results in complement activation. The mechanism of immune complex formation (in situ versus circulating) is unknown. IgAN is the most common form of glomerulonephritis in the world and primarily affects young men (peak age 15–30 years). IgAN is frequently exacerbated by respiratory and gastrointestinal infections, and a major histocompatability complex (MHC)–linked susceptibility and abnormal glycosylation of IgA have been hypothesized to play a role in disease pathogenesis.

Light microscopy may reveal a variety of appearances, ranging from normal-appearing glomeruli to diffusely hypercellular glomeruli. IF demonstrates the presence of IgA, often other immunoglobulins, and C3. EM demonstrates immune complexes typically in the mesangium, but involving capillary loops in approximately 25% of cases.

IgAN is a slowly progressive disease, with 20% of patients developing ESRD after 10 years. Treatment includes control of hypertension. Renal transplantation may result in recurrence of IgA deposition within the tissue.

Antiglomerular Basement Membrane (Anti-GBM) Glomerulonephritis

Antiglomerular basement membrane (anti-GBM) glomerulonephritis is an uncommon, aggressive form of glomerulonephritis. This disease is caused by an autoimmune response against type IV collagen, and antibodies may crossreact with collagen in the pulmonary alveolar capillary basement membrane, leading to pulmonary hemorrhage (Goodpasture syndrome). The onset of anti-GBM glomerulonephritis frequently occurs after an upper respiratory viral infection.

Light microscopy typically demonstrates tuft necrosis and the presence of crescents within Bowman's space. Linear IF staining for IgG and C3 along the glomerular basement membrane are characteristic of this lesion. These complexes are not identified by EM.

Patients with anti-GBM may rapidly progress to renal failure, and treatment involves high-dose corticosteroids and plasmapheresis. Renal transplant is often successful in these patients.

Antineutrophil Cytoplasmic Antibody Glomerulonephritis

ANCA glomerulonephritis is an aggressive type of glomerulonephritis that is manifested by glomerular necrosis and crescents by light microscopy. This disease is associated with circulating ANCAs that frequently target myeloperoxidase or proteinase 3, which can be involved in activation of neutrophils and can lead to endothelial damage. Patients with ANCA glomerulonephritis may rapidly progress to renal failure; however, less than 25% of patients develop ESRD after 5 years. Other systemic manifestations of vasculitis may be present. Figure 16-6 summarizes four common types of renal disease present with the nephritic syndrome.

Vascular Diseases of the Kidney

Renal Vasculitis

Vasculitis is an inflammation of small, medium, or large blood vessels that present with specific symptoms based on vessel size (Table 16-3).

- Small-vessel vasculitis: small arteries, arterioles, capillaries, and venules; often presents with glomerulonephritis, purpura, arthralgias, myalgias, peripheral neuropathy, and pulmonary hemorrhage; may be caused by immune complex formation, anti-GBM antibodies, or ANCAs.
- Medium-sized vessel vasculitis: arteries; may present with necrotizing arteritis, pseudoaneurysm formation, renal thrombosis, infarction, and hemorrhage
- Large vessel vasculitis: aorta and its major branches; may cause renovascular hypertension or renal ischemia

By light microscopy, lymphocytes and fibrinoid necrosis are identified within the wall of the blood vessel.

Hypertensive Nephrosclerosis (Benign Nephrosclerosis)

Hypertensive nephrosclerosis is caused by mild to moderate hypertension, reflected by a sustained systolic pressure of greater than

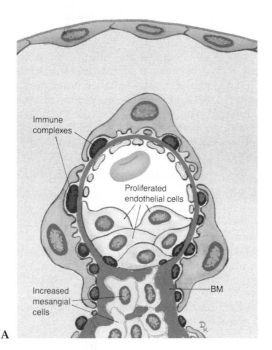

A

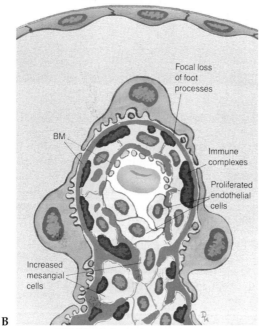

B

F I G U R E   16-6
Postinfectious glomerulonephritis (A), type I MPGN (B), (*continues*)

474

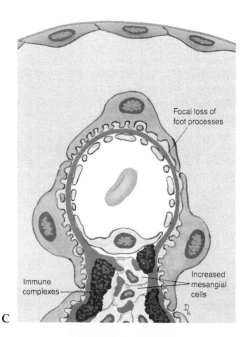

C

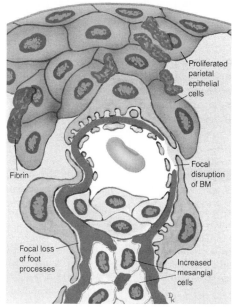

D

F I G U R E   16-6 (*continued*)
IgA nephropathy (C), and crescentic rapidly progressive glomerulo-nephritis (D). (From Rubin E, Gorstein F, Rubin R, et al. Rubin's Pathology, 4th ed. Philadelphia: Lippincott Williams & Wilkins, 2005, part A, p. 850; part B, p. 852, part C, p. 857; part D, p. 858.)

Table 16-3

Renal Vasculitic Disease

Type of Vasculitis	Age	Major Target Vessels	Major Renal Manifestations
Small-vessel vasculitis			
Immune-complex vasculitis			
Henoch-Schonlein purpura	Childhood	Glomeruli (IgA deposition)	Nephritis (IgA nephropathy)
Cryoglobulinemic vasculitis	Adult	Glomeruli	Nephritis (type I membranoproliferative glomerulonephritis) Hyaline thrombi seen in capillary lumina
Anti-GBM vasculitis			
Goodpasture syndrome	Adult	Glomeruli (anti-GBM Ab)	Nephritis (anti-GBM glomerulonephritis)
ANCA-vasculitis syndromes			
Wegener granulomatosis	Adult	Glomeruli, arterioles, lobular AA	Nephritis with necrotizing granulomatous
Churg-Strauss syndrome	Adult	Glomeruli, arterioles, lobular AA	Nephritis with eosinophilia and asthma
Microscopic polyangiitis	Adult	Glomeruli, arterioles, lobular AA	Nephritis without granulomatous inflammation, eosinophilia or asthma

Medium-sized-vessel vasculitis			
Polyarteritis nodosa	Adult	Interlobar and arcuate arteries	Infarcts and hemorrhage
Kawasaki disease	Childhood	Interlobar and arcuate arteries	Infarcts and hemorrhage
Large-vessel vasculitis			
Giant cell arteritis	Adult	Main renal artery	Renovascular hypertension
Takayasu arteritis	Adult	Main renal artery	Renovascular hypertension

AA, arteries; ANCA, antineutrophil cytoplasmic autoantibody; GBM, glomerular basement membrane.
Modified from Rubin E, Gorstein F, Rubin R, et al. Rubin's Pathology, 4th ed. Philadelphia: Lippincott Williams & Wilkins, 2005, p. 860.

140 mm Hg and a diastolic pressure greater than 90 mm Hg. This condition is most prevalent in African Americans. A small proportion of patients may develop progressive renal failure and ESRD.

On gross examination, the kidneys appear atrophic bilaterally, with a fine surface granularity and a thinning of the cortex. On microscopic examination, some glomeruli may appear normal, whereas other glomeruli appear acellular, densely eosinophilic, and solid (end result of ischemic change). Tubular atrophy, interstitial fibrosis and chronic inflammation are present. Large arteries demonstrate fibrotic intimal thickening and multilayering of the internal elastic lamina. Arterioles demonstrate a concentric hyaline thickening of the wall with loss of smooth muscle cells, termed hyaline arteriolosclerosis.

Malignant Hypertensive Nephropathy

Malignant hypertension is a condition defined as a diastolic pressure greater than 130 mm Hg associated with retinal vascular changes, papilledema, and renal functional impairment. Common symptoms include headache, dizziness, and visual disturbances. Hematuria and proteinuria are frequent findings. Malignant hypertension is more common in men older than 40 years of age, and 50% of affected patients have a prior history of benign hypertension.

Kidney size varies based on the course of prior disease. The cut surface is mottled red and yellow, often with cortical infarcts. On microscopy, a hypertensive nephrosclerotic background with infarcts is identified. The arteries demonstrate edematous intimal expansion and layering ("onion skinning") and fibrinoid necrosis.

Renovascular Hypertension

This disorder is caused by stenosis or complete occlusion of a main renal artery, evidenced clinically as a bruit heard over the renal artery. The most frequent cause in older adults is atherosclerosis, whereas fibromuscular dysplasia accounts for the majority of cases in children and young adults.

Patients often present with mild to moderate elevations in blood pressure caused by increased production of renin, angiotensin II, and aldosterone. Men are more frequently affected than women. Sampling of blood from the renal veins identifies elevated renin levels from the stenotic kidney and normal renin levels from the contralateral kidney.

On gross examination, the affected kidney is reduced in size. On microscopic examination, the glomeruli appear normal, but tubular ischemic atrophy without prominent interstitial fibrosis is present. In addition, the J-G apparatus appears prominent.

Treatment options include surgery, angioplasty, or nephrectomy.

Renal Atheroembolism

Renal atheroembolism occurs when atheromatous debris embolizes into the renal vasculature and is most common in patients with severe aortic atherosclerosis. The process may be spontaneous or more commonly initiated by catheterization procedures. Microscopy reveals cholesterol clefts within vessel lumens. Early lesions are surrounded by thrombus, whereas late lesions are surrounded by fibrosis and a foreign body reaction.

Thrombotic Microangiopathy

Thrombotic microangiopathy affects the kidney as well as other organs, and causes include agents that lead to endothelial damage, such as malignant hypertension. Endothelial damage allows plasma constituents to enter vessel walls, leading to luminal narrowing and ischemia. A cycle of thrombosis and worsening ischemia ensues, leading to focal ischemic necrosis. The end result may be microangiopathic hemolytic anemia, characterized by a nonimmune (Coombs negative) hemolytic anemia with misshapen and disrupted erythrocytes (schistocytes) and thrombocytopenia.

Two common types of thrombotic microangiopathy follow:

- Hemolytic-uremic syndrome (HUS): limited to the kidney; presents with acute, rapidly progressive renal failure and hemorrhagic diarrhea; most common cause of acute renal failure in children; caused by Shiga-like toxin produced by enterohemorrhagic *Escherichia coli*
- Thrombotic thrombocytopenic purpura: systemic microvascular thrombosis; presents with thrombocytopenia, purpura, fever, anemia, and changes in mental status; more severe bleeding tendency than in HUS; renal involvement may be minimal or absent

On microscopic examination, arteriolar fibrinoid necrosis, edematous arterial intimal expansion, and glomerular collapse, necrosis, or congestion may be seen. Fibrin thrombi are present within the preglomerular arterioles. By EM, flocculent material is present between the endothelial cell and the GBM.

Pre-eclampsia

Pre-eclampsia occurs during the third trimester of pregnancy and presents with the triad of hypertension, proteinuria, and edema. The term eclampsia denotes pre-eclampsia associated with seizures. Microscopy reveals enlarged glomeruli, an increased number and size of mesangial cells, and swollen endothelial cells with large irregular vacuoles.

Mild to moderate disease can be treated with antihypertensive therapy and bed rest. However, severe cases may require induction of delivery, which alleviates the disease process.

Sickle Cell Nephropathy

This disease is the most common organ manifestation of sickle cell disease and may present as the nephrotic syndrome. Low oxygen tension in the vasa recta causes red blood cells to sickle, occluding the lumen and resulting in medullary infarcts and occasionally papillary necrosis. The glomeruli may appear congested, or demonstrate an FSGS appearance. Over time, ischemic scarring of the medulla leads to focal tubular loss and atrophy.

Renal Infarction

Renal infarcts are caused by arterial obstruction, especially embolization to the large interlobar branches of the renal artery. These emboli may originate from mural thrombi in the heart, infected cardiac valves, or atherosclerotic plaques in the aorta. Small emboli may result in renal infarction when superimposed on underlying renal disease. Patients present with sharp flank or abdominal pain and hematuria.

The kidneys demonstrate well-defined, wedge-shaped regions of pallor, often adjacent to the renal capsule. On microscopy, all structures contained within the infarct demonstrate coagulative necrosis. A surrounding hemorrhagic border is frequently present. The histologic response progresses through inflammation, granulation tissue formation and fibrosis. Healed infarcts appear as sharply circumscribed cortical scars.

Hemorrhagic renal infarction caused by renal vein thrombosis can occur during dehydration (infants) or septic thrombophlebitis and hypercoagulable states (adults).

Cortical Necrosis

Cortical necrosis represents widespread ischemic necrosis of part or all of the renal cortex with sparing of the medulla. In contrast, an infarction affects only one or a few areas within the kidney.

Cortical necrosis occurs after occlusion of the outer cortical vessels and presents as acute renal failure. The extent ranges from patchy to confluent. Causes of cortical necrosis include the following:

- Premature placental separation (placental abruption)
- Hypovolemic shock
- Endotoxic shock
- Hemolytic uremic syndrome

On gross examination, the cortex is pale yellow and soft. Microscopy reveals necrotic proximal and distal tubules. Over time, dystrophic calcification of the necrotic areas may occur.

Recovery is determined by the extent of the disease. There is a significant risk of hypertension among surviving patients.

Diseases of the Tubules and Interstitium

Acute Tubular Necrosis and Injury

Acute tubular necrosis (ATN) and acute tubular injury (ATI) is most commonly caused by ischemic or nephrotoxic agents. ATN presents with rapidly rising serum creatinine level and decreased urine output (oliguria), and represents the leading cause of acute renal failure. Milder forms may demonstrate polyuria. Examination of the urine reveals dirty brown granular casts.

Microscopy reveals a flattening and simplification of the tubular epithelium and epithelial cell loss, often with intratubular cell debris. Specific histologic and pathophysiologic findings associated with ischemic and nephrotoxic ATN include the following:

- Ischemic ATN: rapid depletion of ATP in renal tubular epithelial cells caused by reduced renal perfusion (hypotension) in cases of massive hemorrhage, shock, severe burns, dehydration, or congestive heart failure; swollen kidneys with a pale cortex and a congested medulla; flattened, paucicellular tubular cells with loss of the brush border; absence of widespread necrosis of tubular epithelium; interstitial edema; or granular casts in the urine (sloughed epithelium)
- Nephrotoxic ATN: tubular cells absorb and concentrate toxins from antibiotics, contrast agents, heavy metals, organic solvents, and poisons; hemoglobin and myoglobin may induce nephrotoxic ATN (pigment nephropathy); more widespread necrosis than ischemic ATN; proximal tubular cells often most prominently affected

In all cases, recovery generally depends on the removal of provoking factors.

Pyelonephritis

Pyelonephritis is a bacterial infection of the kidney that may be acute or chronic.

Acute pyelonephritis often is preceded by a bladder infection and occurs after an ascending infection. The patient presents with fever, chills, sweats, malaise, flank pain, and costovertebral angle tenderness. Leukocytosis with neutrophilia is common, and leukocyte casts may be identified in the urine. Approximately 80% of cases are caused by fecal gram-negative bacteria (often *E. coli*). Acute pyelonephritis occurs more frequently in women (short urethra, lack of antibacterial secretions, sexual intercourse). Predisposing factors are pregnancy, urinary outflow obstruction, catheterization, and the reflux of urine during micturition. In addition, acute bacterial nephritis also may occur with hematogenous spread of bacteria and fungus.

Grossly, small white abscesses may be present on the subcapsular and cut surface of the kidney. Purulent material also may be present in the calyces and pelvis, although these findings may be focal. An inflammatory infiltrate of the cortex, with focal peritubular and intratubular neutrophils, and destruction and sparing of the vessels and glomeruli, are present.

Chronic pyelonephritis is caused by recurrent or persistent bacterial infection and most commonly occurs secondary to urinary tract obstruction or urine reflux. Patients present with episodic symptoms. On gross examination, chronic pyelonephritis demonstrates broad, depressed regions of cortical fibrosis and atrophy overlying a dilated calyx. The medulla and overlying cortex are scarred from recurrent acute and chronic inflammation. Lymphoid infiltrates and even germinal centers may be seen. Severe tubular epithelial atrophy with diffuse, eosinophilic hyaline casts (thyroidization) may be present.

Xanthogranulomatous pyelonephritis, a form of chronic pyelonephritis, often is caused by *Proteus* species and results in a yellow nodular appearance of the kidney owing to the presence of lipid-laden foamy macrophages.

Analgesic Nephropathy

Analgesic nephropathy is caused by chronic analgesic overuse, often after an ingestion of more than 2 kg of analgesics. The analgesics that carry a risk of nephropathy include (in order of decreasing risk) phenacetin, acetaminophen, and aspirin or nonsteroidal anti-inflammatory drugs (NSAIDs); however, phenacetin has been banned in the United States.

Analgesic nephropathy presents in late stages with an inability to concentrate urine, distal tubular acidosis, hematuria, hypertension, and anemia. Progressive renal failure may result.

Microscopy reveals a homogeneous thickening of the capillary walls immediately beneath the urothelium. Ischemic changes with fibrosis are seen in the overlying cortex. Papillary necrosis with subsequent dystrophic calcification may occur.

Drug-induced (Hypersensitivity) Acute Tubulointerstitial Nephritis

Drug-induced acute tubulointerstitial nephritis is most commonly caused by NSAIDs, diuretics, and antibiotics (especially β-lactam antibiotics) and is a cell-mediated immune reaction. This disease often presents as acute renal failure approximately 2 weeks after drug administration. Urine analysis identifies the presence of erythrocytes, eosinophils leukocytes, and leukocyte casts. Tubular defects, including sodium wasting, glucosuria, aminoaciduria, and renal tubular acidosis, also occur.

On microscopic analysis, patchy infiltrates of activated T lymphocytes and eosinophils are found primarily within the cortex. Eosinophils are often present within tubular lumens, and the proximal and distal tubules are infiltrated by leukocytes (tubulitis). Granulomas may be seen in response to some drugs. Glomeruli and blood vessels often are spared from the inflammatory process.

Most patients recover after removal of the inciting drug.

Light-chain Cast Nephropathy

Light-chain cast nephropathy is the most common form of renal disease associated with multiple myeloma. Renal damage occurs after accumulation of monoclonal immunoglobulin light chains within the tubules, leading to acute or chronic renal failure. Light chains bind to Tamm-Horsfall glycoproteins of the distal tubular epithelial cells to form dense, eosinophilic casts in the distal tubules and collecting ducts. Immunolabeling of these casts reveals a strong reaction for either kappa or lambda light chains, but not both. Interstitial edema, chronic interstitial inflammation, and a foreign-body reaction may be present.

Urate Nephropathy

Elevation of blood uric acid levels leads to urate nephropathy. The acute form of this disease is caused by increased cellular turnover, such as in leukemia, polycythemia, or tumor lysis syndrome, and results in acute renal failure. Grossly, precipitated uric acid appears as yellow streaks in the renal papillae. Frozen tissue analysis reveals amorphous tubular deposits containing birefringent crystals. The tubules proximal to the obstruction appear dilated.

The chronic form of urate nephropathy is caused by gout and presents with chronic renal tubular defects. The prolonged course of the disease results in extensive urate crystal deposition in the interstitium, leading to interstitial fibrosis and renal cortical atrophy.

Focal urate crystal accumulation in the soft tissue results in surrounding inflammation and the appearance of a nodular growth, referred to as a gouty tophus.

Nephrocalcinosis

Nephrocalcinosis results from a deposition of calcium in the renal parenchyma and is caused by increased calcium levels within the urine (hypercalcinuria). Nephrocalcinosis may lead to tubular defects, including renal tubular acidosis and salt wasting, interstitial calcium deposits, and calcification of the renal tubular basement membrane. If severe, nephrocalcinosis may result in interstitial fibrosis and parenchymal atrophy. Metastatic calcification occurs in association with hypercalcemia.

Renal Calculi

The presence of renal calculi/stones within the collecting system of the kidney is referred to as *nephrolithiasis*, whereas the presence of stones outside of the kidney is referred to as *urolithiasis*. Renal stones are more common in men and can vary in size from less than 1 mm to stones large enough to lodge within the urinary tract. Renal stones may erode the mucosa of the urinary tract, leading to hematuria, or may obstruct urinary outflow, leading to hydronephrosis and pyelonephritis. Renal colic is the characteristic symptom of renal stones and describes excruciating pain along the flank caused by the passage of stones along the urinary outflow tract. Calculi may serve as a nidus for bacterial infection. A variety of materials make up renal stones:

- Calcium: 75% of stones; radiodense; calcium oxalate stones are hard, occasionally dark from hemorrhage; calcium phosphate stones are softer and paler
- Infectious: 15% of stones; urea-splitting bacteria, such as *Proteus* and *Providencia*, induce alkaline urine, which leads to the precipitation of magnesium ammonium phosphate (struvite) and calcium phosphate (apatite); staghorn calculi are caused by a castlike formation of the renal pelvis and calyces; frequently result in intractable urinary tract infections, pain, bleeding, perinephric abscess, and urosepsis
- Uric acid: less than 10% of stones; radiolucent; hard, yellow, <2 cm diameter; common in patients with hyperuricemia and gout
- Cystine: 1% of stones; most often occur in childhood in association with hereditary cystinuria

Although smaller stones often pass through the urinary tract spontaneously, larger stones are frequently eliminated by lithotripsy (ultrasonic disintegration).

Obstructive Uropathy and Hydronephrosis

An impedance of urine outflow may lead to either renal dysfunction (obstructive uropathy) or hydronephrosis (dilation of the collecting system). Both of these end results of urinary tract obstruction predispose the kidney to infection. In general, hydronephrosis progresses from distal to proximal, with initial dilation of the collecting ducts and ultimate dilation of the proximal tubule. The end stage of hydronephrosis is an atrophic kidney, with relative sparing of the glomeruli. Unilateral obstruction may be asymptomatic; however, bilateral obstruction may lead to acute renal failure.

Renal Transplantation

Renal transplantation is used as treatment for many patients with ESRD. The transplanted kidney may undergo subsequent injury from a variety of sources, including the following:

- Immunosuppressive drugs cyclosporine and tacrolimus (FK506): Inhibit calcineurin; may cause arteriolopathy (arteriolar smooth muscle cell degeneration and necrosis), which leads to interstitial fibrosis and tubular atrophy; may cause thrombotic microangiopathy
- Recurrent primary renal disease: Type II membranoproliferative glomerulonephritis and diabetic glomerulosclerosis
- Rejection (Table 16-4) (graded by the Banff classification that scores interstitial inflammation, tubular inflammation [tubulitis], and vasculitis)

The two most common groups of tissue antigens inciting rejection are the following:

- ABO blood group antigens expressed on endothelial cells and erythrocytes: mismatch between donor and recipient incite preformed antibodies against the foreign blood group that bind to endothelial cells in the transplanted kidney, leading to hyperacute rejection
- Human leukocyte antigens (HLAs/MHCs) expressed on most cell membranes: may induce acute or chronic rejection caused by either cell-mediated or antibody-mediated reactions

Renal Tumors

Both benign and malignant tumors affect the kidney (Table 16-5). A subset of malignant lesions are described.

Wilms Tumor (Nephroblastoma)

Wilms tumor often occurs in children between 1 and 3 years of age. Patients frequently present with an abdominal mass, as well as abdominal pain, intestinal obstruction, hypertension, hematuria, and traumatic rupture of the kidney. The majority of cases (90%)

Table 16-4

Classification of Renal Rejection

Rejection Category	Frequency	Characteristic Findings
Hyperacute (humoral)	<0.5%	Occurs within 48 hours Neutrophils in glomerular and peritubular capillaries; fibrin thrombi in the preglomerular arterioles; ischemic collapse of glomeruli
Acute (cellular)		
Acute tubulointerstitial	Most common	Tubulitis (mononuclear leukocytes in tubules) and interstitial inflammation
Acute cellular vascular		Intimal arteritis (mononuclear leukocytes in intima)
Acute (humoral)		
Acute humoral capillary	More common	Neutrophils and C4d in capillaries
Acute necrotizing vascular	<1%	Arterial fibrinoid necrosis
Chronic		Intimal fibrosis and thickening of arteries, partially with splintering of elastica; ischemic changes within glomeruli, tubules, and interstitium; cortical atrophy; multilayering of capillary basement membrane

Table 16-5
Renal Tumors

Type	Gross Appearance	Microscopic Appearance
Benign lesions		
Adenoma	Well-circumscribed, <1 cm	Small cuboidal cells with round, regular nuclei
Oncocytoma	Well-circumscribed, variable size, mahogany-brown, central scar	Plump cells, finely granular pink cytoplasm, (mitochondria-rich), and round nuclei
Medullary fibroma	Well-circumscribed, <0.5 cm, pale gray	Small stellate/polygonal cells in a loose stroma
Angiomyolipoma*	Well-circumscribed, variable size, yellow, bosselated	Mixture of adipose tissue, smooth muscle cells, and thick-walled vessels
Mesoblastic nephroma	Irregular appearance, variable size	Spindle cells of fibroblastic/ myofibroblastic lineage
Malignant lesions		
Clear cell (conventional)	Yellow-orange, hemorrhage, necrosis, well-circumscribed	Clear cells in rounded/tubular collections; graded by Fuhrman grading system
Papillary	Yellow-brown, well-circumscribed	Cuboidal cells on fibrovascular stalks; stromal macrophages often present; graded by Fuhrman grading system
Chromophobe	Light-brown, lobulated, turns pale gray following fixation, well-circumscribed	Mixture of pink granular and pale cells with sharply demarcated borders; cells stain blue with Hale's colloidal iron stain
Collecting duct	Poorly circumscribed, firm, white, ± cysts	Tubular and papillary structures lined by a single layer of cuboidal cells with a hobnail appearance and desmoplastic stroma

* Association with tuberous sclerosis.

are sporadic and unilateral, whereas subsets are inherited and frequently bilateral.

Alterations in the Wilms tumor gene *WT1* occur in a subset of sporadic and inherited lesions. *WT1* is a tumor suppressor gene that regulates transcription of the growth factors IGF-2 and PDGF. In addition to sporadic forms, 5% to 6% of Wilms tumors are familial without associated syndrome, and 5% arise in association with one of three syndromes:

- WAGR syndrome: Wilms tumor, aniridia, genitourinary anomalies, and mental retardation; 11p13 *deletion* of *WT1*, *PAX6*
- Denys-Drash syndrome (DDS): Wilms tumor, sexual disorders, and glomerulopathy; mutations of the *WT1* gene
- Beckwith-Wiedemann syndrome (BWS): Wilms tumor, large physical stature, visceromegaly, and macroglossia: LOH or paternal gene duplication of the *WT2* gene on 11p15 (*IGF-2* locus)

On gross examination, lesions often are large and demonstrate a bulging, pale tan cut surface surrounded by a thin cortex and renal capsule. Microscopic examination reveals a mixture of blastemal (small ovoid cells), stromal (spindle cells), and epithelial (small tubular structures) elements.

Patients have a better prognosis if Wilms tumor occurs before 2 years of age and demonstrates lack of capsular invasion and anaplasia. With current therapy, the survival of patients with Wilms tumor is greater than 90%.

Renal Cell Carcinoma

Renal cell carcinoma (RCC) is a malignant neoplasm of the renal tubular epithelium that occurs in adulthood and account for 90% of all renal cancers. RCC is twice as common in men as in women. Tobacco use has been implicated as a risk factor for the development of RCC. Approximately 50% of all patients present with hematuria, flank pain, and a palpable abdominal mass. Occasionally, RCC may be associated with ectopic hormone production leading to hypercalcemia, polycythemia, or gynecomastia. The majority of RCC cases are sporadic, although approximately 5% are familial. Familial forms may demonstrate an earlier onset and often may be bilateral.

Subtypes of RCC include clear cell (conventional), papillary, and chromophobe among others. Documented genetic alterations in RCC include loss of heterozygosity of the von-Hippel Lindau *VHL* gene (chromosome 3p) in clear cell RCC and *MET* gene mutations in papillary RCC. Syndromes associated with RCC development include Birt-Hogg-Dubé syndrome, von-Hippel Lindau disease, and hereditary papillary RCC. The development of sarcomatoid features in any form of RCC portends a worsened prognosis.

Grading of RCC follows the Fuhrman system:

- Grade I: round, uniform nuclei with inconspicuous or absent nucleoli
- Grade II: irregular nuclei with inconspicuous or absent nucleoli
- Grade III: irregular, enlarged nuclei with nucleoli prominent at low magnification
- Grade IV: bizarre, large nuclei with prominent nucleoli

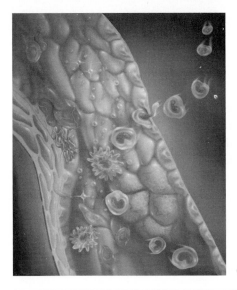

CHAPTER 17

The Lower Urinary Tract and Male Reproductive Tract

THE LOWER URINARY TRACT

Normal Anatomy and Histology

The lower urinary tract is made up of the ureters, urinary bladder, and urethra. The ureters are retroperitoneal structures that conduct urine from the kidneys to the bladder; the ureterovesical valves allow one-way passage of urine into the bladder, thereby preventing urinary reflux. The bladder is also located in the retroperitoneum and resides anterior to the rectum in males and anterior to the lower uterine corpus in females. The bladder is subdivided into the apex (dome), midportion, and trigone, which leads to the urethra. The male urethra, approximately 20 cm in length, is divided into the prostatic urethra, the membranous urethra (penetrates pelvic floor), and spongy (penile) urethra. The male urethra receives inflow from the ejaculatory ducts. The female urethra averages 3 to 4 cm in length and receives secretions from surrounding mucous glands (Fig. 17-1). The lower urinary tract is lined by urothelium (previously described as transitional epithelium). The layers of the bladder include:

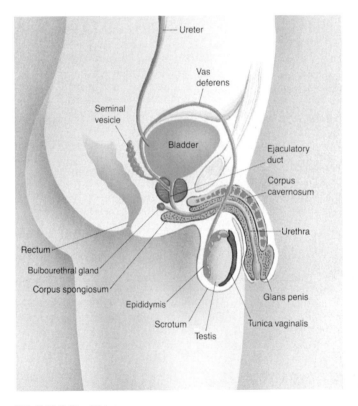

F I G U R E   17-1

The lower urinary tract in relation to the male reproductive system. (From Rubin E, Gorstein F, Rubin R, et al. Rubin's Pathology, 4th ed. Philadelphia: Lippincott Williams & Wilkins, 2005, p. 886.)

- Urothelium: composed of the basement membrane, the basal cell layer (dividing cells), an intermediate zone (3–4 layers of mature polygonal cells), and umbrella cells (a single layer of surface epithelium resistant to damage by urine)
- Lamina propria: loose connective tissue and blood vessels
- Muscularis mucosa: incomplete thin muscle layer
- Muscularis propria (detrusor muscle)
- Adventitia

THE URETERS

Congenital Anomalies of the Renal Pelvis and Ureters

Congenital anomalies of the urinary system occur in 2% to 3% of the population and are often asymptomatic. The most common anomalies include agenesis, ectopia (incorrect location), duplications, and obstructions. In rare cases, anomalies may lead to urinary tract obstruction and infection. Abnormalities in the vesicoureteral valves may lead to severe urine reflux into the ureter, resulting ultimately in dilation of the renal pelvis and ureter (hydronephrosis) and destruction of renal parenchyma.

Ureteritis and Ureteral Obstruction

Ureteritis is an inflammation of the ureter that may be caused by descending renal infections or ascending bladder infection caused by incompetent vesicoureteric valves leading to reflux of urine. Often, ureteritis is caused by obstruction of urine outflow secondary to calculi, inflammatory strictures, benign prostatic hyperplasia, pregnancy, endometriosis, and prostate cancer.

Ureteral Cancer

The majority of ureteral cancer is composed of *urothelial cell carcinoma* and is histologically similar to that found in the bladder (see following section). Patients often present in their sixth and seventh decades with hematuria and flank pain. Treatment involves surgical resection of the involved renal pelvis and ureter (radical nephroureterectomy).

THE URINARY BLADDER

Congenital Anomalies of the Urinary Bladder

The most frequently identified congenital anomalies of the bladder include:

- *Diverticula*: outpouchings of the bladder wall due to incomplete muscular layer formation
- *Urachal remnants*: incomplete involution of the fetal allantoic stalk; may lead to fistula formation or adenocarcinoma
- *Congenital incompetence of the vesicoureteral valve*: caused by an abnormal junction between the ureters and the urinary bladder; may lead to vesicoureteric reflux
- *Bladder exstrophy*: absence of the anterior wall of the bladder and a portion of the anterior abdominal wall, leaving the posterior wall of the bladder externally exposed; may be associated with epispadias (see "The Testis, Epididymis, and Vas Deferens" below).

Cystitis

Cystitis is an inflammation of the bladder that may be acute or chronic. Cystitis often occurs following infection of the lower urinary tract with organisms, including *Escherichia coli, Proteus vulgaris, Pseudomonas aeruginosa,* and *Enterobacter*. In special circumstances, colonization with fungi (immunosuppressed patients), gas-forming bacilli (diabetic patients), or schistosomiasis (North Africa and Middle East) may occur.

The risk of cystitis is increased in patients with:

- Female gender: short urethra
- Bladder calculi
- Bladder outlet obstruction
- Prior instrumentation or catheterization
- Radiation or chemotherapy
- Medical conditions: diabetes mellitus, immunodeficiency

Patients present with urinary frequency, pain on urination (dysuria), and lower abdominal or pelvic pain. Evaluation of the urine reveals inflammatory cells; the inciting organism may be cultured. Cystitis is treated by antibiotic administration.

Ongoing inflammation with a predominance of lymphocytes and fibrosis of the lamina propria are hallmarks of chronic cystitis. *Follicular cystitis* is a form of chronic cystitis that contains lymphoid follicles within the lamina propria. Additional forms of chronic cystitis include:

- *Granulomatous cystitis*: may occur with tuberculosis or schistosomiasis
- *Eosinophilic cystitis*: dense eosinophils in the lamina propria
- *Hemorrhagic cystitis*: focal petechial hemorrhages in the mucosa caused by acute infection, cytotoxic drugs, disseminated intravascular coagulation
- *Ulcerative cystitis*: ulceration and focal mucosal hemorrhage caused by indwelling catheters or traumatic cystoscopy

- *Suppurative cystitis*: purulent exudate caused by sepsis, pyelo-nephritis, local infection
- *Pseudomembranous cystitis*: shaggy gray material covering bladder surface with underlying hemorrhagic ulcerated mucosa caused by infection following cytotoxic drugs

Chronic interstitial cystitis affects middle-aged women. Presenting symptoms include long-standing suprapubic pain and urinary frequency and urgency. On cystoscopy, the mucosa contains focal hemorrhages. On microscopy, transmural inflammation of the bladder and occasional mucosal ulceration (Hunner ulcer) are evident. This disease is resistant to therapy, and organisms are typically not cultured from the urine.

Malakoplakia is characterized by soft, yellow mucosal plaques that are composed of an accumulation of macrophages. This disease is uncommon, may occur in all age groups, and most frequently affects women. Often a clinical history of cancer, immunosuppression, or chronic infections is obtained. Microscopically, the lamina propria demonstrates a histiocytic infiltrate; the histiocytes often contain cytoplasmic inclusions termed *Michaelis-Guttman bodies*.

Benign Lesions

Reactive and Metaplastic Urothelial Lesions

Although these lesions may affect any portion of the urinary tract, they most frequently affect the bladder. Common associations include urinary calculi, infections, and neurogenic bladder. Benign proliferative and metaplastic lesions include:

- *Von Brunn's nests*: invaginations of the urothelium into the lamina propria
- *Cystitis cystica*: fluid-filled grouped cysts lined by urothelium
- *Cystitis glandularis*: glandular structures within the lamina propria lined by epithelium-containing goblet cells
- *Squamous metaplasia*
- *Nephrogenic metaplasia (adenoma)*: papillary exophytic nodule identified microscopically as numerous small clustered tubules within the lamina propria

Urothelial Cell Papilloma

Urothelial cell papilloma is an uncommon, benign lesion that is encountered incidentally or after examination for painless hematuria. Generally, this condition affects men older than 50 years of age. Papillomas occur as one of two subtypes:

- *Exophytic papilloma*: 2- to 5-cm diameter lesions made up of papillary fronds covered by normal urothelium

- *Inverted papilloma*: nodular mucosal lesions lined by normal urothelium that involute into the lamina propria

Urothelial Cell Carcinoma

The most common urinary tract neoplasm is *urothelial cell carcinoma*, which may arise at any location containing urothelium, including the renal pelvis, ureters, bladder, and urethra. Additional types of carcinomas that arise within the urinary tract, most commonly the bladder, include squamous cell carcinoma, adenocarcinoma, and neuroendocrine carcinoma.

Urothelial cell carcinoma affects predominantly male patients older than 65 years of age and accounts for 3% to 5% of cancer-related deaths in the United States. Although urothelial cell carcinoma may occur at any site within the urinary tract, the bladder is most commonly affected. Patients may present with sudden hematuria and occasionally dysuria. Risk factors for urothelial cell carcinoma development include:

- Cigarette smoking
- Industrial exposure to azo dyes
- Infection with *Schistosomiasis haematobium* (primarily squamous cell carcinoma)
- Drugs, including cyclophosphamide and analgesics
- Regional radiation therapy

In certain instances, multiple urothelial carcinomas may arise at different sites of the urinary tract; these lesions appear to arise from the same clone of cells. Fifty percent of urothelial carcinomas contain specific cytogenetic abnormalities, including abnormalities of:

- Tumor suppressor gene *p16*: low-grade tumors
- Tumor suppressor gene *p53*: high-grade and invasive tumors

Urothelial cell carcinomas may be in situ or invasive. In situ urothelial carcinoma may be flat or papillary. *Flat urothelial cell carcinoma* does not show any papillary structures microscopically but is characterized by full-thickness cellular atypia of the urothelium, including nuclear enlargement and hyperchromasia, irregular nuclear shape, prominent nucleoli, and coarse chromatin. By cystoscopy, multiple red, velvety, flat patches are identified. Flat urothelial cell carcinoma may occur in concurrence with papillary urothelial cell carcinoma. *Papillary urothelial cell carcinoma* often arises from the lateral walls of the bladder, although any region of the bladder may be affected. By cystoscopy, these lesions range in appearance from delicate frondlike structures to solid, ulcerated lesions. Microscopically, these lesions demonstrate papillary fronds with a fibrovascular stalk lined by urothelium with varying degrees of dysplasia. These lesions are further categorized by histologic grade (Fig. 17-2).

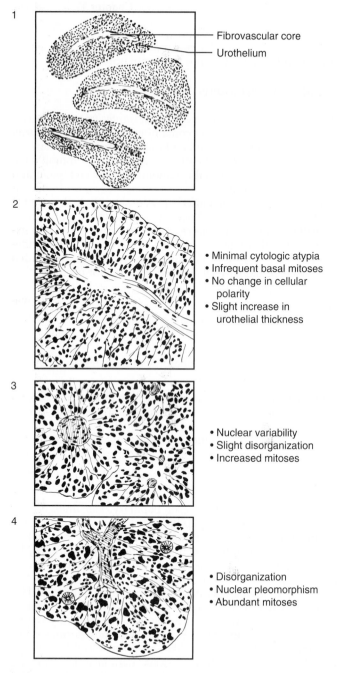

1
— Fibrovascular core
— Urothelium

2
- Minimal cytologic atypia
- Infrequent basal mitoses
- No change in cellular polarity
- Slight increase in urothelial thickness

3
- Nuclear variability
- Slight disorganization
- Increased mitoses

4
- Disorganization
- Nuclear pleomorphism
- Abundant mitoses

FIGURE 17-2
Grading of papillary urothelial cell carcinoma.

- Low grade (grade 1): increased thickness of the urothelium with minimal nuclear pleomorphism and low mitotic index
- High grade (grades 2 and 3): increased nuclear stratification, loss of nuclear polarization, moderate nuclear pleomorphism, frequent mitotic activity.

Treatment of these lesions includes the use of intravesical chemotherapy agents or bacillus Calmette Guerin (BCG).

Invasive urothelial carcinoma demonstrates invasion into the tissue underlying the epithelium, including the lamina propria and detrusor muscle. Invasion often initially occurs within the fibrovascular stalk of a papillary lesion or immediately below the location of flat carcinoma in situ, with subsequent invasion into the lamina propria, followed by detrusor muscle invasion. The depth and extent of invasion is important in the staging and prognosis of urothelial carcinoma. Lesions that are noninvasive or invade the lamina propria may be conservatively treated by transurethral resection (TURP) and/or BCG administration; removal of the bladder (radical cystectomy) is performed in lesions with more extensive invasion. The 5-year survival ranges from 80% for minimally invasive lesions to less than 20% for lesions with extension into the detrusor muscle and beyond.

THE URETHRA

Urethritis

Urethritis is an inflammation of the urethra that may be acute or chronic.

Sexually Transmitted Urethritis

Urethritis may be caused by a sexually transmitted disease, such as *Neisseria gonorrhoeae*, *Chlamydia trachomatis*, or *Ureaplasma urealyticum*. This form of urethritis has an acute onset, and onset is related to sexual intercourse. Patients often experience pain or tingling at the meatus of the urethra and pain on urination (dysuria), and there is a greenish-yellow urethral discharge.

Nonspecific Infectious Urethritis

This form of urethritis may be associated with cystitis, prostatitis, or vaginitis. Causative organisms include *E. coli* and *Pseudomonas*. Symptoms include urinary urgency and a burning sensation during urination. Often, no discharge is present.

Urethral Caruncles

These lesions occur most commonly in postmenopausal women and are inflammatory 1 to 2 cm diameter polypoid lesions at the urethral meatus. Symptoms include pain and bleeding. The cause of caruncles is unknown. Treatment is via surgical excision.

Reiter Syndrome

Reiter syndrome is defined as urethritis, conjunctivitis, and arthritis of weight-bearing joints. Reiter syndrome often affects young adults with an HLA-B27 haplotype. Urethritis occurs following infection with a variety of pathogens and may be caused by an inappropriate immune reaction to antigen. Symptoms often disappear spontaneously in 3 to 6 months.

Urethral Cancer

Urethral carcinoma occurs twice as frequently in women and may be associated with strictures or bladder cancer. Elderly persons are most commonly affected and may present with urethral bleeding and dysuria. The most common urethral cancer is squamous cell carcinoma; urothelial cell carcinoma may also occur. Treatment is via radical surgery.

THE MALE REPRODUCTIVE TRACT

Normal Anatomy and Histology

The male reproductive system includes the testes, epididymis, ductus (vas) deferens, seminal vesicles, prostate, and penis. Spermatogenesis occurs in the testes within the seminiferous tubules, which occurs under the guidance of the gonadotrophins follicle-stimulating hormone (FSH) and luteinizing hormone (LH), regulated by inhibin produced by Sertoli cells and testosterone produced by Leydig cells (Figs. 17-3 and 17-4).

THE PENIS, URETHRA, AND SCROTUM

Congenital Disorders of the Penis

Hypospadias

In *hypospadias*, the urethra opens onto the underside (ventral side) of the penis, secondary to incomplete closure of the urethral folds

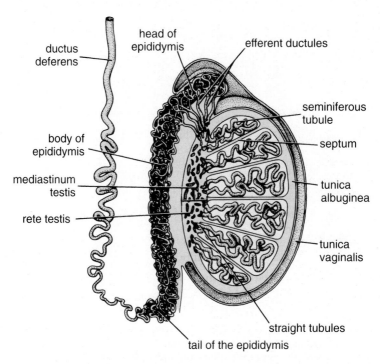

FIGURE   17-3
Anatomy of the testis. (From Ross MH, Kaye GI, Pawlina W. Histology: A Text and Atlas, 4th ed. Philadelphia: Lippincott Williams and Wilkins, 2003, p. 686.)

of the urogenital sinus. This condition occurs in 1 of 350 male neonates. Occasionally, it is associated with multisystem developmental syndromes.

Epispadias

This is a rare congential anomaly in which the urethra opens on the upper side (dorsal side) of the penis. If severe, *epispadias* may be associated with bladder exstrophy.

Phimosis

In *phimosis*, the orifice of the prepuce may be too narrow to allow retraction over the glans penis, predisposing to infection. Treatment is via circumcision.

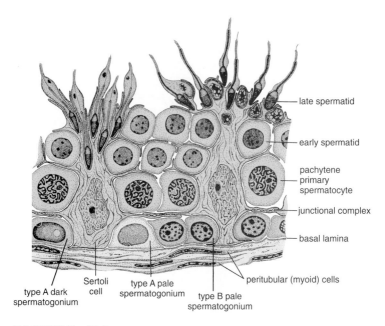

FIGURE   17-4
**The human seminiferous epithelium. Maturation of sperm pro-
gresses through numerous stages including spermatogonia, primary
spermatocytes, early spermatids and late spermatids. (From Ross
MH, Kaye GI, Pawlina W. Histology: A Text and Atlas, 4th ed. Philadelphia: Lippincott Williams and Wilkins, 2003, p. 686.)**

Scrotal Masses

Scrotal masses reflect abnormalities occurring within the testicle,
epididymis, and surrounding tissues. A *hydrocele* is the most common cause of scrotal swelling in infants and may be diagnosed by
transilluminating the fluid in the cavity by ultrasound. Additional
causes of scrotal masses are listed in Table 17-1.

Circulatory Disturbances

Scrotal Edema

Accumulation of lymph (*lymphedema*) or serous fluid may occur
secondary to outflow obstruction of lymphatic or venous drainage.
Lymphedema may occur in association with pelvic or abdominal
tumors, surgical scars, or infections. Plasma accumulation may
occur with heart failure, cirrhosis, or the nephrotic syndrome.

Table 17-1

Scrotal Masses

Disease entity	Findings	Cause
Hydrocele		Patent processus vaginalis testis
Congenital hydrocele	Collection of serous fluid between the two layers of tunica vaginalis; associated with inguinal hernia	
Acquired hydrocele	Collection of serous fluid between the two layers of tunica vaginalis	Infection, tumor, trauma
Hematocele	Accumulation of blood between the two layers of tunica vaginalis	Trauma, hemorrhage into hydrocele
Spermatocele	Hilar paratesticular nodule filled with milky fluid; spermatozoa at various stages of degeneration	Protrusion of efferent ducts of rete testis or epididymis
Varicocele	Asymptomatic; nodularity on lateral side of scrotum; common cause of infertility and oligospermia	Dilation of testicular veins
Scrotal inguinal hernia	Mass; long-standing; may be associated with testicular atrophy	Protrusion of intestines into scrotum

Erectile Dysfunction (Impotence)

The inability to achieve or maintain an erection sufficient for satisfactory sexual performance describes *impotence*. The prevalence of impotence increases with age from 20% at age 40 years to 50% by age 70 years. A combination of hormonal, vascular, and neural factors influences the filling of the corpora cavernosa and spongiosa of the penis, necessary to maintain an erection. Several disor-

From Rubin E, Gorstein F, Rubin R, et al. Rubin's Pathology, 4th ed. Philadelphia: Lippincott Williams & Wilkins, 2005, p. 902.

Table 17-2	
Causes of Erectile Dysfunction	
Neuropsychiatric	Drugs
Psychiatric disorders (e.g., depression)	Antihypertensives
Spinal cord injury	Psychotropic drugs
Nerve injury during surgery (e.g., pelvic	Estrogens
or perineal surgery)	Anticancer drugs
Endocrine	Idiopathic
Hypogonadism	"Performance anxiety"
Pituitary disease (e.g., hyperpro-	Age-related "impotence"
lactinemia)	
Hypothyroidism, Cushing syndrome,	
Addison disease	
Vascular	
Diabetic microangiopathy	
Hypertension	
Atherosclerosis	

ders may lead to erectile dysfunction (Table 17-2). Treatment of this condition may be achieved with medications that prevent the degradation of cGMP, such as sildenafil (Viagra).

Priapism

Priapism is the continued painful erection of the penis unrelated to sexual excitation. Often, the cause of priapism is unknown. Secondary priapism occurs with interference of blood outflow from the penis (pelvic tumors), hematological disorders (sickle cell anemia), or brain and spinal cord diseases (syphilis).

Inflammatory Disorders of the Penis

Inflammatory disorders of the penis occur in the setting of sexually transmitted diseases, infections, dermatoses, and dermatitis. *Balantitis* refers to an inflammation of the glans penis specifically. Occasionally, the cause of inflammation is unknown. Table 17-3 provides a description of penile inflammatory disorders.

Penile Cancer and Precursor Lesions

Squamous carcinoma of the penis is an uncommon lesion, which is more prevalent in less developed countries. The average age of pre-

Table 17-3

Inflammatory Lesions of the Penis

Disease	Findings
Sexually transmitted diseases	
Herpes genitalis (HSV-2)	Grouped vesicles that ulcerate and form crusts
Syphilis (*Treponema pallidum*)	Solitary, soft ulcer (chancre)
Chancroid (Haemophilus ducreyi)	Papule that transforms into a pustule that ulcerates
Granuloma inguinale (*Calymmatobacterium granulomatus*)	Tropical disease; raised ulceration filled with exudate and granulation tissue
Lymphogranuloma venereum (*Chlamydia trachomatis*)	Small vesicle that ulcerates; tender inguinal lymph node enlargement that may form sinuses and drain pus
Human papillomavirus infection	Flat-topped warts (condylomata acuminata)
Nonspecific infectious balanoposthitis	
Bacterial, fungal, viral	
Diseases of unknown etiology	
Balanitis xerotica obliterans	White, indurated glans; fibrosis, sclerosis of subepithelial connective tissue
Circinate balanitis	Circular, linear, plaquelike discoloration; occurs in Reiter syndrome
Plasma cell balanitis (Zoon balanitis)	Macular discoloration or painless papules on the glans; plasma cell infiltrate of the connective tissue
Peyronie disease	Focal, asymmetric fibrosis of the shaft of the penis; penile curvature
Dermatitis involving the penile shaft and scrotum	
Infectious (bacterial, viral, fungal)	
Noninfectious (e.g., lichen planus, bullous skin disease)	

Modified from Rubin E, Gorstein F, Rubin R, et al. Rubin's Pathology, 4th ed. Philadelphia: Lippincott Williams & Wilkins, 2005, p. 902.

sentation is 60 years. Although the cause is unknown, proposed etiologic agents include accumulation of keratin under the prepuce (smegma), phimosis, and human papillomavirus (HPV) types 16 and 18.

The preinvasive form of squamous cancer (carcinoma in situ) occurs in two forms:

- *Bowen disease*: sharply demarcated, erythematous gray-white plaque on the shaft
- *Erythroplasia of Queyrat*: solitary or multiple, shiny, soft, erythematous plaques on the glans and foreskin

Microscopically, both forms demonstrate full-thickness cytological atypia of the keratinocytes, but no invasion of the underlying lamina propria. Parakeratosis and hyperkeratosis may be present.

Bowenoid papulosis is a squamous lesion caused by HPV that affects young, sexually active men. Bowenoid papulosis appears as multiple brownish or violaceous papules. Microscopically, these lesions demonstrate similar transdermal atypia of the keratinocytes, although they tend to be more sharply demarcated than in situ squamous carcinoma and often contain giant, multinucleated keratinocytes. These lesions generally regress spontaneously.

Invasive squamous cell cancer may present as an ulcer, indurated lesion, friable hemorrhagic mass, or exophytic, fungating papillary tumor. The glans and prepuce are most commonly affected. Often, the lesions are well-differentiated, focally keratinizing cancers with the potential to metastasize. Treatment often involves amputation of the penis.

Verrucous carcinoma is a form of squamous cell carcinoma that appears grossly and microscopically like condyloma acuminatum, although it demonstrates local invasion. The risk of metastases from this subtype of cancer is low. Treatment is by local surgical resection.

THE TESTIS, EPIDIDYMIS, AND VAS DEFERENS

Cryptorchidism (Undescended Testis)

This congenital abnormality occurs when one or both testes are not found within their normal position in the scrotum. Undescended testes are described by their location internally, including abdominal, inguinal, and upper scrotal. At birth, 5% of full-term males and 30% of premature males demonstrate an undescended testis; by 1 year of age, the majority of these cases resolve. Cryptorchidism is the most common cause of urologic surgery in infants

Overall, undescended testes are smaller than normal and demonstrate parenchymal fibrosis. Even if they are surgically replaced into the scrotum (orchiopexy), a progressive loss of seminiferous tubules occurs in affected patients. In addition, hyaline thickening of the tubular basement membrane and prominent stromal fibrosis are apparent.

Patients with cryptorchidism are at increased risk for infertility and germ cell neoplasia. Men with bilateral cryptorchid testes have azoospermia and are infertile; men with a unilateral cryptorchid testis have oligospermia in 40% of cases. Cryptorchidism is also associated with a 20- to 40-fold increased risk of testicular cancer, especially in patients with intra-abdominal testes. Orchiopexy does not reduce this risk.

Abnormalities of Sexual Differentiation

This class of disorders encompasses abnormalities in gonadogenesis, development of the external genitals, and secondary sex characteristics (Table 17-4).

Hermaphroditism

This is a rare developmental disorder characterized by ambiguous genitalia in a person with both male and female gonads. The gonads in these patients may have a variety of compositions, including one male and one female gonad, or a combination ovary-testis

Table 17-4

Disorders of Sexual Differentiation

Sex chromosomal abnormalities	Prenatal hormonal effects
Klinefelter syndrome and its variants	Exogenous hormones during pregnancy
Turner syndrome	Maternal hormone-producing tumors
46,XX males	Idiopathic conditions
Single-gene defects	Hermaphroditism
Adrenogenital syndrome	Gonadal dysgenesis
Androgen insensitivity syndromes	
Müllerian inhibitory substance deficiency	

From Rubin E, Gorstein F, Rubin R, et al. Rubin's Pathology, 4th ed. Philadelphia: Lippincott Williams & Wilkins, 2005, p. 908.

(ovotestes). Half of all patients are 46,XX; the remainder are 46,XY or 45,X.

Female Pseudohermaphroditism

These patients are genetically normal females (46,XX) with normal ovaries and genital organs but virilization of the external genital organs. Findings include fusion of the scrotal folds and clitoromegaly. This condition may occur in adrenogenital syndrome caused by 21-hydroxylase deficiency.

Male Pseudohermaphroditism

These patients have a normal male (46,XY) karyotype but demonstrate cryptorchid testes and feminine or ambiguous external genital organs. This condition often occurs in concurrence with androgen insensitivity syndromes due to a congenital deficiency of the androgen receptor.

Male Infertility

Infertility is described as the inability to conceive after 1 year of coital activity with the same sexual partner without contraception. Infertility affects approximately 15% of couples in the United States. Causes of male infertility may be supratesticular, testicular, or posttesticular. Supratesticular causes often demonstrate immature seminiferous tubules without evidence of spermatogenic differentiation. Posttesticular causes often reflect a blockage of the excretory duct outflow. Causes of male infertility are listed in Table 17-5 and Figure 17-5.

Inflammatory Disorders

Epididymitis

Inflammation of the epididymis may be acute or chronic and is often caused by bacterial infection. Acute inflammation demonstrates neutrophilic infiltration, whereas chronic inflammation demonstrates plasma cell, lymphocyte, and macrophage infiltration. Infection in younger men often occur secondary to *Chlamydia* or gonorrhea, whereas older men experience epididymitis secondary to *E. coli* infection of the urinary tract. Patients present with intrascrotal pain, tenderness, and occasionally fever.

Specific forms of epididymitis include *tuberculous epididymitis* and *spermatic granuloma*. Tuberculous epididymitis occurs in the setting of established tuberculosis and contains caseating granu-

Table 17-5

Causes of Male Infertility

Supratesticular causes
  Disorders of the hypothalamic–pituitary–gonadal axis
  Endocrine disease of the adrenal, thyroid; diabetes
  Metabolic disorders
  Major organ diseases (e.g., renal hepatic, cardiopulmonary diseases)
  Chronic infections and debilitating diseases (e.g., tuberculosis, AIDS)
  Drugs and substance abuse
Testicular causes
  Idiopathic hypospermatogenesis or azoospermia
  Developmental (cryptorchidism, gonadal dysgenesis)
  Genetic disease affecting gonads (Klinefelter syndrome)
  Orchitis (immune and infectious)
  Iatrogenic testicular injury (radiation, cytotoxic drugs)
  Trauma of the testis and surgical injury
  Environmental (phytoestrogens)
Posttesticular causes
  Congential anomalies of the excretory ducts
  Inflammation and scarring of excretory ducts
  Iatrogenic or posttraumatic lesions of excretory ducts

From Rubin E, Gorstein F, Rubin R, et al. Rubin's Pathology, 4th ed.
Philadelphia: Lippincott Williams & Wilkins, 2005, p. 908.

lomas microscopically. Spermatic granuloma occurs when sperm enter the interstitium of the epididymis, resulting in a robust inflammation lasting up to several months. The outcome of spermatic granuloma is often fibrosis, ductal obstruction, and infertility.

Orchitis

Orchitis is an acute or chronic inflammation of the testis that often occurs secondary to hematogenous pathogen spread, ascending infection, or as a part of immune-mediated disease. Orchitis frequently presents with testicular pain and swelling. The most common form of orchitis is gram-negative orchitis, which occurs with urinary tract infections and is often associated with epididymitis. Additional forms of orchitis include syphilitic orchitis, mumps orchitis, granulomatous orchitis of unknown cause, and malakoplakia.

Tumors

Testicular tumors are rare, accounting for less than 1% of all adult malignancies. The majority of testicular tumors occur between the

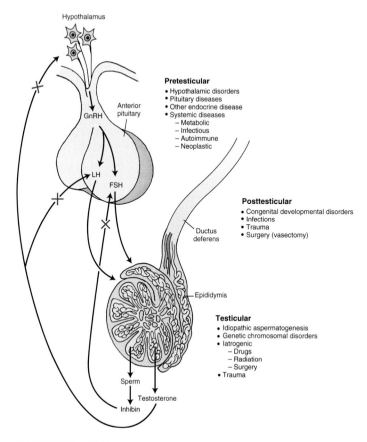

F I G U R E   17-5
Causes of male infertility. Pretesticular infertility, testicular infertility, and posttesticular (obstructive) infertility. (From Rubin E, Gorstein F, Rubin R, et al. Rubin's Pathology, 4th ed. Philadelphia: Lippincott Williams & Wilkins, 2005, p. 909.)

ages of 25 and 45 years and often present as a testicular mass. Many of these tumors demonstrate an isochromosome 12 and may release markers detectable in the serum, which allows for monitoring of relapses. The incidence of testicular tumors is highest in the countries Denmark, Sweden, and Norway, although no specific environmental risk factors have been identified. The only known risk factors to date include cryptorchidism and gonadal dysgenesis.

Testicular tumors include the general categories of germ cell tumors, sex-cord stromal tumors (nongerm cell tumors) and metastasic lesions to the testicles (Table 17-6).

Table 17-6
Testicular Tumors

Tumor	Frequency (%)	Gross Appearance	Histology	Immunostain	Serum Marker
Germ cell tumors	90				
Seminatous					
Seminoma	40	Solid, rubbery, bosselated	Nests, sheets of uniform cells Fibrous septa containing lymphocytes	PLAP	None
Nonseminomatous					
Embryonal carcinoma	5	Solid, cystic, necrosis, hemorrhage	Undifferentiated, atypical cells Large, hyperchromatic nuclei Prominent nucleoli	AFP, HCG	AFP, HCG
Teratocarcinoma	35	Solid, cystic, necrosis, hemorrhage	Foci of embryonal carcinoma Multiple somatic elements	AFP, HCG	AFP, HCG
Choriocarcinoma	<1	Solid, cystic, necrosis, hemorrhage	Syntio- and cytotrophoblasts	AFP, HCG	AFP, HCG
Yolk sac tumor	2	Homogeneous, white, mucinous	Cuboidal cells, eosinophilic foci of embryonal carcinoma, Schiller-Duval bodies	AFP, α1-AT	AFP
Mixed germ cell tumors	15	Hemorrhage, necrosis	Combination of germ cell tumors		

(continues)

Table 17-6
(continued)

Tumor	Frequency (%)	Gross Appearance	Histology	Immunostain	Serum Marker
Teratoma	1	Heterogeneous, cartilage	Collections of differentiated cells		None
Spermatocytic seminoma	1	Pale gray, soft, friable	Medium and small cells, giant cell globules		
Sex cord-stromal tumors	5				
Leydig cell tumors	60	Well-circumscribed, lobular	Cells resemble Leydig cells Uniform cells with round nuclei Cytoplasmic inclusions (Reinke crystals)		Testosterone, estrogen
Sertoli cell tumors	40	Well-circumscribed, small	Columnar cells in tubules or cords Fibrous trabecular background		None
Metastases	5				

Germ Cell Tumors

Germ cell tumors have been proposed to arise from malignant transformation occurring either during fetal development or during the peripubertal period, although the exact sequence of events of early carcinogenesis is currently unknown. Most frequently, germ cell tumors progress through an in situ stage, termed *intratubular testicular germ cell neoplasia* (ITGCN). Of note, certain testicular tumors do not demonstrate ITGCN (spermatocytic seminoma) and have therefore been hypothesized to arise via different developmental sequences. Figure 17-6 illustrates the pathogenesis of testicular tumors

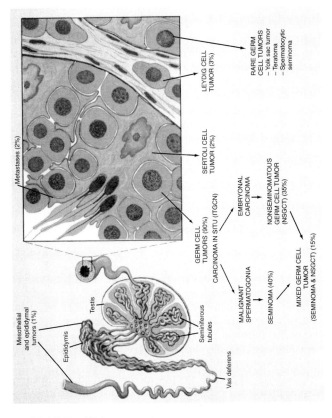

F I G U R E   17-6

Tumors of the testis, epididymis, and related structures. (From Rubin E, Gorstein F, Rubin R, et al. Rubin's Pathology, 4th ed. Philadelphia: Lippincott Williams & Wilkins, 2005, p. 912.)

Germ cell tumors are primarily separated into *seminomatous (SGCT)* and *nonseminomatous (NSGCT)* subsets. The seminomatous subtype includes the classic seminoma, whereas the nonseminomatous subtypes include embryonal carcinoma, yolk sac tumor, teratocarcinoma (malignant teratoma), and choriocarcinoma. A mixture of at least two histologic patterns is termed a mixed germ cell tumor.

In general, NSGCTs tend to grow more rapidly than SGCTs and have a greater tendency to metastasize. Seminomas are often readily cured by surgical excision and are extremely sensitive to radiation therapy. In contrast, NSGCTs require surgical excision, lymph node dissection, and adjuvant chemotherapy. The overall cure rate for patients with germ cell tumors is approximately 90%.

Intratubular Germ Cell Neoplasia (ITGCN)

ITGCN is an in situ form of germ cell neoplasia that may be present adjacent to an existing lesion or may be an isolated change within a testicular biopsy examined for infertility. Often, ITGCN is patchy, affecting 10% to 30% of the tubules. Microscopically, the affected tubules contain a thickened basement membrane and lack sperm. These tubules are filled with neoplastic germ cells that are larger than normal spermatogonia and contain large, centrally located nuclei with finely dispersed chromatin and prominent nucleoli and clear cytoplasm. These cells stain for placental alkaline phosphatase (PLAP).

THE PROSTATE

Prostatitis

Prostatitis may present as a variety of forms, including acute, chronic bacterial, nonbacterial, and granulomatous. *Acute prostatitis* occurs in the setting of a urinary tract infection when infected urine refluxes into the prostate. Patients with acute prostatitis present with fever, chills, perineal pain, and dysuria; occasionally, serum prostate-specific antigen (PSA) may be elevated. Microscopically, neutrophils are present within the prostatic glands.

Chronic bacterial prostatitis occurs in the context of repeated bouts of acute prostatitis or in the setting of prostatic calculi and duct obstruction. Patients present with dysuria and burning at the urethral meatus. Treatment of both acute and chronic prostatitis is by antibiotic administration.

Nonbacterial prostatitis is a diagnosis of exclusion. Typically, no organism is identified and no specific therapy is available. Similarly, in granulomatous prostatitis a causative organism is frequently not identified.

Nodular Hyperplasia of the Prostate (Benign Prostatic Hyperplasia)

Benign prostatic hyperplasia (BPH) is a common disorder that increases in incidence with age. The proliferation of glands and stroma that occur in BPH initially affects the transitional zone of the prostate (involving the submucosa of the proximal urethra) and leads to an obstruction of urine outflow (clinical prostatism). The pathogenesis of BPH is not understood, although the administration of sex steroid combinations in dogs appears to mimic BPH.

Patients with BPH often describe decreased intensity of the urinary stream and urinary frequency. Rectal examination identifies a firm, enlarged, nodular prostate.

Gross pathologic examination of the prostate in BPH demonstrates large, firm, centrally located nodules surrounded by a fibrous pseudocapsule. In large nodules that have outgrown their blood supply, hemorrhage and necrosis may be present. Microscopically, proliferation of acinar and ductal cells, smooth muscle cells, and stromal fibroblasts are identified in variable proportions.

The most common form of BPH nodule, the fibromyoadenomatous nodule, demonstrates variably sized hyperplastic prostatic acini that retain an overall lobular configuration. The epithelium is made up of a double layer of tall columnar cells overlying a thin, elongated basal cell layer. Often, the epithelium may demonstrate papillary hyperplasia. In addition, chronic inflammatory cells and corpora amylacea (eosinophilic lamellated concretions) are present. Other forms of BPH nodules include stromal, fibromuscular, muscular, and fibroadenomatous subtypes. Treatment of BPH may involve transurethral resection of the prostate or the administration of drugs that inhibit 5α-reductase (finasteride).

Adenocarcinoma

Prostate cancer is the most common cancer affecting men in the United States. The vast majority of men with prostate cancer are older 50 years of age, with 75% of patients between 60 and 80 years of age. The highest frequency of prostate cancer occurs in the United States and Scandinavia. Additional risk factors may include African-American race, increasing age, hereditary influences, endocrine effects, and possibly dietary factors, such as specific forms of dietary fat. Prostate cancer is often initially identified in patients by digital rectal examination or elevated serum PSA.

Prostatic adenocarcinoma appears to arise in many cases from intraductal dysplastic foci termed *prostatic intraepithelial neoplasia* (PIN). PIN describes prostatic acini lined by atypical epithelial cells with hyperchromatic nuclei and prominent nucleoli. The presence of a basal cell layer is maintained in PIN, in contrast to invasive carcinoma. The evidence that supports the likelihood that PIN is a precursor lesion to prostate cancer includes the peripheral distri-

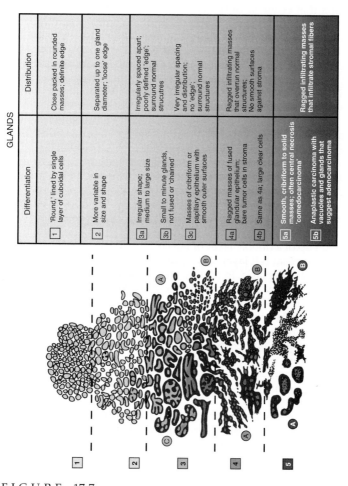

GLANDS	Differentiation	Distribution
1	'Round', lined by single layer of cuboidal cells	Close packed in rounded masses; definite edge
2	More variable in size and shape	Separated up to one gland diameter; 'loose' edge
3a	Irregular shape; medium to large size	Irregularly spaced apart; poorly defined 'edge'; surround normal structures
3b	Small to minute glands, not fused or 'chained'	
3c	Masses of cribriform or papillary epithelium with smooth outer surfaces	Very irregular spacing and distribution; no 'edge'; surround normal structures
4a	Ragged masses of fused glandular epithelium; bare tumor cells in stroma	Ragged infiltrating masses that overrun normal structures; No smooth surfaces against stroma
4b	Same as 4a; large clear cells	
5a	Smooth, cribriform to solid masses; often central necrosis 'comedocarcinoma'	Ragged infiltrating masses that infiltrate stromal fibers
5b	Anaplastic carcinoma with vacuoles and glands that suggest adenocarcinoma	

FIGURE 17-7
Prostate carcinoma. Gleason grading system. (From Rubin E, Gorstein F, Rubin R, et al. Rubin's Pathology, 4th ed. Philadelphia: Lippincott Williams & Wilkins, 2005, p. 922.)

bution of both lesions, the cytological similarity between PIN and prostate cancer, the close topographical proximity of high-grade PIN and invasive cancer, and similar molecular changes between the two lesions.

PIN is classified as low-grade PIN or high-grade PIN. Low-grade PIN demonstrates cellular crowding and overlap, variation in nuclear size, and the presence of nucleoli. High-grade PIN describes epithelial cells with more prominent cellular crowding, nuclear enlargement, prominent enlarged nucleoli, and decreased numbers of basal cells (identified by high molecular weight cytokeratin and p63 immunostains).

Prostatic adenocarcinoma (>98% of all prostatic cancers) is often localized to the periphery of the gland and is frequently multicentric. Grossly, prostate cancer appears as an irregular, yellow-white region. Microscopically, the majority of prostatic adenocarcinoma arises from acini and demonstrates small to medium-sized glands that infiltrate the stroma of the prostate. These glands are lined by a single layer of epithelium and lack a basal cell layer. Nucleoli are prominent. Prostate adenocarcinoma stains for PSA and prostate-specific acid phosphatase (PSAP), similar to the normal epithelium of the prostate.

Prostatic adenocarcinoma is microscopically graded according to the Gleason grading system, which is based on five histologic patterns of gland formation and infiltration. The Gleason score is the summation of the most prominent histologic patterns and is reported as such (3 + 4 = 7). When combined with tumor stage, the Gleason score has a prognostic value, with lower scores demonstrating a better outcome (Figure 17-7).

Local and distant spread of prostate adenocarcinoma influences the pathologic staging and outcome of patients with this disease. Commonly, perineural invasion is identified, which allows local spread of the disease. Other factors that influence local spread include invasion of the prostatic capsule and invasion of the seminal vesicles. The earliest metastases occur to the obturator lymph node, with subsequent spread to the iliac and periaortic lymph nodes. Metastases to the lung and to the spine, which induce prominent bony pain, may occur. Immunostaining for PSA and PSAP may help identify metastases that arise from a prostatic primary.

Treatment of prostate adenocarcinoma includes surgical resection (radical prostatectomy) for localized disease or radiation and hormonal therapy for patients with advanced or metastatic disease.

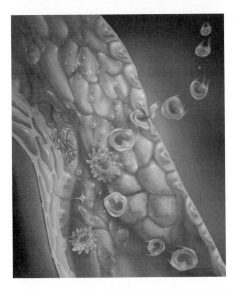

CHAPTER *18*

The Female Reproductive Tract

Chapter Outline

Development of the Female Reproductive Tract

The formation of the male and female reproductive tracts progresses similarly during the initial weeks of embryonic development. The wolffian (mesonephric) ducts, which give rise to the male reproductive organs, begin to form at embryonic day 25, whereas the müllerian (paramesonephric ducts), which give rise to the female reproductive tract, arise at day 37. The influence of a variety of factors in the male directs the evolution of the male reproductive organs:

- Testis-determining gene (Y chromosome): formation of seminiferous tubules
- Testosterone: produced by Leydig cells; converted to dihydrotestosterone; promotes the formation of the vas deferens, epididymis, and seminal vesicles from the wolffian ducts (day 70)
- Müllerian-inhibiting substance: produced by Sertoli cells; induce regression of the müllerian ducts

In the female embryo, lack of testosterone induces involution of the wolffian ducts (day 84). In general, the formation of the

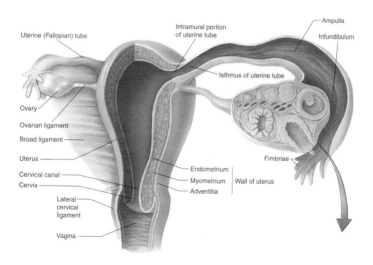

Female reproductive tract. (From Gartner LP, Hiatt JL. Color Atlas of Histology, 3rd ed. Philadelphia: Lippincott Williams & Wilkins, 2000, p. 342.)

female reproductive tract, completed by day 120, does not require the presence of additional influencing factors produced during the embryonic period (Fig. 18-1).

Sexually Transmitted Genital Infections

Bacterial Infections

Bacterial infections of the female reproductive tract often occur in combination and frequently present with vaginal discharge. The majority of bacterial infections are sexually transmitted diseases (Table 18-1).

Pelvic inflammatory disease (PID) is an infection of the fallopian tubes and ovaries that can cause acute salpingitis, pyosalpinx, and tubo-ovarian abscesses. Common organisms in PID include gonorrhea and chlamydia; most infections in PID are polymicrobial. Patients with PID present with lower abdominal pain and severe discomfort with manipulation of the cervix ("chandelier sign") during physical examination. Long-term sequelae of PID include rupture of a tubo-ovarian abscess, sterility, ectopic pregnancy secondary to scarring, and intestinal obstruction due to fibrous adhesions.

Table 18-1

Infectious Diseases of the Female Genital Tract

Organism	Disease	Diagnostic Feature
Sexually transmitted diseases		
Gram-negative rods and cocci		
Calymmatobacterium granulomatis	Granuloma inguinale	Donovan body
Gardnerella vaginalis	Gardnerella infection	Clue cell
Haemophilus ducreyi	Chancroid (soft chancre)	
Neisseria gonorrhoeae	Gonorrhea	Gram-negative diplococcus
Spirochetes		
Treponema pallidum	Syphilis	Spirochete
Mycoplasmas		
Mycoplasma hominis	Nonspecific vaginitis	
Ureaplasma urealyticum	Nonspecific vaginitis	
Rickettsiae		
Chlamydia trachomatis type D–K	Various forms of pelvic inflammatory disease	
Chlamydia trachomatis type L₁₋₃	Lymphogranuloma venereum	
Viruses		
Human papillomavirus (HPV)	Condyloma acuminatum/planum	Koilocyte
	Neoplastic potential	
Types 6, 11, 40, 42, 43, 44, 57	Low risk	
Types 16, 18, 31, 33, 35, 39, 45, 51, 52, 56, 58, 66	High risk	

(continues)

523

Table 18-1
(continued)

Organism	Disease	Diagnostic Feature
Herpes simplex, type 2	Herpes genitalis	Multinucleated glial cell with intranuclear inclusion bodies
Cytomegalovirus (CMV)	Cytomegalic inclusion disease	Bulbous intranuclear inclusion body
Molluscum contagiosum	Molluscum infection	Molluscum body
Protozoa		
Trichomonas vaginalis	Trichomoniasis	Trichomonad
Selected Nonsexually Transmitted Diseases		
Actinomyces and related organisms		
Actinomyces israelii	Pelvic inflammatory disease (one of many organisms)	"Sulfur" granules
Mycobacterium tuberculosis	Tuberculosis	Necrotizing granulomas
Fungi		
Candida albicans	Candidiasis	*Candida* species

From Rubin E, Gorstein F, Rubin R, et al. Rubin's Pathology, 4th ed. Philadelphia: Lippincott Williams & Wilkins, 2005, p. 930.

Gonorrhea

The causative organism in gonorrhea is *Neisseria gonorrhoeae* (gram-negative diplococcus), which causes an ascending infection of the female reproductive tract. Localized complications include purulent discharge, acute endometritis, acute salpingitis, and tubo-ovarian abscess. Systemic complications include septicemia and septic arthritis. Microscopic lesions demonstrate purulent exudates and granulation tissue. Diagnosis of gonorrhea is established by culture; treatment involves antibiotic administration.

Syphilis

Syphilis is caused by *Treponema pallidum* (motile, spiral-shaped bacterium), which enters the body at mucosal membranes or sites of skin abrasions. Interaction with the host immune system induces progressive stages of infection if untreated:

- Primary syphilis: chancre (painless, indurated papule, 1 cm to several centimeters) arising at site of infection after 3-week incubation period; persists for 2 to 6 weeks
- Secondary syphilis: occurs weeks to months postinfection; low-grade fever, headache, malaise, lymphadenopathy, macules on the buccal mucosa, palms and soles, macules on the genitals (condylomata lata/syphilitic warts); resolves after 2 to 6 weeks
- Tertiary syphilis: usually occurs months to years postinfection; nervous system and cardiovascular damage

Syphilitic lesions demonstrate plasma cell infiltration and obliterative endarteritis. When transmitted to the fetus, congenital syphilis may result in stillbirth, osteochondritis, rash, or fibrosis of the lung. Diagnosis is established by identification of the organism by Warthin-Starry stain or serologic positive titers for rapid plasma reagin test.

Granuloma Inguinale

Infection with *Calymmatobacterium granulomatis* (gram-negative, encapsulated rod) occurs via invasion of the organism through skin abrasions. *C. granulomatis* spreads by local extension with associated tissue damage and lymphatic invasion. The primary lesion is a painless, ulcerated nodule at the site of infection. Microscopically, vacuolated macrophages containing intracellular bacteria (Donovan bodies) are identified. The disease frequently recurs following antibiotic treatment.

Chancroid

Chancroid presents as single or multiple small, vesiculopustular lesions in the anogenital area 3 to 5 days following exposure. This infection is caused by *Haemophilus ducreyi* (gram-negative bacillus) and is most common in underdeveloped countries. Lesions often rupture to form a painful, purulent ulcer that bleeds. Patients may present with inguinal lymphadenopathy, fever, chills, and malaise. Microscopically, a granulomatous inflammation is present.

Gardnerella vaginalis

G. vaginalis (gram-negative coccobacillus) infection often presents with a thin, homogeneous, milklike discharge and a fishy odor following application of 10% potassium hydroxide. The organism does not penetrate the mucosa and biopsy specimens appear normal without inflammation. Diagnosis is established on a wet-mount specimen or Papanicolaou (Pap) smear by the presence of a clue cell, which is a squamous cell covered by coccobacilli. Gardnerella is often accompanied by other bacteria (polymicrobial) and referred to as bacterial vaginosis.

Mycoplasma

These organisms, which include *Ureaplasma urealyticum* and *Mycoplasma hominis*, are minute organisms that are commensals of the oropharyngeal and urogenital tracts and are spread via sexual contact to the genital tract. Microscopic evaluation of tissue appears normal. These organisms often occur in conjunction with other sexually transmitted diseases.

Chlamydia

Chlamydia trachomatis (gram-negative obligate, intracellular rickettsia) is a common sexually transmitted disease that results in severe inflammation of the cervix, occasionally complicated by an ascending infection of the endometrium, fallopian tube, and ovary, as well as acute urethritis and Bartholin gland abscess. Transmission to the fetus may result in conjunctivitis, otitis media, and pneumonia. Microscopically, metaplastic squamous cells demonstrate small perinuclear cytoplasmic inclusions. Diagnosis of chlamydia infection is by culture and treatment involves antibiotic administration.

Lymphogranuloma Venereum

The L form of *C. trachomatis* (serotypes L1 through L3) is endemic in tropical countries and is responsible for this disease. The initial infection presents with a small, painless vesicle at the site of infection that rapidly heals. Later, bilaterally enlarged, painful, inguinal lymph nodes may form that can rupture and form fistulas to the overlying skin. A chronic form may occur that causes scarring of the lymphatics, resulting in genital elephantiasis and rectal strictures. Microscopically, necrotizing granulomas and neutrophilic infiltrates are identified.

Viral Infections

Human Papillomavirus (HPV)

HPV is a DNA virus that consists of over 100 strains. Infection with HPV is common, occurring in approximately two-thirds of women by the time of college graduation.

Infection with HPV types 6 and 11 predispose to the formation of condylomata acuminata (genital warts) in the perianal and vulvar region. Condylomata appear as papules, plaques, nodules, or cauliflowerlike growths on the skin surface. Microscopically, a papillomatous proliferation of squamous epithelium demonstrating koilocytes (infected epithelial cells with perinuclear halos and wrinkled, raisinlike nuclei) are identified.

Infection with HPV types 16, 18, 31, and 45 predispose to the formation of low- and high-grade intraepithelial neoplasia. Although many cases of cervical dysplasia resolve, a small proportion progress to invasive squamous carcinoma of the cervix. Detection of these high-risk types may be performed by in situ hybridization on cervical biopsy or Pap smear specimens. Treatment of high-grade dysplastic lesions may involve excision of the affected cervix by curettage (loop electrosurgical excision procedure [LEEP]) or conization.

Herpesvirus

Following an incubation period of 1 to 3 weeks, infection with the double-stranded DNA virus herpes simplex type 2 (HSV2) leads to the development of multiple small vesicles in the anogenital region. These vesicles ultimately erode into painful ulcers. Following resolution of the lesions, the virus remains latent in the sacral ganglia, where it may reactivate under certain conditions. Microscopically, squamous epithelial cells demonstrate intraepithelial vesicles and large, lobulated nuclei with intranuclear inclusions. Immunostaining for HSV2 reveals the presence of virus in the specimen. Transmission of herpes to the fetus during delivery may result in death of the newborn.

Cytomegalovirus

Cytomegalovirus (CMV) is a double-stranded DNA virus that is ubiquitous and rarely causes genital infections in women. When present, infections may cause spontaneous abortion or infection of the newborn. Microscopically, CMV infected cells appear large with eosinophilic, intranuclear inclusions and occasionally cytoplasmic inclusions.

Molluscum Contagiosum

Molluscum contagiosum belongs to the poxvirus family and consists of a double-stranded DNA virus. Lesions often appear in the genital region, but may occur at other skin sites as well. These lesions appear as multiple, smooth, gray-white nodules that are centrally umbilicated and exude a cheesy material. Most lesions regress spontaneously, but some may persist for years if untreated. Microscopically, infected epithelial cells demonstrate large, cytoplasmic viral inclusions (molluscum bodies).

Protozoan Infection: Trichomoniasis

Trichomonas vaginalis is a large, pear-shaped, flagellated protozoan that causes vaginitis but may be asymptomatic in 25% of infected women. Symptoms include a heavy, yellow-gray, thick, foamy discharge associated with severe itching, painful intercourse, and dysuria. Diagnosis is established by wet mount preparation demonstrating motile organisms.

Nonsexually Transmitted Genital Infections

Tuberculous salpingitis and tuberculous endometritis occur secondary to hematogenous dissemination of *Mycobacterium tuberculosis* from the lungs. Within the endometrium, noncaseating, poorly formed granulomas are identified secondary to the rapid turnover of the endometrium during the reproductive cycle. Long-term sequelae include fibrosis of the fallopian tube and complications thereof.

Candida albicans, a common commensal organism in the vagina, may cause a clinically apparent vulvovaginitis presenting as vulvar itching and a white, cheeselike discharge. Physical examination reveals adherent white plaques in the vagina. Organisms are identified on wet mount or Pap smear. Treatment consists of topical or systemic antifungals.

Actinomyces israelii is also a commensal organism in 4% of women. Genital tract actinomycosis is found most commonly in association with the use of an intrauterine device (IUD), when the bacteria ascend to the uterus along the tail of the IUD. Infection with this organism may lead to extensive scarring of the female genital tract.

Colonization of the female genital tract by *Staphylococcus aureus*, often from the use of long-acting tampons, may lead to toxic shock syndrome. Patients with toxic shock syndrome present with fever, shock, and a desquamative erythematous rash. Additional symptoms include vomiting, diarrhea, myalgias, neurological signs, thrombocytopenia, and disseminated intravascular coagulation. If untreated, this disease may be fatal.

THE VULVA

Developmental Anomalies and Cysts

Anomalies of the vulva include:

- *Bartholin gland cyst*: obstruction of the mucoid outflow of the Bartholin glands may produce a cyst; infection by various organisms may lead to an abscess that requires incision, drainage, and antibiotics
- *Follicular cyst (epithelial inclusion cyst)*: lined by stratified squamous epithelium with a granular cell layer and filled with keratinaceous material
- *Mucinous cyst*: lined by columnar cells; may become infected

Vulvar Dermatoses

Acute Dermatitis

Acute dermatitis presents as reddened vesicles that ultimately rupture to form an overlying crust. Common causes of acute dermatitis include atopic (hypersensitivity) dermatitis and seborrheic dermatitis. Common causes of acute or chronic dermatitis include irritant dermatitis and contact allergic dermatitis. Microscopically, lesions may demonstrate inflammation and spongiosis of the epithelium as well as dermal perivascular lymphocytic and eosinophilic infiltrate and edema.

Chronic Dermatitis (Lichen Simplex Chronicus)

Chronic dermatitis may occur at an end stage of acute dermatoses, including lichen planus, psoriasis, and lichen sclerosis. Following chronic scratching of a pruritic lesion, the skin of the vulva becomes thickened, scaled, and white (hyperkeratotic), and demonstrates prominent skin markings (lichenification).

A specific subtype of chronic dermatitis is *lichen sclerosis*, which occurs in association with certain autoimmune diseases. Grossly, the vulva demonstrates white patches, atrophic skin, and contractures. Microscopically, the squamous epithelium demonstrates hyperkeratosis, loss of rete ridges, and a pale, acellular zone in the upper dermis under which a band of chronic inflammatory cells

are present. These women have a 15% chance of developing squamous cell carcinoma.

Neoplasms

Benign Tumors

The most common benign vulvar lesions include hidradenoma and
syringoma. A *hidradenoma* appears as a small, sharply circumscribed nodule on the labia majora and is a tumor of apocrine sweat
glands. A *syringoma* appears as a flesh-colored papule on the labia
majora and is an adenoma of eccrine glands.

Premalignant and Malignant Lesions of the Vulva

Vulvar Intraepithelial Neoplasia (VIN)

VIN is a precursor of invasive squamous cancer of the vulva and
in 30% to 40% of cases is caused by HPV. VIN occurs as a progression of lesions, categorized as VIN-1, -2, and -3, corresponding with
increasing severity of dysplasia (atypical mitoses, enlarged nuclear
size and nuclear atypia, loss of orientation toward the surface of
the epithelium). On physical examination, VIN appears as single
or multiple macular, popular, or plaquelike lesions, and may be
associated with lesions in other regions of the female reproductive
tract. Lesions of VIN recur in 25% of patients following excision.

Squamous Cell Carcinoma

Squamous cell carcinoma accounts for the majority (86%) of vulvar
carcinoma and occurs following progression of VIN. Two thirds
of these lesions appear exophytic, whereas the remainder appears
ulcerative and infiltrative. An early symptom is pruritus, which
ultimately results in ulceration, bleeding, and infection. Squamous
cell carcinoma spreads by local invasion and metastases to inguinal,
femoral, and pelvic lymph nodes. Factors affecting survival include
tumor size, metastases, and tumor grade.

A specific subtype of squamous cell carcinoma of the vulva is
termed *verrucous carcinoma*; this lesion appears large and fungating
on gross examination. Microscopically, the tumor is well differentiated, with maturing squamous epithelium producing keratin
pearls, and broad tongues of invasion with few mitoses. These
tumors demonstrate HPV types 6 and 11 (similar to condyloma
acuminata). They are treated by wide local excision.

Extramammary Paget Disease

Extramammary Paget disease occurs on the labia majora of elderly
women and appears grossly as a large, red, sharply demarcated
lesion. Patients frequently complain of vulvar pruritus or burning

for several years. Microscopically, these lesions generally demonstrate single, large cells with pale, vacuolated cytoplasm percolating through the epithelium. These cells are periodic acid–Schiff positive and stain by immunohistochemistry for carcinoembryonic antigen. This disease is rarely associated with metastatic disease and is often cured by wide local excision.

THE VAGINA

The vagina is a hormonally sensitive organ that responds to steroid hormone during the reproductive cycle and can undergo atrophy in postmenopausal women due to loss of estrogen. Benign and malignant conditions of the vagina are presented in Table 18-2. Malignant conditions of the vagina account for only 2% of all genital tract tumors and often present with vaginal discharge and bleeding during coitus.

THE CERVIX

The cervix makes up the lower portion of the uterus and is microscopically separated into the endocervix, which is lined by columnar epithelium, and the ectocervix, which is lined by squamous epithelium. The junction of columnar and squamous epithelium, termed the *squamocolumnar junction*, migrates with age and level of sexual activity. The distal portion of the squamocolumnar junction is termed the *transformation zone*, which is primarily examined in Pap smear specimens.

Cervicitis

Acute and chronic cervicitis occur secondary to infection with endogenous vaginal bacteria (*Streptococcus, Staphylococcus*) and sexually transmitted diseases (*C. trachomatis*). *Acute cervicitis* presents as a swollen, red cervix with purulent fluid extruding from the os. Microscopically, polymorphonuclear leukocytes infiltrate the cervical epithelium and stroma. *Chronic cervicitis* demonstrates a reddened (hyperemic) cervix with surface erosions. Microscopically, lymphocytes and plasma cells are present within the stroma and the epithelium demonstrates squamous metaplasia.

Benign Tumors and Tumorlike Conditions

Endocervical Polyps

Endocervical polyps are often single smooth or lobulated lesions less than 3 cm in greatest dimension that may protrude from the cervi-

Table 18-2
Benign and Malignant Conditions of the Vagina

Disease	Gross Appearance	Microscopic Appearance
Congenital anomalies		
Absence of the vagina	May be associated with uterine and urinary tract anomalies	
Septate vagina	Persistent median wall of vagina	
Vaginal atresia/imperforate hymen	Attenuation of the vagina with a persistent vaginal orifice membrane	Glandular epithelium lining the vagina
Nonneoplastic conditions		
Atrophic vaginitis	Thinning of vaginal epithelium; abrasions, secondary infections	Decreased thickness of epithelium
Vaginal adenosis	Red, granular patches on the mucosa; fetal defect caused by DES	Combination of mucinous columnar epithelium and ciliated cells with eosinophilic cytoplasm lining the vagina
Fibroepithelial polyp	Single, gray-white, polypoid	Connective tissue core lined by squamous epithelium
Leiomyoma	Submucosal firm nodule	Whorls of benign smooth muscle cells
Neoplastic conditions		
Squamous cell carcinoma	Ulcerating or polypoid lesion	Nests of invading squamous epithelium at various stages of maturation; adjacent vaginal intraepithelial neoplasia (VAIN) may be present
Clear cell adenocarcinoma	Mass on anterior vaginal wall; fetal DES exposure	Cancer cells with abundant clear cytoplasm, occasional hobnail cells are present lining glandular lumens
Embryonal rhabdomyosarcoma	Girls younger than 4 years; confluent grapelike mass	Primitive spindle cells with cross-striations in the lamina propria, round rhabdomyoblasts, myxomatous stroma

DES, diethylstilbestrol.

cal os. Patients often present with vaginal bleeding. Microscopically, endocervical polyps have a fibrovascular core and are lined by columnar epithelium with foci of squamous metaplasia. Excision is curative.

Microglandular Hyperplasia

This condition is typically asymptomatic and occurs via progestin stimulation with oral contraceptives and pregnancy. Microscopic analysis reveals closely packed superficial glands lacking an intervening stroma and demonstrating a neutrophilic infiltrate.

Premalignant and Malignant Lesions of the Cervix

Squamous Cell Neoplasia

Cervical Intraepithelial Neoplasia (CIN)

The development of squamous cancer of the cervix progresses through a distinct series of events termed *CIN lesions* that are primarily activated through infection with HPV, especially types 16 and 18. Precancerous changes occur predominantly within regions of the transformation zone that demonstrate squamous metaplasia. CIN often occurs in women younger than 40 years of age, although infection may occur at any age. HPV infection is considered a sexually transmitted disease and risk factors include multiple sexual partners and early age at first coitus.

The earliest change, termed *CIN-1* (also called low-grade squamous intraepithelial lesion [SIL]), is evidenced by koilocytes within the upper layers of the epithelium. Koilocytes, as described previously, demonstrate perinuclear halos (due to accumulation of viral particles within the cytoplasm) and a wrinkled, raisinlike nucleus.

Worsening dysplasia, categorized as *CIN-2* or *CIN-3* (both considered high-grade SIL/HSIL), demonstrate decreased maturation of the squamous epithelium, increased numbers of mitotic figures that extend above the basal cell layer, and decreased orientation of nuclei to the surface of the epithelium. In these lesions, it has been suggested that the HPV virus has integrated into the host DNA and suppresses the function of the tumor suppressor proteins p53 and Rb. Cellular changes associated with CIN progression are depicted in Figure 18-2.

CIN lesions are typically asymptomatic and are identified by colposcopy (acetowhite changes) and Pap smear during annual gynecologic examinations. At colposcopy, the altered blood vessels that are associated with CIN-2 and -3 (HSIL) appear as a mosaic or punctate pattern. Definitive diagnosis is established on biopsy.

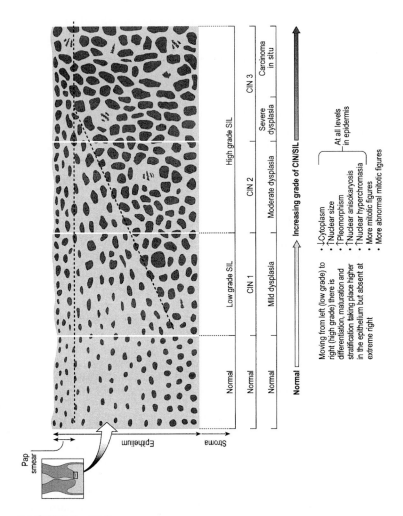

FIGURE   18-2

Interrelations of naming systems in preneoplastic cervical disease. This complex chart integrates multiple aspects of the disease complex. It lists the qualitative and quantitative features that become increasingly abnormal as the preneoplastic disease advances in severity. It also illustrates the changes in progressively more abnormal disease states and provides translation nomenclature for the dysplasia/CIS system, CIN system, and Bethesda system. CIN, cervical intraepithelial neoplasia. (Modified from Rubin E, Gorstein F, Rubin R, et al. Rubin's Pathology, 4th ed. Philadelphia: Lippincott Williams & Wilkins, 2005, p. 946.)

Difficult cases may require the additional technique of in situ hybridization for viral messenger RNA.

Approximately half of all CIN-1 lesions resolve spontaneously and are therefore followed conservatively. CIN-2 and -3 lesions more frequently progress to invasive squamous carcinoma and are therefore more aggressively treated by LEEP or cervical conization (excision of a cone-shaped wedge of cervix surrounding the os). Patients are subsequently followed by Pap smears and examination for vaginal or vulvar squamous carcinoma arising from latent HPV infection.

Microinvasive Squamous Cell Carcinoma

Microinvasive squamous carcinoma occurs in approximately 7% of specimens removed because of a high-grade SIL. Microinvasive squamous carcinoma demonstrates minimal invasion, with a depth less than 3 mm below the basement membrane and a maximum lateral extension of less than 7 mm. Patients are generally treated with cervical conization or simple hysterectomy.

Invasive Squamous Cell Carcinoma

Invasive squamous cell carcinoma is the most common form of cervical cancer (approximately 70% to 80% of cervical cancers). It is a major cause of death in underdeveloped countries, where Pap smears are not readily available. Patients often present with vaginal bleeding following intercourse or douching. If localized spread has occurred, hydronephrosis, hydroureter, renal failure, and bladder or rectal stricture may also be evident. More advanced stages may demonstrate lymphatic spread to the paracervical, hypogastric, and external iliac lymph nodes.

On gross examination, cervical squamous carcinoma may appear as a poorly defined, eroded lesion or as an exophytic mass. Microscopic examination reveals invasive nests of squamous epithelium, often with limited keratinization.

Screening for cervical squamous carcinoma is readily accomplished via Pap smear. The best prognostic indicator of patient survival is the clinical stage of cervical cancer, which considers depth of invasion and localized extension. Treatment consists of radical hysterectomy for localized cancer; radiotherapy is also used for more advanced tumors.

Adenocarcinoma

The second most common cervical cancer is *adenocarcinoma*, which accounts for approximately 20% of all cervical cancers. The mean age of presentation is 56 years. Lesions are often associated with the presence of the HPV types 16 and 18 and, occasionally, adjacent squamous cell lesions may be identified due to the presence of high-risk HPV.

Adenocarcinoma in situ, which demonstrates tall columnar cells with eosinophilic or mucinous cytoplasm, resembling goblet cells, is a precursor of invasive adenocarcinoma. On gross examination, adenocarcinoma appears as a fungating polypoid or papillary mass that demonstrates papillary, tubular, or glandular patterns microscopically. Extension of cervical adenocarcinoma is via local spread and lymphatic metastases. Treatment includes radical hysterectomy and possible radiation therapy.

THE UTERUS

Normal Anatomy and Histology

The uterus increases in size following puberty due to the influence of estrogen and progesterone. The endometrium comprises the zona functionalis (superficial two thirds) and the zona basalis (deep one third). The zona functionalis responds to hormonal stimulation and is shed during menses. The zona basalis remains and supplies the regenerating cells that reform the zona functionalis. The endometrium is supplied by basal arteries (zona basalis) and spiral arteries (zona functionalis).

The menstrual cycle comprises several phases, including the following:

- Proliferative phase: day 0 to 14; mitotic activity and pseudostratification of glands
- Secretory phase: follows ovulation; day 15 to 27; coiled glands, prominent luminal secretions, stromal edema, spiral arteries present
- Menstrual phase: begins day 28; spiral arteries collapse and necrotic endometrium (zona functionalis) is shed; lasts 3 to 7 days

Figure 18-3 describes the changes evident in the endometrium during the menstrual cycle. In addition, specific endometrial alterations may occur at other times. Following menopause, the endometrium becomes atrophic, demonstrating decreased numbers of glands, mitotically inactive epithelium and a collagenous stroma. During pregnancy, the endometrium becomes hypersecretory, demonstrating widely dilated glands lined by cells containing large amounts of glycogen. Stimulation during pregnancy may cause

Day of Cycle	Before 14	15–16	17	18	19–22	23	24–25	26–27	28+
Post-ovulatory day		1–2	3	4	5–8	9	10–11	12–13	14+
Cycle phases	Proliferative	Interval	Early secretory		Mid-secretory			Late secretory	Menstrual
Key feature	Mitoses	Mitoses and subnuclear vacuoles	Maximum subnuclear vacuoles	Subnuclear vacuoles present	Stromal edema	Focal decidua around spiral arteries	Patchy decidua	Extensive decidua	Stromal crumbling
Microscopic features of functional zone — Stroma	Loose stroma. Mitoses	Same as proliferative	Loose stroma. Scanty mitoses	Loose stroma	Stromal edema	Focal decidua around spiral arteries. Edema prominent	Decidua throughout stroma. Some edema	Extensive decidua. Prominent granulated lymphocytes	Stromal crumbling. Hemorrhage
Microscopic features of functional zone — Glands	Straight to tightly coiled tubules. Mitoses	Some subnuclear vacuoles, otherwise as proliferative	Extensive subnuclear vacuoles	Dilated glands. Some subnuclear vacuoles	Dilated glands with irregular outline. Luminal secretion		'Saw tooth' glands	Prominent 'saw tooth' glands	Disrupted glands. Secretory exhaustion. Regenerating epithelium
Appearances	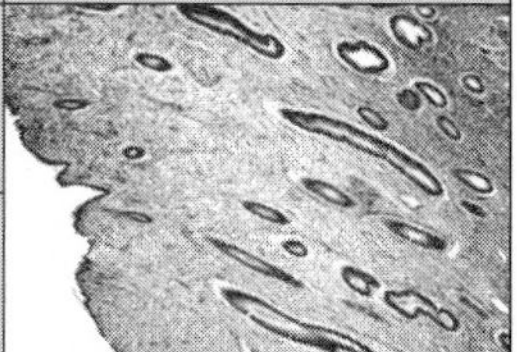 A				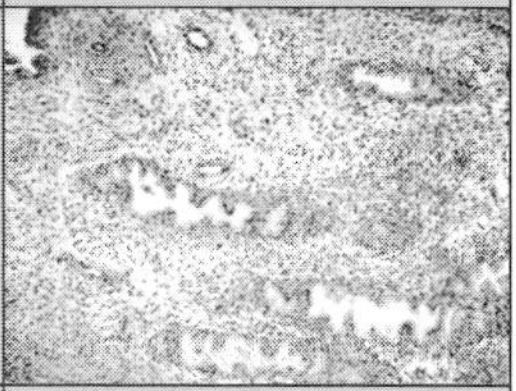 B			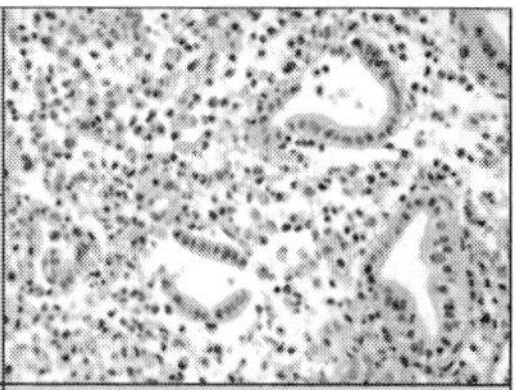 C	

FIGURE 18-3

Main histological features of the endometrial phases of the normal menstrual cycle. A: Proliferative phase. Straight tubular glands are embedded in a cellular monomorphic stroma. B: Secretory phase, day 24. Dilated tortuous glands with serrated borders are situated in a predecidual stroma. C: Menstrual endometrium. Fragmented glands, dissolution of the stroma, and numerous neutrophils are evident. (Modified from Rubin E, Gorstein F, Rubin R, et al. Rubin's Pathology, 4th ed. Philadelphia: Lippincott Williams & Wilkins, 2005, p. 952.)

endometrial cells to increase chromosome number without doubling, lending a distinct, hobnail cellular appearance with prominent, protruding nuclei termed an *Arias-Stella reaction*.

Contraceptive steroids, which also alter the endometrium, primarily comprise combinations of potent progestins and low-dose estrogens. Over time, endometrial glands atrophy, but can reconstitute following discontinuation of contraceptive therapy. Use of contraceptive steroids is associated with reduced rates of endometrial and ovarian cancer.

Congenital Anomalies of the Uterus

These anomalies are rare and include:

- *Congenital absence of the uterus*: failure of müllerian ducts to develop; often associated with other urogenital anomalies
- *Uterus didelphys* (double uterus): failure of the two müllerian ducts to fuse; often associated with a double vagina
- *Uterus duplex bicornis*: double uterus with fused common wall between endometrial cavities
- *Uterus septus*: single uterus with partial remaining septum
- *Bicornuate uterus*: single uterus with two cornua and a common cervix

Endometritis

Inflammation of the endometrium is termed *endometritis* and may be acute or chronic. Patients may complain of pelvic pain, vaginal bleeding, or both.

Acute Endometritis

Acute endometritis signifies the presence of polymorphonuclear leukocytes in the endometrium not associated with menstrual changes. Often, a nidus of necrotic tissue is present. Acute endometritis may be caused by an ascending infection of the cervix. Diagnosis is by endometrial curettage and microscopy. Treatment includes curettage and antibiotic therapy.

Chronic Endometritis

The finding of plasma cells within the stroma of the endometrium characterizes *chronic endometritis*. This disease may be associated with the presence of IUDs, pelvic inflammatory disease, or retained products of conception. Culture is necessary to determine an infectious etiology.

Pyometra

Pyometra indicates pus in the uterine cavity that may be secondary to cervical stenosis.

Adenomyosis

Adenomyosis describes the presence of endometrial glands and stroma within the myometrium of the uterus. Adenomyosis occurs in approximately 20% of women. Patients often may be asymptomatic or present with pelvic pain, dysmenorrhea, menorrhagia, or dyspareunia. Gross examination demonstrates an enlarged uterus with a uniformly thickened myometrium containing small, red, soft areas. Microscopically, the embedded glands contain proliferative or inactive endometrium surrounded by stroma. Adenomyosis is hormonally responsive, and lesions often regress following menopause.

Abnormal Uterine Bleeding

Abnormal uterine bleeding (AUB) describes excessive or reduced menstrual flow, or bleeding that occurs outside of the normal menstrual cycle. AUB may have intrauterine (leiomyoma) or extrauterine (coagulation abnormality) causes. Table 18-3 describes possible causes of abnormal uterine bleeding by age.

Dysfunctional uterine bleeding (DUB) is abnormal uterine bleeding that is not attributable to a distinct intra- or extrauterine cause; many cases occur secondary to endocrine disturbances. The most common cause of DUB is anovulatory bleeding, in which there is an absence of ovulation during the reproductive years. Lack of ovulation induces excessive and prolonged estrogen stimulation without a subsequent postovulatory rise in progesterone; this hormonal mismatch results in a continuously proliferative endometrium that appears disordered and fragmented with intermittent stromal breakdown and bleeding.

Tumors and Tumorlike Lesions of the Uterus

Leiomyomas

The most common uterine tumor is the *leiomyoma* ("fibroid"), which is an estrogen-dependent, benign smooth muscle neoplasm.

Table 18-3
Causes of Abnormal Uterine Bleeding (Uterine and Extrauterine) by Age

Age	Cause
Newborn	Maternal estrogen
Childhood	Iatrogenic (trauma, foreign body, infection of vagina) Vaginal neoplasms (sarcoma botryoides) Ovarian tumors
Adolescence	Hypothalamic immaturity Psychogenic and nutritional problems Inadequate luteal function
Reproductive age	Anovulatory Central: psychogenic, stress Systemic: nutritional and endocrine disease Gonadal: functional tumors End-organ: endometrial hyperplasia Pregnancy: ectopic, retained placenta, abortion, mole Ovulatory Organic: neoplasia, infections (PID), leiomyomas Polymenorrhea: short follicular or luteal phases Iatrogenic: anticoagulants, IUD Irregular shedding
Menopause	Organic: carcinoma, hyperplasia, polyps
Postmenopause	Organic: carcinoma, hyperplasia, polyps Endometrial atrophy

IUD, intrauterine device; PID, pelvic inflammatory disease.

From Rubin E, Gorstein F, Rubin R, et al. Rubin's Pathology, 4th ed. Philadelphia: Lippincott Williams & Wilkins, 2005, p. 956.

Leiomyomas commonly develop after age 30 years and frequently regress following menopause. These lesions are described by location within the uterus (submucosal, intramural, or subserosal). Although many patients are asymptomatic, some patients demonstrate a variety of symptoms:

- Bleeding: ulceration of the overlying endometrium in a submucosal leiomyoma
- Mass effect: interference with bowel or bladder function (rare)
- Pain: infarction may occur in a large leiomyoma

On gross examination, leiomyomas are well-circumscribed (but nonencapsulated), white-gray, firm, and whorled in appearance. Microscopically, interlacing fascicles of uniform spindled cells with elongated, blunt-ended nuclei with rare mitoses are identified. Rarely, malignant transformation may occur, leading to a *leiomyosarcoma*. Leiomyosarcomas often appear grossly similar to leiomyomas, but contains geographic necrosis, cellular atypia, and increased mitoses microscopically.

Endometrial Polyps

Endometrial polyps vary in size from a few millimeters to many centimeters and generally occur during the perimenopausal period. These benign growths often occur within the fundus of the uterus and may be single or multiple. Patients often present with intermenstrual bleeding. Microscopically, these polyps are superficially lined by endometrial epithelium. Their cores are made up of dilated glands surrounded by a fibrotic stroma that contains thick-walled, enlarged blood vessels. Approximately 0.5% of these polyps contain a focus of adenocarcinoma.

Endometrial Hyperplasia and Adenocarcinoma

Endometrial Hyperplasia

Endometrial hyperplasia reflects a spectrum of changes, often induced by estrogenic stimulation, that may ultimately result in endometrioid adenocarcinoma of the uterus. Causes of increased estrogen include:

- Anovulatory cycles
- Polycystic ovary syndrome
- Estrogen-producing tumor
- Obesity

Hyperplasia of the endometrium varies from simple glandular crowding to atypical gland proliferation. The presence of cytologic atypia is most important prognostic feature in endometrial hyperplasia. Types of endometrial hyperplasia include the following (Fig. 18-4):

- *Simple hyperplasia*: minimal glandular crowding, minimal glandular complexity, no cytologic atypia
- *Complex hyperplasia*: glandular crowding and complexity, no cytologic atypia
- *Atypical hyperplasia*: glandular crowding with back-to-back glands and cytologic atypia; used to describe either simple or

Simple hyperplasia   Complex hyperplasia

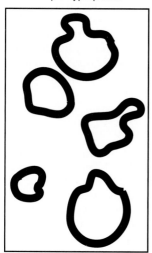 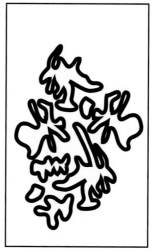

FIGURE 18-4
Simple and complex hyperplasia of the endometrium. Simple hyperplasia is characterized by cystically dilated gland containing pink secretions and no atypia. Complex hyperplasia is characterized by complex, budding, irregular glands.

complex hyperplasia although simple atypical hyperplasia is extremely rare

Endometrial intraepithelial neoplasia (EIN), a new type of endometrial hyperplasia, describes increased numbers of glands that occupy a greater proportion of the endometrium than the stromal component (measuring at least 1 mm in greatest dimension). A monoclonal growth, EIN is subject to malignant transformation. The majority of EIN lesions demonstrate loss of function of the *PTEN* tumor suppressor gene.

Treatment of endometrial hyperplasia may involve high-dose progestins or hysterectomy in women who do not desire continued fertility.

Figure 18-5 demonstrates the relation between endometrial proliferation, hyperplasia, and carcinoma.

Endometrial Adenocarcinoma

Endometrial adenocarcinoma is the most common gynecological cancer and occurs most commonly in perimenopausal and post-

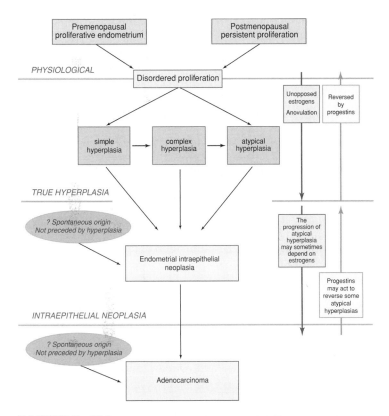

FIGURE   18-5
Relations among proliferation, hyperplasia, atypical hyperplasia, and carcinoma of the endometrium. (From Rubin E, Gorstein F, Rubin R, et al. Rubin's Pathology, 4th ed. Philadelphia: Lippincott Williams & Wilkins, 2005, p. 957.)

menopausal women. Patients with endometrial adenocarcinoma often present with abnormal uterine bleeding. Pelvic examination may be unremarkable or may reveal an enlarged uterus. Transvaginal ultrasound is used to detect luminal masses or thickened endometrial "stripes" (endometrial thickness) greater than 5 mm. Endometrial curettage is necessary for a preoperative diagnosis of endometrial adenocarcinoma.

On gross examination, endometrial adenocarcinoma may appear as multiple nodules that "carpet" the endometrium or appear as a polypoid growth protruding into the uterine lumen. Hemorrhage and necrosis may be present. Adenocarcinoma of the endometrium occurs as a variety of histologic subtypes, including endo-metrioid, serous, clear cell, and secretory.

The most common form of endometrial adenocarcinoma is *en-dometrioid adenocarcinoma of the endometrium*, which accounts for 60% of endometrial carcinomas. The remaining types of endome-trial adenocarcinoma include:

- *Serous adenocarcinoma*: epithelium appears similar to that found in the fallopian tube
- *Clear cell adenocarcinoma*: composed of large cells with copious cytoplasmic glycogen and cells with bulbous nuclei that pro-trude into the glandular lumens (hobnail cells)
- *Secretory adenocarcinoma*: cells with subnuclear vacuolization that respond to progesterone; most favorable outcome of all endometrial cancers.

Endometrioid adenocarcinoma of the endometrium occurs sec-ondary to increased estrogen stimulation of the uterus. Risk factors for increased estrogen include:

- Obesity: enhanced aromatization of androstenedione to es-trone in adipocytes
- Diabetes
- Nulliparity
- Early menarche
- Late menopause
- Family history of breast and ovarian cancer
- Hereditary nonpolyposis colon cancer syndrome

Protective factors include cigarette smoking (affects hepatic conversion of estrone to active metabolic forms).

Endometrioid adenocarcinoma of the endometrium is com-posed of glands containing atypical cells with pleomorphic nuclei, prominent nucleoli, and abnormal mitotic figures. This cancer is graded according to the International Federation of Gynecology and Obstetrics system, with worsening grade corresponding to areas of solid growth (Fig. 18-6). In certain instances, squamous epithelium may be present in these lesions.

Treatment of endometrial carcinomas involves simple hyster-ectomy if the lesion is confined to the endometrium. More ad-vanced cases require the addition of postoperative radiation.

Endometrial Stromal and Smooth Muscle Tumors

Endometrial stromal tumors account for less than 2% of all uterine cancers and may be composed of stromal components alone or a combination of stromal and epithelial components. Each compo-nent within the lesion is separately evaluated for cancerous trans-formation. A listing of stromal and smooth muscle tumors of the uterus is presented in Table 18-4.

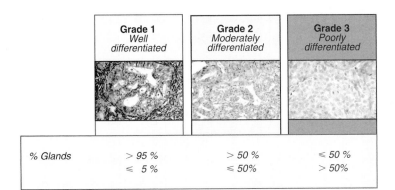

	Grade 1 *Well differentiated*	Grade 2 *Moderately differentiated*	Grade 3 *Poorly differentiated*
% Glands	*> 95 %* *≤ 5 %*	*> 50 %* *≤ 50%*	*≤ 50 %* *> 50%*

Significant
NUCLEAR ATYPIA
if present
increases the grade

Nuclear atypia
Round nuclei
Variation in shape and size
Variation in staining
Hyperchromasia
Coarsely clumped chromatin
Prominent nucleoli
Frequent mitoses
Abnormal mitoses

F I G U R E   18-6
Grading of endometrial adenocarcinoma. The grade depends primarily on the architectural pattern. but significant nuclear atypia changes a grade 1 tumor to grade 2, and a grade 2 to grade 3. (From Rubin E, Gorstein F, Rubin R, et al. Rubin's Pathology, 4th ed. Philadelphia: Lippincott Williams & Wilkins, 2005, p. 960.)

THE FALLOPIAN TUBE

Normal Anatomy and Histology

The fallopian tube contains different anatomical regions that extend from the uterus towards the ovary and include (respectively) the isthmus, ampulla, infundibulum, and fimbriated end. The fallopian tube is lined by ciliated cells that facilitate the passage of the ovum from the ovary towards the uterus.

Salpingitis

Inflammation of the fallopian tube may be acute or chronic. *Acute salpingitis* often occurs in the context of an ascending genital tract

Table 18-4
Endometrial Stromal Tumors

Tumor	Components	Histology	Clinical Behavior
Epithelial-stromal tumors			
Endometrial stromal nodule	Benign stroma	Expansile lesion; benign appearing stroma	Benign
Endometrial stromal sarcoma	Malignant stroma	Infiltrative lesion; spindled cells with scanty cytoplasm; highly vascular; cells arranged around blood vessels; nuclear atypia; minimal mitoses (low grade) or robust mitoses (high grade)	Malignant
Uterine adenosarcoma	Benign epithelium, malignant stroma	Polypoid lesion; proliferative endometrial glands and cellular, mitotically active stroma surrounding glands (periglandular cuffing)	Malignant
Carcinosarcoma (malignant mixed Müllerian tumor)	Malignant epithelium, malignant stroma	Infiltrative; atypical glands and stroma; may contain mesenchymal elements, bone, muscle)	Malignant

(continues)

Table 18-4
(continued)

Tumor	Components	Histology	Clinical Behavior
Smooth muscle tumors			
Leiomyoma ("fibroid")			
Intravenous leiomyomatosis	Benign stroma	Worklike growth within vessels; originates from leiomyoma or venous smooth muscle growth into vessels	Benign
Leimyosarcoma	Malignant stroma	Soft leiomyomalike growth, irregular borders; increased mitotic activity (>10 mitoses/HPF), geographic necrosis, cellular atypia	Malignant

infection caused by *N. gonorrhoeae*, *E. coli*, *Chlamydia*, or *Mycoplasma*. Patients with acute salpingitis are often asymptomatic, although pelvic inflammatory disease and peritonitis may occur.

Chronic salpingitis occurs following repeated episodes of acute salpingitis and may lead to severe complications due to chronic inflammation, fibrosis, and adhesions within the fallopian tube. Complications of chronic salpingitis include:

- *Hydrosalpinx*: watery fluid collection within a dilated fallopian tube
- *Pyosalpinx*: purulent material collected within a dilated fallopian tube
- *Tuboovarian abscess*: purulent inflammation of the fallopian tube and ovary
- *Ectopic pregnancy*: implantation of embryo outside of the uterine cavity

Ectopic Pregnancy

Ectopic pregnancy refers to embryonic implantation outside of the uterine cavity, such as in the fallopian tube and peritoneum. Approximately 95% of ectopic pregnancies occur in the fallopian tube. Ectopic pregnancies are caused by processes that interfere with tubal motility, including chronic salpingitis and endometriosis.

Patients with ectopic pregnancy often present with abdominal pain secondary to expansion of the fallopian tube and intratubal bleeding that ultimately extends into, and irritates, the peritoneum. The diagnosis is confirmed by elevated serum β-HCG levels and absence of an intrauterine pregnancy. This condition requires emergent treatment by surgery or methotrexate administration to prevent rupture and exsanguination into the peritoneal cavity.

On gross examination, the fallopian tube appears dilated. Microscopically, placental villi may be found within the lumen of the fallopian tube and cytotrophoblasts are identified invading the tubal wall. Often, a background of serosal adhesions is identified, suggestive of chronic salpingitis.

Tumors

The fallopian tubes are most commonly involved by metastatic cancers or implants from associated ovarian tumors. The most common primary fallopian tube tumor is the *adenomatoid tumor*, which arises from the mesothelium. This lesion is small, circumscribed, and demonstrates benign mesothelial cells surrounding slitlike spaces on microscopic examination.

THE OVARY

Normal Anatomy and Histology

The ovaries are attached to the posterior surface of the broad ligament, between the internal iliac vessels and the ureter. The ovaries have an outer cortex (epithelial surface, stromal cells, follicles) and inner medulla (blood vessels, fibroblasts). At birth, approximately 1 million primordial follicles are present, of which 15% persist to age 25 years. Only approximately 450 ova mature and are shed during a female's lifetime.

The maturation of the follicles occurs under the direction of luteinizing hormone and follicle-stimulating hormone from the pituitary, as well as the steroid-producing cells of the stroma, which ultimately form the theca interna and externa layers of the maturing follicle. Figure 18-7 illustrates the development and regulation of maturing female germ cells.

Cystic Lesions

The ovaries are most commonly enlarged secondary to cystic lesions, which include:

- *Serous cyst*: invaginated surface epithelium filled with serous fluid
- *Follicle cyst*: unilocular, thin-walled cysts filled with serous fluid and lined internally by granulosa cells and externally by theca interna cells; arise from ovarian follicles; may be luteinized; may cause precocious puberty or menstrual irregularities if filled with estrogen or progesterone containing contents; less than 5 cm in size
- *Corpus luteum cyst*: unilocular, yellow-appearing cyst filled with serous fluid or blood (*hemorrhagic corpus luteum cyst*); lined by large, luteinized granulosa cells; may cause menstrual irregularities due to progesterone synthesis; 3 to 5 cm in size
- *Theca lutein cyst*: multiple thin-walled cysts filled with serous fluid and lined by a luteinized layer of theca interna; often bilateral; caused by high levels of circulating gonadotropin (pregnancy, choriocarcinoma); surrounding ovary with edema and luteinized stromal cells; may replace ovarian parenchyma

Polycystic Ovary Syndrome

A relatively common syndrome that leads to multiple small, bilateral, subcapsular cysts in the ovary is *polycystic ovary syndrome*

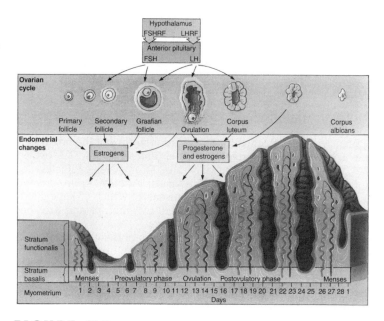

FIGURE 18-7
Normal ovarian histology and ovarian changes in response to hormonal stimulation. (From Gartner LP, Hiatt JL. Color Atlas of Histology, 3rd ed. Philadelphia: Lippincott Williams & Wilkins, 2000, p. 342.)

(Stein-Leventhal syndrome), which affects up to 7% of women. Patients may present with amenorrhea or, in extreme cases, also present hirsutism (excess hair growth) and obesity. Infertility is common in these patients.

The primary abnormality is proposed to be abnormal regulation of 17α-hydroxylase in the ovary (and possibly adrenal), leading to increased androgen production. An associated abnormality is an increase in circulating levels of luteinizing hormone, although it is unclear whether this represents a causative or secondary pathophysiological effect. Symptoms related to polycystic ovary syndrome are caused generally by increased androgens and increased estrone, as well as decreased progesterone (Fig. 18-8).

On gross examination, the ovaries of patients with polycystic ovary syndrome appear enlarged and with a smooth surface (lack of ovulation). On cut section, the cortex is thickened and contains numerous 2- to 8-mm cysts arranged around a dense core of stroma. Microscopically, the following features define polycystic ovary syndrome:

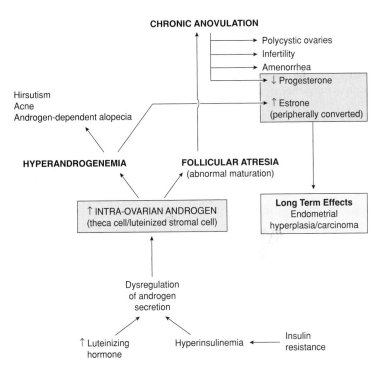

F I G U R E   18-8
Pathogenesis of the polycystic ovary syndrome. (From Rubin E, Gorstein F, Rubin R, et al. Rubin's Pathology, 4th ed. Philadelphia: Lippincott Williams & Wilkins, 2005, p. 968.)

- Numerous follicles in early stages of development
- Follicular atresia
- Increased stroma with occasional luteinization
- Lack of ovulatory signs (smooth capsule, no corpora albicans)

   Treatment primarily involves hormone therapy.

Stromal Hyperthecosis

This condition affects postmenopausal women and is caused by focal luteinization of the ovarian stromal cells. Consequently, patients often present with signs of virilization (malelike features such as increased hair growth and deepened voice). On gross examination, the ovaries appear enlarged and demonstrate a homogeneous, brown-yellow appearance. Microscopically, nests of luteinized stromal cells with eosinophilic, vacuolated cytoplasm are present.

Tumors

Ovarian cancers are the second most common group of gynecologic malignancies (following endometrial cancer) but account for the most cancer-related mortality of the gynecologic tract. The high rate of mortality from ovarian cancer often reflects late-stage detection of these lesions. The general cell types involved in ovarian cancer include:

- Surface epithelial cells (85%–90%)
- Sex cord/stromal cells (10%)
- Metastatic cells (3%)
- Germ cells (rare)

A summary of these lesions is presented in Figure 18-9.

Epithelial Tumors (Carcinomas)

Tumors of epithelial origin account for greater than 90% of ovarian cancers. These tumors most frequently arise from the surface epi-

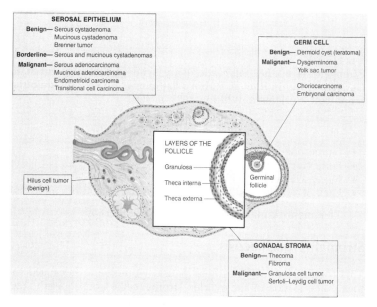

FIGURE 18-9
Classification of ovarian neoplasms based on cell of origin. (From Rubin E, Gorstein F, Rubin R, et al. Rubin's Pathology, 4th ed. Philadelphia: Lippincott Williams & Wilkins, 2005, p. 970.)

thelium (serosa) of the ovary, but may occasionally arise from intra-ovarian epithelial rests. Tumors arising from the ovarian serosa have been hypothesized to occur secondary to the increased cellular turnover of the surface epithelium that occurs following repeated ovulation. In support of this, ovarian carcinoma occurs more frequently in nulliparous women and less frequently in women on long-term oral contraceptive therapy or who have had multiple pregnancies. In addition, gynecologic irritants, such as talc, have been proposed to promote the formation of ovarian carcinoma.

A subset of patients also demonstrates a family history of ovarian cancer; women with a first-degree relative with ovarian carcinoma have a 3.5-fold increased risk of developing the same disease. Additional associations that have an increased risk of ovarian carcinoma include:

- *BRCA-1* mutation (17q12–q23): increased risk of ovarian and breast carcinoma
- Hereditary nonpolyposis colon cancer (NHPCC): increased risk of ovarian and colon carcinoma

The most common epithelial tumors, in order of decreasing frequency, include:

- *Serous* tumors: resemble epithelium of the fallopian tube
- *Mucinous* tumors: resemble mucosa of the endocervix (columnar) or colon
- *Endometrioid* tumors: resemble endometrial glands
- *Clear cell* tumors: resemble endometrial glands in pregnancy (glycogen-rich cells)
- *Transitional cell* tumors: resemble urothelium of the bladder
- *Mixed*

Table 18-5 identifies defining features of benign and malignant epithelial lesions of the ovary.

Serous and mucinous tumors are classified as benign, borderline, or malignant lesions. Borderline tumors, also termed tumors of low malignant potential or atypical proliferative tumors, demonstrate microscopic features that suggest cancer, yet these patients have an excellent prognosis. These lesions demonstrate unique chromosomal abnormalities that are not shared with classic ovarian cancers. Although these patients may demonstrate late recurrences, surgical cure is possible. Most borderline tumors occur in women between 20 and 40 years of age. Similar to their benign counterparts, borderline tumors may have serous or mucinous epithelium; however, borderline tumors differ in that they demonstrate:

- Epithelial stratification
- Nuclear atypia
- Mitotic activity

Table 18-5
Epithelial Tumors (Carcinomas) of the Ovary

Lesion	Age	Gross Appearance	Histology
Benign Lesions			
Serous cystadenoma	20–60 years	15–30 cm diameter; serous contents; commonly unilocular, bilateral	Single layer tall columnar epithelium; +/− papillary structures
Mucinous cystadenoma	20–60 years	15–50 cm diameter; mucinous contents; commonly multilocular, unilateral	Single layer columnar epithelium with mucin; +/− papillary structures
Brenner tumor	All ages; 1/2 > 50 years	Up to 8 cm; solid lesion	Solid nests of urothelial-like cells in a dense, fibrous stroma
Malignant Lesions			
Serous adenocarcinoma	40–60 years	Most common ovarian malignancy; unilocular or paucilocular; soft, delicate papillae; often solid areas with hemorrhage and necrosis; two thirds are bilateral	Papillary structures (well-differentiated) to sheetlike (poorly-differentiated); 1/3 with psammoma bodies; stromal and capsular invasion common
Mucinous adenocarcinoma	40–60 years	10% of ovarian cancers; multilocular (up to thousands of cysts); often solid and papillary regions; one-sixth are bilateral	Well- to poorly-differentiated; tall, columnar, mucin-producing cells; malignant features most common in solid areas; stromal invasion
Endometrioid adenocarcinoma	Postmenopause	20% of ovarian cancers; mostly solid with necrosis; 2–30 cm diameter; one-half are bilateral	Endometrial glandlike appearance; grade as endometrial adenocarcinoma; ↑ risk of endometrial adenocarcinoma
Clear cell adenocarcinoma	Postmenopause	5%–10% of ovarian cancers; partially cystic; solid areas with hemorrhage and necrosis; two-fifths are bilateral; 2–30 cm in diameter	Tubules or sheets of atypical cells with clear cytoplasm; protruding nuclei may form "hobnail" cells; often associated endometriosis

- Occasional microinvasion (less than 3 mm of invasion into the ovarian stroma)
- May have peritoneal implants and lymph node metastases

In general, the majority of ovarian carcinomas are hormonally inactive, but may produce the antigen CA-125. Serum CA-125 can be detected in 50% of patients with ovarian-confined cancer and up to 90% of patients with extragonadal spread.

Patients with ovarian carcinoma often present with advanced disease and symptoms that reflect the large size of the lesion (pain, pelvic pressure, regional organ compression). Ovarian carcinomas often spread by implantation into the peritoneum, diaphragm, paracolic gutters, and omentum and by lymphatic dissemination. Due to the frequent late-stage presentation, the overall 5-year survival is 35%. The most important prognostic factor is surgical stage.

Treatment of ovarian carcinoma is surgical, with adjuvant chemotherapy.

Germ Cell Tumors

Ovarian germ cell tumors may present at any age, although lesions in children are more commonly malignant than those in adults. Stages of differentiation categorize types of germ cell tumors, as demonstrated in Figure 18-10.

Ovarian tumors may present in a pure form or as a combination of different tumor types; care should be taken to categorize all components present within a lesion. One of the most common forms of ovarian tumor is the *teratoma*, which may be *mature* or

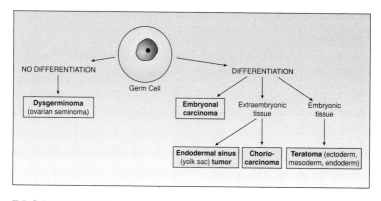

FIGURE 18-10
Classification of germ cell tumors of the ovary. (From Rubin E, Gorstein F, Rubin R, et al. Rubin's Pathology, 4th ed. Philadelphia: Lippincott Williams & Wilkins, 2005, p. 976.)

immature. Although both mature and immature teratomas demonstrate potential to form all three germ layers (endoderm, mesoderm, and ectoderm), the immature teratoma never demonstrates fully matured somatic tissue. In addition, immature teratomas frequently demonstrate immature neuronal tissue, seen forming "rosette"-like structures and having an increased likelihood of metastases.

In contrast, mature teratomas demonstrate mature somatic tissue, often as grossly identifiable hair and bone, and are typically benign. However, malignant transformation may occur in any tissue present (squamous cell carcinoma is the most common malignancy).

Table 18-6 summarizes the different types of ovarian germ cell tumors.

Sex Cord/Stromal Tumors

These lesions arise from either the primitive sex cords or the developing gonadal stroma and may differentiate toward male (Sertoli or Leydig cell) or female (granulosa or theca cell) elements. *Sex cord/stromal tumors* are generally benign or low-grade malignant lesions. These lesions are most common around or following menopause and are frequently hormonally active. A summary of sex cord/stromal tumors is presented in Table 18-7.

Metastatic Lesions

The vast majority of metastatic lesions to the ovary present as multiple, bilateral lesions. The most common sites of origin of tumors metastatic to the ovary include (in descending order):

- Breast (often small lesions)
- Large intestine (often large lesions)
- Endometrium
- Stomach

Krukenberg tumors are metastatic tumors to the ovary that demonstrate nests of signet-ring cells (mucinous cytoplasm with a compressed nucleus that resembles a signet ring) embedded in a cellular stroma. The majority (75%) of Krukenberg tumors arise from gastric cancer, and the remainder (25%) often arise from metastatic colon cancer.

THE PERITONEUM

Normal Anatomy and Histology

The peritoneum lines the peritoneal cavity and is made up of a single layer of cuboidal cells called *mesothelium*. In females, the

Table 18-6
Ovarian Germ Cell Tumors

Tumor	Age (years)	Gross Appearance	Histology	Other
Dysgerminoma	10–30	Large, fleshy, bosselated	Nests of uniform cells with clear cytoplasm and flattened nuclei; fibrous septa with lymphocytes (like seminoma in males)	Highly radiosensitive
Mature teratoma (dermoid cyst)	20–30	Cystic; may have hair, keratin, teeth	Somatic elements form ectoderm, mesoderm, endoderm (hair, skin, muscle, gut, bone, teeth); when thyroid tissue prominent = struma ovarii	Autofertilization of germ cell (46,XX); most are benign
Immature teratoma	<20	Solid, lobulated, small cysts	Immature (embryonic) somatic elements; primitive neuronal tissue with rosettes; immature glia	Metastases are often embryonal; survival correlates with grade
Yolk sac tumor	<30	Large with necrosis and hemorrhage	Multiple patterns; reticular, honeycombed pattern; Schiller-Duval bodies (papillae that protrude into space lined by tumor cells)	α-fetoprotein (AFP) detectable in serum
Choriocarcinoma	20–40	Unilateral, solid, hemorrhagic	Mixture of cytotrophoblasts and syncytiotrophoblasts; occasional bilateral theca lutein cysts	hCG detectable in serum; +/− precocious puberty
Gonadoblastoma	<30	Solid, extensively calcified	Nests of cells comprising germ cells and sex cord derivatives (Sertoli and granulosa cells); may demonstrate prominent dysgerminoma	Associated with gonadal dysgenesis; virilizing effect

Table 18-7
Sex Cord/Stromal Tumors of the Ovary

Tumor	Age (years)	Gross Appearance	Histology	Other
Benign				
Fibroma	All, perimenopausal	Solid, firm, white	Similar to mature ovarian stroma; fibroblasts, variable	May be associated with ascites (Meigs syndrome if ascites + pleural effusions)
Thecoma	Postmenopausal	Solid, yellow	Large, oblong to round cells with vacuolated cytoplasm (lipid); bands of hyalinized collagen	Estrogen production; risk of endometrial hyperplasia, cancer; irregular menses
Steroid cell tumor	Postmenopausal	Fleshy, yellow-brown	Cells resemble lutein cells, Leydig cells, adrenal cortical	Secretes weak androgens, testosterone
Hilus cell tumor	Postmenopausal	Small	Leydig cells, Reinke crystals in cytoplasm	Secretes testosterone
Low-grade malignant				
Granulosa cell tumor (adult)	Postmenopausal	Focally cystic to solid with yellow regions (lipid), hemorrhage	Various patterns (sarcomatoid, trabecular, insular); follicle-like formation of tumor cells around a central space (Call-Exner body)	Majority secrete estrogen: risk of endometrial carcinoma; may secrete inhibin; associated with oocyte loss
Sertoli-Leydig cell tumor	Childbearing age	Unilateral, lobulated solid, brown-yellow	Large Leydig cells (eosinophilic, round central nucleus), sarcomatoid stroma	Secretes weak androgens; large size required for

peritoneum is interrupted at the fallopian tubes, permitting agents from the female genital tract access to the peritoneal cavity.

Endometriosis

Endometriosis is the presence of benign, functional endometrial glands and stroma outside of the uterus. Patients often present between the ages of 20 and 40 years with symptoms of dysmenorrhea (intense pain during menstruation) or infertility (affecting one third of women with endometriosis). Endometriosis responds to hormone production and may regress following menopause, during pregnancy, or with oral contraceptive therapy. Endometriotic tissue commonly involves the ovaries, uterine adnexa, or occasionally distant sites such as the lung and bones. In approximately 1% to 2% of lesions, malignant transformation occurs, primarily in the form of clear cell or endometrioid carcinomas.

Theories that attempt to explain the pathophysiology of endometriosis include:

- Transplantation theory: most widely accepted theory; menstrual endometrium refluxes through the fallopian tube into pelvis; instrumentation may influence lymphatic and hematogenous spread to distant sites
- Celomic metaplasia theory: peritoneum or other serosalike structures may differentiate into endometrial tissue
- Induction theory: endometrial-derived substance induces endometrial differentiation at ectopic sites

On gross examination, endometriotic lesions vary in color from red to yellow-black, depending on the stage of blood (hemosiderin) metabolism. Black implants on the ovaries or serosa are frequently termed "mulberry" lesions. Over time, endometriotic lesions may scar and form fibrous adhesions, which can lead to complications such as intestinal obstruction. Within the ovaries, enlargement of endometriotic foci may lead to the formation of large cysts (up to 15 cm) filled with dark-brown hemorrhage, termed "chocolate" cysts.

On microscopic examination, endometrial glands and stroma are present. Often, surrounding hemosiderin-laden macrophages may be identified. Resolved foci may demonstrate only fibrotic tissue and hemosiderin-laden macrophages.

Tumors

Mesothelial Tumors

Mesothelial tumors are rare and include adenomatoid tumor, well-differentiated papillary mesothelioma, and diffuse malignant mesothelioma.

Diffuse malignant mesothelioma is one of the most common mesothelial lesions and arises in middle-aged to postmenopausal women. Symptoms include ascites, abdominal discomfort, digestive disturbances, and weight loss. Grossly, the peritoneum may appear thickened. On microscopic evaluation, the lesion demonstrates a tubulopapillary to solid pattern and commonly contains polygonal or cuboidal cells with abundant cytoplasm. The prognosis for patients with this lesion is poor.

Serous Tumors

Primary peritoneal tumors are commonly serous and are classified as serous tumor of borderline malignancy or serous adenocarcinoma. In all cases of a serous lesion, a primary ovarian lesion with secondary peritoneal spread must be excluded from the diagnosis.

Serous tumor of borderline malignancy appears as a fine nodularity of the peritoneum. Microscopically, papillary processes, cell stratification, detached cellular clusters, nuclear atypia, and mitotic activity are identified. Psammoma bodies are frequently encountered. Invasion is absent in this lesion.

Serous adenocarcinoma, in contrast to serous tumor of borderline malignancy, demonstrates more pronounced cellular atypia and invasion.

Pseudomyxoma Peritonei

Pseudomyxoma peritonei describes a condition wherein the pelvic or peritoneal cavity is filled with gelatinous mucin. The primary lesion in this disease is often an appendiceal adenocarcinoma. Microscopically, clusters of mucin-producing epithelial cells are present floating within a mucinous background. Treatment involves extensive surgical debulking and intraperitoneal chemotherapy.

THE PLACENTA AND GESTATIONAL DISEASE

Normal Anatomy and Histology

The development of the placenta begins when the fertilized ovum implants in the endometrium approximately 5 days after ovulation. The blastocyst gives rise to the three layers of trophoblast:

- Cytotrophoblast: small, mononuclear cells; germinative layer of placenta
- Syncytiotrophoblast: large multinucleated cells; produce hCG and human placental lactogen (hPL)
- Intermediate trophoblastic cells: mononuclear cells with eosinophilic cytoplasm; produce primarily hPL and minimal hCG

The chorionic villi of the placenta develop on embryonic day 21. The basic form of the placenta is formed by the fourth month of gestation, after which the placenta primarily increases in size.

The placenta consists of a placental disk, placental membranes, and umbilical cord. The fetus is in direct contact with the amnion, which consists of a single layer of cuboidal cells. Fetal blood enters the placenta through two umbilical arteries and exits via a single umbilical vein. The functional unit of the placenta that functions in fetal blood oxygenation is the terminal villus, which contains an inner layer of cytotrophoblast cells, a middle layer of intermediate trophoblast cells, and an outer layer of syncytiotrophoblasts. By the third trimester, the syncytiotrophoblasts have developed syncytial knots. Figure 18-11 demonstrates the normal placental structure and positioning of the fetus within the uterus.

Infections

Chorioamnionitis

Acute chorioamnionitis is an inflammation of the placental membranes that involves both the amnion and the chorion. Most commonly, the infection is caused by an ascending infection, often caused by premature rupture of membranes. Common organisms include *Mycoplasma, Bacteroides,* and aerobes such as group B streptococci. An increased risk of preterm labor, neonatal infections, and intrauterine hypoxia is associated with acute chorioamnionitis. At delivery, the placental membranes are thickened, yellow, and malodorous. The amniotic fluid is cloudy. Microscopically, neutrophils are identified invading the amnion and chorion. In more advanced cases, the umbilical cord may also be involved (funisitis).

Effects of acute chorioamnionitis in newborns include pneumonia, skin or eye infections, and neonatal gastritis or enteritis. Maternal complications include intrapartum fever, postpartum endometritis, and pelvic sepsis with venous thrombosis.

Villitis

Villitis reflects a hematogenous spread of organisms to the placenta, rather than an ascending infection as is the case with acute chorioamnionitis. Diverse organisms may cause villitis, including bacteria (*T. pallidum*), viruses (rubella, herpes), parasites, and fungi. An increased risk of fetal infection is present in cases of villitis.

Pre-eclampsia and Eclampsia

Pre-eclampsia and eclampsia are hypertensive disorders that occur during pregnancy, especially during the last trimester of pregnancy and in association with a first pregnancy. *Pre-eclampsia* is defined

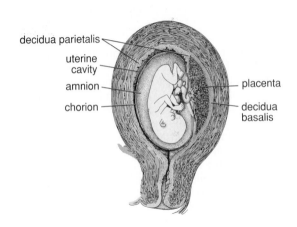

decidua parietalis

uterine cavity

amnion

chorion

placenta

decidua basalis

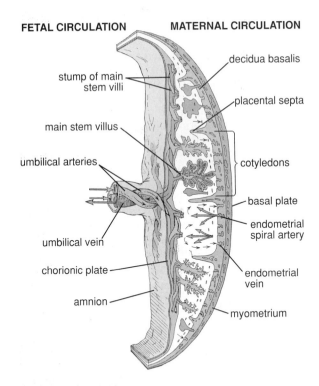

FETAL CIRCULATION

MATERNAL CIRCULATION

stump of main stem villi

decidua basalis

placental septa

main stem villus

umbilical arteries

cotyledons

basal plate

endometrial spiral artery

umbilical vein

chorionic plate

endometrial vein

amnion

myometrium

FIGURE 18-11

The developing embryo situated within the uterus and the structure of the placenta (From Ross MH Kaye GI, and Pawlina W. Histology: A Text and Atlas, 4th ed. Philadelphia: Lippincott Williams & Wilkins, 2003, p. 754.)

as a combination of hypertension, proteinuria, and edema. Often, disseminated intravascular coagulation is present. *Eclampsia* is a more advanced stage, characterized by the findings of pre-eclampsia in conjunction with seizures.

The pathophysiology of pre-eclampsia and eclampsia is complicated and may involve immunologic and genetic factors, as well as altered vascular reactivity, endothelial injury, and coagulation abnormalities. The proposed source of the underlying pathophysiology in this disease is the trophoblast, which fails to invade the maternal spiral arteries. Ultimately, failure of the spiral arteries to fully dilate leads to reduced maternal blood flow to the placenta and subsequent placental ischemia. The pathophysiology of these disorders is diagrammed in Figure 18-12.

The definitive treatment for these disorders is delivery of the placenta as soon as the fetus is viable. Prior to delivery, patients with pre-eclampsia are treated with antihypertensive and antiplatelet drugs. Patients with eclampsia are treated with magnesium sulfate to reduce cerebrovascular tone.

On examination, the placenta may demonstrate infarction and retroplacental hemorrhage (see following section). Microscopically, the cytotrophoblastic cells are hyperplastic and the basement membrane is thickened along the chorionic villi secondary to hypoperfusion. In addition, the spiral arteries may demonstrate acute atherosis (fibrinoid necrosis and accumulation of lipid-laden macrophages) and thrombosis.

Placental Abruption (Retroplacental Hematoma)

Retroplacental hematoma is an accumulation of blood between the basal plate of the placenta and the uterine wall. The most common causes of retroplacental hematoma include a ruptured maternal artery or a premature separation of the placenta from the uterus. In the absence of clinical hemorrhage, this condition is termed *placental abruption*. Risk factors include smoking, advanced maternal age, acute chorioamnionitis, and cocaine abuse. Retroplacental hematoma represents one of the most common causes of perinatal mortality (8%) due to placental infarction.

Abnormalities of Placental Implantation

The abnormal adherence of the placenta to the uterus, without intervening decidua, is described as placenta accreta, increta, or percreta, depending on the depth of invasion. In these instances, the placental villi are histologically normal, but separation from the uterus following delivery may be impossible. Complications of these disorders include hemorrhage, retained placental prod-

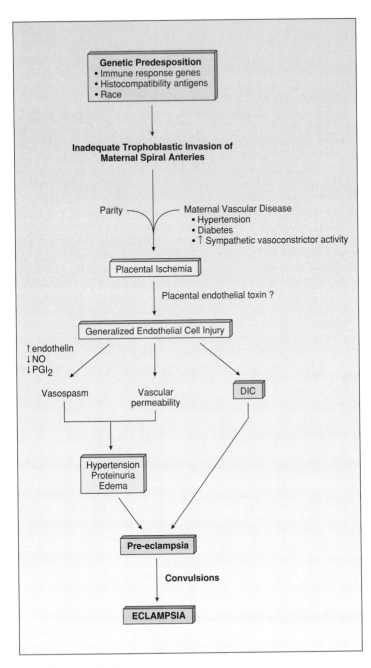

FIGURE 18-12
Pathogenesis of pre-eclampsia and eclampsia. (From Rubin E, Gorstein F, Rubin R, et al. Rubin's Pathology, 4th ed. Philadelphia: Lippincott Williams & Wilkins, 2005, p. 987.)

ucts, and uterine rupture. The types of abnormal implantation include:

- *Placenta accreta*: villi attach directly to myometrium without invasion
- *Placenta increta*: villi invade the myometrium
- *Placenta percreta*: villi penetrate through the entire uterine wall

Multiple Gestations

Multiple gestations occur in less than 1% of pregnancies. *Dizygotic twins* occur when two separate ova are fertilized, leading to two genetically distinct embryos that may be the same or opposite sex. Dizygotic twinning demonstrates a maternal hereditary tendency and may occur in women administered hormone treatment for infertility. Dizygotic placentas may be separate or fused, depending on the sites of implantation. Examination of the intervening membranes reveals a dual amnion and chorion (diamnionic, dichorionic).

Monozygotic twinning occurs when a single ova divides following fertilization. The embryos derived from this event are genetically identical and therefore the same sex. The time of ova division determines placental findings:

- Division within 2 days of fertilization: diamnionic, dichorionic
- Division between 3 and 8 days: diamnionic, monochorionic
- Division between 8 and 13 days: monoamnionic, monochorionic
- Division after 13 days: conjoined (Siamese) twins

Figure 18-13 summarizes gestational placentas.

Spontaneous Abortion

A *spontaneous abortion* refers to a natural termination of pregnancy prior to fetal viability outside of the uterus (<22 weeks). The overall spontaneous abortion rate is approximately 45%, with up to 30% of women undergoing spontaneous abortion without knowledge of a pregnancy. Underlying causes of spontaneous abortion include:

- Fetal congenital or chromosomal abnormalities
- Infection
- Immunologic factors
- Endocrine factors
- Uterine mechanical factors

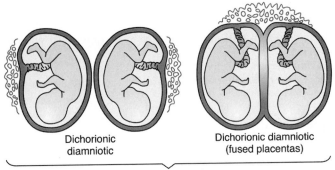

Dichorionic   Dichorionic diamniotic
diamniotic   (fused placentas)

13% monozygotic
56% dizygotic

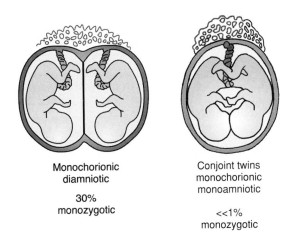

Monochorionic   Conjoint twins
diamniotic   monochorionic
                      monoamniotic
30%
monozygotic   <<1%
                      monozygotic

FIGURE 18-13
Placental structure in twin pregnancies. The percentages in the figure refer to the proportion of total twin pregnancies (100%) accounted for by each variant. (From Rubin E, Gorstein F, Rubin R, et al. Rubin's Pathology, 4th ed. Philadelphia: Lippincott Williams & Wilkins, 2005, p. 989.)

Gestational Trophoblastic Disease

Complete and Partial Molar Pregnancy

Molar pregnancies occur secondary to abnormal fertilization events, described below. Treatment of a molar pregnancy involves evacuation of the uterine contents by suction curettage and subsequent hCG monitoring. Complications of a molar pregnancy include uterine hemorrhage, disseminated intravascular coagulation, uterine perforation, trophoblastic embolism, and infection. The differences between these two entities are described in Table 18-8.

Invasive Hydatidiform Mole

Penetration of molar villi into the myometrium, whether superficially or deep, constitutes an *invasive mole*. Invasion into uterine veins leads to distant spread of molar cells, often to the lungs; however, these cells do not invade at the distant site. Microscopically, occasional hydropic villi and prominent trophoblast growth is identified. The ovaries may also demonstrate theca lutein cysts due to hCG stimulation.

Choriocarcinoma

Choriocarcinoma is a malignant lesion of trophoblasts that often presents with abnormal uterine bleeding or metastases to the lungs or brain. Choriocarcinoma may present years after the last pregnancy. Increased risk includes a prior history of molar pregnancy (50% of cases) and possibly Asian descent.

On gross examination, choriocarcinoma is markedly hemorrhagic. Microscopically, rims of syncytiotrophoblasts are found surrounding cores of cytotrophoblasts, with variable amounts of intermediate cells and associated hemorrhage. No true villous structures are identified.

Treatment of choriocarcinoma involves resection and administration of chemotherapy. Even with metastatic spread, survival rates are over 70%. Serial monitoring of serum hCG is used to monitor tumor recurrence.

Placental Site Trophoblastic Tumor (PSTT)

PSTT is the most common trophoblastic disease and is primarily made up of intermediate trophoblastic cells. Patients with PSTT may present with abnormal vaginal bleeding or amenorrhea. A preceding molar pregnancy is documented in only 5% of patients with PSTT.

On gross examination, PSTT appears as an ill-defined, yellow uterine mass without hemorrhage. Microscopically, monomorphous intermediate trophoblasts are identified invading the myo-

Table 18-8
Complete versus Partial Molar Pregnancies

Features	Complete Mole	Partial Mole
Karyotype	46,XX (paternal DNA)	47,XXY or 47,XXX
Pathophysiology	Fertilization of empty ovum	Fertilization of normal ovum by two haploid sperm or one diploid sperm
Maternal age	<15 years, >40 years	No association
Risk factors	Maternal age, Asian ethnicity, prior molar pregnancy	None
Symptoms	Marked vaginal bleeding, Enlarged uterus	Modest vaginal bleeding, Small uterus
Serum hCG	Very high	Less high
Gross appearance	Bunches of grapes (hydropic villi)	Focal grapelike structures
Microscopic findings	Cisterns in villi, cellular atypia Diffuse trophoblast growth No blood vessels in villi	Two villous populations: normal and with cisterns Focal trophoblast growth Blood vessels in villi
Embryo present	No	Sometimes
Nucleated erythrocytes	No	Sometimes
Persists after initial therapy	20% of cases	7% of cases
Choriocarcinoma risk	2%	Rare

From Rubin E, Gorstein F, Rubin R, et al. Rubin's Pathology, 4th ed. Philadelphia: Lippincott Williams & Wilkins, 2005, p. 992.

metrium, similar to that seen in normal placental implantation sites. No necrosis or placental villi are identified. The cells in this lesion are positive for hPL, but rarely hCG.

PSTT is generally a benign tumor, although rare lesions can metastasize and prove fatal. Risk factors for malignant transformation include increased mitotic rate and large tumor size. If the PSTT appears to demonstrate aggressive behavior, hysterectomy and chemotherapy are warranted. Serial monitoring of serum hCG is used to monitor tumor recurrence (short hPL half-life makes this a less useful marker).

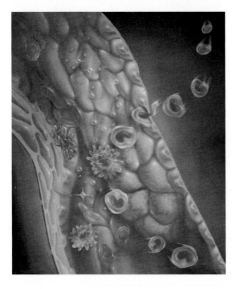

CHAPTER 19

The Breast

Chapter Outline

Normal Anatomy and Histology

The breast is a modified, hormonally sensitive sweat gland comprisingconnective tissue stroma, adipose tissue, a branching ductal

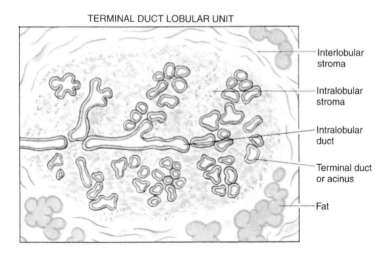

TERMINAL DUCT LOBULAR UNIT

Interlobular stroma

Intralobular stroma

Intralobular duct

Terminal duct or acinus

Fat

FIGURE 19-1
The normal terminal duct lobular unit. (From Rubin E, Gorstein F, Rubin R, et al. Rubin's Pathology, 4th ed. Philadelphia: Lippincott Williams & Wilkins, 2005, p. 1003.)

system, and terminal duct lobular units (TDLUs). The TDLUs are made up of the terminal ductules that differentiate into acini, intralobular collecting ducts, within a specialized intralobular stroma. Histologically, the terminal ductules are made up of an inner, luminal epithelial cell layer and an outer, myoepithelial cell layer, surrounded by a basement membrane. The intralobular ducts converge onto the intermediate and larger ducts of the breast that ultimately empty into the orifices of the nipple (Fig. 19-1).

Lymphatic drainage of the breast occurs via the lower pectoralis group of axillary nodes (75%) and the parasternal (internal mammary) nodes (25%).

Hormonal Control of Breast Development and Function

The breast undergoes maturation with development of TDLUs at menarche, when estrogen and progesterone levels increase. Hormonal changes also affect the breast during:

- Postovulation/luteal phase: increased number of terminal ducts within a lobule; vacuolated basal epithelium; edematous intralobular stroma

- Menstruation
- Pregnancy: increased number of terminal ducts such that the lobular units make up the majority of breast tissue; darkened pigmentation of the areola
- Lactation: vacuolated epithelial cells; duct lumens distended with secretions
- Postmenopause: atrophy of TDLUs; intermediate and larger ducts remain unchanged; increased fat content of breast

Congenital Anomalies

Accessory breast tissue may be found along the original "milk line," which occurs on the anterior trunk along the vertical plane of the nipple. *Inversion* of the nipple may lead to difficulties in nursing and must be distinguished from secondary inversion caused by breast carcinoma.

Benign Proliferative and Reactive Disorders of the Breast

Breast Hypertrophy

Breast hypertrophy is a clinical term that describes an increased breast size. Microscopically, this finding represents a benign hyperplastic change evidenced by increased numbers of ducts lined by hyperplastic epithelial cells and an expansion of the fibrous stroma (see "Fibrocystic Change"). In neonates, hypertrophy is caused by maternal hormones. During puberty, males and females may experience unilateral or bilateral hypertrophy due to hormonal changes. Secondary hypertrophy occurs due to abnormally high hormone levels produced by functioning tumors (ovarian, adrenal, pituitary).

Gynecomastia

Gynecomastia refers to an enlargement of the adult male breast with morphologic changes similar to that seen in hypertrophic breast tissue. This condition is often idiopathic and unilateral; there is no increased risk of breast cancer. Gynecomastia may occur secondary to increased estrogen or decreased androgen levels. Causes of increased estrogen production include the following:

- Exogenous estrogens: digitalis, opiates
- Hormone-secreting tumors: pituitary, adrenal
- Paraneoplastic syndromes: lung or liver cancer
- Metabolic disorders: hyperthyroidism, liver disease

Decreased androgen production may occur in the setting of:

- Inadequate testicular secretion of testosterone: Klinefelter syndrome, orchitis, castration
- Androgen insensitivity: testicular feminization

Acute Mastitis

Acute mastitis is a painful bacterial infection of the breast that occurs most commonly during lactation or involution. This condition is often caused by *Staphylococcus* or *Streptococcus* infection distal to a duct obstructed by secretions. Abscess formation may complicate this disease. Treatment includes hot compresses, antibiotics, and/or surgical drainage.

Duct Ectasia

Duct ectasia occurs in elderly women and demonstrates dilated intermediate and large ducts filled with pasty, inspissated material and macrophages. These ducts are commonly surrounded by chronic inflammation and, if they rupture, they are associated with a foreign-body giant cell reaction.

Fat Necrosis

Fat necrosis may occur at any age and is generally associated with trauma to the breast. Clinically, a firm, fixed mass may be present. On microscopic examination, early lesions demonstrate adipocyte necrosis and hemorrhage. Later stages are characterized by prominent macrophages and giant cells, as well as fibrosis. Due to the irregular, firm character of the mass and the occasional associated calcification, this lesion is often biopsied to rule out the possibility of breast carcinoma.

Granulomatous Mastitis

The formation of granulomas within the breast may occur secondary to silicone breast implants when silicone slowly leaks from the implant capsule or with mycobacterial infection. *Granulomatous lobular mastitis* is an idiopathic condition that typically affects parous women.

Fibrocystic Change

This condition is common, affecting up to 75% of women in the United States, predominantly between 30 and 55 years of age. Although most women are asymptomatic, symptoms may present secondary to the presence of a large, dilated cyst. *Fibrocystic change* affects the TDLUs and may be either proliferative or nonproliferative. Common features shared by both forms of fibrocystic change include cystic dilation of terminal ducts and a relative increase in fibrous stroma.

Nonproliferative fibrocystic change often occurs in multiple regions of both breasts and demonstrates the microscopic appearance of cystically dilated terminal ducts and increased dense, fibrous stroma. The cysts are lined by columnar or flatted epithelium. Apocrine metaplasia may occur in the cyst epithelium, which shows large, eosinophilic, granular cells with apical cytoplasm that protrudes into the lumen of the cyst. Occasionally, cysts become enlarged and filled with dark watery fluid, appearing blue on gross examination; these cysts are termed *blue-domed cysts of Bloodgood*.

Sclerosing adenosis is a form of proliferative fibrocystic change. Sclerosing adenosis is caused by a proliferation of small ducts and myoepithelial cells in the TDLU and is often accompanied by fibrosis. Microscopically, these lesions demonstrate a lobulocentric proliferation of small acini with central sclerosis. *Usual duct hyperplasia* is a common histologic finding in breast biopsies and is not identified by physical examination or radiography. On microscopic examination, usual duct hyperplasia appears as slightly dilated ducts filled with epithelial cells that form irregular, slitlike lumens within the main duct structure. These cells are polymorphous and cytologically identical to the normal epithelial cells of the ducts.

The fibrocystic lesions described in this section do not demonstrate a significantly increased risk for the development of breast carcinoma.

Neoplasms

Benign Tumors

Fibroadenomas

Fibroadenomas are the most common benign breast neoplasms and typically occur in women between the ages of 20 and 35 years. These lesions are usually solitary and are hormonally responsive, growing rapidly during pregnancy and slowing in growth following menopause. These lesions are derived from the TDLUs in the lobular stroma. Fibroadenomas pose no significant increased risk of breast cancer.

On physical examination, fibroadenomas are firm, mobile masses. Gross examination reveals a round, rubbery, sharply demarcated lesion that appears gray-white. Although these lesions are typically 2 to 4 cm in greatest dimension, they may achieve tremendous size and are then termed *giant fibroadenomas*.

Microscopic examination demonstrates primarily dense connective tissue with compressed epithelial elements that appear curved and slitlike. Occasionally, rounded ducts may be seen within this lesion.

Intraductal Papilloma

Intraductal papillomas are typically solitary lesions of middle-aged to elderly women that occur within the large, subareolar ducts. Occasionally, symptoms include a serous or bloody nipple discharge. Intraductal papillomas appear at low magnification as papillary projections attached to the duct wall by a fibrovascular stalk. High magnification reveals a luminal layer of cuboidal or columnar cells and an outer layer of myoepithelial cells. Intraductal papilloma does not pose an increased risk of invasive carcinoma.

In Situ Carcinoma of the Breast

Proliferative Ductal Abnormalities and Ductal Carcinoma in Situ

Proliferative ductal abnormalities of the breast include the following:

- Atypical ductal hyperplasia (ADH)
- Ductal carcinoma in situ (DCIS)
- Invasive ductal carcinoma (discussed under the "Breast Cancer" section)

Atypical ductal hyperplasia (ADH) demonstrates epithelial cells that fill the lumen of an intralobular duct and orient around "punched-out" appearing lumens within the lumen of the main duct structure (in contrast to the irregular, slitlike lumens in usual duct hyperplasia discussed previously). The cells demonstrate minimal atypia. ADH is distinguished from low grade DCIS by lesser size.

DCIS is best classified by nuclear grade. In *high nuclear grade ductal carcinoma in situ (DCIS)*, the terminal ducts are markedly dilated and are filled with cells that appear cytologically malignant, with pleomorphism, prominent nucleoli, and mitoses. DCIS is noninvasive (hence, in situ) and demonstration of a surrounding layer of myoepithelial cells and basement membrane is possible in these cases by immunostains. High grade DCIS often incites a prominent surrounding desmoplastic reaction. In contrast, *low-grade DCIS* is characterized by a monotonous population of evenly placed, uniform ductal cells, often forming "punched out" lumens, over an area of greater than 3 mm. Approximately 20% to 30% of cases of low grade DCIS progress to invasive carcinoma, whereas most high grade DCIS progresses to invasive carcinoma if untreated. DCIS may be identified by radiographic analysis if microcalcifications are present.

Multiple patterns of DCIS exist and are described by their architectural features; these forms include micropapillary, cribriform, solid, and comedo. The comedo type of DCIS is distinct in that the cells are large and pleomorphic and contain abundant eosinophilic cytoplasm, prominent nucleoli, and central necrosis.

Proliferative Lobular Abnormalities and Lobular Carcinoma in Situ

Lobular lesions of the breast include the following:

- Atypical lobular hyperplasia (ALH)
- Lobular carcinoma in situ (LCIS)
- Invasive lobular carcinoma (discussed under the "Breast Cancer" section)

Lobular lesions also involve the TDLU, although these epithelial cells appear smaller and more monotonous than those identified in ductal lesions. In addition, these cells have round, regular nuclei with minute nucleoli. The cells are dyscohesive and often have intracytoplasmic mucin vacuoles.

Atypical lobular hyperplasia demonstrates partial filling of the lobules with dyscohesive cells demonstrating minimal atypia.

Lobular carcinoma in situ (LCIS) appears as a solid cluster of cells within the lumen of the ductal and lobular structure, without the formation of new lumens. These cells are confined within the basement membrane of the lobule and contain an outer layer of myoepithelial cells. Occasionally, microcalcifications are present, though LCIS is usually an incidental finding. LCIS does not demonstrate a surrounding prominent desmoplastic reaction. Women with LCIS have an increased risk of developing breast cancer in both breasts.

Breast Carcinoma

Breast cancer is the most common cancer of women in the United States and the second leading cause of cancer death in women. In the United States, approximately 1 in 9 women will develop breast cancer at some point in their lives; one-third of them will die of the disease.

Etiology and Epidemiology

Risk factors that influence the development of breast cancer include the following:

- Family history of breast cancer in a first-degree relative (mother, sister): strongest association
- Increasing age: rare in patients younger than 35 years of age
- *BRCA1* gene mutation or deletion: tumor suppressor gene on chromosome 17; increased risk breast cancer before age 50 years; increased risk of ovarian cancer

- *BRCA2* gene mutation: tumor suppressor gene on chromosome 13; increased risk of ovarian cancer; increased risk of breast cancer in males carrying a mutation
- *P53* gene mutation in Li-Fraumeni syndrome: associated with brain and adrenal tumors in children; 90% of women develop breast cancer
- *CHEK2* gene mutation: interacts with the *BRCA1* pathway; doubles the risk of breast cancer development
- Increased lifetime hormone exposure: early menarche, late menopause, older age at first-term pregnancy
- Radiation
- History of prior breast cancer
- Dietary factors: increased fat ingestion (controversial)

Clinical Features

The detection of breast cancer may be made by monthly breast examination and annual mammography in women older than 40 years of age. Tissue diagnosis is established by core biopsy (in which a small needle is inserted into the mass) or by open biopsy. Findings that may indicate the presence of breast cancer include the following:

- Firm, immobile mass
- Inverted nipple
- Bloody nipple discharge
- Indentation or "puckering" of the skin
- Enlarged axillary lymph nodes
- Radiographic findings of an ill-defined, spiculated mass or calcifications

Pathology

In general, gross examination often reveals a spiculated, infiltrative, white, firm mass. Occasionally, enlarged lymph nodes may be identified in a resected axillary tail of breast tissue, suggesting the presence of metastasis.

Breast cancer spreads primarily via the lymphatic system. Some of the earliest lymph nodes affected include the axillary, internal mammary and supraclavicular nodes. The probability of lymph node spread is related to the size of the lesion. A "sentinel node" is the first lymph node drained by the lesion and is often surveyed intraoperatively for lymphatic tumor spread. Distant metastases may involve the brain, lung, liver, bone, adrenals, and skin.

Management

Treatment of breast cancer generally involves surgical excision with negative tissue margins. Small lesions may be excised by lumpectomy. Larger cancers are removed by modified radical mastectomy, which spares the chest wall muscles, and concomitant axillary lymph node dissection may be performed in instances of a positive sentinel node. Adjuvant therapy may include radiation therapy or chemotherapy. Patients may receive tamoxifen if the carcinoma is positive for the estrogen receptor or monoclonal antibody treatment if the lesion contains an *HER2/neu* amplification.

Factors that influence the prognosis of breast cancer include the following:

- Stage (I-IV) at diagnosis: stage is determined by tumor size, lymph node metastases, immobile lymph nodes (extranodal spread), and distant metastases; smaller tumors without metastases carry the best prognosis. Stage is by far the most important prognostic factor.
- Histological grade (I-III): breast cancers receive an Elston grade that encompasses degree of glandular differentiation, degree of nuclear atypia, and mitotic index. Lower scores reflect a better prognosis.
- Estrogen and progesterone receptors: the presence of these receptors indicates increased survival rates and may be used as a target for antiestrogen therapy
- Proliferative capacity and ploidy: increased proliferation and aneuploidy are associated with poorer prognosis
- Lymphatic and vascular invasion: associated with a poorer prognosis
- Oncogene expression: overexpression of *HER2/neu* due to gene amplification is an adverse prognostic factor; these patients may benefit from monoclonal antibody treatment directed against this gene product

Types of Breast Cancer

The vast majority of breast cancers are adenocarcinomas derived from the epithelium of the TDLU. The majority of breast cancers are either ductal or lobular carcinomas, and are preceded by a series of defined lesions. *Invasive ductal carcinoma* is the most common form of breast carcinoma. Additional types of breast cancer are discussed later in this section and in Table 19-1. The absence of a basal cell layer by immunohistochemistry can help identify invasive breast cancer in difficult cases. In a subset of cases, *Paget disease* of the nipple may occur, which often accompanies an invasive carcinoma and appears microscopically as single, large, atypical cells with clear cytoplasm that are present throughout the epidermis.

Invasive Ductal Carcinoma

Invasive ductal carcinoma contains malignant glandular cells that have invaded through the basement membrane into the stroma. Microscopically, invasive ductal carcinoma demonstrates irregular nests and glands made up of a single layer of malignant

Table 19-1

Breast Carcinoma Subtypes

Carcinoma	Gross Appearance	Microscopic Appearance	Prognosis
Ductal	Firm, white, irregular	Irregular infiltrating ducts, atypical cells, mitoses, desmoplastic stroma; microcalcifications	Moderate-poor
Lobular	Firm, white, irregular May be soft	Single columns of cells infiltrating stroma (Indian files); minimal desmoplasia; microcalcifications	Moderate-poor
Colloid	Glistening, mucinous	Small clusters of cells floating in mucin	Good-moderate
Tubular	Firm, white, irregular	Small, well-formed ducts of one cell layer; no cellular atypia	Good
Medullary	Well-circum-scribed Fleshy, pale gray	Sheet of pleomorphic cells with many mi-toses; surrounding plasmacytic infiltrate	Good-moderate
Metaplastic	Variable	Often admixed with other subtypes; formation of cartilage, bone, squamous epithelium	Depends on grade
Inflammatory	Irregular; skin with peau d'orange (erythema)	Dermal lymphatic invasion	Poor

epithelial cells. Cellular atypia, mitoses, and surrounding desmoplasia are common.

Rarely, invasive ductal carcinoma extends to the epidermis of the nipple and areola, leading to nipple ulceration.

Invasive Lobular Carcinoma

Invasive lobular carcinoma appears microscopically as single strands of epithelial cells invading the stroma ("Indian filing"). Desmoplasia is less prominent than with invasive ductal carcinoma. The cytologic features of these cells, including round nuclei, intracytoplasmic mucin and scant mitoses, are identical to those of LCIS.

Colloid (Mucinous) Carcinoma

This invasive carcinoma occurs in older women and appears grossly as a glistening lesion with a mucoid consistency. Microscopically, small clusters of epithelial cells are seen floating in pools of extracellular mucin. Patients with colloid carcinoma in its pure form have a better prognosis than ductal or lobular carcinoma.

Tubular Carcinoma

Tubular carcinoma is an extremely well-differentiated carcinoma composed of infiltrating small ducts formed by one layer of small, regular cells. Patients with tubular carcinoma in its pure form have an excellent prognosis.

Medullary Carcinoma

On gross examination, *medullary carcinoma* is well-circumscribed and has a fleshy, pale-gray appearance. Microscopically, this lesion appears as a sheet of pleomorphic cells with a high mitotic rate surrounded by a plasmacytic infiltrate. This lesion carries a better prognosis than usual invasive ductal or lobular carcinoma.

Metaplastic Carcinoma

A subtype of other invasive forms of breast carcinoma, *metaplastic carcinoma* demonstrates areas of squamous differentiation, spindle cell differentiation, or heterologous differentiation (into such substances as cartilage and bone).

Phyllodes Tumor

Phyllodes tumors occur as benign and malignant variants. These tumors represent a neoplastic proliferation of stromal elements accompanied by a benign proliferation of ductal structures. These lesions occur in women between 30 and 70 years of age, and patients often present with a breast mass.

On gross examination, phyllodes tumor is sharply circumscribed, firm, and the cut surface is glistening and gray-white. These lesions average 5 cm in greatest dimension. Microscopically, the stroma appears hypercellular and demonstrates mitoses. The stroma indents the epithelium to give a "leafy pattern." A *malignant phyllodes tumor* demonstrates a malignant transformation of the stroma into a sarcomatous component, which overgrows the epithelium and demonstrates local invasion.

Treatment of benign phyllodes tumor is by local excision. Malignant phyllodes tumor requires a wider excision but without lymph node dissection. Malignant lesions often recur, and 15% may ultimately metastasize.

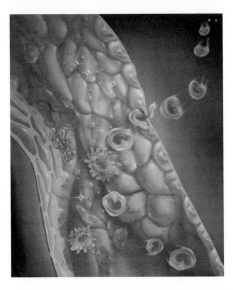

CHAPTER *20*

Hematopathology

Chapter Outline

Bone Marrow

Development

Normal Anatomy and Histology

Red Blood Cells

Normal Structure and Function

Anemia

Anemia Caused by Decreased Red Blood Cell Production

Anemia Caused by Ineffective Red Blood Cell Production

Anemia Caused by Increased Red Blood Cell Destruction (Hemolytic Anemias)

Anemia Caused by Acute Blood Loss

Polycythemia (Erythrocytosis)

Platelets and Hemostasis

Hemostatic Disorders

Blood Vessel Dysfunction

Platelet Disorders

Coagulation Factor Disorders

Hypercoagulable States

White Blood Cells

Neutrophil Abnormalities
    Neutropenia
    Neutrophilia
    Chronic Granulomatous Disease
    Chédiak-Higashi syndrome

Eosinophil Abnormalities

Basophil Abnormalities

Monocyte Abnormalities

Langerhans Cell Histiocytosis

Mast Cell Abnormalities

Techniques in the Diagnosis of Myeloid and Leukemic Disorders

Leukemias and Myelodysplastic Syndromes
    Chronic Myeloproliferative Diseases
    Myelodysplastic Syndromes
    Acute Myeloid Leukemia

Lymphopoietic System

Lymphoid Cells

Lymph Nodes

Reactive Alterations in the Lymphopoietic System
    Lymphocytosis
    Plasmacytosis
    Lymphocytopenia
    Lymph Node Hyperplasia
    Sinus Histiocytosis
    Infection-induced Hemophagocytic Syndrome

Malignant Lymphomas
    Precursor B-cell Neoplasms
    Precursor T-cell Neoplasms
    Mature (Peripheral) B-cell Lymphomas
    Mature T-cell and NK-cell Lymphomas
    Hodgkin Lymphoma
    Posttransplant Lymphoproliferative Disorder

The Spleen

The Thymus

Hyperplasia

Thymic Tumors

The development of normal hematopoietic elements is a complex process that involves numerous organs, including the bone marrow, lymph nodes, thymus, spleen, and mucosal-associated lymphoid tissues. Furthermore, the correct maturation and activation of these elements can occur at various sites throughout the body and involves many cell types. Dysregulation at any of these steps can lead to disease.

BONE MARROW

Development

The earliest hematopoiesis occurs in the fetal yolk sac. By the third week of embryogenesis, hematopoiesis shifts to the liver and spleen and persists in these organs until birth. In neonates and adults, hematopoiesis occurs in the bone marrow, primarily in the vertebrae, sternum, and ribs. In cases of hematologic malignancies that involve and replace the bone marrow, the formation of hematopoietic elements may take place outside of the bone marrow, termed *extramedullary hematopoiesis*.

Normal Anatomy and Histology

The bone marrow is situated between thin trabeculae of cancellous bone and is composed of a network of cords (containing hematopoietic elements and stroma) and sinuses. The marrow cords and sinuses are separated by semipermeable endothelial cells, a thin basement membrane, and reticular adventitial cells that aid in the support and development of maturing hematopoietic elements (Fig. 20-1). With increasing age, the marrow is gradually replaced by adipose tissue, leading to the appearance of "yellow" marrow, in contrast to the hematopoietic-rich "red" marrow of younger persons. A general rule that is useful for calculating the percentage of the bone marrow filled by hematopoietic elements is 100 minus age in years.

The development of hematopoietic elements involves differentiation of self-renewing, pluripotent stem cells in the bone marrow into mature, terminally differentiated elements in the blood. Activation of subsets of cells within the blood, such as monocytes or lymphocytes, can lead to further specification of cellular function in peripheral tissues.

Elements of the bone marrow include the following:

- Stem cells: self-renewing; pluripotential or multipotential; small mononuclear cells difficult to identify morphologically; can form colony-forming units (CFUs) when injected into irradiated mice
- Progenitor cells: limited self-renewal capacity; unipotential; small- to medium-sized mononuclear cells difficult to identify

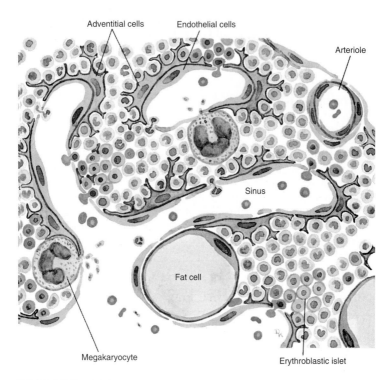

F I G U R E   20-1
Structure of normal bone marrow. (From Rubin E, Gorstein F, Rubin R, et al. Rubin's Pathology, 4th ed. Philadelphia: Lippincott Williams & Wilkins, 2005, p. 1021.)

morphologically; can form CFUs when injected into irradiated mice

- Precursor cells ("blasts"): no capacity for self-renewal; nearly fully differentiated; cells are recognizable as specific early hematopoietic elements

The *precursor cells* identified in the bone marrow are primarily four types:

- Erythroid precursor cell/proerythroblast/pronormoblast: large cell with intense blue cytoplasm, round homogenous nucleus, few nucleoli; matures through several stages, including the following:
  - ➤ Basophilic erythroblast: lacks nucleoli
  - ➤ Polychromatic erythroblast: gray cytoplasm and nucleus with coarsely clumped chromatin

> ➤ Orthochromatic erythroblast: red hemoglobin-containing cytoplasm and dense pyknotic nuclei
> ➤ Reticulocyte: non-nucleated cell with cytoplasmic polyribosomes; last step before a mature red blood cell

- Granulocytic precursor cell/myeloblast: round to oval nucleus with delicate chromatin and blue-gray cytoplasm; precursor to neutrophils, basophils, and eosinophils; matures through several stages, including the following:

> ➤ Promyelocyte: development of primary cytoplasmic granules
> ➤ Specific precursor: development of specific granules and nuclear lobation

- Monocytic precursor cell
- Megakaryocytic precursor cell

Figure 20-2 illustrates the development of the hematopoietic lineage within the bone marrow.

The bone marrow is examined by bone marrow biopsy and aspiration, commonly from the posterior iliac crest. The bone marrow obtained is assessed for cellularity (percentage of hematopoietic elements within the marrow space), myeloid (gametocyte) to erythroid ratio, and number of cellular components. The normal values determined on adult biopsy are presented in Table 20-1.

A variety of growth factors influence the components of the bone marrow:

- Interleukin-1 (IL-1), IL-3, IL-6, IL-11, and stem cell factor (SCF): Support survival and proliferation of stem cells
- Erythropoietin: promotes the early growth of erythroid progenitor cells and the transformation of late erythroid progenitor cells to erythroblasts; produced by the kidney in response to hypoxia
- Thrombopoietin: promotes the production and maturation of megakaryocytes

A brief summary of the function of mature hematopoietic elements is described in the following.

Lymphocyte, erythrocyte, and monocyte functions are discussed in further detail in this chapter; however, the following presents a summary:

- Erythrocyte: Carries oxygen to tissue
- Platelets: aid in blood clotting
- Monocyte: activated peripherally transform into mononuclear phagocytes (i.e., alveolar macrophages) and immunoregulator effector cells (i.e., Langerhans cells)
- Neutrophils: pink, finely granulated cytoplasm; react to microorganisms

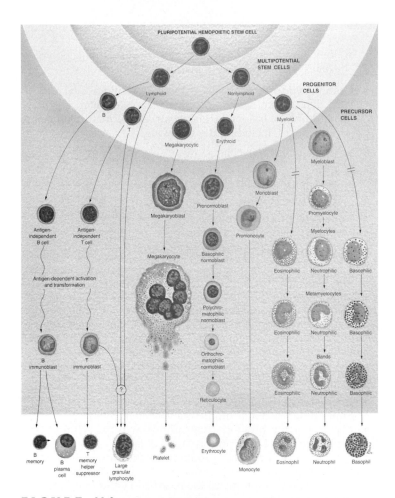

FIGURE 20-2
Cellular differentiation and maturation of the lymphoid (left) and myeloid (right) components of the hematopoietic system. Only the precursor cells (blasts and maturing cells) are identifiable by light microscopic evaluation of the bone marrow. (From Rubin E, Gorstein F, Rubin R, et al. Rubin's Pathology, 4th ed. Philadelphia: Lippincott Williams & Wilkins, 2005, p. 1018.)

Table 20-1	
Normal Adult Bone Marrow (Age 18–70 years)	
Fat-to-cell ratio, 50:50 ± 15%	Megalokaryocytes, 2–5/high-power field
Myeloid-to-erythroid ratio, 2:1 to 7:1	Plasma cells, <3% of nucleated cells

Cell distribution (percent surface area)
  Fat cells, 35%–65%
  Erythroid series, 10%–20%
  Granulocytic (myeloid) series, 40%–65%
	Lymphocytes, <20% of nucleated cells
	
	No fibrosis

From Rubin E, Gorstein F, Rubin R, et al. Rubin's Pathology, 4th ed. Philadelphia: Lippincott Williams & Wilkins, 2005, p. 1025.

- Eosinophils: large, red cytoplasmic granules; react to parasites and allergens
- Basophils: prominent blue-black cytoplasmic granules that contain histamine; participate in certain allergic disorders
- Lymphocytes: B and T cells that participate in host immune defense

RED BLOOD CELLS

Normal Structure and Function

Red blood cells are nonnucleated, deformable cells that transport oxygen to tissues. The red hue imparted by Wright-stained specimens reflects the presence of hemoglobin within the cell. The central pallor of these cells is caused by the biconcave shape of the cell. Red blood cells are released from the bone marrow as reticulocytes, which are larger than mature red blood cells and contain a basophilic gray cytoplasm that results from the residual presence of cytoplasmic ribosomes.

The cytoskeleton of the red blood cell is formed by a network of spectrin dimers, ankyrin, actin, and band 4.1, which allows the red blood cell to deform and pass through narrow capillary spaces. Some membrane proteins contain specific carbohydrate groups, which serve as the basis for the formation of red cell antigen groups (Fig. 20-3).

Because of the lack of prominent cytoplasmic organelles, red blood cells use the anaerobic pathway, primarily the glycolytic

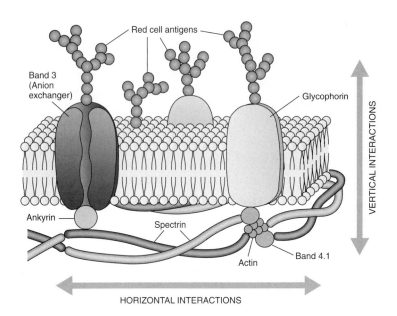

F I G U R E   20-3

Structure of the erythrocyte plasma membrane. The membrane is stabilized by a number of interactions. The two vertical interactions are spectrum-ankyrin–band 3 and spectrin-protein 4.1–glycophorin. The two horizontal interactions are spectrin heterodimer assembly and spectrin-actin–protein 4.1. (From Rubin E, Gorstein F, Rubin R, et al. Rubin's Pathology, 4th ed. Philadelphia: Lippincott Williams & Wilkins, 2005, p. 1027.)

pathway, as a source of energy. Red blood cells use the hexose monophosphate shunt to obtain the additional metabolic energy they need.

The majority of the red blood cell cytoplasm is hemoglobin. Hemoglobin is composed of four globin chains (generally two alpha and two beta chains), four heme groups, and up to four molecules of oxygen. The heme portion of the molecule is a porphyrin ring (protoporphyrin IX) into which a ferrous iron atom (Fe^{2+}) has been inserted. Each heme portion interacts with a hydrophobic pocket of one of the globin chains. The saturation of the hemoglobin molecule is influenced by oxygen tension (Fig. 20-4). Deoxygenated hemoglobin has a low oxygen affinity and requires increased oxygen tension for oxygen binding to occur. When aninitial oxygen molecule binds, the hemoglobin molecule undergoes a conformational change to more readily bind addi-

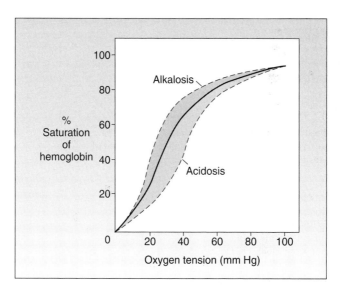

F I G U R E   20-4
Oxygen dissociation curve of hemoglobin. With decreasing pH (acidosis) the oxygen affinity declines (shifts right); with increasing pH (alkalosis) the affinity increases (shifts left). (From Rubin E, Gorstein F, Rubin R, et al. Rubin's Pathology, 4th ed. Philadelphia: Lippincott Williams & Wilkins, 2005, p. 1027.)

tional molecules of hemoglobin (up to four). This progressive increase in oxygen affinity results in the S-shaped binding curve shown below. The overall slope of this curve can be altered by acidosis or increased 2,3-DPG levels (right shift, more readily releases oxygen at tissues) or alkalosis (left shift, more tightly binds oxygen).

The average life span of a red blood cell is 120 days. Analysis of red blood cell parameters includes evaluation of a complete blood count (CBC) and peripheral blood smear. Normal results for a CBC are presented in Table 20-2. Abnormalities of red blood cell volume, structure, or life span account for the majority of red blood cell disorders.

Anemia

Anemia is a reduction in the total circulating red blood cell mass, which is identified by a reduction in hemoglobin, hematocrit, or

Table 20-2

Complete Blood Count: Normal Adult Values

Erythrocytes

Hemoglobin (HGB)	Male, 14–18 g/dL
	Female, 12–16 g/dL
Hematocrit (5 MCV × RBC)	Male, 40%–54%
	Female, 35%–47%
Red blood cell (RBC) count	Male, 4.5–6 3 106/μL
	Female, 4–5.5 3 106/μL
Reticulocytes	0.5–2.5%

Indices

Mean corpuscular volume (MCV)	82–100 μm³
Mean corpuscular hemoglobin (= HGB/RBC)	27–34 pg
Mean corpuscular hemoglobin concentration (= HGB/HCT)	32%–36%

Leukocytes

	Absolute count/mL	Differential count (%)
White blood cells	4,000–11,000	
Neutrophil granulocytes	1,800–7,000	50–60
Neutrophil bands	0–700	2–4
Lymphocytes	1,500–4,000	30–40
Monocytes	0–800	1–9
Basophils	0–200	0–1
Eosinophils	0–450	0–3

Platelets—

Quantitative normal value:
    150,000–400,000/μL
Qualitative estimation on smear:
    Number of platelets/oil immersion
    field × 10,000 = estimated platelet count
Normal ratio of RBC to platelets = 15:1 to 20:1

Modified from Rubin E, Gorstein F, Rubin R, et al. Rubin's Pathology, 4th ed. Philadelphia: Lippincott Williams & Wilkins, 2005, p. 1028.

red blood cell count. This decrease in the red blood cell volume ultimately results in decreased oxygen transport and tissue hypoxia. The classification of anemia may be performed based on morphologic or pathophysiologic criteria.

Morphologic classification of anemias reflects the appearance of red blood cells by peripheral blood smear or automated blood counters. In general, the morphologic appearance is reflected by the mean corpuscular volume (MCV), or size of the red blood cell. There are three morphologic classifications of anemia:

- Macrocytic: increased MCV
- Normocytic: normal MCV
- Microcytic: decreased MCV

Table 20-3 presents an overview of the anemias within a morphologic classification scheme. In addition to the red blood cell size, the morphologic classification accounts for the shape and color of the red blood cell. Abnormally shaped red blood cells are termed poikilocytes, and certain shapes reflect specific underlying disease processes (Fig. 20-5).

A second classification scheme of the anemias reflects the pathophysiology underlying the disease process.

On the basis of underlying pathophysiology, anemia can be classified into four categories:

- Decreased production of red blood cells by the bone marrow
- Ineffective production of red blood cells by the bone marrow
- Increased destruction of red blood cells in the blood
- Acute blood loss

Table 20-4 presents a summary of the pathophysiologic classification of anemia.

Table 20-3

Morphologic Classification of Anemia

Macrocytic	Normocytic
Megaloblastic	Anemia of chronic disease/in-
Alcohol use	flammation
Liver disease	Anemia of renal disease
Hypothyroidism	Acute blood loss
Reticulocytosis	
Primary bone marrow disease	
Microcytic	
Iron deficiency	
Anemia of chronic disease	
inflammation	
Thalassemias	
Sideroblastic anemias	

From Rubin E, Gorstein F, Rubin R, et al. Rubin's Pathology, 4th ed. Philadelphia: Lippincott Williams & Wilkins, 2005, p. 1028.

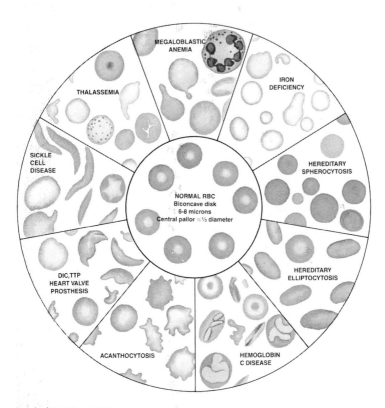

F I G U R E   20-5

Anemias. The pathophysiology of characteristic morphologic features of the various anemias is shown. The morphology of normal erythrocytes is contrasted in the central circle. (From Rubin E, Gorstein F, Rubin R, et al. Rubin's Pathology, 4th ed. Philadelphia: Lippincott Williams & Wilkins, 2005, p. 1029.)

In general, the destruction of red blood cells leads to a compensatory increase in red blood cell production in the bone marrow with subsequent increased numbers of circulating reticulocytes. In contrast, decreased or ineffective red blood cell production does not demonstrate increased numbers of circulating reticulocytes. The clinical presentation of anemia is similar, irrespective of the underlying cause. Classically, patients present with signs and symptoms that reflect decreased oxygen delivery to the tissues, including a rapid heart rate (tachycardia), shortness of breath, and systolic murmurs. If severe, anemia may result in easy fatigability,

Table 20-4

Pathophysiologic Classification of Anemia

Decreased Production	Increased Production
Stem cell- and progenitor cell-based	Intracorpuscular
Aplastic anemia	Membrane defect
Pure red cell aplasia	Enzyme deficiency
Paroxysmal nocturnal hemoglobinuria	Hemoglobinopathies
Leukemia	Extracorpuscular
Myelodysplastic syndromes	Immunologic
Marrow infiltration	Autoimmune
Anemia of chronic disease/inflammation	Alloimmune
Anemia of renal disease	Nonimmunologic
Nutritional deficiency	Mechanical
Megaloblastic anemia (vitamin B_{12}	Hypersplenism
and folic acid)	Infectious
Iron deficiency	Chemical
	Acute blood loss

From Rubin E, Gorstein F, Rubin R, et al. Rubin's Pathology, 4th ed. Philadelphia: Lippincott Williams & Wilkins, 2005, p. 1028.

faintness, angina, and dyspnea on exertion. To increase oxygen delivery to tissues, the body compensates by increasing the cardiac output, respiratory rate, and red blood cell production in the bone marrow, decreasing hemoglobin-oxygen affinity to more readily release oxygen to the tissues, and by shunting blood to more readily perfuse vital organs such as the brain.

The remaining discussion of anemias is based on the pathophysiologic classification scheme.

Anemia Caused by Decreased Red Blood Cell Production

Iron Deficiency Anemia

Iron deficiency anemia is the most common cause of anemia worldwide. Lack of iron interferes with normal hemoglobin synthesis, which leads to impaired red blood cell production and subsequent anemia. Iron is acquired from dietary sources, absorbed by the duodenum and jejunum, transported in the blood by transferrin, and ultimately incorporated into developing red blood cells by surface transferrin receptors (Table 20-5). Iron also is retained by the body after senescent red blood cell breakdown and is stored as hemosiderin (large aggregates) or ferritin (organized in a complex with apoferritin).

Table 20-5
Anemia Caused by Decreased Red Blood Cell Production

Anemia Type	Description	Bone Marrow	Blood
Aplastic anemia	Disorder of pluripotent stem cells; chemotherapy, radiation, viral	Variably reduced cellularity; decrease in myeloid, erythroid, and megakaryocyte precursors	Anemia, leukopenia, thrombocytopenia (pancytopenia)
Pure red cell aplasia	Idiopathic, parvovirus B19, thymic lesion	Normocellular; selective lack of erythroid precursors; 6 nuclear viral inclusions	Anemia, no reticulocytosis
Iron deficiency anemia	↓ Hemoglobin production resulting from ↓ dietary iron, chronic bleeding, menstruation	Normocellular; ↑ erythroid precursors	Microcytic, hypochromic anemia; pencil cells; no reticulocytosis
Anemia of renal disease	↓ Renal erythropoietin production	Lack of erythroid precursors	Normocytic, normochromic; burr cells, ± schistocytes
Anemia of chronic disease	Block in use of storage iron; malignancy; chronic inflammation	Increased iron stores in macrophages	Mild to moderate normocytic to microcytic anemia
Myelophthisic anemia	Bone marrow infiltration	Infiltration by processes such as carcinoma and granulomas	Normocytic anemia; teardrop cells; immature granulocytes, nucleated red blood cells
Anemia of lead poisoning	Ingestion of lead paint, exposure; ↓ hemoglobin synthesis	Ringed sideroblasts (impaired iron use by red blood cell precursors)	Microcytic, hypochromic red blood cells with basophilic stippling

Iron deficiency may result from the following:

- Inadequate dietary iron
- Pregnancy, lactation
- Chronic blood loss, often caused by gastrointestinal tumors or vascular lesions
- Menstruation, parturition, vaginal bleeding

Microscopically, the bone marrow demonstrates erythroid hyperplasia with red blood cell precursors demonstrating a ragged border. Decreased Prussian blue staining for iron is demonstrated. Examination of the blood reveals a normocytic to microcytic, hypochromic anemia. Anisopoikilocytosis, a variation in the size and shape of red blood cells, is reflected by an increased red blood cell distribution width (RDW). Oval- to pencil-shaped erythrocytes may be identified. No reticulocytosis is present. Blood values demonstrate decreased serum iron and ferritin levels, increased total iron-binding capacity, and decreased percent transferring saturation.

In addition to the classic symptoms of anemia, severe cases also may demonstrate atrophic glossitis, angular stomatitis, and koilonychias (spoon-shaped deformity of the fingernails). Treatment involves iron supplementation and correction of the source of chronic bleeding.

Aplastic Anemia

Aplastic anemia is characterized by a disorder of pluripotential stem cells that leads to bone marrow failure, with a reduction of all precursor elements within the bone marrow. Although most cases of aplastic anemia are idiopathic, a number of etiologic factors have been identified in a subset of cases, including radiation exposure, chemotherapeutic agents, viruses, and genetic abnormalities. A list of causative agents is provided in Table 20-6.

The mechanisms of stem cell injury in aplastic anemia appear to occur by either a predictable, dose-dependent toxic injury (often secondary to chemotherapeutic drugs) or an idiosyncratic, dose-independent, immunologic reaction (often secondary to certain drug exposures or viruses).

On microscopic examination, the bone marrow demonstrates variably reduced cellularity, with a notable decrease in the number of myeloid, erythroid, and megakaryocytic cells. In addition, an increase in the amount of fat and numbers of identifiable plasma cells and lymphocytes is present. Examination of the blood reveals anemia, leukopenia (primarily granulocytopenia) and thrombocytopenia. Red blood cells demonstrate a normal shape, but are often mildly macrocytic. Circulating reticulocytes are not identified.

Etiology of Aplastic Anemia

Idiopathic (two thirds of cases)	Viruses
Ionizing radiation	Hepatitis C virus (HCV)
Drugs	Epstein-Barr virus (EBV)
Chemotherapeutic agents	HIV
Chloramphenicol	Parvovirus B19
Anticonvulsants	Hereditary
Nonsteroidal antiinflammatory	Fanconi anemia (germline *FAC*
agents	mutation leading to chromosomal
Gold	instability)
Chemicals	
Benzene	

From Rubin E, Gorstein F, Rubin R, et al. Rubin's Pathology, 4th ed. Philadelphia: Lippincott Williams & Wilkins, 2005, p. 1031.

Clinically, patients demonstrate weakness, fatigue, infections, and bleeding. Fanconi anemia presents within the first decade of life in association with hypoplastic thumbs, absent radii, skin pigmentation, and renal anomalies. The treatment of aplastic anemia involves immunosuppressive therapy, and most patients undergo subsequent bone marrow or stem cell transplantation.

Pure Red Cell Aplasia

Pure red cell aplasia (PRCA) is the selective lack of erythroid precursor production in the bone marrow. PRCA may be idiopathic or may occur secondary to viral infections or thymic lesions. In idiopathic forms, immunologic suppression of red blood cell production appears to play a role. In a heritable form known as Diamond-Blackfan syndrome, in which PRCA appears in the first year of life, decreased red blood cell formation occurs because of a diminished response to erythropoietin.

Microscopically, the bone marrow is normocellular and demonstrates only a selective absence of erythroid precursors. In cases of parvovirus B19 infection, nuclear inclusions may be found. Examination of the blood reveals moderate to severe anemia and increased erythropoietin levels, but no increase in reticulocyte numbers.

PRCA may be an acute self-limited process, often caused by parvovirus B19 infection; a chronic relapsing process, often caused by thymic lesions; or may appear in idiopathic cases. Treatment involves transfusion and, in cases of thymic lesion, thymectomy.

Anemia of Renal Disease

Chronic renal insufficiency results in decreased erythropoietin production and subsequent lack of erythroid production. In addition, a uremic toxin has been suggested to additionally suppress the formation of erythroid precursors. Microscopically, the bone marrow demonstrates a lack of erythroid precursors. Examination of the blood reveals a normocytic, normochromic anemia with cells containing scalloped membranes (echinocytes, burr cells). If hypertension underlies the renal disease, red cell fragments and schistocytes may be identified. Treatment involves administration of recombinant erythropoietin.

Anemia of Chronic Disease

Chronic inflammatory conditions or malignancies may cause anemia of chronic disease. The pathophysiology underlying this condition reflects an ineffective use of iron stored within bone marrow macrophages, as well as possible contributory effects from inflammatory cytokines. The bone marrow demonstrates increased amounts of stored iron by Prussian blue staining. Examination of the blood reveals a mild to moderate microcytic anemia and decreased serum iron levels. However, in contrast to iron deficiency anemia, the total iron binding capacity is decreased because of decreased serum albumin levels. Treatment involves control of the underlying disease.

Anemia Associated with Marrow Infiltration (Myelophthisic Anemia)

Myelophthisic anemia is caused by any process that infiltrates and replaces the normal bone marrow, including metastatic carcinoma, granulomatous disease, myelofibrosis, or hematologic malignancies. Anemia results, as well as leukopenia and thrombocytopenia. Often, extramedullary hematopoiesis may occur in the liver and spleen. Examination of the blood often reveals anisopoikilocytosis, teardrop cells, nucleated red blood cells, and immature granulocytes.

Anemia Caused by Lead Poisoning

Lead poisoning often occurs with ingestion of lead-based paint or occupational exposure to lead. Lead interferes with several enzymes essential to heme synthesis, including aminolevulinic acid (ALA) dehydratase and ferrochelatase. Lead also inhibits pyrimidine 5′-nucleotidase, which leads to basophilic stippling in circulating red blood cells. Examination of the bone marrow reveals ringed sideroblasts caused by the impaired use of iron in erythroid precursors. Examination of the blood reveals microcytic, hypochromic red blood cells with prominent basophilic stippling.

Anemia Caused by Ineffective Red Blood Cell Production
Megaloblastic Anemia

Megaloblastic anemia is caused by impaired DNA synthesis, which often is secondary to vitamin B_{12} or folate deficiency. Both vitamin B_{12} and folate are required for the formation of thymidylate, which is necessary to form DNA molecules (Fig. 20-6).

Ineffective DNA synthesis leads to impaired nuclear development, resulting in large nuclei relative to volume of cytoplasm (megaloblasts). Megaloblasts undergo intramedullary destruction within the bone marrow. The most common causes of megaloblastic anemia are vitamin B_{12} and folate deficiency (Table 20-7). Other

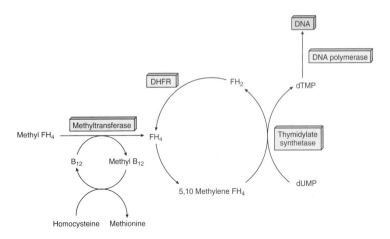

FIGURE 20-6
Relationship of folic acid to vitamin B_{12}. A one-carbon transfer mediated by folic acid, methylates dUMP to dTMP, which is then used for the synthesis of DNA. To enter this cycle, folate (methyl FH_4) is demethylated to FH_4, vitamin B_{12} acting as the cofactor. Thus, both vitamin B_{12} and folic acid deficiencies lead to impaired DNA synthesis and megaloblastic anemia. DHFR, dihydrofolate reductase; dTMP, deoxythymidine monophosphate; dUMP, deoxyuridine monophosphate; FH_2, dihydrofolate; FH_4, tetrahydrofolate. (From Rubin E, Gorstein F, Rubin R, et al. Rubin's Pathology, 4th ed. Philadelphia: Lippincott Williams & Wilkins, 2005, p. 1034.)

Table 20-7
Anemia Caused by Ineffective Red Blood Cell Production

Anemia Type	Description	Blood
Megaloblastic anemia	Impaired DNA synthesis; ↓ vitamin B_{12}, folate levels	Pancytopenia; oval macrocytes; teardrop cells; hypersegmented neutrophils
β *Thalassemias*		
Homozygous β thalassemia (β thalassemia major)	Absence of β hemoglobin chains	Moderate to severe microcytic, hypochromic anemia; target cells; basophilic stippling
Heterozygous β thalassemia (β thalassemia minor)	Absence of single β hemoglobin chain	Mild microcytic, hypochromic anemia; target cells; basophilic stippling
α *Thalassemias*		
Silent carrier α thalassemia	One α gene deleted	Normal; patients asymptomatic
α Thalassemia trait	Two α genes deleted	Mild microcytic anemia; minimal anisopoikilocytosis; erythrocytosis; patients asymptomatic
Hemoglobin H disease	Three α genes deleted	Moderate microcytic anemia; anisopoikilocytosis; target cells; patients symptomatic
Homozygous α thalassemia (hydrops fetalis)	Four α genes deleted	Fatal in utero; severe anemia; anisopoikilocytosis; large amounts of hemoglobin Bart

causes include chemotherapeutic agents (methotrexate, hydroxyurea), antiretroviral drugs (azidothymidine), and inherited defects.

Vitamin B_{12} is found in many animal food sources and is synthesized by intestinal organisms. After ingestion, vitamin B_{12} binds to intrinsic factor (IF) secreted by gastric parietal cells and is ultimately absorbed in the distal ileum and transferred to the carrier molecule transcobalamin II in the blood. Any process that interferes with vitamin B_{12} absorption or use may lead to megaloblastic anemia, including the following:

- Inadequate intake: rare; may occur in strict vegetarians
- Lack of intrinsic factor: loss of parietal cells with prior gastric surgery; *pernicious anemia* in which antibodies are directed against intrinsic factor and parietal cells (autoimmune disease)
- Decreased ileal absorption of vitamin B_{12}-IF complex: primary intestinal disorders (inflammatory bowel disease), ileal bypass surgery, bacterial overgrowth, inherited defect in vitamin B_{12} receptor (*Imerslund-Grasbeck syndrome*)

Folic acid is found in leafy vegetables, meat, and eggs. After ingestion, folic acid is converted to a monoglutamate form, absorbed in the jejunum, reduced and methylated to form 5-methyl tetrahydrofolate, and transported in the blood by folate-binding protein. Folic acid deficiency occurs in the following:

- Inadequate dietary intake: most common cause; alcoholics
- Increased demands: pregnancy, lactation, chronic hemolytic processes
- Intestinal processes: inflammatory bowel disease, sprue
- Medications: phenytoin, methotrexate

Microscopically, the bone marrow in megaloblastic anemia is hypercellular and all lineages demonstrate cellular enlargement with asynchronous maturation of the nucleus and cytoplasm. Examination of the blood reveals pancytopenia (secondary to intramedullary destruction of precursors), macrocytic red blood cells with an oval or teardrop shape, hypersegmented neutrophils (more than five lobes), and no increase in reticulocytes. Elevated levels of serum lactate dehydrogenase (LDH) occur because of the massive destruction of intramedullary elements.

A distinction between folic acid and vitamin B_{12} deficiencies usually can be established by measurement of serum levels. Further evaluation of vitamin B_{12} deficiency includes identification of elevated homocysteine and methyl malonic acid in the serum, circulating antibodies against intrinsic factor in pernicious anemia, or decreased absorption of vitamin B_{12} by the Schilling test (administration of radioactive vitamin B_{12} with or without intrinsic factor followed by an evaluation of urinary radioactivity).

Patients with megaloblastic anemia demonstrate signs and symptoms of anemia. However, megaloblastic anemia caused by vitamin B_{12} deficiency also may present with neurologic symptoms secondary to the degeneration of the posterior and lateral columns of the spinal cord, which may become irreversible over time. Figure 20-7 illustrates the absorption of vitamin B_{12} and folate.

Thalassemias

Defects in hemoglobin chains results in thalassemia, which is classified according to the hemoglobin chain affected. Normal hemoglo-

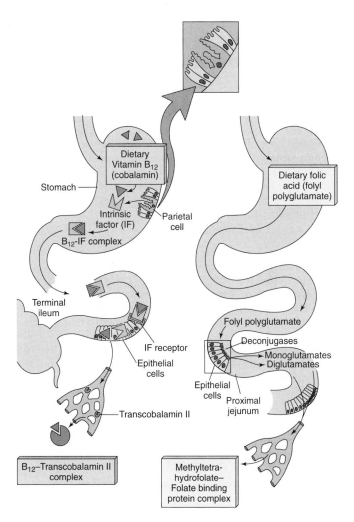

F I G U R E   20-7

Absorption of vitamin B_{12}, folic acid, and iron. Absorption of vitamin B_{12} requires initial complexing with intrinsic factor (IF), which is produced by the parietal cells of the gastric mucosa. Absorption then occurs in the terminal ileum, where there are receptors for the IF–B_{12} complex. Dietary folic acid is conjugated by conjugase enzymes to polyglutamate. Absorption occurs in the jejunum after deconjugation in the intestinal lumen. Reduction and methylation result in the generation of methyl tetrahydrofolate, which then is transported by folate-binding protein. Dietary ferric iron is reduced to ferrous iron in the stomach and absorbed principally in the duodenum. Iron is transported by transferrin in the circulation. (From Rubin E, Gorstein F, Rubin R, et al. Rubin's Pathology, 4th ed. Philadelphia: Lippincott Williams & Wilkins, 2005, p. 1035.)

bin comprises four globin chains, two of which are alpha (α) and two of which are non-alpha in the adult. The most common form of hemoglobin is hemoglobin A ($\alpha2\beta2$), which accounts for up to 98% of all hemoglobin. Additional uncommon forms include hemoglobin F ($\alpha2\gamma2$) and hemoglobin A$_2$ (α 2δ2). Four α genes exist on chromosome 16, whereas the non-α genes are located on chromosome 11 and consist of two γ, one δ, and one β gene. The assembly of hemoglobin subunit chains is summarized in Figure 20-8. The most common forms of thalassemia are α and β thalassemia. Thalassemia is most common in Italy, Greece, and regions with a high incidence of malaria, for which a heterozygous thalassemic state may provide a protective effect.

Beta Thalassemias

Beta thalassemias are a heterogeneous group of disorders in which a point mutation of the β globin gene on chromosome 11 leads to partial to no transcription of the β globin gene.

Homozygous β thalassemia (Cooley anemia, β thalassemia major) results in a marked excess of α chains that precipitate in the cytoplasm of erythroid precursors. In instances of absent β chain formation, fetal hemoglobin makes up the majority of erythrocyte hemoglobin. The presence of hemoglobin F (α 2γ2), which has an increased oxygen affinity and therefore a decreased oxygen delivery capacity, leads to an increase in erythropoietin production.

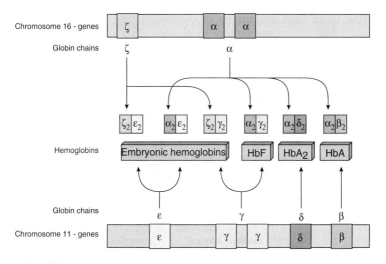

FIGURE 20-8
Assembly of subunit chains to form different hemoglobins. (From Rubin E, Gorstein F, Rubin R, et al. Rubin's Pathology, 4th ed. Philadelphia: Lippincott Williams & Wilkins, 2005, p. 1037.)

Therefore, the bone marrow demonstrates an increased number of erythroid precursor cells with expansion of the marrow space, leading to facial and cranial bone deformities. In addition, extramedullary hematopoiesis occurs, leading to hepatosplenomegaly.

Examination of the peripheral blood reveals a moderate to severe microcytic and hypochromic anemia, anisopoikilocytosis with target cells, basophilic stippling, and circulating normoblasts (red blood cell precursors).

Patients with homozygous β thalassemia require frequent blood transfusions and may therefore develop morbidity associated with iron overload.

Heterozygous β thalassemia (β thalassemia minor) is often asymptomatic. The bone marrow demonstrates a mild increase in red blood cell precursors. Examination of the peripheral blood reveals mild microcytic, hypochromic anemia, minimal anisocytosis, target cells, and basophilic stippling.

Alpha Thalassemias

The α thalassemias demonstrate a broader symptomatic presentation, because as many as four α chains may be affected (versus only two β chains). α Thalassemias occur secondary to gene deletions of the a chain on chromosome 16. In certain cases, α thalassemia may be associated with excess β or γ chains, which may form hemoglobin H (β_4) or hemoglobin Bart (γ_4). Hemoglobin H and hemoglobin Bart are unstable hemoglobin molecules that have high oxygen affinities and decrease oxygen delivery to tissues, as well as precipitate in the red blood cell cytoplasm, leading to the formation of Heinz bodies. The various forms of α thalassemia include the following:

- Silent carrier α thalassemia (one gene affected): asymptomatic, no anemia, no hematologic abnormalities (slight hemoglobin Bart in infancy only)
- α Thalassemia trait (two genes affected): mild microcytic anemia, erythrocytosis, minimal anisopoikilocytosis; no elevation of hemoglobin A2
- Hemoglobin H disease (three genes affected): moderate microcytic anemia; moderate anisopoikilocytosis; some target cells; increased amounts of hemoglobin Bart; variable levels of hemoglobin H; Heinz bodies on peripheral blood smear
- Homozygous α thalassemia (four genes affected): incompatible with life; results in fetal hydrops; die in utero or early neonatal life with severe anemia, marked anisopoikilocytosis, large amounts of hemoglobin Bart

Anemia Caused by Increased Red Blood Cell Destruction (Hemolytic Anemias)

The hemolytic anemias encompass processes that result in red blood cell destruction (hemolysis) after release from the bone marrow. Broad categories encompassed within hemolytic anemia include defects in the erythrocyte membrane, enzymatic defects, hemoglobinopathies, immune hemolytic anemias, cold agglutinin disease, hemolytic transfusion reactions, hemolytic disease of the newborn, mechanical red cell fragmentation syndromes, paroxysmal nocturnal hemoglobinuria, and hypersplenism (Table 20-8).

Hemolytic anemias are classified according to site of red blood cell destruction. Extravascular hemolysis occurs in the spleen and liver by cells of the monocyte/macrophage system. Intravascular hemolysis involves the destruction of cells within the circulation. In general, a common compensatory change that accompanies hemolytic anemias is an increase in production of red blood cell precursors, manifested by polychromasia of red blood cells and increased reticulocyte count. Additional findings include increased unconjugated (indirect) bilirubin, decreased haptoglobin, increased LDH, free hemoglobin in the blood and urine, increased urobilinogen, and urine hemosiderin.

Hereditary Spherocytosis

Hereditary spherocytosis (HS) is a diverse group of inherited disorders of the erythrocyte cytoskeleton characterized by a deficiency of a cytoskeletal component such as spectrin, ankyrin, protein 4.2, or band 3. HS is primarily autosomal dominant, although rare autosomal recessive forms may occur. Loss of any of the components of the cytoskeleton results in a dissociation of the cytoskeleton from the lipid bilayer membrane, with subsequent loss of membrane surface area and deformation of the red blood cell into a spheroid shape (spherocytes). Destruction of the red blood cells occurs in the spleen (extravascular hemolysis).

Microscopically, the bone marrow of these patients demonstrates erythroid hyperplasia. Examination of the blood reveals a moderate normocytic anemia, with conspicuous spherocytes lacking central pallor. In addition, polychromasia and reticulocytosis are present.

Patients with HS demonstrate splenomegaly because of chronic extravascular hemolysis, jaundice, cholelithiasis with bilirubin gallstones and, rarely, aplastic crises often secondary to infection by parvovirus B19. Patients generally do not require transfusions and may be managed by splenectomy.

Hereditary Elliptocytosis

Hereditary elliptocytosis (HE) is an autosomal dominant disorder of the cytoskeletal components of the red blood cell. In general, these disorders reflect a defect in the self-assembly of the cytoskeleton, resulting in an elliptical shape of the red blood cell (elliptocytes). However, in contrast to HS, the membrane remains intact; therefore, the cells maintain a zone of central pallor. Patients with

Table 20-8

Anemia Caused by Increased Red Blood Cell Destruction (the Hemolytic Anemias)

Anemia Type	Description	Blood
Extravascular hemolysis		
Hereditary spherocytosis (membrane defect)	Heritable deficiency of cytoskeletal protein; uncoupling of membrane from cytoskeleton	Normocytic anemia; spherocytes; reticulocytosis
Hereditary elliptocytosis (membrane defect)	Heritable deficiency of cytoskeleton; problem with cytoskeletal assembly	Mild normocytic anemia; elliptocytes; minimal reticulocytosis
Acanthocytosis (membrane defect)	Intrinsic defects of the lipid bilayer of red blood cells	Spur cells (irregular surface projections); mild anemia
G6PD deficiency (enzyme deficiency)	X-linked; abnormal sensitivity of red blood cells to oxidative stress	Normal if no oxidative stress; Heinz bodies during oxidative stress; bite cells
Sickle cell disease (hemoglobinopathy)	Point mutation of β globin chain; glutamic acid $\rightarrow$ valine position 6; homozygous hemoglobin S	Severe anemia; sickled and target cells; Howell-Jolly bodies
Sickle cell trait	Heterozygous hemoglobin S	Occasional target cells
Hemoglobin C disease	Point mutation of β globin chain; glutamic acid $\rightarrow$ lysine position 6	Mild normocytic anemia; numerous target cells; rhomboid crystals (HbC)
Hemoglobin E disease	Point mutation of β globin chain; glutamic acid $\rightarrow$ lysine position 26	Mild microcytic anemia; $\downarrow$ MCV; erythrocytosis; target cells
Extravascular or intravascular hemolysis		
Warm antibody autoimmune hemolytic anemia (AIHA)	IgG antibody against Rh determinants on erythrocytes	Normocytic or macrocytic anemia; spherocytes; polychromasia

(*continues*)

Table 20-8

(continued)

Anemia Type	Description	Blood
Cold agglutinin disease (cold AIHA)	IgM antibodies against I/i system on red blood cells	Erythrocyte agglutination at room temperature; falsely ↓ HCT
Intravascular hemolysis		
Cold hemolysin disease (cold AIHA; paroxysmal cold hemoglobinaria)	IgG antibodies against P antigen system on erythrocytes	Severe anemia; no agglutination of erythrocytes
Alloimmune hemolytic anemia	ABO, Rh, minor blood product incompatibility	Severe hemolysis
Mechanical red cell fragmentation syndrome	Abnormal vascular surface; disturbances in blood flow	Mild to moderate anemia; reticulocytosis; schistocytes
Paroxysmal nocturnal hemoglobinuria	Somatic mutation of *PIG-A* gene; ↑ sensitivity of RBCs to complement-mediated lysis	Episodic normocytic or macrocytic anemia; reticulocytosis

HE may be asymptomatic or demonstrate only mild normocytic anemia. Blood smear reveals elliptocytes and only minimal reticulocytosis. Splenectomy is warranted in patients with severe disease.

Acanthocytosis

Acanthocytosis results from defects of the lipid bilayer of red blood cells, such as in chronic liver disease (increased deposition of free cholesterol in the membrane) or abetalipoproteinemia. Red blood cells in acanthocytosis develop spiny surface projections and a centrally dense cytoplasm that lacks central pallor (spur cells). Mild hemolytic anemia is associated with this condition.

Glucose-6-phosphate Dehydrogenase Deficiency

Glucose-6-phosphate dehydrogenase (G6PD) catalyzes the conversion of glucose-6-phosphate to 6-phosphogluconate in the glycolytic pathway and is involved the recycling of reduced glutathione. G6PD deficiency is an X-linked disorder that results in the abnormal sensitivity of red blood cells to oxidative stress (e.g., infections, drugs, fava bean ingestion). Females are asymptomatic carriers, whereas males demonstrate hemolytic anemia with oxidative stress.

Two forms of G6PD deficiency occur. The A-variant of G6PD deficiency affects African Americans and demonstrates reduced enzyme activity, whereas the Mediterranean version demonstrates absent enzyme activity with more severe, sustained hemolytic anemia. Examination of the blood during periods of normal oxidation reveals normal-appearing red blood cells. However, during periods of oxidative stress, precipitation of methemoglobin results in the formation of cytoplasmic Heinz bodies. In addition, red blood cells may lose portions of their membranes during periods of oxidative stress as they pass through the spleen, leading to the formation of "bite cells."

Hemoglobinopathies

The hemoglobinopathies are caused by point mutations of the β globin chain gene. Hundreds of hemoglobin variants have been described; only the most common hemoglobinopathies are discussed in this chapter.

Sickle Cell Disease

Sickle cell disease is caused by a point mutation resulting in a substitution of a valine for the normal glutamic acid at the sixth amino acid position in the β globin chain gene (hemoglobin S). This substitution leads to a polymerization of the β globin chain within the cytoplasm of red blood cells during deoxygenation, resulting in characteristic sickling of the cells. Sickled red blood cells are less deformable and may lead to obstruction of the microcirculation with resultant tissue hypoxia and ischemic injury. In addition, the rigid nature of these cells promotes their destruction as they pass through the spleen (extravascular hemolytic anemia).

Sickle cell disease demonstrates highest incidence in persons of African ancestry, and heterozygosity for hemoglobin S may offer some protection against infection by malaria. On examination of the blood, patients with sickle cell disease have severe normocytic or macrocytic anemia. Reticulocytosis may be present secondary to chronic hemolysis. Marked anisopoikilocytosis, polychromasia, sickled cells, target cells, and Howell-Jolly bodies (nuclear remnants) also may be identified on blood smear. Patients who are homozygous for hemoglobin S (hemoglobin SS) demonstrate the full manifestation of sickle cell disease.

During the first several months of life, patients with sickle cell disease are asymptomatic because of the high levels of hemoglobin F present in the circulation. However, over time, patients primarily have circulating hemoglobin SS and develop an adaptive response to lifelong hemolysis. Patients may frequently develop repeated vasoocclusive disease manifested by episodes of severe pain in the chest, abdomen, and bones, often triggered by infections, acidosis, or dehydration. In addition, patients may develop aplastic crisis and sequestration crisis. Aplastic crisis occurs when the bone marrow no longer compensates for the chronic blood loss, and patients demonstrate a rapid drop in hemoglobin levels and absence of reticulocyte formation. Aplastic crisis may be caused by infection with parvovirus B19 or other viruses.

Sequestration crisis often affects young children and reflects a sudden pooling of erythrocytes, predominantly in the spleen. This sequestration results in a rapid drop in hemoglobin levels, circulating blood volume, and hypovolemic shock.

Multiple medical problems may arise in sickle cell patients, which reflect the outcomes of repeated vasoocclusive disease and include the following:

- Myocardial ischemia, cardiomegaly, congestive heart failure
- Acute chest syndrome with pulmonary infiltrates and decreased respiratory function
- Functional autosplenectomy after repeated infarcts with increased susceptibility to *Streptococcus pneumoniae*
- Transient ischemic attacks, strokes, and cerebral hemorrhages
- Inability to form concentrated urine, renal infarcts, and papillary necrosis
- Priapism
- Pigmented bilirubin gallstones secondary to increased unconjugated bilirubin, cholecystitis
- Cutaneous ulcers on the lower extremities, osteomyelitis with *Salmonella typhimurium*

Sickle Cell Trait

Heterozygosity for the hemoglobin S mutation is referred to as sickle cell trait. Patients with sickle cell trait are asymptomatic, except for instances of extreme oxidative stress such as deep sea diving. In these patients, the presence of hemoglobin A prevents polymerization of hemoglobin S and therefore sickling. In contrast, patients who are double heterozygotes for hemoglobin S and another structurally abnormal hemoglobin (e.g., hemoglobin C or thalassemia) may not prevent the polymerization of hemoglobin S and therefore lead to sickling crises or persistent splenomegaly.

Hemoglobin C Disease

Hemoglobin C disease results from a homozygous inheritance of hemoglobin that contains a substitution of a lysine for the normal glutamic acid molecule at the sixth amino acid position of the β globin gene. Hemoglobin C precipitates within red blood cells, making them less deformable and therefore susceptible to removal by the spleen. Patients may experience a mild chronic hemolytic anemia and splenomegaly. Examination of the blood reveals a mild normocytic anemia, numerous target cells, mild polychromasia and dense, rhomboid crystals (precipitated hemoglobin C). More than 90% of the hemoglobin is hemoglobin C, and no hemoglobin A is present.

Hemoglobin E Disease

Hemoglobin E disease results from a homozygous inheritance of a hemoglobin that contains a substitution of a lysine for the normal glutamic acid at position twenty-six of the β globin gene. This mutation occurs at a splice site, which leads in addition to decreased gene transcription and an unstable messenger RNA. Hemoglobin E may also precipitate within the cell and has been proposed to serve a protective role against malaria. Patients with homozygous EE have a mild microcytic anemia, decreased MCV, erythrocytosis, and target cells. Greater than 90% of the hemoglobin is made up of hemoglobin E.

Immune Hemolytic Anemias

This group of diseases is characterized by increased red blood cell destruction secondary to antibodies directed against antigens on the red blood cell surface. These antibodies may be alloantibodies or autoantibodies.

Autoimmune Hemolytic Anemias

The autoimmune hemolytic anemias (AIHAs) demonstrate antibodies directed against red blood cells are categorized by the temperature of antibody reactivity.

Warm Antibody Autoimmune Hemolytic Anemias

Warm antibody AIHA accounts for 80% of AIHA. In this disease, predominantly IgG antibodies are directed against Rh determinants on the red blood cell, with optimal reactivity at 37°C. Warm antibodies do not bind complement but are recognized by Fc receptors on splenic macrophages, which remove portions of the red blood cell membrane, ultimately resulting in spherocyte formation and hemolysis. Warm antibody AIHA more commonly affects women and may be idiopathic or caused by infection, collagen vascular disease, lymphoproliferative disorders, and drug reactions. Examination of the blood reveals a normocytic or macrocytic anemia, spherocytes, and polychromasia. A direct antiglobulin (Coombs) test often is positive; this test involves an incubation of patients' red blood cells with anti-human globulin serum with agglutination as a positive test result. Patients are treated with corticosteroids primarily, with splenectomy or transfusion for refractory cases.

Cold Antibody Autoimmune Hemolytic Anemias

Cold antibody AIHA accounts for the remainder of AIHA and is characterized either by IgM antibodies directed against the I/i antigen system on red blood cells (cold agglutinins) or by IgG antibodies directed against the P antigen on red blood cells (cold hemolysins). Maximal reactivity of these antibodies occurs at 4°C. *Cold agglutinins* bind to and agglutinate red blood cells in the cooler peripheral blood and can fix complement. The thermal amplitude of the antibody determines whether the red blood cells ultimately undergo extravascular hemolysis because of binding by complement receptors in the liver or intravascular hemolysis because of complement activation (Fig. 20-9).

Cold agglutinins may be idiopathic or secondary to infections or lymphoproliferative disorders. Blood examination reveals erythrocyte agglutination at room temperature (which can lead to falsely lowered hematocrit and falsely elevated MCV and MCHC); warming the blood to 37°C reverses the agglutination. Patients generally do not demonstrate prominent hemolysis and most commonly develop peripheral vascular symptoms on cold exposure (*Raynaud phenomenon*).

Cold hemolysins (Donath-Landsteiner antibodies) rarely cause AIHA. In *cold hemolysin disease (paroxysmal cold hemoglobinuria)*, antibodies bind to red blood cells at low temperatures and fix complement but do not induce agglutination. As the blood warms, the antibody remains attached and complement is activated, leading to intravascular hemolysis. Paroxysmal cold hemoglobinuria often occurs after a viral illness. Patients experience a severe anemia, decreased haptoglobin levels, and hemoglobinuria secondary to intravascular hemolysis. The direct Coombs test is positive for complement but may be negative for IgG because of the rapid dissociation from red blood cells in vitro. Treatment is primarily supportive.

Alloimmune Hemolytic Anemia

Alloimmune hemolytic anemia refers to the destruction of circulating foreign red blood cells by alloantibodies. Alloimmune hemolytic anemia may be caused by an immediate or delayed hemolytic transfusion reaction to foreign, incompatible blood products. An *immediate hemolytic transfusion reaction* occurs when ABO incompatible blood is erroneously administered to a patient and results in severe hemolysis that can lead to hypotension or death. *A delayed hemolytic transfusion reaction* occurs to minor blood antigens and may be undetectable clinically.

Alloimmune hemolytic anemia also occurs in *hemolytic disease of the newborn* (HDN), in which an incompatibility between fetal and maternal blood types occurs. Generally, the mother lacks an antigen displayed by the fetus and therefore develops an alloim-

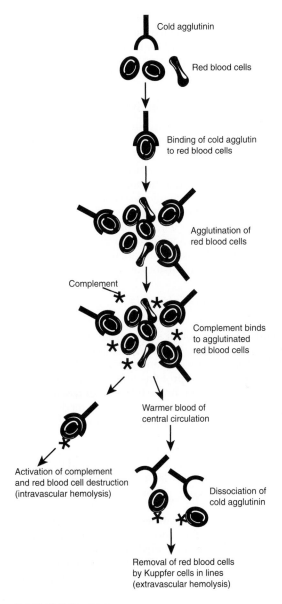

FIGURE 20-9
Cold agglutinin reaction.

mune response against the "foreign" antigen. The two most common forms are *ABO-type HDN* in which the mother is type O and the fetus is type A, and *Rh-type HDN* in which the mother is Rh-negative and the fetus is Rh-positive. The Rh-type HDN requires preexposure to the antigen, whereas the ABO-type does not.

Mechanical Red Cell Fragmentation Syndrome

Mechanical red cell fragmentation syndrome occurs when normal red blood cells are fragmented within the blood vessels (intravascular hemolysis). Fragmentation may occur in larger vessels *(macroangiopathic hemolytic anemia)* containing a synthetic vascular graft or prosthetic valve because of absence of normal endothelium. Fragmentation of red blood cells within smaller vessels *(microangiopathic hemolytic anemia)* occurs secondary to turbulent flow patterns as result from disseminated intravascular coagulation (DIC), malignant hypertension, or thrombocytopenic purpura (TTP). Examination of the blood reveals a mild to moderate anemia, reticulocytosis, and fragmented red blood cells (schistocytes).

Paroxysmal Nocturnal Hemoglobinuria

Paroxysmal nocturnal hemoglobinuria (PNH) is an acquired abnormality of multipotential hematopoietic stem cells. A mutation of the phosphatidylinositol glycan-class A (PIG-A) gene on chromosome Xp22.1 leads to a disruption of protein anchoring on the red blood cell membrane. The most crucial proteins affected include decay acceleration factor (CD55) and membrane inhibitor of reactive lysis (CD59), loss of which leads to episodic, complement-mediated, intravascular hemolysis. PNH may be idiopathic or evolve from preexisting aplastic anemia.

Examination of the blood reveals episodic normocytic or macrocytic anemia and reticulocytosis; often, leukopenia and thrombocytopenia are present. Hemoglobinuria occurs secondary to intravascular hemolysis. Loss of GPI-anchored protein in PNH is diagnosed by flow cytometry.

Patients with PNH develop intermittent intravascular hemolysis, and are at an increased risk for venous and arterial thrombosis and bleeding. PNH may progress to myelodysplasia or acute leukemia, and abnormalities in leukocytes and platelets also may occur. Treatment is primarily supportive, and bone marrow transplantation is curative.

Hypersplenism

Enlargement of the spleen results in a pooling of blood within the organ and prolonged exposure of red blood cells to splenic macrophages, which results in their destruction. Patients generally experience a mild hemolytic anemia and congestive splenomegaly. The bone marrow demonstrates a compensatory hyperplasia of all lineages. Examination of the blood reveals occasional mild leukopenia and thrombocytopenia. Treatment includes splenectomy for symptomatic patients.

Anemia Caused by Acute Blood Loss

The final category of anemias, acute anemia, is caused by an acute loss of whole blood from the intravascular component. Rapid blood loss results in volume depletion, hypotension, and decreased tissue perfusion. A redistribution of fluid from extravascular to intravascular sites occurs during the first 24 to 48 hours, at which time the true magnitude of anemia becomes apparent. In response to acute blood loss, erythropoietin is released from the kidney and the bone marrow undergoes erythroid hyperplasia in response.

Polycythemia (Erythrocytosis)

Polycythemia denotes an increase in red blood cell mass, reflected by a hematocrit greater than 54% in men and 47% in women. As red cell mass increases over 50%, peripheral blood flow is impaired, and increases over 60% result in tissue hypoxia. Several types of polycythemia exist:

- Relative polycythemia: dehydration; reduction in plasma volume
- Gaisbock syndrome: middle-aged, overweight, hypertensive smokers; decreased plasma volume and increased red blood cell production
- Absolute polycythemia: true increase in red blood cell mass; divided into primary (polycythemia vera) or secondary (neoplasms, renal cysts, hydronephrosis) forms

PLATELETS AND HEMOSTASIS

Approximately 1,000 to 40,000 anucleated platelets are derived from megakaryocytes in the bone marrow. Each platelet measures 2 to 3 μm in diameter and circulates for approximately 10 days. Platelets contain mitochondria, glycogen particles, dense granules (nucleotides such as ADP), and alpha granules (polypeptides such as fibrinogen and von Willebrand factor [vWF]). Platelets are the earliest elements in hemostasis, which is achieved via a stepwise process of adherence to the vascular endothelium, aggregation with the aid of fibrin, and ultimately dissolution by the fibrinolytic system. The hemostatic cascade is diagrammed in Figure 20-10.

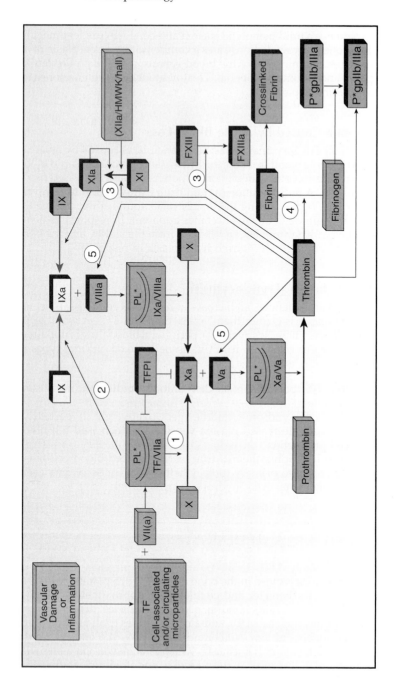

The activation of platelets (adherence and aggregation) includes the following sequential steps (diagrammed in Fig. 20-11):

- Adhesion to the subendothelial matrix proteins (collagen, vWF) of the blood vessels by specific glycoprotein receptors on the platelet surface (GP Ib/IX, GP Ia/IIa)
- Discoid to stellate shape change: protects the procoagulant surface membrane
- Secretion of platelet granule contents (ADP, epinephrine, calcium, vWF, platelet-derived growth factor): activates additional platelets
- Generation of thromboxane A_2 by cyclooxygenase 1: activates additional platelets
- Conformational membrane change to expose P-selectin and procoagulant anionic phospholipids: binds and localizes leukocytes
- Aggregation of platelets by fibrinogen receptor GP IIb/IIIa cross-linking

Under normal conditions, endothelial cells synthesize nitric oxide and the potent vasodilator prostacyclin, which together inhibit platelet function. When the endothelium is damaged, the subendothelial matrix, which consists of collagen, elastin, laminin, fibronectin, vWF, and tissue factor, is exposed. This subendothelial matrix is highly thrombogenic and promotes activation of platelets. Effective coagulation requires both activated platelets as well as activated coagulation proteins, which normally are present in the circulation as inactive zymogen forms. Disorders of clotting are termed *hemostatic disorders*.

F I G U R E   20-10

Hemostasis and thrombosis. After injury to a vessel, rupture of an atherosclerotic plaque, or the presence of major inflammation, coagulation is initiated when tissue factor (TF) binds to circulating factor VII. The TF/VIIa complex is activated by localizing to an activated phospholipid surface (PL*) such that provided by activated platelets. TF/VIIa activates factor X to form Xa (1) and IX to form IXa (2). Sustained amplification is achieved through the actions of factors XI, IX, and VIII. Factor IX is activated through the small amount of initial thrombin formed and, to a limited extent, by autoactivation of factor XIIa. Cofactors II and VIII, when activated by thrombin, form complexes with X (Xa/Va) and IX (IXa/VIIIa), respectively, on activated PL surfaces. Fibrinogen binds to the gpIIb/IIIa integrin receptor on activated platelets (P*). The combined result is the platelet–fibrin thrombus. (From Rubin E, Gorstein F, Rubin R, et al. Rubin's Pathology, 4th ed. Philadelphia: Lippincott Williams & Wilkins, 2005, p. 1049.)

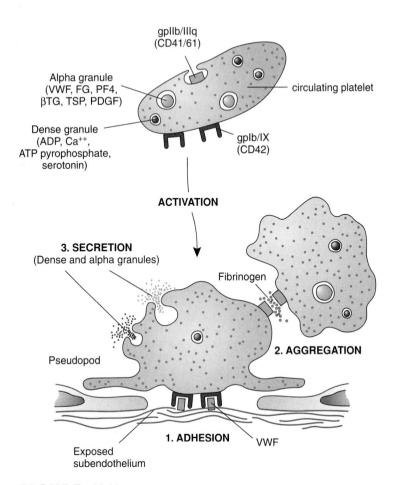

F I G U R E 20-11

Platelet activation involves three overlapping mechanisms. *(1)* Adhesion to the exposed subendothelium is mediated by the binding of von Willebrand factor (vWF) to gpIb/IX (CD42) and is the initiation signal for activation. *(2)* Exposure of gpIIb/IIIa (CD41/61) to the fibrinogen (FG) receptor on the platelet surface allows for platelet aggregation. *(3)* At the same time, platelets secrete their granule contents, which facilitates further activation. α-Granules contain vWF, fibrinogen, platelet factor 4 (PF4), thromboglobulin (TG), thrombospondin (TSP), and platelet-derived growth factor (PDGF). (From Rubin E, Gorstein F, Rubin R, et al. Rubin's Pathology, 4th ed. Philadelphia: Lippincott Williams & Wilkins, 2005, p. 1050.)

After the thrombus is formed, additional growth is controlled by removal of platelet-activating factors and coagulation proteins. Fibrinolysis, or dissolution of the thrombus, is activated by endothelial cells, which produce plasminogen activators that convert plasminogen to plasmin. The two major plasminogen activators are tissue plasminogen activator (t-PA) and urokinase-type plasminogen activator (u-PA). Conversion of plasminogen also is regulated by various inhibitors, including plasminogen activator inhibitor-I (PAI-I), antiplasmin, and thrombin-activatable fibrinolysis inhibitor (TAFI). Fibrolysis occurs with wound repair, which involves migration of fibroblasts into the wound, extracellular matrix formation, and recanalization of occluded blood vessel. Disorders of anticoagulation are termed *hypercoagulable states*.

Hemostatic Disorders

Disorders of clotting can be placed in two categories: *hemostatic disorders*, in which failure to repair damaged blood vessels results in bleeding; and *thrombotic disorders*, in which the fluidity of the blood is not maintained and obstructive vascular events occur. Several conditions may result in hemostatic disorders with consequent bleeding, including vascular disorders (purpura), platelet abnormalities (petechiae and purpuric hemorrhage), and coagulation factor deficiencies (hemorrhage into muscles, viscera, and joint spaces) (Table 20-9).

Blood Vessel Dysfunction

Blood vessel dysfunction may be caused by defects in supporting structures (extravascular dysfunction) or defects in the vessels directly (vascular dysfunction) (Table 20-10).

Extravascular dysfunction may occur in the following conditions:

- Senile purpura: age-related atrophy of supporting connective tissues
- Purpura simplex: occurs at time of menstruation; resolves quickly
- Scurvy: vitamin C deficiency resulting in defective collagen synthesis

Deposition of immunoglobulin fragments may occur in amyloidosis, cryoglobulinemia, and other paraproteinemias. Additional forms of vascular dysfunction include immunologic damage to the vessel such as in arteritis and allergic purpura, as well as heritable syndromes (e.g., hereditary hemorrhagic telangiectasia).

Table 20-9

Principal Causes of Bleeding

Vascular disorders
  Senile purpura
  Purpura simplex
  Glucocorticoid excess
  Dysproteinemias
  Allergic (Henoch-Schönlein)
    purpura
  Hereditary hemorrhagic
    telangiectasia
Platelet abnormalities
  Thrombocytopenia
  Qualitative disorders
    Inherited
      Glycoprotein IIb/IIIa deficiency
        (Glanzmann thrombasthenia)
      Glycoprotein Ib/IX/V deficiency
        (Bernard-Soulier syndrome)
      Storage pool disease (α and Δ)
      Abnormal arachidonic acid
        metabolism
    Acquired
      Uremia
      Drugs
      Cardiopulmonary bypass
      Myeloproliferative disorders
      Liver disease
Coagulation factor deficiencies
  Inherited
    von Willebrand disease
    Hemophilia A
    Hemophilia B
  Acquired
    Vitamin K deficiency/antagonism
    Liver disease
    Disseminated intravascular
      coagulation

From Rubin E, Gorstein F, Rubin R, et al. Rubin's Pathology, 4th ed. Philadelphia: Lippincott Williams & Wilkins, 2005, p. 1051.

Hereditary Hemorrhagic Telangiectasia

Hereditary hemorrhagic telangiectasia, also termed *Rendu-Osler-Weber syndrome,* is an autosomal dominant disorder of venules and capillaries that results in tortuous, dilated blood vessels. The vessels have inadequate elastic tissue and smooth muscle surrounding the vessels, which results in thinning and vascular dilation. Telangiectasias are reddish nodules that appear on the lips and nose and can subsequently transform into arteriovenous malformations or aneurysmal dilations at multiple sites throughout the body. Patients demonstrate recurrent hemorrhage, recurrent epistaxis (nosebleeds), anemia, and gastrointestinal hemorrhage with advancing age.

Allergic Purpura

Allergic purpura, also termed *Henoch-Schönlein purpura* (HSP), occurs in children after viral infection as a self-limited disease or in adults after drug exposure, and may be chronic. Microscopically,

Table 20-10

Hemostatic Disorders Leading to Increased Bleeding

Anemia Type	Description	Blood
Extravascular dysfunction		
Senile purpura	Age-related atrophy of supporting tissues	Superficial, sharply demarcated purpura on forearms
Purpura simplex	Menstruation	Purpura of deeper dermis resolves quickly
Scurvy	Vitamin C deficiency; defective collagen	Perifollicular hemorrhages
Vascular dysfunction		
Amyloidosis, arteritis	Vessel wall weakening	
Hereditary hemorrhagic telangiectasia (Rendu-Osler-Weber syndrome)	Autosomal dominant; thinning of vascular wall because of inadequate surrounding smooth muscle	Tortuous, dilated vessels (telangiectasias) that may progress to arteriovenous malformations
Allergic purpura (Henoch-Schönlein Purpura)	Follows viral illness or drug exposure; immuno logical damage to blood vessels	Purpura with associated raised urticarial lesions; ± gastrointestinal and renal disease
Platelet disorders		
Leukemia	Replacement of bone marrow by leukemic cells; decreased numbers of megakaryocytes	Petechiae to severe hemorrhage
Idiopathic thrombocytopenic purpura	Antibodies against platelet/megakaryocyte antigens	Self-limited hemorrhagic form (children); chronic bleeding disorder (adults)
Drug-induced thrombocytopenia	Immune-mediated platelet destruction (quinine, heparin) or decreased production (chemotherapy)	Petechiae to severe hemorrhage

(continues)

Table 20-10
(continued)

Anemia Type	Description	Blood
Pregnancy-associated thrombocytopenia	Often dilutional during third trimester; may be severe in pre-eclampsia/eclampsia syndromes	HELLP syndrome in eclampsia includes hemolysis, elevated liver enzymes, and low platelets
Neonatal thrombocytopenia	Inherited (e.g., Wiskott-Aldrich syndrome) or acquired (e.g., neonatal alloimmune thrombocytopenia)	± Congenital abnormalities
Thrombotic thrombocytopenic purpura	Possible introduction of platelet-aggregating substance into the blood	Thrombocytopenia, microangiopathic hemolytic anemia, neurologic symptoms, fever, renal impairment; platelet microthrombi in end organs
Hemolytic-uremic syndrome	Enteric infection (children), unclear in adults	Platelet microthrombi in the renal vasculature, leading to renal failure
Splenic sequestration of platelets	Splenomegaly	Mild thrombocytopenia; platelet life span normal or only slightly reduced
Bernard-Soulier syndrome (giant platelet syndrome)	Autosomal recessive; defect in membrane glycoprotein complex GPIb/IX (CD42) or GPV	Platelets vary widely in size and shape; giant platelets; childhood onset of ecchymoses, epistaxis, gingival bleeding; GI bleeding
Glanzmann thrombasthenia	Autosomal recessive; defect in membrane glycoprotein complex GPIIb/IIIa (CD41/61)	Mucocutaneous bleeding, epistaxis shortly after birth

(continues)

Table 20-10

(continued)

Anemia Type	Description	Blood
Alpha storage pool disease	Absence of α granules in platelets	Thrombocytopenia; mild bleeding; large, pale platelets
Delta storage pool disease	Abnormality of dense granules in platelets	Mild to moderate bleeding; associated with other hereditary disorders (e.g., Chediak-Higashi syndrome)
Thrombocytosis	Iron-deficiency anemia, splenectomy, cancer, chronic inflammation, polycythemia vera	Increased platelets; may lead to thrombosis
Coagulopathies		
Hemophilia A	Factor VIII deficiency; X-linked	Mild to severe hemorrhage
Hemophilia B	X-linked disorder of factor IX	15% of hemophilia cases; similar clinically to hemophilia A
von Willebrand disease	Deficiency of abnormality of vWF; 20 subtypes	Mild bleeding diathesis in types I and III; severe hemorrhage in type III

HSP demonstrates leukocytoclastic vasculitis with a perivascular neutrophilic and eosinophilic infiltrate. In addition, the vessel wall demonstrates fibrinoid necrosis and platelet plugging. Immunofluorescence reveals IgA and complement in the vessel wall. Patients have purpuric spots with raised urticarial lesions as well as occasional renal failure and gastrointestinal bleeding.

Platelet Disorders

Platelet disorders are associated frequently with bleeding, ranging from easy bruisability to severe hemorrhage, and commonly occur in the mucocutaneous tissues, leading to menorrhagia, epistaxis, and gingival bleeding. Petechiae also are often associated with platelet disorders and appear as small (<2 mm) red lesions that do not blanch; frequently they are found on the buccal mucosa, soft palate, lower extremities, and pressure points.

Thrombocytopenia

Thrombocytopenia is a platelet count of greater than $150,000/\mu L$ (normal $150,000-400,000/\mu L$), with the risk of hemorrhage inversely associated with platelet count. Thrombocytopenia may be caused by decreased platelet production, increased platelet destruction, or impaired platelet function. Table 20-11 describes the most common forms of thrombocytopenia.

Decreased production of platelets within the bone marrow may be caused by loss of megakaryocytes (infiltrating *leukemia* cells, *metastatic cancer*, and *aplastic anemia*) or intrinsic abnormalities of the megakaryocytes (*myelodysplasia*). *Mary-Hegglin anomaly* is a hereditary defect in megakaryocyte maturation associated with thrombocytopenia and circulating giant platelets.

Increased destruction of platelets occurs after immune-mediated damage, such as in *idiopathic thrombocytopenic purpura (ITP)* and *drug-induced thrombocytopenia*.

Idiopathic (Immune) Thrombocytopenic Purpura

ITP is caused by antibodies directed against platelet or megakaryocyte antigens. The bone marrow demonstrates a compensatory increase in megakaryocytes. Peripheral blood examination reveals decreased platelet counts ($<20,000/\mu L$ in acute ITP), nu-

---

Table 20-11

Principal Causes of Thrombocytopenia

Decreased production	Increased destruction
Aplastic anemia	Immunologic (idiopathic, HIV,
Bone marrow infiltration	drugs, alloimmune, posttransfusion
(neoplastic fibrosis)	purpura, neonatal)
Bone marrow suppression by	Nonimmunologic (DIC, TTP, HUS,
drugs or radiation	vascular malformations, drugs)
Ineffective production	Increased sequestration: splenomegaly
Megaloblastic anemia	Dilutional: blood and plasma transfusions
Myelodysplasias	

From Rubin E, Gorstein F, Rubin R, et al. Rubin's Pathology, 4th ed. Philadelphia: Lippincott Williams & Wilkins, 2005, p. 1053.

merous large platelets, and commonly, IgG bound to the surface of the platelets.

Acute ITP is a self-limited hemorrhagic disease of children that occurs after a viral illness. Affected patients present with the sudden onset of petechiae and purpura, often without additional symptoms. Severe cases may be at risk for intracranial hemorrhage. Severe cases of acute ITP are managed with corticosteroids and gamma globulin administration.

Chronic ITP is a chronic bleeding disorder of adults that is associated with collagen vascular disease, chronic lymphocytic leukemia, and human immunodeficiency virus (HIV). Patients with chronic ITP present with repeated episodes of bleeding, including epistaxis, menorrhagia, or ecchymoses. This disease is treated with corticosteroids, danazol, and intravenous gamma globulin; splenectomy may produce remission in severe cases.

Neonatal Thrombocytopenia

Neonatal thrombocytopenia may be inherited or acquired. Inherited forms include the following:

- Wiskott-Aldrich syndrome: X-chromosome WASP gene defect; affected boys have small platelets, eczema, and immunodeficiency
- Amegakaryocytic thrombocytopenia
- Thrombocytopenia-absent radius syndrome
- Fanconi anemia: genetic bone marrow failure; thrombocytopenia and red blood cell macrocytosis; associated congenital anomalies including skin hypopigmentation, short stature, microcephaly, microphthalmia, and radial/thumb abnormalities

Acquired forms of neonatal thrombocytopenia include the following:

- Neonatal alloimmune thrombocytopenia (NAIT): caused by alloimmunization to platelet antigens such as HPA-1a during pregnancy. NAIT leads to destruction of fetal platelets, predisposing the fetus or neonate to intracranial hemorrhage.
- Additional causes: birth asphyxia, necrotizing enterocolitis, and thrombosis

Thrombotic Thrombocytopenic Purpura

TTP most likely occurs after the introduction of platelet-aggregating substances into the circulation (e.g., large vWF multimers), which leads to widespread platelet deposition in the microvasculature as evidenced by hyaline thrombi. TTP may occur as a rare heritable form or secondary to autoimmune collagen vascular disease, drug administration, infections, and pregnancy.

Microscopically, PAS-positive hyaline microthrombi are present in the arterioles and capillaries of end organs, such as the kidney, brain, and heart. No inflammation is associated with these thrombi. Blood examination reveals fragmented erythrocytes (schistocytes) and numerous reticulocytes.

TTP most commonly affects women in the fourth and fifth decades and may occur as an acute, fulminant, often fatal disease or as a chronic, recurrent disease. The classical presentation of TTP is the pentad of thrombocytopenia (often $<20,000/\mu L$), microangiopathic hemolytic anemia, neurologic symptoms, fever, and renal impairment. Widespread purpura is present. Despite platelet aggregation, the coagulation cascade is not activated; therefore, the prothrombin time, partial thromboplastin time (PTT), and fibrinogen concentration is normal. Treatment involves plasma infusion and plasmapheresis, with a cure rate of 80%.

Hemolytic-uremic Syndrome

Hemolytic-uremic syndrome (HUS) may represent a variant of TTP and is primarily characterized by platelet microthrombi in the renal glomerulus, which ultimately leads to renal failure. The additional findings of TTP are not present in HUS. HUS occurs in both children and adults. In children, the disease often occurs after an enteric infection with *Escherichia coli* or *Shigella dysenteriae*.

Inherited Platelet Disorders

Bernard-Soulier Syndrome

Bernard-Soulier syndrome, also known as giant platelet syndrome, is an autosomal recessive disorder in which a defect in the membrane glycoprotein complex GPIb/IX (CD42) or GPV that binds vWF. Examination of the blood reveals thrombocytopenia and circulating giant platelets. The disease becomes symptomatic during childhood with ecchymoses, epistaxis, and gingival bleeding. During later ages, the disease is manifested by menorrhagia and gastrointestinal bleeding

Glanzmann Thrombasthenia

Glanzmann thrombasthenia is an autosomal recessive disorder in which a defect occurs in the glycoprotein complex IIb/IIIa (CD41/61), which binds fibrinogen and vWF. Platelets fail to aggregate or retract, leading to impaired hemostasis. Patients present shortly after birth with mucocutaneous or gingival hemorrhage, epistaxis, or bleeding after circumcision.

Acquired Platelet Disorders

A variety of causes may lead to acquired platelet disorders, including the following:

- Drugs: aspiring, nonsteroidal analgesics, β-lactam antibiotics, ticlopidine
- Renal failure: heterogeneous abnormality; aggravated by uremia
- Cardiopulmonary bypass surgery: Extracorporeal circuit
- Hematologic malignancies: chronic myeloproliferative disorders, dysproteinemias (platelets coated by plasma paraprotein)

Coagulation Factor Disorders

Many coagulation factors are produced in the liver. Any disease process that interferes with hepatic function, such as liver failure, can lead to widespread decreases in the levels of coagulation factors. In addition, a subset of coagulation factors produced by the liver are vitamin K–dependent and include factors II, VII, IX, and X; the activities of this subset of coagulation factors is decreased in cases of vitamin K deficiency. Vitamin K deficiency may occur secondary to reduced dietary intake, antibiotic use, or colonic resection, because intestinal bacteria are necessary for vitamin K conversion to a highly absorbable form.

Coagulation factor abnormalities often may be detected as increased prothrombin time (PT) and partial thromboplastin time (PTT). Increased thrombin time indicates an abnormality of fibrinogen, which can lead to bleeding with fibrinogen deficiencies and either bleeding or thrombosis with fibrinogen dysfunction.

Hereditary and acquired disorders of all of the coagulation factors have been identified. The most common abnormalities involve factor VIII (hemophilia A), factor IX (hemophilia B), and vWF (vWD). Hemophilia A is discussed in Chapter 6.

Acquired inhibitors of coagulation factors (also termed circulating anticoagulants), contribute to hemostatic disorders. These antibodies are often IgG autoantibodies directed against factor VIII and vWF and may occur after administration of plasma concentrates and with autoimmune disorders. Lupus anticoagulants are antiphospholipid antibodies that occur in many autoimmune diseases and most commonly presents with thrombotic events rather than bleeding disorders.

Hemophilia B

Hemophilia B is an X-linked deficiency of factor IX, which accounts for 15% of all cases of hemophilia (hemophilia A accounts for the remainder). Factor IX is a vitamin K–dependent protein that is synthesized in the liver. Factor IX is activated by tissue factor/VIIa and functions together with VIIIa, PL, and calcium on activated platelet surfaces to activate factor X, which subsequently leads to clotting. The clinical manifestations of hemophilia B include a mild, moderate, or severe bleeding tendency.

von Willebrand Disease

vWF disease (vWD) is a heterogeneous group of hereditary diseases characterized by a deficiency or abnormality of vWF. vWF is synthesized by megakaryocytes and endothelial cells. Following endothelial injury, vWF undergoes polymerization and binding to platelet glycoprotein receptors GPIIb/IX (D42) and GPIIb/IIIa (CD41/61) to promote platelet aggregation. In the plasma, vWF binds to and protects factor VIII; vWF absence is associated with a deficiency in factor VIII activity.

There are three subtypes of vWD, which are listed as follows:

- Type I: 75% of cases; autosomal dominant; quantitative vWF deficiency
- Type II: 20% of cases; qualitative vWF defect; vWF and endothelial cell interaction is defective; decreased plasma vWF and factor VIII activity
- Type III: autosomal recessive; least common; most severe form, near or total absense of vWF

The majority of cases of vWD, with the exception of type III, is associated with mild bleeding diathesis. The most common presenting symptom is excessive hemorrhage after trauma or surgery. Other symptoms include easy bruising, epistaxis, menorrhagia, and gastrointestinal bleeding. vWD can be treated with factor VIII, vWF concentrates, or cryoprecipitate. Administration of the vasopressin analogue DDAVP, which increases the release of preformed vWF from endothelial cells, is of use in types I and II vWD.

Disseminated Intravascular Coagulation

DIC originates with activation of the clotting cascade by tissue damage or damage to the endothelium. The substantial amounts of thrombin produced in these cases, as well as failure of thrombin neutralization, lead to uncontrolled intravascular coagulation that ultimately results in consumption of clotting factors, platelets, and fibrinogen and a consequent hemorrhagic diathesis (Fig. 20-12). DIC may occur in many settings, including massive trauma, septicemia, and obstetric emergencies, all of which lead to the release of tissue factor.

The endothelium itself plays an important role in the pathogenesis of many cases of DIC (Fig. 20-13). Microscopically, microthrombi composed of fibrin and platelets are identified in arterioles,

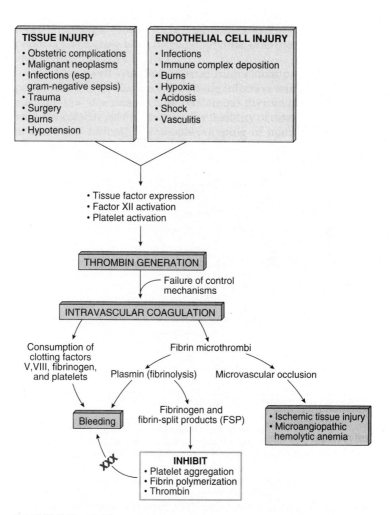

FIGURE 20-12
The pathophysiology of disseminated intravascular coagulation
(DIC). The DIC syndrome is precipitated by tissue injury, endothelial cell injury, or a combination of the two. These injuries trigger
increased expression of tissue factor on cell surfaces and activation
of clotting factors (including XII and V) and platelets. With the failure of normal control mechanisms, generation of thrombin leads to
intravascular coagulation. (From Rubin E, Gorstein F, Rubin R, et
al. Rubin's Pathology, 4th ed. Philadelphia: Lippincott Williams &
Wilkins, 2005, p. 1059.)

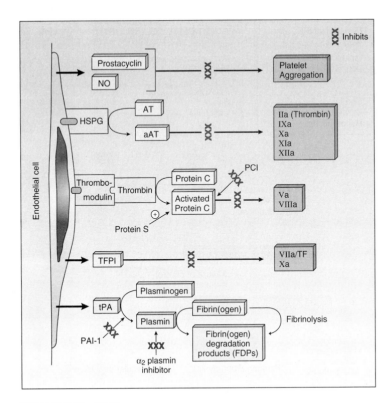

F I G U R E   20-13

The role of endothelium in anticoagulation, platelet inhibition, and thrombolysis. The endothelial cell plays a central role in the inhibition of various components of the clotting mechanism. Heparan sulfate proteoglycan potentiates the activation of antithrombin (AT) 15-fold. Thrombomodulin stimulates the activation of protein C by thrombin 30-fold. NO, nitric oxide; HSPG, heparan sulfate proteoglycan; PCI, protein C inhibitor; TFPI, tissue factor pathways inhibitor; tPA, tissue plasminogen activator; PAI-I, plasminogen activator inhibitor-I. *Arrows*, products secreted by the endothelial cell; *bars*, molecules bound to the cell surface; +, potentiation; *XXX*, inhibition. (From Rubin E, Gorstein F, Rubin R, et al. Rubin's Pathology, 4th ed. Philadelphia: Lippincott Williams & Wilkins, 2005, p. 1060.)

capillaries, and venules throughout the body. Obstruction by microthrombi leads to tissue ischemia, which is most evident in the end organs such as the brain, kidneys, and heart. Bleeding also occurs at these sites because of the consumption of clotting factors in this cascade. Examination of the blood reveals fragmented erythrocytes (schistocytes). DIC can lead to microangiopathic hemolytic anemia, thrombocytopenia, and depletion of clotting factors. Increased levels of D-dimers and fibrin degradation products are present.

The clinical features of DIC reflect microvascular thrombosis as well as a bleeding tendency. Symptoms may include seizures, coma, acute renal failure, acute respiratory distress syndrome, and gastrointestinal tract hemorrhages. Treatment involves the administration of heparin (to interrupt intravascular coagulation) and replacement of platelets and clotting factors (to control bleeding).

Hypercoagulable States

A hypercoagulable state is defined as an increased risk of thrombosis in circumstances that would not cause thrombosis in a normal person. In some cases, the thrombotic event may be arterial. Clinically, hypercoagulable states may be suspected in patients who have unexplained thrombotic episodes and one or more of the following:

- Recurrence of thrombotic event
- Thrombosis at a young age
- Family history of thrombotic episodes
- Thrombosis in unusual anatomical locations
- Difficulty in controlling thrombosis with anticoagulants

A summary of hypercoagulable states is presented in Table 20-12.

Table 20-12

Principal Causes of Hypercoagulability

Inherited	Therapy
Activated protein C resistance	Factor concentrates
(factor V Leiden)	Heparin
Antithrombin deficiency	Oral contraceptives
Protein C deficiency	Hyperlipidemia
Protein S deficiency	Thrombotic thrombocytopenia
Dysfibrinogenemias	purpura
Acquired	
Lupus inhibitor	
Malignancy	
Nephrotic syndrome	

From Rubin E, Gorstein F, Rubin R, et al. Rubin's Pathology, 4th ed. Philadelphia: Lippincott Williams & Wilkins, 2005, p. 1061.

Inherited Hypercoagulability

Inherited forms of a hypercoagulability state often are caused by mutations in components of the fibrinolytic cascade. These heritable forms include:

- Activated protein C (APC) resistant-factor V Leiden: point mutation in factor V becomes resistant to actions of APC and there is an increased risk of deep venous thrombosis (DVT) by sevenfold in heterozygotes and 80-fold in homozygotes
- Antithrombin deficiency: autosomal dominant with an increased risk of venous thrombosis
- Protein C and protein S deficiencies: increased risk of venous thrombosis and homozygous protein C deficiency results in life-threatening neonatal thrombosis with purpura fulminans
- Prothrombin genetic variants

Acquired Hypercoagulability

Acquired forms of hypercoagulability occurs in conditions such as the following:

- Venous stasis: prolonged immobility, congestive heart failure
- Myeloproliferative disorders
- Heparin-associated thrombocytopenia
- TTP
- Antiphospholipid antibody syndrome

The *antiphospholipid antibody syndrome* occurs when IgG antibodies are formed against proteins that interact with anionic phospholipids such as phosphatidylserine (PS) or cardiolipin, which are exposed on activated platelets. Antiphospholipid antibody syndrome is the leading acquired cause of thrombosis. A subtype of antibody formed in this syndrome is lupus anticoagulant. Laboratory workup for this syndrome includes the detection of lupus-type anticoagulant activity, anticardiolipin antibodies, and antibodies to β2-GPI in the presence of cardiolipin. Patients with this syndrome develop thromboembolic events, thrombocytopenia, and spontaneous abortions.

Impaired Platelet Function

Impaired platelet function also may lead to a hypercoagulable state and has been implicated in recurrent arterial thrombosis and post-coronary angioplasty stenosis. Antiplatelet treatment includes aspirin, ticlopidine, and ReoPro (a GPIIa/IIIb inhibitor).

Vascular Injury

Vascular injury may lead to a hypercoagulable state. Atherosclerosis, arteritis, aneurysms, and arteriovenous malformations may lead to arterial thrombotic events. Venous thrombosis may occur with vasculitis, tortuous veins, or venous stasis.

WHITE BLOOD CELLS

White blood cells (WBCs) encompass the neutrophils, eosinophils, basophils, lymphocytes, monocytes, and mast cells. Normal WBC counts range from 4,000 to 11,000 cells/μL, with the differential made up of 50% to 60% neutrophils, 2% to 4% neutrophil bands (immature forms), 30% to 40% lymphocytes, 1% to 9% monocytes, and usually less than 2% eosinophils and basophils (see Table 20-1).

Each component of the WBC panel may be reduced or increased in number or undergo neoplastic change.

Neutrophil Abnormalities

Neutrophils are responsible for the destruction of microorganisms at sites of infection by phagocytosis of organisms and intraphagosome release of hydrogen peroxide and lysosomal myeloperoxidase. Normal neutrophil levels range from 1,800 to 7,000/μL. Abnormalities may occur in neutrophil function in conjunction with altered absolute neutrophil counts or with intrinsic neutrophil dysfunction.

Neutropenia
Neutropenia is a reduction in number of neutrophils, which leads to impaired defenses against microorganisms, especially when neutrophil counts drop to <500/μL. Neutrophil levels may be reduced because of decreased production or increased peripheral destruction by hypersplenism, overwhelming infections, or antibody-mediated removal. The majority of cases of neutropenia are asymptomatic, but severe cases may result in widespread bacterial infections. Table 20-13 lists common causes of neutropenia.

Neutrophilia
Neutrophilia is defined as an absolute neutrophil count greater than 7,000/μL and occurs secondary to increased mobilization from the bone marrow storage pool, enhanced release from the peripheral blood marginal pool, or stimulation of granulopoiesis in the bone marrow. In acute infections, the neutrophil level may

Table 20-13

Principal Causes of Neutropenia

Decreased production	Increased destruction
Irradiation	Isoimmune neonatal
Drug induced (long and short term)	Autoimmune
	Idiopathic
Viral infections (HIV)	Drug induced (e.g., zidovudine, sulfonamides)
Congenital (Kostmann syndrome, infantile genetic agranulocytosis)	Felty syndrome
Cyclic (decreased production every 21 days)	Systemic lupus erythematosus
	Dialysis (complement activation induced)
Ineffective production	
Megaloblastic anemia	Splenic sequestration
Myelodysplastic syndromes	Increased margination

Modified from Rubin E, Gorstein F, Rubin R, et al. Rubin's Pathology, 4th ed. Philadelphia: Lippincott Williams & Wilkins, 2005, p. 1062.

be elevated to such levels that it may be mistaken for chronic myeloid leukemia; this condition is termed leukemoid reaction. However, unlike leukemic states, the leukemoid reaction contains mature appearing neutrophils with cytoplasmic granules. Table 20-14 lists common causes of neutrophilia.

Chronic Granulomatous Disease

Chronic granulomatous disease (CGD) is a rare, X-linked or autosomal recessive disease characterized by a failure of the respiratory

Table 20-14

Principal Causes of Neutrophilia

Infections	Drugs
Primarily bacterial	Glucocorticoids
Immunologic inflammatory	Colony-stimulating factors (CSFs)
Rheumatoid arthritis	Lithium
Rheumatic fever	Hereditary: CD18 deficiency
Vasculitis	Metabolic
Neoplasia	Acidosis
Hemorrhage	Uremia

From Rubin E, Gorstein F, Rubin R, et al. Rubin's Pathology, 4th ed. Philadelphia: Lippincott Williams & Wilkins, 2005, p. 1062.

Table 20-15	
Principal Causes of Eosinophilia	
Allergic disorders	Collagen vascular disorders
Skin diseases	Miscellaneous
Parasitic (helminth) infestations	Hypereosinophilic syndromes
Malignant neoplasms	Eosinophilia–myalgia syndrome
Hematopoietic	IL-2 therapy
Solid tumors	

From Rubin E, Gorstein F, Rubin R, et al. Rubin's Pathology, 4th ed. Philadelphia: Lippincott Williams & Wilkins, 2005, p. 1064.

burst and hydrogen peroxide formation after phagocytosis of organisms. Therefore, these neutrophils and macrophages are unable to kill catalase-positive microorganisms such as *Staphylococcus aureus* and *Salmonella*, which are able to neutralize hydrogen peroxide by their own catalase. CGD manifests at any age with recurrent infections that lead to widespread microabscesses and granulomas. The diagnosis is established by measuring the respiratory burst by nitroblue tetrazolium (NBT) test.

Chédiak-Higashi syndrome

Chédiak-Higashi syndrome is a rare autosomal recessive disease characterized by giant lysosomes in many cell types. It results in neutropenia, decreased chemotaxis, impaired degranulation, and ineffective bactericidal activity. Patients have recurrent bacterial and fungal infections of the skin, mucous membranes, and respiratory tract, as well as prolonged bleeding times and oculocutaneous albinism.

Eosinophil Abnormalities

Eosinophils differentiate in the bone marrow, circulate briefly in the peripheral blood, and migrate preferentially to the gastrointestinal and respiratory tracts and the skin. Eosinophils participate in IgA-mediated responses such as parasitic, dermatologic, and allergic conditions. Normal absolute eosinophil counts range from 0 to 450/μL. Causes of eosinophilia are listed in Table 20-15.

An increase in circulating eosinophils greater than 1,500/mL for more than 6 months, without known underlying disease, results in the *idiopathic hypereosinophilic syndrome*. Eosinophil degranulation can lead to myocardial necrosis and neurologic dysfunction. Aggressive treatment with corticosteroids increases 5-year survival to 70%.

Basophil Abnormalities

Basophils differentiate in the bone marrow, circulate briefly in the peripheral blood and pass into tissues. Normal absolute eosinophil counts range from 0 to 200/μL. Basophils contain histamine and chondroitin sulfate granules and can synthesize leukotriene. Basophilia often occurs in immediate-type hypersensitivity reactions and chronic myeloproliferative syndromes. Additional causes of basophilia are listed in Table 20-16.

Monocyte Abnormalities

Monocytes are derived from precursor cells in the bone marrow and are found in many tissues throughout the body. Normal absolute monocyte levels range from 0 to 800/μL. Elevated levels of monocytes, or *monocytosis*, occurs in many conditions including:

- Hematologic disorders: accounts for 50% of monocytosis; may be a component of acute or chronic myelogenous leukemia
- Immunologic and inflammatory conditions: may occur with neutropenia as a compensatory mechanism
- Infectious disease
- Solid cancers

Table 20-16
Principal Causes of Basophilia

Allergic (drug, food)	Neoplasia
Inflammation	Myeloproliferative syndromes
Juvenile rheumatoid arthritis	Basophilic leukemia
Ulcerative colitis	Carcinoma
Infection	Endocrine
Viral (chickenpox, influenza)	Diabetes mellitus
Tuberculosis	Myxedema
	Estrogen administration

From Rubin E, Gorstein F, Rubin R, et al. Rubin's Pathology, 4th ed. Philadelphia: Lippincott Williams & Wilkins, 2005, p. 1065.

Langerhans Cell Histiocytosis

Langerhans cells are components of the mononuclear phagocyte system and are found in the epidermis, lymph nodes, spleen, thymus, and mucosal tissues. Langerhans cells ingest, process, and present antigens to T lymphocytes. Langerhans cell histiocytosis (LCH) is believed to represent a neoplastic proliferative disorder that affects children and young adults and demonstrates a broad manifestation from asymptomatic involvement of a single site to an aggressive systemic disorder. Various subtypes of LCH include the following:

- Eosinophilic granuloma: 75% of LCH; localized, self-limited disorder; older children (5–10 years) and young adults (<30 years); male predominance; bones and lungs affected
- Hand-Schüller-Christian disease: 25% of LCH; multifocal indolent disorder; children between 2 and 5 years; involvement of bones and endocrine glands; classic triad of diabetes insipidus, proptosis, and defects in membranous bones in 15% of patients
- Letterer-Siwe disease: less than 10% of LCH; acute disseminated variant; infants and children under 2 years of age; involvement of skin, visceral organs, and hematopoietic system; poor outcome

The LCH cells are large with abundant pink cytoplasm and round to indented nuclei with nuclear creases or grooves, delicate vesicular chromatin, and small nucleoli. Electron microscopy demonstrates rod-shaped Birbeck granules in the cytoplasm. These cells stain for CD1a and S100.

LCH cells infiltrate numerous organs and are accompanied by a mixed population of eosinophils, neutrophils, and plasma cells. Foci of necrosis may be seen. Organ infiltration demonstrates specific patterns, including sinusoidal infiltration of the lymph nodes and liver, alveolar septa of the lung, the red pulp of the spleen, the superficial papillary dermis of the skin, and the bone marrow stroma. Patients demonstrate various findings based on site of involvement, including seborrheic dermatitis, painless lymphadenopathy, hepatosplenomegaly, painful lytic bone lesions, and diabetes insipidus.

Mast Cell Abnormalities

Mast cells are derived from precursors in the bone marrow and subsequently are localized adjacent to blood vessels within connective tissues. Mast cells may range in shape from elongated, spindled cells to stellate cells and contain a centrally situated, round, frequently indented nucleus. The cytoplasm is pale pink and finely granular, with prominent granules identified by special stains. These granules contain histamine, heparin, chemotactic factors, and proteases; extensive release of these substances may cause flushing, pruritus, and hives as is evident in mast cell proliferative disorders. Increased levels of mast cells (*mastocytosis*) occur in the following conditions:

- Mast cell hyperplasia: reactive mastocytosis; immediate- and delayed-type hypersensitivity reactions; associated with Waldenström macroglobulinemia, osteoporosis, and myelodysplastic syndromes
- Mastocytoma: localized mastocytosis; cutaneous nodule in children; spontaneously resolves
- Urticaria pigmentosa: multiple, symmetric cutaneous nodules in children; spontaneously resolves
- Systemic mastocytosis: infiltration of many organs including skin, lymph nodes, spleen, liver, bones, bone marrow, and gastrointestinal tract by mast cells; results in gastrointestinal pain, diarrhea, anaphylactic episodes, and occasionally secondary pancytopenia caused by marrow involvement
- Mast cell leukemia: complicates 15% of systemic mastocytosis cases
- Mast cell sarcoma: anaplastic mast cell variants infiltrate many sites; poor prognosis

Techniques in the Diagnosis of Myeloid and Leukemic Disorders

The remainder of this chapter is dedicated to hematologic malignancies arising from myeloid or leukemoid cells, which include leukemias and lymphomas. Common techniques are used to categorize surface marker expression and cellular morphology in these disorders.

- Flow cytometry: uses the passage of single cells labeled with a panel of fluorescent antibodies through various detectors to determine cell size (forward scatter), granularity (side scatter), and surface molecules.
- Immunohistochemistry: used on paraffin-embedded tissue to determine cellular expression of various molecules
- Cytogenetics (including conventional banding techniques and fluorescence in situ hybridization [FISH]): used to detect chromosomal aberrations and translocations
- Molecular diagnostics (with polymerase chain reaction [PCR]–based techniques): used to determine Ig heavy chain

rearrangements for B-cell clonality and T-cell receptor rear-rangements for T-cell clonality.

Leukemias and Myelodysplastic Syndromes

Chronic Myeloproliferative Diseases

Chronic myeloproliferative diseases are defined as clonal hematog-enous stem cell disorders with increased proliferation of one or more myeloid lineages (granulocytic, erythroid, or megakaryocytic cells). The diseases affect adults 40 to 80 years of age. A summary of bone marrow, liver, and spleen findings, as well as laboratory values, is presented in Tables 20-17 and 20-18.

Chronic Myelogenous Leukemia

Chronic myelogenous leukemia (CML) is a disease of transformed pluripotent stem cells in the bone marrow, resulting in prominent increases in neutrophilic cells over the full range of maturation in the bone marrow and blood. The most common myeloproliferative disease, CML accounts for 15% to 20% of all cases of leukemia, with peak onset during the fifth and sixth decades.

More than 95% of all cases contain the Philadelphia chromo-some, which is a t(9:22),(q34:q11) translocation resulting in the for-mation of the *BCR/ABL* fusion gene. *BCR/ABL* encodes the p210 protein, which acts as a constitutively activated tyrosine kinase. Exposure to benzene or radiation has been suggested to represent risk factors for CML.

CML may present in chronic, accelerated, or blast phases.

- Chronic phase: increased levels of maturing neutrophils; less than 10% blasts; elevated levels of basophils, eosinophils, and platelets in the blood; completely hypercellular bone marrow filled with myeloid and myeloid precursor cells; abnormal-appearing megakaryocytes may be present
- Accelerated phase: follows chronic phase; 10% to 20% blasts in the blood or bone marrow; greater than 20% blood basophils; may be associated with persistent thrombocytopenia or throm-bocytosis; splenomegaly; increasing white blood cell count un-responsive to therapy, additional chromosomal abnormalities
- Blast phase: final outcome; greater than 20% blasts in the bone marrow; clusters of blasts in the bone marrow; extramedullary proliferation of blasts in the skin, lymph nodes, spleen, other sites; 70% of patients show residual myeloid features; remain-ing patients appear lymphoblastic and contain features of B- or T-precursor cells

Table 20-17

Chronic Myeloproliferative Syndromes: Morphologic Features

	Polycythemia Vera	Chronic Myelogenous Leukemia	Chronic Idiopathic Myelofibrosis	Essential Thrombocythemia
Bone marrow				
Histopathology	Panhyperplasia (predominantly erythroid)	Panhyperplasia (predominantly granulocytic)	Panhyperplasia with fibrosis	Atypical megakaryocytes predominate
M:E ratio	≤2:1	10:1 to 50:1	2:1 to 5:1	2:1 to 5:1
Marrow iron	↓ or absent	Normal or ↑	Normal or ↑	Normal to absent
Marrow fibrosis	15%–20%	<10%	90%–100%	<5%
Liver, spleen				
Extramedullary hematopoiesis (myeloid metaplasia)	Moderate (predominantly erythroid)	Moderate to marked (predominantly granulocytic)	Moderate to marked	Slight (predominantly megakaryocytic)

From Rubin E, Gorstein F, Rubin R, et al. Rubin's Pathology, 4th ed. Philadelphia: Lippincott Williams & Wilkins, 2005, p. 1070.

Table 20-18

Chronic Myeloproliferative Syndromes: Laboratory Features

	Polycythemia Vera	Chronic Myelogenous Leukemia	Chronic Idiopathic Myelofibrosis	Essential Thrombocythemia
Hemoglobin	>20 g/dL	Mild anemia	Mild anemia	Mild anemia
RBC morphology	Slight anisocytosis and poikilocytosis	Slight anisocytosis and poikilocytosis	Immature erythrocytes, marked anisocytosis, poikilocytosis, and tear drop cells	Hypochromic microcytes
Granulocytes	Normal to mildly increased; may show a few immature forms	Moderate to markedly increased with spectrum of maturation	Normal to moderately increased; some immature WBCs	Normal to slightly increased
Platelets	Normal to moderately increased	Normal to moderately increased	Increased to decreased	Markedly increased with abnormal forms
Leukocyte alkaline phosphatase (LAP)	Normal to increased	Decreased to absent	Variable	Variable
Cytogenetics	Nonspecific	Philadelphia chromosome (Ph¹); *BCR/ABL* gene rearrangement	Nonspecific	Nonspecific

From Rubin E, Gorstein F, Rubin R, et al. Rubin's Pathology. 4th ed. Philadelphia: Lippincott Williams & Wilkins, 2005, p. 1071.

The median survival time for CML is 5 to 7 years. The treatment involves specific targeting of the *BCR/ABL* gene product using Gleevec, although cure may be achieved in certain cases only by allogenic bone marrow transplantation.

Polycythemia Vera

Polycythemia vera (PCV) is caused by an uncontrolled production of erythropoietin-independent red blood cells by a clonal hematopoietic stem cell, which undergoes proliferation in the bone marrow and occasionally extramedullary sites (e.g., spleen, lymph nodes, liver). PCV often is diagnosed at 60 years of age, and a specific set of major and minor criteria must be satisfied for diagnosis (Table 20-19).

The bone marrow in PCV appears homogenously red-purple and microscopically is hypercellular, with hyperplasia of all elements, although the erythroid precursor cells predominate. Erythroid and granulocytic maturation is normal; megakaryocytes tend to cluster. A decrease in bone marrow iron is present in 90% of patients; many patients show an increase in fibrosis. Examination of the peripheral blood reveals normal erythrocytes with hypochromia and microcytosis in certain patients secondary to iron deficiency. Elevations in serum hemoglobin, hematocrit (often >60%), total iron-binding capacity, and leukocyte, neutrophil, eosinophil, basophil, and platelets numbers are present. Platelets often appear abnormal and aggregate readily on exposure to ADP, epinephrine, and collagen.

Table 20-19

Criteria Used in the Diagnosis of Polycythemia Vera

Major criteria

Increased blood cell mass: Hgb>18.5 g/dL in men, >16.5 g/dL in women
No elevation of erythropoietin
No cause of secondary erythrocytosis
Splenomegaly
Demonstration of a clonal genetic abnormality other than *BCR/ABL*
Erythroid colony formation in vitro in the absence of growth factors

Minor criteria

Thrombocytosis: platelets >400 × 10^9/L
Leukocytosis: >12 × 10^9/L
Prominent erythropoiesis and megakaryopoiesis in the bone marrow
Low serum erythropoietin levels

Patients with PCV demonstrate symptoms related to the increased red blood cell mass, such as splenomegaly because of accumulation of red cells in the red pulp and sinuses, headache, dizziness, visual problems, angina pectoris, intermittent claudication, gastric ulcers, and thrombotic events leading to stroke and myocardial infarction.

PCV occurs in distinct phases, which include the following:

- Proliferative phase: prolonged phase of erythroid proliferation and increased red blood cell mass; one third of patients progress
- Spent phase: proliferation ceases; stable or decreased erythrocyte mass
- Postpolycythemic myelofibrosis with myeloid metaplasia: severe myelofibrosis with progressive anemia and myeloid metaplasia (immature erythroid, granulocyte and megakaryocyte forms) in the spleen; mean survival of 2 years in this stage
- Acute myelogenous leukemia (AML): Occurs in 5% to 10% of PCV cases; increased risk if prior ^{32}P or alkylating agent treatment

The average survival of patients with PCV is 13 years, although because of the late onset of disease, many patients succumb to diseases related to advanced age rather than PCV.

Chronic Idiopathic Myelofibrosis

Chronic idiopathic myelofibrosis represents a clonal myeloproliferative disorder in which marrow fibrosis is accompanied by prominent megakaryopoiesis and granulopoiesis. This disease occurs most frequently in the seventh decade of life.

The malignant megakaryocytes produce PDGF and TGF-α that stimulate proliferation of fibroblasts, leading to myelofibrosis. After myelofibrosis overwhelms the marrow space, the malignant cells enter the circulation and give rise to extramedullary hematopoiesis at multiple sites.

Most patients are diagnosed at the prefibrotic stage and have a hypercellular marrow with neutrophil and abnormal megakaryocyte predominance. In the fibrotic phase, the peripheral blood demonstrates leukopenia or marked leukocytosis, as well as immature myeloid and erythroid precursors. The bone marrow in this phase is extensively fibrotic.

Patients present with signs of extramedullary hematopoiesis, including hepatosplenomegaly and lymphadenopathy. In addition, patients may experience fatigue, night sweats, fever, and weight loss. A subset of patients (approximately 15%) may progress to AML.

Essential Thrombocythemia

Essential thrombocythemia is a neoplastic proliferation of mega-karyocytes that results in a marked increase in circulating platelets (>600,000/µL) and recurrent episodes of thrombosis and hemor-rhage. This disease primarily affects middle-aged adults. A diagno-sis of essential thrombocythemia may not be made in the presence of other underlying myeloproliferative disease, chromosomal ab-normality, dysplastic change, or reactive thrombocytosis.

The bone marrow in essential thrombocythemia is hypercellu-lar with increased numbers of megakaryocytes. Rarely, hyperplasia of all lineages is seen. Megakaryocytes often are clustered and dem-onstrate abnormal morphology, including large, bizarre, hyperch-romatic, hyperlobulated nuclei as well as smaller micromegakaryo-cyte forms. Large clusters of free platelets are identified.

The spleen is mildly enlarged and demonstrates a homogene-ous red-purple cut surface with expansion of the red pulp and myeloid metaplasia. Because platelets accumulate in the spleen, splenectomy (which enhances thrombocytosis leading to worsened thrombotic events) is contraindicated.

Patients have a median survival of 10 years, with a course complicated by mild bleeding, small vessel thrombosis, and rarely thrombosis of large arteries and veins. Recurrent hemorrhage in the gastrointestinal tract also may lead to iron deficiency anemia. AML may occur in 5% of patients. Treatment involves plate-letpheresis and myelosuppressive chemotherapy.

Chronic Neutrophilic Leukemia

Features of this rare disease include sustained peripheral blood neutrophilia, bone marrow hypercellularity, neutrophilic granulo-cyte proliferation, and hepatosplenomegaly. More than 80% of the peripheral blood must contain mature, segmented neutrophils, and no BCR/ABL gene rearrangement may be present. All other forms of neutrophilia must be excluded before this diagnosis may be made.

Chronic Eosinophilic Leukemia and Hypereosinophilic Syndrome

Chronic eosinophilic leukemia features a clonal proliferation of eosinophils with elevated blood eosinophils (>1,500/µL). In-creased eosinophils also involve the bone marrow and peripheral tissues, resulting in cardiac and pulmonary damage. This disease also may be diagnosed after exclusion of secondary eosinophilia. If no clonal origin or abnormal phenotype can be established, chronic elevation of eosinophils is designated *hypereosinophilic syndrome*.

Myelodysplastic Syndromes

Myelodysplastic syndromes (MDS) are clonal hematopoietic stem cell disorders that predominantly affect elderly people. Dysplastic morphologic features in one or more hematopoietic lineages are accompanied by ineffective hematopoiesis. The diseases demonstrate a surprising discrepancy between the paucity of peripheral blood elements and the marked hyperplasia in the bone marrow in contrast to the myeloproliferative diseases, in which increased marrow cellularity leads to increased circulating elements.

All forms of MDS are characterized by *refractory anemia* but may have additional types of cytopenia. Depending on the subtype, increased myeloblasts may be identified in the bone marrow. When the number of myeloblasts reaches 20% (determined by flow cytometry), a diagnosis of AML is established. Risk factors for MDS include the following:

- Prior chemotherapy with alkylating agents or radiation
- Viral infection
- Benzene exposure
- Cigarette smoking
- Fanconi anemia

The classification of MDS is based on the number of myeloblasts and the presence of morphologically dysplastic features in at least one hematopoietic lineage; the erythroid lineage is most commonly affected. Dysplastic features include the following:

- Erythroid lineage: megaloblastoid change, multinucleation, nuclear budding, bridging between nuclei, karyorrhexis and ringed sideroblasts (iron stain)
- Granulocyte lineage: nuclear hypersegmentation or hyposegmentation, cytoplasmic hypogranulation
- Megakaryocyte lineage: mononuclear or hypolobated forms (may be seen in a variety of conditions; not specific for MDS)

The number of blasts is categorized as less than 5% (refractory anemia), 5% to 9% (refractory anemia with excess blasts-1/RAEB-1) and 10% to 19% (RAEB-2). Blast counts of 20% or greater in the bone marrow is classified as AML.

Patients with MDS present with anemia, neutropenia, and thrombocytopenia. A specific subtype of MDS affects predominantly women and demonstrates isolated deletion of chromosome 5 (5q-). *MDS associated with isolated del(5q)* features normal or increased platelet counts and is associated with a more favorable prognosis. Table 20-20 lists the various subtypes of MDS.

Acute Myeloid Leukemia

AML is characterized by clonal expansion of myeloblasts in the bone marrow and their subsequent appearance in the blood and

Table 20-20

World Health Organization Classification Peripheral Blood and Bone Marrow Findings in Myelodysplastic Syndromes

Disease	Blood Findings	Bone Marrow Findings
Refractory anemia (RA)	Anemia No or rare blasts	Erythroid dysplasia only <5% blasts <15% ringed sideroblasts
Refractory anemia with ringed sideroblasts (RARS)	Anemia No blasts	≥15% ringed sideroblasts Erythroid dysplasia only <5% blasts
Refractory cytopenia with multilineage dysplasia (RAMD)	Cytopenia (bicytopenia or pancytopenia) No or rare blasts No Auer rods <1 × 10⁹/L monocytes	Dysplasia in ≥10% of the cells of two or more myeloid cell lines <5% blasts in marrow No Auer rods <15% ringed sideroblasts
Refractory cytopenia with multilineage dysplasia and ringed sideroblasts (RCMD-RS)	Cytopenia (bicytopenia or pancytopenia) No or rare blasts No Auer rods <1 × 10⁹/L monocytes	Dysplasia in ≥10% of the cells of two or more myeloid cell lines ≥15% ringed sideroblasts <5% blasts No Auer rods
Refractory anemia with excess blasts (RAEB-1)	Cytopenias <5% blasts No Auer rods <1 × 10⁹/L monocytes	Unilineage or multilineage dysplasia 5%–9% blasts No Auer rods
Refractory anemia with excess blasts (RAEB-2)	Cytopenias 5%–19% blasts Auer rods ± <1 × 10⁹/L monocytes	Unilineage or multilineage dysplasia 10%–19% blasts Auer rods ±
Myelodysplastic syndrome -unclassified (MDS-U)	Cytopenias No or rare blasts No Auer rods Anemia	Unilineage dysplasia: one myeloid cell line <5% blasts No Auer rods
MDS associated with isolated del(5q)	Usually normal or increased platelet count <5% blasts	Normal to increased megakaryocytes with hypolobated nuclei <5% blasts Isolated del(5q) cytogenetic abnormality No Auer rods

From Rubin E, Gorstein F, Rubin R, et al. Rubin's Pathology, 4th ed. Philadelphia: Lippincott Williams & Wilkins, 2005, p. 1076.

tissues. At least 20% of blasts must be present in the bone marrow for a diagnosis of AML, and myeloblasts must demonstrate cytochemical and immunophenotypic characteristics of myeloid cells. AML accounts for 70% of acute leukemias (the remainder are lymphoblastic leukemias). Onset of AML occurs near 60 years of age. Risk factors for AML include cigarette smoking; radiation exposure; chemotherapy; or the presence of certain myeloproliferative or myelodysplastic conditions, including polycythemia vera, essential thrombocytopenia, chronic idiopathic myelofibrosis, and RAEB-1 and -2.

The bone marrow demonstrates prominent hypercellularity and is filled with monotonous medium to large-sized cells with round or slightly irregular nuclei. The presence of Auer rods, which are specific for the myeloid lineage, may be present in certain types of AML. Flow cytometry identifies myeloblasts by the presence of CD13, CD15, CD33, CD34, and CD117. Immunostaining reveals reactivity for myeloperoxidase and for nonspecific esterase.

AML may be subdivided into four categories:

- AML with recurrent genetic abnormalities
- AML evolving from multilineage dysplasia
- AML related to treatment
- AML not otherwise specified

The major clinical problems associated with AML are related to the rapid growth of certain cells within the bone marrow at the expense of others. Patients often demonstrate granulocytopenia, thrombocytopenia, and anemia.

Acute Promyelocytic Leukemia

Acute promyelocytic leukemia (APL) is a form of AML that demonstrates a distinct underlying translocation involving chromosomes 15 and 17. It accounts for 5% to 10% of all cases of AML, which primarily affects middle-aged patients. APL results from a translocation involving the *PML1* gene and the retinoic acid receptor (*RAR*) gene, which encodes a functional retinoic acid receptor. This receptor can be specifically targeted by treatment with all-*trans*-retinoic acid (ATRA), which facilitates the maturation of the leukemic cells.

The bone marrow is markedly hypercellular and filled with cells that have promyelocytic morphologic features. Abundant Auer rods are present. These cells demonstrate strong reactivity for myeloperoxidase, CD13, and CD33. Patients with APL often present with DIC when senescent leukemia cells degranulate and activate the coagulation cascade.

Therapy-induced Acute Myeloid Leukemia

The most common chemotherapeutic drugs that give rise to AML are alkylating agents and topoisomerase II inhibitors.

Acute Myeloid Leukemia Evolving from Multilineage Dysplasia

Acute myeloid leukemia may arise in the context of a myelodysplastic syndrome

Acute Myeloid Leukemia Not Otherwise Specified

These varieties of AML do not demonstrate recurrent cytogenetic abnormalities and have been previously classified in the French-American-British (FAB) classification scheme as M0-M7 and L1–L3. These AML forms are categorized as the following:

- Minimally differentiated (M0): immature myeloblasts with no defining morphologic criteria; identified by flow cytometry; unfavorable prognosis
- AML without maturation (M1): less than 10% of cells are promyelocytes or more mature forms
- AML with maturation (M2): greater than 10% of cells are promyelocytes or more mature forms
- Acute myelomonocytic leukemia (AMML; M4): 20% to 80% of cells show monocytoid features; extramedullary infiltration common
- Acute monoblastic/monocytic leukemia (AmoL; M5): at least 80% of cells show monocytoid features; common in younger patients and infants; masses in the skin, gingival, and CNS; aggressive disease
- Acute erythroid leukemia (M6): greater than 50% of nucleated cells in the bone marrow are erythroid precursors with remaining population as at least 20% myeloblasts; aggressive disease
- Acute megakaryoblastic leukemia (AmegL; M7): at least 50% of blasts have a megakaryocytic phenotype; childhood leukemia associated with t(1;22) and hepatosplenomegaly; late complication of mediastinal germ cell tumors; dismal prognosis

LYMPHOPOIETIC SYSTEM

The lymphopoietic system comprises the B and T lymphocytes, lymph nodes, spleen, thymus, and mucosal-associated lymphoid tissues (MALT) of the intestine and bronchus.

Lymphoid Cells

Lymphocytes are derived from bone marrow precursor cells but, unlike the myeloid lineages, undergo maturation at variable sites.

T lymphocytes mature in the thymus, where recombination of the T-cell receptor genes leads to the production of different receptors that each recognizes a specific antigen. T cells express CD2 (earliest marker), CD3, and CD5 with variable expression of CD4 (helper T cells) or CD8 (suppressor T cells). After maturation, T cells migrate to the lymph nodes, spleen, and peripheral blood. $CD4^+$ T cells are activated by HLA class II molecules and subsequently induce differentiation and antibody production by B cells. $CD8^+$ T cells are activated by HLA class I molecules and subsequently limit the expansion of activated B cells and terminate their immune response.

B lymphocytes mature within the bone marrow and demonstrate the markers CD19 (earliest), CD20, CD22, and CD79a. Early B cells also express CD10 and TdT. Like all cells, B cells demonstrate surface HLA class I molecules; however, because of their antigen-presenting nature, these cells also demonstrate surface HLA class II molecules. During B-cell maturation, the immunoglobulin heavy chains undergo gene rearrangement in preparation for the synthesis of IgM, as well as demonstrate kappa and lambda light chains. When activated by antigen and T cells, B cells undergo differentiation into plasma cells that can synthesize and secrete antibodies. *Null cells* or *natural killer (NK) cells* are a small percentage of lymphocytes that do not require antigenic recognition for their function. NK cells are recognized by their granular cytoplasm and also termed large granular lymphocytes.

Lymphocytes that have not been activated appear as small- to medium-sized cells. Following activation by antigen, both B and T cells undergo transformation to large, protein-synthesizing cells, called atypical lymphocytes, in the peripheral blood and immunoblasts in tissue sections, where they demonstrate a round nucleus with vesicular chromatin and one to several nucleoli apposed to the nuclear membrane. Terminally differentiated B cells are termed *plasma cells* and demonstrate a clock-face chromatin pattern, eccentric nuclei, moderate amounts of cytoplasm, and a clear paranuclear zone that represents the Golgi complex. In the peripheral blood, approximately 60% to 80% of lymphocytes are T lymphocytes and 10% to 15% are B lymphocytes.

Lymph Nodes

Lymph nodes are organized collection of lymphoid tissue located along the lymphatic vessels. The lymph node contains an outer cortex, which contains B and T cell populations, and an inner medulla. The B-cell–dependent cortex contains primary (inactive) follicles and secondary (active) follicles. Secondary follicles contain germinal centers, which demonstrate a mixed of small cleaved lymphocytes (centrocytes) and large lymphocytes (centroblasts). Scattered "tingible body" macrophages are present in the germinal centers to phagocytose apoptotic debris. Follicular dendritic cells form a meshwork within the follicular center and serve to present antigens to follicular B cells. The interdigitating reticulum cells (IDCs) present antigen to T cells in this region. Lymphatic fluid enters the lymph node via afferent vessels, passes through the subcapsular sinuses, and exits via the efferent lymphatics (Fig. 20-14).

Aggregates of lymphoid tissue are also present in the gastrointestinal tract, oropharynx and nasopharynx (Waldeyer ring), and bronchial tree. These MALTs are important in protection of the host from potential invaders.

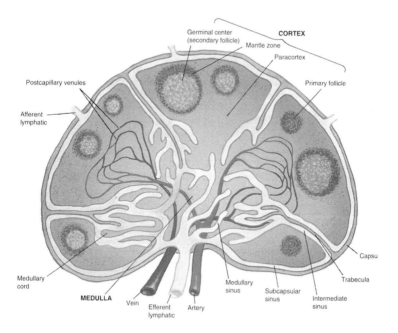

FIGURE   20-14
Structure of a normal lymph node. (From Rubin E, Gorstein F, Rubin R, et al. Rubin's Pathology, 4th ed. Philadelphia: Lippincott Williams & Wilkins, 2005, p. 1084.)

Reactive Alterations in the Lymphopoietic System

Lymphocytosis

Peripheral blood lymphocytosis is defined as an absolute peripheral blood lymphocyte count of greater than $4,000/\mu L$ in adults. Lymphocytosis may occur with the following:

- Acute infections: infectious mononucleosis, whooping cough
- Chronic bacterial infections: tuberculosis, brucellosis
- Lymphoproliferative diseases

Viral infections often present with lymphocytosis and are characterized by atypical lymphocytes, which are large cells with round to irregular nuclei, coarsely clumped chromatin, one to several nucleoli, and abundant blue cytoplasm. The majority of atypical lymphocytes are $CD8^+$ T cells.

Acute infectious lymphocytosis is a rare, self-limited childhood disorder that is often asymptomatic but may manifest with mild fever, abdominal pain, and diarrhea and demonstrates increased levels of circulating T cells.

Plasmacytosis

Peripheral blood plasmacytosis (increased levels of circulating plasma cells) may occur in plasma cell neoplasia (multiple myeloma) and some viral infections.

Reactive bone marrow plasmacytosis occurs when marrow plasma cells account for more than 3% of the marrow cellularity. This condition is seen with many infectious, inflammatory, and neoplastic disorders. Increased production of immunoglobulins may lead to the presence of cytoplasmic eosinophilic aggregates termed Russell bodies. The invagination of immunoglobulin-containing cytoplasm into the nucleus creates an impression of an eosinophilic nuclear inclusion on cut section and is termed a Dutcher body.

Lymphocytopenia

Lymphocytopenia reflects decreased peripheral blood lymphocytes to less than $1,500/\mu L$ in adults, which is generally reflected as a decrease in $CD4^+$ T cells (the most numerous lymphocyte in the circulating blood).

Lymphocytopenia occurs in the following conditions:

- Decreased production of lymphocytes: Hodgkin lymphoma, acquired immunodeficiency syndromes
- Increased destruction of lymphocytes: radiation, chemotherapy, ACTH, steroids, AIDS

- Loss of lymphocytes: damage to lymphatics in the gastrointestinal tract, as in Whipple disease

Lymph Node Hyperplasia

The lymph nodes may demonstrate a variety of patterns reflective of the underlying disease process that can affect all cellular components present. Hyperplasia of the secondary follicles and medullary cords indicate B-cell immunoreactivity (germinal centers), whereas hyperplasia of the deep cortex or paracortex reflects T-cell immunoreactivity (interfollicular or diffuse hyperplasia). Figure 20-15 illustrates the various forms of lymph node reactivity.

Follicular Hyperplasia

This nonspecific reaction demonstrates expansion of the germinal centers in the cortex. The cells contained within the germinal centers may be small, cleaved cells (centrocytes) or larger cells with vesicular chromatin and prominent nucleoli (centroblasts). Numerous macrophages with pale cytoplasm give the germinal centers a "starry sky" appearance. In addition, numerous mitotic figures and apoptotic debris within the germinal center and a well-defined surrounding mantle of normal small B lymphocytes are present. Lymphadenopathy, or enlargement of the lymph nodes, may be localized or generalized in many diseases.

For instance, in *Castleman disease* (angiofollicular lymph node hyperplasia), which is a disorder of unknown etiology, the lymph nodes and extranodal tissue are involved and associated with follicular hyperplasia. Hyaline-vascular angiofollicular lymph node hyperplasia (90% of cases) commonly presents in the mediastinum of young men; demonstrates numerous small follicularlike structures with penetrating hyalinized thick-walled vessels, concentrically arranged small lymphocytes around the follicles (onion-skinning),

---

FIGURE   20-15

Lymph nodes. Patterns of benign reactive hyperplasia are contrasted with the structure of a normal lymph node. *Follicular hyperplasia* **with prominent enlarged and irregular benign follicles is characteristic of B-cell immunoreactivity.** *Interfollicular hyperplasia* **is typical of T-cell immunoreactivity. The** *sinusoidal pattern* **with expansion of sinuses by benign macrophages is seen in reactive proliferations of the mononuclear–phagocyte system. Mixed patterns of follicular, interfollicular, and sinusoidal hyperplasia are common in a variety of complex immune reactions. In** *necrotizing lymphadenitis,* **variable** *(continues)*

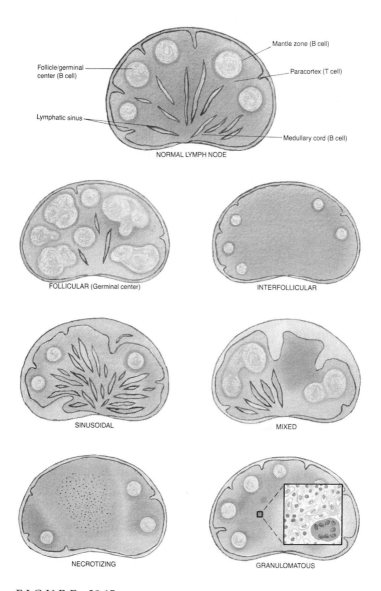

F I G U R E   20-15
(continued) necrosis of the lymph node architecture with residual cell debris is present. In *granulomatous inflammation,* cohesive clusters of macrophages and occasional multinucleated glial cells are characteristic. (From Rubin E, Gorstein F, Rubin R, et al. Rubin's Pathology, 4th ed. Philadelphia: Lippincott Williams & Wilkins, 2005, p. 1087.)

and prominent vascularity. Castleman disease termed Plasma cell angiofollicular lymph node hyperplasia: localized or generalized disease is pronounced interfollicular plasmacytosis and prominent vascularity. Patients with the multicentric form have a more aggressive course and are at increased risk for Kaposi sarcoma or immunoblastic lymphoma.

Interfollicular Hyperplasia

This disorder is an expansion of the paracortex by a heterogeneous cell population consisting of small T lymphocytes, variably activated lymphocytes, immunoblasts, scattered macrophages, and prominent postcapillary venules. Interfollicular hyperplasia may be nonspecific and occur in a variety of viral infections or as a result of specific etiologic factors, which are listed in Table 20-21.

Mixed Patterns of Reactive Hyperplasia

Mixed patterns of reactive hyperplasia may occur in variety of conditions, including toxoplasmosis and cat scratch disease.

Sinus Histiocytosis

Sinus histiocytosis is an increased number of tissue macrophages (histiocytes) in the subcapsular and trabecular sinuses of the lymph node. It occurs in lymph nodes draining sites of cancer or near sites of inflammation or infection. Often, material may be identified in the cytoplasm of the macrophages, such as hemosiderin or anthracotic pigment.

Rosai-Dorfman Disease

Rosai-Dorfman disease is a rare, benign, self-limited disorder that causes bilateral painless cervical lymphadenopathy. This disorder most commonly affects African Americans during the first two decades of life. Microscopically, Rosai-Dorfman disease demonstrates capsular and pericapsular fibrosis and chronic inflammation, sinus histiocytosis, and prominent intersinusoidal plasmacytosis. Often, lymphocytes may be identified within the cytoplasm of the histiocytes. The histiocytes are immunoreactive for CD68 and S100.

Infection-induced Hemophagocytic Syndrome

This syndrome occurs in immunodeficient patients and is characterized by generalized activation of tissue macrophages and ingestion of red blood cells. Clinically, patients experience acute onset

Table 20-21

Patterns of Reactive Lymph Node Hyperplasia

Disease	Etiology	Lymph Node Appearance	Associated Findings
Follicular hyperplasia			
Rheumatoid arthritis	Autoimmune disease	Prominent follicular hyperplasia and interfollicular plasmacytosis	Systemic disease; Swan-neck deformities of hands
Castleman disease (hyaline-vascular	Unknown	Numerous small follicles with penetrating thick-walled vessels; onion-skinning of follicles	Mediastinal mass in young men
Castleman disease (plasma cell form)	Unknown	Large hyperplastic follicles; interfollicular plasmacytosis; prominent vessels	Localized or multicentric disease
AIDS lymphadenopathy	HIV virus	Loss of mantle zones; infiltration of follicles by small lymphocytes; interfollicular hemorrhage	High risk of neoplasia; many other findings
Interfollicular hyperplasia			
Infectious mononucleosis	EBV virus	Immunoblastic cells in lymph node sinuses; ± bizarre binucleated or multinucleated immunoblasts	Fever, sore throat, splenomegaly, generalized lymphadenopathy

(continues)

Table 20-21
(continued)

Disease	Etiology	Lymph Node Appearance	Associated Findings
Varicella-herpes zoster	Varicella zoster virus	Endothelial cells with eosinophilic nuclear inclusions	Painful vesicular lesion in dermatome pattern
Measles	Rubeola	Scattered multilobed or mutinucleated lymphoid cells (Warthin-Finkeldey cells)	Rash, ulcerated mucosal lesions, subacute sclerosing panencephalitis
Cytomegalovirus	Cytomegalovirus	Large endothelial cells with intranuclear inclusions	Often immunocompromised patients
Kikuchi disease	Unknown	Focal infiltrates of immunoblasts and macrophages in cortex and paracortex; cellular debris	Cervical nodes of young women; self-limited
Phenytoin-induced	Phenytoin (Dilantin)	Infiltrate of small lymphocytes, immunoblasts, eosinophils, and plasma cells	Fever, rash, polyclonal agammaglobulinemia, peripheral eosinophilia
Systemic lupus erythematosus	Autoimmune	Infiltration by immunoblasts and plasma cells; focal to extensive necrosis	Systemic disease; multiple additional findings
Mixed pattern			
Toxoplasmosis	*Toxoplasma gondii*	Prominent follicular hyperplasia; foci of epitheliod macrophages in interfollicular regions; perisinusoidal B-cell hyperplasia	Mild disease in healthy patients; severe disease in immunocompromised and
Cat-scratch	*Bartonella* species	Follicular hyperplasia; suppurative granulomatous foci; stellate abscesses with central necrosis	Axillary and cervical lymphadenopathy

of fever, hepatosplenomegaly, lymphadenopathy, rash, pulmonary infiltration, and pancytopenia. Often, this disease is self-limited.

Malignant Lymphomas

Malignant lymphomas are malignant proliferations of lymphocytes or lymphoblasts and are categorized as Hodgkin lymphoma and B- and T-cell lymphomas. In addition, B- and T-cell neoplasms are subdivided into precursor and mature forms. Tables 20-22 and 20-23 provide a classification of B- and T-cell neoplasms. (Hodgkin disease is discussed at the end of this section.) In general, lymph nodes affected by lymphomas classically demonstrate a fleshy, pale gray to white homogenous cut surface with an appearance similar to fish flesh.

Precursor B-cell Neoplasms

B acute lymphoblastic leukemia/lymphoma (B-ALL/LBL) is a neoplasm of immature, or precursor, B lymphoblasts that can involve

---

Table 20-22

WHO Histological Classification of B-cell Neoplasms

Precursor B-cell neoplasm

  Precursor B lymphoblastic leukemia/lymphoma

Mature B-cell neoplasms

  Chronic lymphocytic leukemia/small lymphocytic lymphoma
  B-cell prolymphocytic leukemia
  Lymphoplasmacytic lymphoma
  Splenic marginal zone lymphoma
  Hairy cell leukemia
  Plasma cell lymphoma
  Monoclonal gammopathy of undetermined significance (MGUS)
  Solitary plasmacytoma of bone
  Extraosseous plasmacytoma
  Primary amyloidosis
  Heavy-chain diseases
  Extranodal marginal zone B-cell lymphoma of mucosa-associated
    lymphoid tissue (MALT lymphoma)
  Nodal marginal zone B-cell lymphoma
  Mediastinal (thymic) large B-cell lymphoma
  Intravascular large B-cell lymphoma
  Primary effusion lymphoma
  Burkitt lymphoma/leukemia

From Rubin E, Gorstein F, Rubin R, et al. Rubin's Pathology, 4th ed. Philadelphia: Lippincott Williams & Wilkins, 2005, p. 1091.

Table 20-23
WHO Histological Classification of T-cell and NK-cell Neoplasms

Precursor T-cell neoplasm

    Precursor T-lymphoblastic leukemia/lymphoma

Mature T-cell neoplasms

Leukemia/disseminated

    T-cell prolymphocytic leukemia
    T-cell large granular lymphocytic leukemia
    Aggressive NK-cell leukemia
    Adult T-cell leukemia/lymphoma

Cutaneous

    Mycosis fungoides
    Sézary syndrome
    Primary cutaneous anaplastic lymphoma
    Large cell lymphoma
    Lymphomatoid papulosis

Other extranodal

    Extranodal NK/T-cell lymphoma, nasal type
    Enteropathy-type T-cell lymphoma
    Hepatosplenic T-cell lymphoma
    Subcutaneous panniculitis-like T-cell lymphoma

Nodal

    Angioimmunoblastic T-cell lymphoma
    Peripheral T-cell lymphoma, unspecified
    Anaplastic large cell lymphoma

Neoplasm of uncertain lineage and stage of differentiation

    Blastic NK cell lymphoma

From Rubin E, Gorstein F, Rubin R, et al. Rubin's Pathology, 4th ed. Philadelphia: Lippincott Williams & Wilkins, 2005, p. 1092.

the peripheral blood and bone marrow (leukemia) or lymph nodes (lymphoma). B-ALL represents the majority of childhood leukemias and often occurs in patients younger than 6 years of age. The bone marrow in B-ALL/LBL contains at least 20% lymphoblasts, which appear as small- to medium-sized cells with increased nuclear-to-cytoplasmic ratio and inconspicuous nucleoli. Precursor B-cell leukemias represent early stage B cells that demonstrate the earliest markers TdT, CD19, and CD79a and lack immunoglobulin surface expression. B-ALL is subdivided into *pre-pre-B (early precur-*

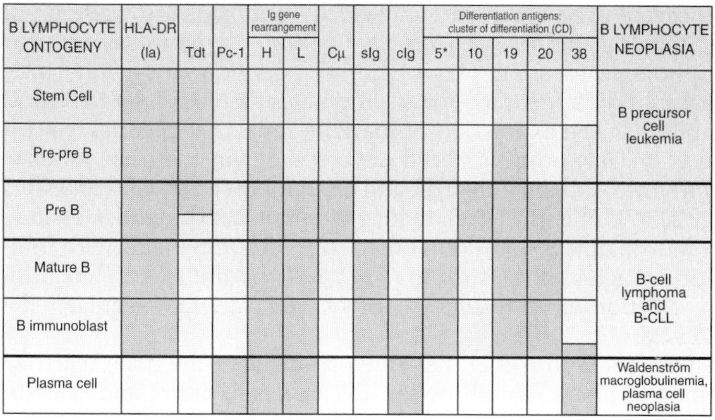

B LYMPHOCYTE ONTOGENY	HLA-DR (Ia)	Tdt	Pc-1	Ig gene rearrangement		Cμ	sIg	cIg	Differentiation antigens: cluster of differentiation (CD)					B LYMPHOCYTE NEOPLASIA
				H	L				5*	10	19	20	38	
Stem Cell														B precursor cell leukemia
Pre-pre B														
Pre B														
Mature B														B-cell lymphoma and B-CLL
B immunoblast														
Plasma cell														Waldenström macroglobulinemia, plasma cell neoplasia

FIGURE 20-16

B-cell maturation: Immunophenotypes and neoplastic counterparts. H, immunoglobulin heavy-chain gene; L, immunoglobulin light-chain gene; Cμ, cytoplasmic μ chain sIg surface immunoglobulin; cIg, cytoplasmic immunoglobulin. (From Rubin E, Gorstein F, Rubin R, et al. Rubin's Pathology, 4th ed. Philadelphia: Lippincott Williams & Wilkins, 2005, p. 1092.)

sor B) leukemia and *pre-B-cell leukemia* based on specific marker expression (Fig. 20-16).

B-ALL demonstrates numeric aberrations and chromosomal translocations that include the Philadelphia chromosome (in a minority of cases). A specific subtype of the Philadelphia chromosome *BCR/ABL* gene product, P190, is produced. Additional chromosomal abnormalities include t(4;11) involving the *MLL* gene at 11q23 and t(1;19) involving *PBX/E2A*.

Patients may demonstrate pancytopenia because of replacement of the bone marrow by neoplastic cells. In addition, organomegaly, CNS involvement, and bony involvement with arthralgias and bone pain may be present. Although highly responsive to chemotherapy, a poorer prognosis is associated with the following characteristics:

- Age less than 1 year or greater than 10 years
- t(9;22), t(1;19), or t(4;11) translocations
- 11q23 translocations involving the MLL gene
- Hypodiploid karyotype (<50 chromosomes)

Precursor T-cell Neoplasms

Precursor T-acute lymphoblastic leukemia (T-ALL) accounts for only 15% of childhood ALL; the remainder is B-ALL. In contrast, the majority of precursor/lymphoblastic lymphomas are made up of precursor *T-lymphoblastic lymphoma (T-LBL)*. T lymphoblasts appear morphologically similar to B lymphoblasts but may demonstrate a "starry sky" appearance of macrophages that is similar to Burkitt lymphoma. The expression of markers reflects sequential expression of markers during T-cell development in the bone marrow and thymus and includes TdT and CD7, followed by CD2 and CD5 (Fig. 20-17). The most common cytogenetic abnormalities include chromosomal translocation of the T-cell receptor chains with transcription factor genes, such as *MYC*, *RBTN1*, and *HOX11*. In addition, deletion of 9p results in loss of *CDKN2A* that regulates the cell cycle.

Patients with T-ALL have involvement of the bone marrow, peripheral blood, lymph nodes, liver, spleen, brain, and gonads. An origin of cells from thymic T cells may manifest as a mediastinal mass.

Mature (Peripheral) B-cell Lymphomas

Mature B-cell lymphomas make up the majority of all lymphomas. The most common are the follicular lymphoma and diffuse large

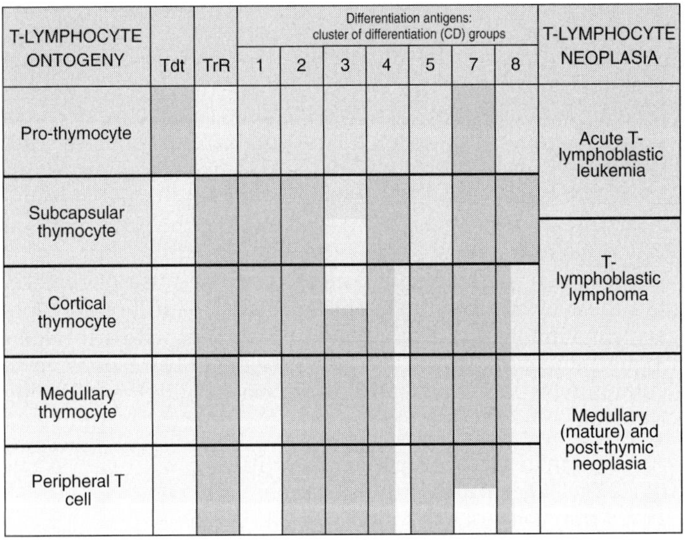

T-LYMPHOCYTE ONTOGENY	Tdt	TrR	Differentiation antigens: cluster of differentiation (CD) groups							T-LYMPHOCYTE NEOPLASIA
			1	2	3	4	5	7	8	
Pro-thymocyte										Acute T-lymphoblastic leukemia
Subcapsular thymocyte										
Cortical thymocyte										T-lymphoblastic lymphoma
Medullary thymocyte										Medullary (mature) and post-thymic neoplasia
Peripheral T cell										

FIGURE 20-17

T-cell maturation: Immunophenotypes and their neoplastic counterparts. TrR, T-cell receptor rearrangement. (From Rubin E, Gorstein F, Rubin R, et al. Rubin's Pathology, 4th ed. Philadelphia: Lippincott Williams & Wilkins, 2005, p. 1094.)

B-cell lymphoma. Most of these lymphomas, except for Burkitt lymphomas and diffuse large B-cell lymphoma, often occur in the sixth and seventh decades of life.

Mature B-cell lymphomas arise from clonal proliferations of peripheral B cells. Risk factors include infection with EBV or HIV, autoimmune diseases such as Hashimoto thyroiditis, or infection with *Helicobacter pylori*; however, the majority of cases are unrelated to these risk factors. Immunophenotyping of mature B-cell lymphomas reflects the developmental stage or maturation index of the malignant B cell and helps subclassify lymphomas.

The World Health Organization (WHO) separates mature B-cell lymphomas into those with predominant involvement of bone marrow, those with predominant extranodal involvement, and those with predominant lymphadenopathy. In general, mature B-cell lymphomas can be subdivided into those with an indolent clinical course (so-called low-grade B-cell lymphomas) and those with a more aggressive course (Table 20-24). Of note, the majority of low-grade lymphomas are not curable, whereas a number of the more highly aggressive lymphomas are sensitive to therapy.

Chronic Lymphocytic Leukemia/Small Lymphocytic Lymphoma

Chronic lymphocytic leukemia/small lymphocytic lymphoma (CLL/SLL) affects elderly persons and represents 7% of all malignant lymphomas. Predominant bone marrow and peripheral blood involvement justifies use of the term leukemia, and lymphadenopathy or solid tumor masses are best considered lymphomas.

CLL/SLL is made up of small, mature-appearing lymphocytes with a variable number of larger cells (prolymphocytes and paraimmunoblasts). Microscopically, the bone marrow exhibits patchy to diffuse involvement by malignant cells and the peripheral blood demonstrates ill-defined nuclear remnants termed "smudge cells." Lymph nodes are effaced and often demonstrate ill-defined follicular-type structures termed pseudofollicles or proliferation centers. The splenic white pulp is expanded and neoplastic cells also may involve the red pulp. Variable numbers of promyelocytes, which are larger cells with prominent nucleoli, may be found and increased promyelocyte numbers indicate a more aggressive course.

SLL/CLL cells express the B cell markers CD19, CD20, CD22, CD43, and CD79a. In addition, these cells express CD23 and the T-cell marker CD5. Expression of the plasma cell marker CD38 (CD138) or ZAP-70 reflects an unfavorable prognosis.

Half of CLL/SLL cases have undergone VH gene mutations. Common karyotypic abnormalities include trisomy 12 and deletions of 13q14 and 11q23.

Table 20-24

Mature (Peripheral) B-cell Lymphomas

Lymphoma	Pathology	Immunophenotype	Cytogenetics
Indolent lymphomas			
CLL/SLL	Ill-defined nodularity; mixture of large and small cells in lymph nodes	BCM, CD23, CD5	*VH* gene mutation, trisomy 12, deletions of 13q14 and 11q23
Lymphoplasmacytic lymphoma/ Waldenström macroglobulinemia	Interfollicular lymphoid infiltrate with plasma cells	BCM	t(9;14), *PAX5* gene rearrangement
Hairy cell leukemia	Marrow with interstitial plasma cells and ↑ reticulin	BCM, CD11c, CD25, FMC7, CD103, TRAP	No specific abnormalities
MALT (marginal zone) lymphomas	Occur in glandular organs or along mucosal surfaces	BCM	Trisomy 3; t(11;18) involving *API2/MLT*; somatic mutation of variable region genes
Follicular lymphoma	Lymph node with follicular pattern; loss of macrophage	BCM, CD10, Bcl-2	t(14;18)(q32;q21) involving *IgH/BCL2*; rearrangements of oncogene *BCL6*
Mantle cell lymphoma	Lymph node with expanded follicular mantle or diffuse infiltrate	BCM, CD5, nuclear Bcl-1, CD43	t(11;14)(q13;q32) involving *cyclin D1* (*BCL1*)/*IgH*

Aggressive lymphomae

Plasma cel neoplasia	Medullary cord or diffuse plasma cell infiltrate	CD79a	*IgH* gene rearrangement; t (11;14); *PAX5* abnormalities
Diffuse large B-cell lymphoma	Large centroblast-like cells or bizarre cells in lymph nodes or extranodal sites	BCM, +/−CD5, +/−CD10	*BCL2* gene rearrangements
Mediastinal (thymic) diffuse large B-cell lymphoma	Fibrotic, locally invasive mediastinal tumor	BCM	Ig gene rearrangements; *MAL* gene overexpression in many cases
Primary effusion lymphoma	HIV-infected patients; tumor cell suspensions in cavities	HHV8 virus; lack of BCM	Clonal *IgH* rearrangements
Burkitt lymphoma	Extranodal tumors, especially jaw	BCM, CD10, Bcl-6, surface IgM	t(8;14) involving *MYC* and *IgH* genes

BCM, B cellmarkers (including CD19, CD20, CD22, and CD79a).

B-CLL is diagnosed on the basis of sustained peripheral blood lymphocytosis (often >15,000/µL) and bone marrow lymphocytosis exceeding 40% of the nucleated elements. Early disease may be asymptomatic with splenomegaly or lymphadenopathy. Advanced disease demonstrates pancytopenia and B- and T-cell immunologic deficiencies leading to infectious complications. In many advanced cases, hypogammaglobulinemia and impaired delayed-type hypersensitivity reactions are present.

The overall mean survival for patients with B-CLL is 6 years. Adverse prognostic indicators include the following:

- Advanced disease (increased tumor burden)
- Diffuse pattern of marrow involvement
- Multiple chromosomal abnormalities
- Trisomy 12
- Lack of the 13q14 deletion
- CD38 expression
- Conversion to *prolymphocytic leukemia*: characterized by marked increase in blood lymphocyte counts, 15% to 50% prolymphocytes, and increasing splenomegaly; mean survival 2 years; increased risk of second cancer
- Development of *Richter syndrome*: rapid onset of fever, abdominal pain, and progressive lymphadenopathy and hepatosplenomegaly; mean survival 2 months; refractory to therapy

Asymptomatic, stable CLL/SLL often is not treated. Patients with advanced disease may receive chemotherapy and antilymphocyte antibodies. Splenectomy may be performed to control hypersplenism, and corticosteroids may be administered to control autoimmune hemolytic anemia.

Lymphoplasmacytic Lymphoma/Waldenström Macroglobulinemia

Lymphoplasmacytic lymphoma (LPL) primarily affects elderly patients and demonstrates a neoplastic proliferation of small lymphocytes and a variable number of IgM-secreting clonal plasma cells. Hepatitis C infection may be a risk factor.

LPL primarily involves the bone marrow but also can involve the lymph nodes, spleen, and peripheral blood. Bone marrow infiltration may be patchy or diffuse and demonstrates prominent numbers of plasma cells. Lymph nodes demonstrate an interfollicular infiltrate with plasma cells. LPL cells express the B antigens CD19, CD20, CD22, and CD79a but not CD23 or CD5. The most common translocation is t(9;14), and rearrangement of the *PAX5* gene, which encodes a B-cell–specific activator protein (BSAP), is common.

The majority of patients present with a monoclonal IgM spike on serum electrophoresis. Symptoms such as visual disturbances and stroke primarily result from hyperviscosity. Rouleaux of the red blood cells are present. Treatment involves plasmapheresis. The outcome is similar to that of B-CLL.

Hairy Cell Leukemia

Hairy cell leukemia affects middle-aged to elderly persons, with a male:female predominance of 5:1. Hairy cell leukemia is a clonal B-cell proliferation of small- to medium-sized lymphocytes that display abundant cytoplasm and hairlike protrusions of the cell membrane, which appear to have a "fried egg" appearance. This disease primarily affects the monocyte/macrophage system of the bone marrow, spleen, and liver. Within the bone marrow, neoplastic cells affect the interstitium without effacing the overall architecture. An increase in reticulin fibers often accompanies this disease, which leads to marrow fibrosis and difficulty in obtaining marrow aspirate material ("dry tap").

The neoplastic cells are immunoreactive for CD19, CD20, CD22, CD79a, as well as CD11c, CD25, FMC7 CD103, and tartrate-resistant acid phosphatase (TRAP).

Patients often present with splenomegaly and peripheral monocytopenia or pancytopenia. Long-term remission may be achieved with deoxycoformycin of 2-chlorodeoxyadenosine (2-CDA).

Extranodal Marginal-zone B-cell Lymphoma of Mucosa-associated Lymphoid Tissue

MALT lymphomas occur within glandular tissue or along mucosal surfaces and have a mean age of onset of 60 years. These lymphomas often arise in the context of autoimmune disease (Sjögren syndrome) or inflammation (H. pylori infection).

MALT lymphomas consist of small- to medium-sized lymphocytes with frequent monocytoid features and variable admixtures of plasma cells. Early lesions demonstrate an expansion of the marginal zone lymphocytes around reactive B-cell follicles. Involvement of the glandular epithelium by malignant lymphocytes is termed lymphoepithelial lesions. Occasionally, MALT lymphomas may transform into diffuse large B-cell lymphomas.

The neoplastic cells express B-cell markers CD19, CD20, CD22, CD79a, and IgM and demonstrate light-chain restriction. The most common cytogenetic abnormalities include trisomy 3 and t(11;18), which involves the apoptosis inhibitor gene *API2* and a novel gene *MLT*. Also, somatic mutation of the variable region genes is common.

MALT lymphomas affect the stomach, respiratory tract, head and neck, and skin, among other regions, and tend to follow an indolent course. Gastric MALT lymphomas respond to antibiotic therapy to treat underlying *H. pylori* infection.

Follicular Lymphoma

Follicular lymphoma (FL) recapitulates follicular formation within lymph nodes. The malignant follicles contain a mixture of smaller cells, with irregular or cleaved nuclei (centrocytes), and larger cells, with prominent nucleoli (centroblasts). FL accounts for 35% of all adult malignant lymphoma and has an average onset of 60 years of age.

FL primarily involves lymph nodes and is distinguished from benign follicular hyperplasia by ill-defined mantle zones, lack of germinal center polarization, absence of "starry sky" macrophages, and extracapsular invasion into the perinodal fat. FL demonstrates B-cell markers, CD10, and surface Ig, and is light-chain restricted. In contrast to normal germinal center B lymphocytes, FL has Bcl-2 expression. The most common cytogenetic abnormality is t(14; 18)(q32;q21), which involves *IgH* and *BCL2*, an inhibitor of apoptosis. A clonal rearrangement of the *BCL6* oncogene also is common.

The majority of cases of FL represent a low-grade, indolent process, although most patients present with advanced disease. FL is divided into grades 1, 2, and 3 based on the number of large cells present, with grade 1 lesions demonstrating few to no large blastic cells. Grade 3 lymphoma, which has more than 15% large cells, is the most aggressive form of FL. One third of patients progress to diffuse large B-cell lymphoma.

Mantle Cell Lymphoma

Mantle cell lymphoma is a B-cell neoplasm consisting of small- to medium-sized lymphocytes with irregular nuclear features. Mantle cell lymphoma affects patients at a median age of 60 years and more commonly affects men. Lymph nodes are diffusely infiltrated by malignant cells. On occasion, an expanded but malignant follicular mantle is present surrounding benign germinal centers (termed mantle zone lymphoma).

Malignant cells express B-cell markers, CD5, CD43, and nuclear Bcl-1 (cyclin D1). The most important cytogenetic abnormality is t(11;14)(q13;q32) involving *IgH* and *cyclin D1/BCL1*, which regulates the cell cycle.

Mantle cell lymphoma is a progressive disease and only 50% of patients survive 3 years.

Plasma Cell Neoplasia

Plasma cell neoplasms are malignant disorders of terminally differentiated B lymphocytes and include the following:

- Multiple myeloma (90%): multifocal infiltration of malignant plasma cells in the bone marrow; lytic bone lesions. Multiple myeloma is defined by a strict set of criteria (Table 20-25).
- Solitary osseous myeloma (5%): single destructive lesion of bone; often ribs, vertebrae, or pelvic bones; treated with radiation; 70% progress to multiple myeloma
- Extramedullary plasmacytoma (5%): soft tissue mass, often in the upper respiratory tract; 20% progress to multiple myeloma; treated by surgical resection or local radiation

Risk factors for the development of plasma cell neoplasia include genetic predisposition, ionizing radiation, or chronic antigenic stimulation. The osseous and extraosseous lesions in plasma cell neoplasia are red, tan, or gray and have a fleshy to gelatinous consistency. The bony lesions are well demarcated and the bone marrow demonstrates diffuse sheets or nodular aggregates of plasma cells that may encircle fat cells. In marrow aspirates, plasma cells generally account for more than 30% of the cellularity. These plasma cells may demonstrate dysplastic features, including binucleation, prominent nucleoli, and irregular chromatin. In addition, cytoplasmic (Russell bodies) and nuclear (Dutcher bodies) inclusions may be identified.

In most cases of plasma cell neoplasia, the cells secrete a homogenous, complete or partial immunoglobulin molecule termed an M-component or paraprotein. A sharp peak representing the paraprotein is present in serum or urine protein electrophoresis.

Table 20-25

WHO Diagnostic Criteria for Plasma Cell Myeloma

The diagnosis of myeloma requires a minimum of one major and one minor criterion or three minor criteria, which must include at least the first two

A. Major criteria
   1. Marrow plasmacytosis (>30%)
   2. Plasmacytoma on biopsy
3. M-component:
      Serum: IgG > 3.5 g/dL, IgA > 2 g/dL
      Urine: >1 g/24 hr of Bence-Jones protein
B. Minor criteria
   1. Marrow plasmacytosis (10%–30%)
   2. M-component present but less than above
   3. Lytic bone lesions
   4. Reduced normal immunoglobulins (<50% normal): IgG <600 mg/dL, IgA, 100 mg/dL, IgM , 50 mg/dL

From Rubin E, Gorstein F, Rubin R, et al. Rubin's Pathology, 4th ed. Philadelphia: Lippincott Williams & Wilkins, 2005, p. 1099.

Immunofixation of immunoglobulins further delineates this abnormal paraprotein. Multiple myeloma is subdivided on the basis of this paraprotein into the following:

- IgG myeloma: mean survival 3 to 4 years; infection common
- IgA myeloma: serum hyperviscosity because of IgA propensity to form dimers
- IgD myeloma: aggressive disorder; mean survival 1 year; extramedullary and renal involvement common; affects middle-aged men
- IgE myeloma: aggressive disorder; affects young adult men
- IgM myeloma
- Light-chain disease: only κ or λ chains synthesized; aggressive disorder
- Biclonal multiple myeloma: two distinct paraproteins secreted; rare
- Nonsecretory myeloma: no paraprotein secreted; rare

The cells in plasma cell neoplasia often secrete IgG or IgA, no surface Ig, and CD79a. Clonal rearrangements of *IgH* are common and multiple chromosomal abnormalities have been described, including t(11;14) of the *BCL1* locus and *PAX5* abnormalities.

Multiple organs are affected by plasma cell neoplasia, including the bones (lytic lesions, osteosclerosis), kidneys (light-chain cast nephropathy, glomerulopathy), lymph nodes, spleen (red pulp infiltrates), and liver (portal triad infiltration). The peripheral blood demonstrates a normocytic, normochromic anemia, hypercalcemia, and hyperuricemia.

Patients often present with bone pain, anemia, hypercalcemia, and renal insufficiency. Amyloidosis of light-chain origin occurs in 15% of cases. The hyperviscosity syndrome is common in IgG and IgA myeloma and results in neurologic abnormalities and spontaneous bleeding episodes. In addition, coagulation abnormalities and humoral immune deficiency often are present.

The clinical course of multiple myeloma is biphasic, with an initial chronic stable phase and a subsequent aggressive/accelerated phase. Patients treated with chemotherapy survive an average of 3 years. An increased risk of MDS or AML development is present in this population because of treatment with alkylating chemotherapeutic agents.

Diffuse Large B-cell Lymphoma

Diffuse large B-cell lymphoma (DLBCL) is a heterogeneous group of aggressive B-cell neoplasms with the highest incidence between 60 and 70 years of age. DLBCL often occurs in the context of EBV and HIV infections, although the exact etiology is unclear. DLBCL involves lymph nodes and extranodal sites. Microscopically, the cells are large and resemble immunoblasts or anaplastic-appearing cells. The malignant cells express B-cell markers and occasionally CD5 and CD10. Patients often present with rapidly evolving, multifocal, nodal and extranodal lesions. A high proliferation rate indicates a poorer prognosis.

Burkitt Lymphoma

Burkitt lymphoma (BL) is a B-cell lymphoma often associated with infection with Epstein-Barr virus (EBV), and patients commonly present with extranodal lesions rather than lymphadenopathy. Specific associations are present in various forms of Burkitt lymphoma. Endemic BL occurs during childhood, is most common in Central Africa, and appears related to EBV infection (virtually ubiquitous in these lesions). Classically it involves destructive lesions of the jaw and facial bones.

- Sporadic BL: affects children and young adults in the Western world, and only approximately 30% of these cases demonstrate EBV infection; often presents with abdominal pain
- Immunodeficiency-associated BL: occurs in HIV-infected persons

Microscopically, BL cells are medium sized and lack cytologic atypia. BL demonstrates a high proliferation rate with numerous mitotic figures and apoptotic cellular debris that is taken up by macrophages, creating a "starry sky" appearance of the cells. Cells express surface IgM, CD22, CD10, Bcl-6, and the B cell antigens CD19, CD20 and CD22. Clonal IgH gene rearrangement is present for heavy and light chains. The translocation t(8;14) involves the *MYC* oncogene and *IgH*, which leads to uncontrolled growth of the cells.

The majority of patients present with bulky extranodal tumors that are responsive to chemotherapy. The endemic and sporadic forms may reach a cure rate of 90%.

Mature T-cell and NK-cell Lymphomas

Mature T- and NK-cell lymphomas arise from postthymic T cells, account for 12% of all non-Hodgkin lymphomas, may be caused in certain instances by the human T-cell leukemia virus (HTLV-1) and have overall a poor prognosis. The immunophenotype expressed by these cells is:

- T cells: CD2, CD3, CD5, CD7 with common loss of one or more markers; cytotoxic T cells express perforin, granzyme B, T-cell intracellular antigen (TIA-1)

- NK cells: CD2, CD7, CD8, CD16, CD56, CD57, perforin, granzyme B, TIA-1

Mature T- and NK-cell lymphomas are subdivided into leukemic or nodal, extranodal, or cutaneous lymphomas. Treatment involves standard chemotherapy. The 5-year survival is only 20% to 30%. Characteristics of common T- and NK-cell lymphomas are described in Table 20-26.

Adult T-cell Leukemia/Lymphoma

Adult T-cell leukemia/lymphoma (ATLL) is caused by HTLV-1, which activates gene transcription through the viral protein P40 tax. ATLL commonly involves the peripheral blood, bone marrow, and skin. The leukemic cells are markedly atypical and contain multilobulated nuclei (flower cells). These cells express CD2, CD3, and CD5, but often lack CD7 expression. The majority of cases consist of the T-cell helper CD4$^+$ phenotype, and some tumor cells express the IL-2 receptor CD25 and CD30. ATLL demonstrates clonal T-cell receptor gene rearrangement and has clonally integrated HTLV-1.

Patients with ATLL have multiorgan manifestations, hypercalcemia, peripheral leukocytosis, and skin involvement. Death often occurs from infectious complications. Chronic and smoldering forms have a better prognosis than acute forms.

Mycosis Fungoides and Sézary Syndrome

Mycosis fungoides is a cutaneous T-cell neoplasm that occurs in adults and elderly persons. Abnormal lymphocytes infiltrate the dermal-epidermal junction (epidermal tropism) and may accumulate within the epithelium (Pautrier microabscesses). Most tumor cells express CD2, CD3, CD5, CD4, and TCRα, β. CD7 and CD8 are usually absent. The T-cell receptor gene demonstrates clonal rearrangement. Mycosis fungoides is an indolent lymphoma and demonstrates the following stages:

- Premycotic or eczematous stage: nonspecific perivascular and periadnexal lymphocytic infiltration with eosinophils and plasma cells
- Plaque stage: well-demarcated raised cutaneous plaques; a definitive diagnosis may be established during this stage; dense subepidermal bandlike infiltrate of lymphocytes with hyperchromatic and cerebriform nuclei (mycosis cells); ± Pautrier abscesses
- Tumor stage: raised cutaneous tumors on face and body folds that ulcerate and become secondarily infected

The spread of mycosis fungoides to the lung, spleen, liver, and peripheral blood is termed Sézary syndrome.

Table 20-26

Cell and NK-Cell Lymphomas

Lymphoma/Leukemia	Pathology	Genetic Abnormalities
T-cell prolymphocytic leukemia (T-PLL)	Medium-sized lymphocytes; hepatosplenomegaly; peripheral leukocytosis	14q32.1 (*TCL1*) abnormalities
T-cell large granular lymphocyte leukemia (T-LGL)	Large granular lymphocytes; involves blood, marrow, liver, spleen; leukopenia, severe anemia	No specific abnormalities
Aggressive NK-cell leukemia	Fever, hepatosplenomegaly, leukemia; associated with EBV infection	Variety of clonal abnormalities; EBV in clonal episomal form
Adult T-cell leukemia (ATLL)	Atypical, multilobulated nuclei (flower cells); associated with HTLV-1 infection	Clonally integrated HTLV-1
Extranodal NK/T-cell lymphoma, nasal type	Angiocentric, necrotizing, vascular infiltrate; often associated with EBV infection; may affect nasal passage, skin, GI tract, testis	Variety of clonal abnormalities; often EBV in clonal episomal form
Enteropathy-associated T-cell lymphoma	Arises from intraepithelial T-cells in persons with celiac disease; expression of CD103	Most have HLA DQA1*0501, DQB1*0201 genotype
Hepatosplenic T-cell lymphoma	Malignant cells express γ,δ T-cell receptor, hepatosplenomegaly, bone marrow involvement	Isochromosome 7q
Subcutaneous panniculitis-like T-cell lymphoma	Malignant cells express α,β T-cell receptor; cells infiltrate around fat; hemophagocytic syndrome common	No specific abnormalities; often TCR genes rearranged

(continues)

671

Table 20-26
(continued)

Lymphoma/Leukemia	Pathology	Genetic Abnormalities
Mycosis fungoides	Cutaneous lymphoma; epidermal tropism; ± Pautrier microabscessed	TCR genes rearranged
Angioimmunoblastic T-cell lymphoma	Generalized lymphadenopathy; t zones expanded by polymorphic T-cell infiltrate and proliferation of high endothelial venules; EBV in B cell component; hypergammaglobulinemia; serosal effusions	Often TCR genes rearranged; may have trisomy 3, trisomy 5, or additional X chromosome
Peripheral T-cell lymphoma, unspecified	May be associated with eosinophilia, pruritus, or hemophagocytic syndrome; no defining features	TCR genes rearranged; complex karyotypes
Anaplastic large cell lymphoma (ALCL)	Large atypical tumor cells with kidney-shaped nuclei and prominent nucleoli; express CD30	t(2;5) involving *NPM* and *ALK*

Anaplastic Large Cell Lymphoma

Anaplastic large cell lymphoma (ALCL) has a bimodal age distribution with the first peak in young adulthood and the second peak in older persons. ALCL is characterized by large atypical tumor cells with kidney- or horseshoe-shaped nuclei and occasionally large multinucleated nuclei with prominent nucleoli. These cells universally express the activation marker CD30. In addition, cytotoxic granule-associated proteins, granzyme B, TIA-1, and perforin are present. Most cases demonstrate the translocation t(2;5) involving nucleophosmin (*NPM*) and anaplastic lymphoma kinase (*ALK*), a tyrosine kinase.

Patients often demonstrate nodal and extranodal disease, as well as fever. ALK-positive ALCL has a favorable prognosis, with a median 5-year survival of 80%.

Hodgkin Lymphoma

Hodgkin lymphoma (HL) is characterized by the presence of large atypical mononuclear or multinucleated tumor cells with prominent nucleoli (Reed-Sternberg cells), which account for only 1% of the cellularity in these lesions. HL is the most common malignant neoplasm of Americans between the ages of 10 and 30 years and demonstrates a bimodal distribution in developed countries, with peaks in age in one's late twenties and one's fifties.

Evidence that HL represents malignant cells of B-cell origin is accumulating. However, HL is still considered a separate disorder because of its unique clinicopathologic properties. Risk factors for HL are controversial and include the following:

- Exposure to unidentified agent of low oncogenic potential in childhood
- Viral etiology because of geographic variation (e.g., EBV)
- Genetic factors such as HLA-B18 subtype
- Decreased immune status, as in autoimmune disease and immunodeficiency

The majority of patients with Hodgkin lymphoma present with lymphadenopathy; after diagnosis, staging of patients is performed, which examines the involvement of lymph nodes, bone marrow, liver, and spleen by HL. Lymphadenopathy often involves a single group or multiple groups of lymph nodes, most commonly in the cervical and mediastinal regions. Initially, HL spreads along nodal regions in a contiguous fashion, although vascular invasion and hematogenous dissemination may be present late in the disease.

Constitutional or "B" symptoms are found in 40% of patients and include low-grade fever, night sweats, and weight loss. As the disease advances, pruritus may be present. An unusual finding is the presence of pain at site of involvement with alcohol use in 10% of patients.

Laboratory findings are generally nonspecific in HL. Deficient T-lymphocyte function, which results in defects of delayed-type hypersensitivity and anergy to skin tests may be noted.

If left untreated, HL has a 10-year survival of only 1%; however, with radiation and chemotherapy, a 70% cure rate can be achieved. The prognosis in HL is more favorable with a younger patient, limited anatomical extent of the disease (stage), and absence of B symptoms. Approximately 15% of treated patients develop secondary malignancies caused by HL therapy.

Hodgkin lymphoma may be subdivided into two overall forms, which include nodular lymphocyte predominant HL and classical HL.

Nodular Lymphocyte Predominant Hodgkin Lymphoma

Nodular lymphocyte predominant Hodgkin lymphoma (NLPHL) is the most indolent type of HL and often affects men younger than 35 years of age. This form of HL contains Reed-Sternberg (R-S) cell variants termed "popcorn" or L&H (lymphohistiocytic) cells that consistently express B cell antigens and lack the characteristic R-S cell expression of CD15 and CD30. EBV is absent in cases of NLPHL. Tumor cells commonly efface lymph nodes in a vaguely nodular pattern, and they demonstrate a background of lymphocytes and an absence of eosinophils and plasma cells, which are common in classical HL.

At the time of diagnosis, NLPHL usually is localized to high cervical, axillary or inguinal lymph nodes and B symptoms often are lacking. NLPHL, in contrast to classical HL, tends to skip anatomical lymph node regions. Mediastinal involvement is rare. The overall survival is excellent (80% 10-year survival). However, NLPHL has a high recurrence rate.

Classical Hodgkin Lymphoma

Classical Hodgkin lymphoma (CHL) is characterized by clonal proliferation of typical mononuclear Hodgkin cells and multinucleated R-S cells with invariable expression of CD30 and common expression of CD15. Common B-cell antigens often are absent. These cells demonstrate prominent nucleoli and, when binucleated, they demonstrate an "owl-eye" appearance. In contrast to NLPHL, CHL has a variably mixed inflammatory background of lymphocytes, eosinophils, macrophages, neutrophils, plasma cells, fibroblasts, and collagen. Four types of CHL have been described:

- Nodular-sclerosis HL: most common HL form; occurs in adolescent and young adult women; characterized by lower cervical, supraclavicular, and mediastinal adenopathy; B symptoms

(40%); background fibrosis and collagen deposition; lacunar cell variants of R-S cells; good prognosis

- Mixed-cellularity HL (MCHL): most common HL in HIV patients; occurs in fourth and fifth decades; left cervical lymph nodes commonly affected; B symptoms (50%); intermediate prognosis; background of mixed inflammation
- Lymphocyte-rich HL (LRHL): abundant lymphocytic background with absence of mixed inflammation and collagen bands
- Lymphocyte-depleted HL (LDHL): most aggressive HL form; middle-aged to elderly men commonly affected; 80% of patients with advanced stage and B symptoms; common retroperitoneal lymphadenopathy and spleen, liver, and bone marrow involvement; profound immunodeficiency; paucity of background lymphocytes

A diagrammatic representation of histologic findings in HL is presented in Figure 20-18.

Posttransplant Lymphoproliferative Disorder

Posttransplant lymphoproliferative disorder (PTLD) results from immunosuppression and is often an EBV-driven monoclonal lymphocyte proliferation with variable morphology. PTLD often occurs in transplant patients and is caused by host lymphocytes in solid organ recipients and donor lymphocytes in bone marrow allograft recipients. PTLD evolves through a series of lesions that include the following:

- Increased plasma cells within lymph nodes
- Polymorphic PTLD that contains a mixture of immunoblasts, plasma cells, and medium-sized lymphocytes in lymph nodes or other organs; clonal *IgH* gene rearrangements are present
- Monomorphic appearance of malignant lymphoma, including DLBCL, HL, and Burkitt lymphoma

PTLD may occur at any nodal or extranodal site. Bone marrow recipients often present within the first 6 months, whereas solid organ recipients present within several years. Early PTLD has an excellent prognosis with decreased levels of immunosuppressive regimens. Late PTLD has a poor prognosis. Treatment with anti-CD20 antibody (Rituxan) can eliminate clonal B-cell proliferations in this population.

THE SPLEEN

The spleen is a lymphoid organ that participates in the removal of senescent cells and immune modulation. The morphology of the spleen is diagrammed in Figure 20-19.

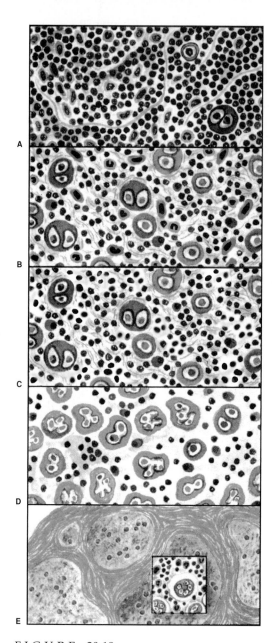

FIGURE 20-18

Histopathologic subtypes of Hodgkin lymphoma. A: Lymphocyte predominant. B: Mixed cellularity. C: Lymphocyte rich. D: Lymphocyte depleted. E: Nodular scleroses. The sequence from lymphocyte-predominant HL to the lymphocyte-depleted variant is characterized *(continues)*

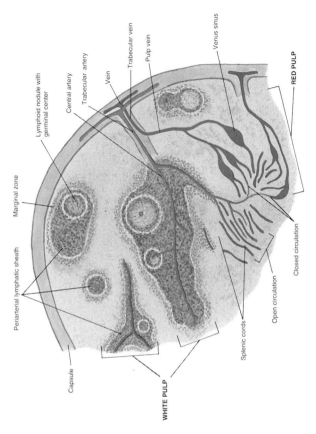

F I G U R E   20-19
Structure of the normal spleen. (From Rubin E, Gorstein F, Rubin R, et al. Rubin's Pathology, 4th ed. Philadelphia: Lippincott Williams & Wilkins, 2005, p. 1118.)

F I G U R E   20-18
(continued) by progressively fewer normal cells. The subtype of lymphocyte-depleted diffuse fibrosis features only a few lymphocytes plus Read-Sternberg cells and abundant loose fibrosis. Nodular sclerosis Hodgkin lymphoma is distinctive because of dense, bandlike, collagenous fibrosis that envelops cellular aggregates that contain lymphoid and inflammatory cells and the specific lacunar cell variant of the Reed-Sternberg cell. (From Rubin E, Gorstein F, Rubin R, et al. Rubin's Pathology, 4th ed. Philadelphia: Lippincott Williams & Wilkins, 2005, p. 1115.)

The spleen contains both red pulp and white pulp, which each serve separate functions:

- White pulp: lymphocyte-rich domain made up of B- and T-cell domains and follicles; protects against blood-borne infections; major site of opsonizing IgM synthesis
- Red pulp: stromal cords and vascular sinuses that filter and screen blood; macrophages uptake debris from red blood cells that are damaged or cannot withstand hypoxic, hypoglycemic or acidotic of the stromal cord microenvironment

One third of the peripheral blood platelet pool and a small fraction of granulocytes are normally sequestered within the spleen.

Splenic conditions include congenital abnormalities of the spleen, such as *congenital absence* or *accessory spleens*, the presence of multiple small spleens. *Acquired asplenia* occurs in sickle cell patients after repeated infarcts of the organ. *Hypersplenism* is a functional disorder characterized by pancytopenia and bone marrow hyperplasia and is associated with hemolytic anemia. Enlargement of the spleen, termed *splenomegaly*, occurs when the weight of the spleen is greater than the average weight of 100 to 170 grams. Causes of splenomegaly are listed in Table 20-27.

Table 20-27

Principal Causes of Splenomegaly

Infections	Primary or metastatic neoplasm
Acute	Leukemia
Subacute	Lymphoma
Chronic	Hodgkin disease
Immunologic inflammatory	Myeloproliferative syndromes
disorders	Sarcoma
Felty syndrome	Carcinoma
Lupus erythematosus	Storage diseases
Sarcoidosis	Gaucher
Amyloidosis	Niemann-Pick
Thyroiditis	Mucopolysaccharidoses
Hemolytic anemias	
Immune thrombocytopenia	
Splenic vein hypertension	
Cirrhosis	
Splenic or portal vein thrombosis	
or stenosis	
Right-sided cardiac failure	

From Rubin E, Gorstein F, Rubin R, et al. Rubin's Pathology. 4th ed. Philadelphia: Lippincott Williams & Wilkins, 2005, p.1119.

THE THYMUS

The thymus is a mediastinal organ that undergoes age-related atrophy.

Hyperplasia

Thymic hyperplasia refers to the presence of lymphoid follicles in the thymus that often have germinal centers containing B lymphocytes expressing IgM and IgD. Thymic hyperplasia occurs in *myasthenia gravis*, as well as other autoimmune diseases including Graves' disease, Addison disease, and scleroderma.

Thymic Tumors

A *thymoma* is a neoplasm of the thymic epithelial cells, without regard to the presence or number of lymphocytes. Thymomas are predominantly benign adult tumors that most commonly affect the anterosuperior mediastinum. Grossly, these lesions appear as encapsulated, firm, lobulated gray-yellow lesions. Foci of hemorrhage, necrosis, and cystic degeneration may be present. Microscopically, thymomas demonstrate neoplastic plump or spindled epithelial cells with vesicular chromatin and vesicular nuclei admixed with variable numbers of benign lymphocytes. Fifteen percent of patients with myasthenia gravis have thymoma. In addition, patients with thymoma may have associated hypogammaglobulinemia, erythroid hypoplasia, myocarditis, dermatomyositis, and other autoimmune diseases.

Malignant thymomas are locally invasive and may metastasize. Two variants of malignant thymoma have been described:

- Type I: most common cancer of the thymus; tumor cells penetrate surrounding capsule and implants on mediastinal organs; metastasizes to lymph nodes, lung, liver, and bone
- Type II (thymic carcinoma): uncommon, invasive tumor; highly variable morphologic appearance including squamous cell and lymphoepitheliallike features; most patients die within 5 years

Malignant thymoma is treated by surgical resection and radiation therapy. Chemotherapy is added for metastatic disease.

Other uncommon tumors of the thymus include carcinoid tumor, small cell carcinoma, and germ cell tumors, especially mature cystic teratoma.

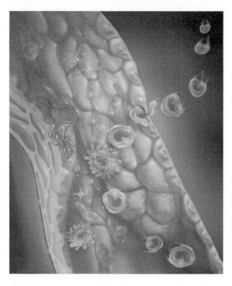

CHAPTER 21

The Endocrine System

Chapter Outline

The Parathyroid Glands

Hypoparathyroidism
  Decreased Secretion of PTH
  Pseudohypoparathyroidism

Primary Hyperparathyroidism
  Parathyroid Adenoma
  Primary Parathyroid Hyperplasia
  Parathyroid Carcinoma

Secondary Hyperparathyroidism

The Adrenal Gland

Normal Anatomy and Histology

Congenital Adrenal Hyperplasia

Adrenal Cortical Insufficiency
  Addison Disease (Primary Chronic Adrenal Insufficiency)
  Acute Adrenal Insufficiency
  Secondary Adrenal Insufficiency

Adrenal Hyperfunction
  Cushing Syndrome
  Conn Syndrome

Other Adrenal Lesions

Adrenal Medullary Tumors
  Pheochromocytoma
  Paraganglioma
  Neuroblastoma
  Ganglioneuroma

The Pineal Gland

Normal Anatomy and Histology

Neoplasms of the Pineal Gland

The endocrine system is formed by a number of organs throughout the body that produce chemical messengers termed hormones that produce local or systemic effects by secretion into the circulation.

THE PITUITARY GLAND

Normal Anatomy and Histology

The pituitary gland is situated in the sella turcica. The anterior portion is known as the adenohypophysis, and the posterior portion is known as the neurohypophysis. Structures that surround the pituitary gland include the optic chiasm and cranial nerves III, IV, V, and VI. Enlargement of the pituitary gland, regardless of cause, can result in compression of these structures.

Adenohypophysis

The adenohypophysis is derived from upward growth of ectoderm from the oral cavity (Rathke duct). Its glandular cells, which are arranged in nests or cords, secrete a variety of hormonal products. The cells are subdivided by staining properties into chromophobe (pale) cells, acidophilic (eosinophilic) cells, and basophilic (blue) cells. Subtypes of cells of the adenohypophysis and regulatory hypothalamic hormones are shown in Figure 21-1. In general, negative feedback loops regulate the amount of hypothalamic hormone released.

Neurohypophysis

The neurohypophysis is derived from a downward projection of the brain and remains connected to the hypothalamus by the hypophyseal stalk. The neurohypophysis contains pituicytes (glial cells without secretory function) and unmyelinated nerve fibers that originate in the hypothalamus and contain antidiuretic hormone (ADH) and oxytocin.

Hypopituitarism

Hypopituitarism is the deficient secretion of one or more pituitary hormones, which is manifested by deficiencies in the target organs. *Panhypopituitarism* refers to a complete failure of pituitary function.

Hypopituitarism occurs in a variety of settings, including the following:

- Pituitary tumors
- Sheehan syndrome: ischemic necrosis of the pituitary often caused by hypotension due to postpartum hemorrhage
- Pituitary apoplexy: hemorrhagic infarction of a pituitary adenoma
- Iatrogenic hypopituitarism
- Trauma
- Infiltrative diseases (e.g., bacterial and viral diseases, hemochromatosis)
- Genetic abnormalities of pituitary development: mutations in Pit-1, PROP1, and HSEX1 have been implicated in decreased transcription of pituitary hormones
- Growth hormone insensitivity (Laron syndrome): rare autosomal condition that results in dwarfism due to resistance to

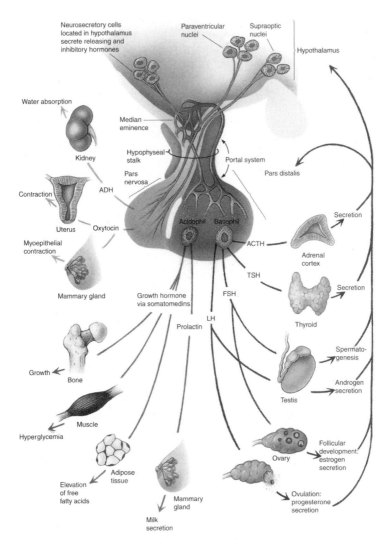

F I G U R E   21-1
The pituitary gland and pituitary hormones. (From Gartner LP, Hiatt JL. Color Atlas of Histology, 3rd ed. Philadelphia: Lippincott Williams & Wilkins, 2000, p. 202.)

growth hormone caused by abnormalities of the growth hormone receptor

- Isolated gonadotrophin deficiency (Kallman syndrome): deficiency of gonadotropin and anosmia that most commonly affects boys
- Empty sella syndrome: radiographic finding of an enlarged sella containing a thin, flattened pituitary at the base

Pituitary Adenomas

Pituitary adenomas are benign neoplasms of the anterior pituitary that are often associated with overproduction of a pituitary hormone. The majority of pituitary adenomas occur in adults between 20 and 50 years of age. The most common pituitary adenomas are nonfunctional or produce prolactin or adrenocorticotropic hormone (ACTH), although many other types of adenomas may occur (Table 21-1). In addition, pituitary adenomas may occur in the context of multiple endocrine neoplasia (MEN) type 1.

Pituitary adenomas may be subclassified by size as microadenomas (<10-mm diameter) or macroadenomas (>10-mm diameter). In general, macroadenomas may result in symptoms not only because they produce pituitary hormone, but also because they compress local structures, leading to bitemporal hemianopsia, loss of central vision, oculomotor palsies, and headaches.

Posterior Pituitary Disorders

The major disorder related to the neurohypophysis is *central diabetes insipidus*, which is caused by a deficiency in ADH (vasopressin). It may be associated with trauma, sporadic mutations, or craniopharyngiomas, or it may occur posthypophysectomy. Central diabetes insipidus leads to chronic water diuresis (polyuria), thirst, and polydipsia.

THE THYROID GLAND

Normal Anatomy and Histology

The thyroid gland originates from the underside of the tongue and descends to its final location in the neck by elongation of the thyroglossal duct, which atrophies in adult life. In the adult, the thyroid is situated anterior to the trachea. The gland is made up of a right and left lobe, isthmus, and occasionally pyramidal lobe, and it weighs approximately 20 grams. The cut surface appears tan-brown and lobulated.

Table 21-1
Pituitary Adenomas

Adenoma	Product	Cell of Origin	Clinical Findings	Specific Pathology of Adenoma Subtype	Selective Treatment of Pituitary Adenoma Subtypes
Prolactinoma	Prolactin	Lactotrope	Women: amenorrhea, galactorrhea, infertility. Men: decreased libido and erectile dysfunction	Amyloid, psammoma bodies	Microadenomas: dopamine agonists (bromocriptine). Macroadenomas: surgery, radiation
Somatotrope adenomas	Growth hormone	Somatotrope	Children: gigantism. Adults: Acromegaly with coarse facial features, often associated neurological and musculoskeletal problems		Growth hormone antagonist, surgery, radiation
Corticotrope adenomas	ACTH	Corticotrope	Cushing disease caused by adrenal cortical hypersecretion	Crooke hyalinization aggregates of intermediate filaments in the cytoplasm)	Surgical resection
Gonadotrope adenoma	LH, FSH	Gonadotrope	Headache, visual disturbances, hypogonadism		Surgical resection
Thyrotrope adenoma	TSH	Thyrotrope	Hyperthyroidism, goiter	Pseudorosettes around blood vessels	Surgical resection

ACTH, adrenocorticotropic hormone; FSH, follicle-stimulating hormone; LH, luteinizing hormone; TSH, thyroid-stimulating hormone.

The thyroid gland contains variably sized follicles lined by cuboidal to columnar cells (follicular cells), a surrounding basement membrane, and luminal pink, glassy, proteinaceous material termed *colloid*. The major constituent of colloid is iodinated thyroglobulin, which can be reabsorbed by the epithelial cells and converted into the thyroid hormones T_3 and T_4 for release into the blood. These thyroid hormones circulate in association with thyronine-binding globulin (TBG). T_4 is ultimately converted in the periphery to the more active T_3 form. Peripheral affects of thyroid hormone include an increased basal metabolic rate and increased hepatic glucose production.

In addition to follicular cells, the thyroid gland also contains scattered interfollicular cells termed *parafollicular*, *clear* or *C cells*. These cells are responsible for the production of calcitonin, which serves to lower the levels of calcium by decreasing osteoclastic resorption and increasing osteoblastic activity.

Congenital Anomalies

Congenital anomalies of the thyroid gland include the following:

- Lingual thyroid: thyroid remains as a nodule at the base of the tongue
- Heterotopic thyroid tissue: thyroid tissue identified along the course of thyroid descent into the neck
- Lateral aberrant thyroid: ectopic thyroid tissue present in the lymph nodes and soft tissue adjacent to the thyroid gland
- Thyroglossal duct cyst: cystic, fluid-filled remnant often lined by squamous or respiratory mucosa; contains associated thyroid tissue that is often identified in children and may ultimately result in squamous cell carcinoma later in life if not removed

Nontoxic Goiter

Nontoxic goiter is an enlargement of the thyroid gland not associated with functional, inflammatory, or neoplastic alterations. The thyroid gland in this condition fails to produce adequate amounts of thyroid hormone, which leads to increased secretion of thyroid-stimulating hormone (TSH) and subsequent enlargement of the gland (up to several hundred grams). This condition affects women more often than men and is generally not associated with symptoms of thyroid dysfunction.

The early stage of the disease is characterized by a diffusely enlarged gland with hyperplasia and hypertrophy of the follicular epithelium, termed *diffuse nontoxic goiter*. The chronic stage of the disease demonstrates a nodular cut surface, termed *multinodular nontoxic goiter.* The nodules may appear soft and filled with reddish colloid when the epithelial component is scarce or appear fleshy and gray when the epithelial component dominates. Microscopically, these lesions are characterized by variably sized follicles that may demonstrate hemorrhage or cystic degeneration.

Clinically, patients do not demonstrate symptoms of thyroid dysfunction, but may present with a neck mass, dysphagia, or inspiratory stridor. The blood concentrations of TSH, T_3, and T_4 are normal. Treatment involves the administration of thyroid hormone to break the feedback loop and reduce TSH levels. Patients are at risk for developing toxic multinodular goiter (see below).

Alterations in Thyroid Function

Hypothyroidism

Hypothyroidism is the clinical manifestation of decreased levels of thyroid hormone, which may be the result of defective thyroid hormone synthesis, inadequate function of the thyroid parenchyma, or inadequate secretion of TSH. Often, the earliest symptoms of hypothyroidism are tiredness, lethargy, cold sensitivity, and inability to concentrate. Additional findings include the following:

- Skin: accumulation of proteoglycans in the skin leads to *myxedema* manifested by boggy facies, puffy eyelids, edema of the hands and feet, and an enlarged tongue; dry, coarse skin
- Nervous system: lethargy, somnolence, depression, paranoid ideation, decreased tendon reflexes, sensory deficits, cerebellar ataxia
- Heart: decreased heart rate and cardiac output, dilated heart
- Gastrointestinal tract: constipation
- Reproductive system: ovulatory failure, progesterone deficiency, and irregular and heavy menstrual bleeding in women and erectile dysfunction and oligospermia in men

Three diseases that result in hypothyroidism are described in Table 21-2. Treatment of most cases of hypothyroidism involves the administration of thyroid hormone (thyroxine).

Primary (Idiopathic) Hypothyroidism

Primary hypothyroidism often occurs in the setting of circulating antibodies to thyroid antigens, suggesting an autoimmune etiology. The majority of cases affect women in the fifth to sixth decades and the thyroid gland is generally not enlarged.

Goitrous Hypothyroidism

Clinical symptoms of decreased thyroid function may occur in the setting of thyroid enlargement and may be subdivided into the following:

Table 21-2
Disorders of Hypothyroidism

Disorder	Sex	Age (years)	Etiology/Association	Gross Pathology
Primary (idiopathic) hypothyroidism	F >M	40s to 50s	Circulating antibodies to thyroid antigens (possible autoimmune etiology)	Variably sized gland (generally not enlarged)
Goiter	Variable with cause	Any age	Iodide deficiency (endemic goiter), lithium or other select drugs, consumption of large amount of iodide (iodide-induced goiter)	Diffusely enlarged gland
Congenital hypothyroidism (cretinism)	F >M	Early weeks of life	Endemic, sporadic, or familial (iodide deficiency in parents; inherited mutations in TRH, TSH, the receptors for both TRH and TSH, the sodium-iodide symporter, thyroglobulin, and thyroid oxidase)	Enlarged gland

TRH, thyroid-releasing hormone; TSH, thyroid-stimulating hormone.

- Endemic goiter: caused by dietary iodine deficiency and may be prevented by iodized salt
- Goiter induced by antithyroid agents: lithium, phenylbutazone, and p-aminosalicylic acid
- Iodide-induced goiter: occurs in patients who consume a large amount of iodide and who have a preexisting thyroid disease

Congenital Hypothyroidism (Cretinism)

Cretinism may be endemic, sporadic, or familial and typically affects females more often than males. A subset of cases occur secondary to mutations in thyroid-releasing hormone (TRH), TSH, the receptors for both TRH and TSH, the sodium-iodide symporter, thyroglobulin, and thyroid oxidase.

Manifestations appear during the first weeks of life and include lethargy, decreased body temperature, pale skin, and often an umbilical hernia. Patients may also develop refractory anemia, heart dilation, mental retardation, stunted growth, and characteristic facies. Serum T_3 and T_4 are low and TSH is elevated. Thyroid hormone replacement is critical to prevent the serious consequences of this disease.

Hyperthyroidism

Hyperthyroidism is caused by increased levels of circulating thyroid hormone that may result from abnormal stimulation of the thyroid in Graves disease, intrinsic disease of the thyroid, or excess production of TSH by a pituitary adenoma. Diseases that result in hyperthyroidism are described in Table 21-3. Manifestations of hyperthyroidism often include nervousness, tremor, weight loss, palpitations, increased heart rate, excessive sweating, and oligomenorrhea.

Graves Disease

Graves disease is an autoimmune disorder in which activating autoantibodies are directed against the TSH receptor on thyrocytes. The antibodies in Graves disease also crossreact with orbital fibroblasts surrounding the eye, which leads to increased numbers of fibroblasts and associated edema within the ocular muscles, resulting in a forward displacement of the eye (proptosis).

Susceptibility loci for Graves disease have been associated with HLA class II molecules (HLA-DR3 and HLA-DQA1). Patients affected with Graves disease have an increased incidence of other autoimmune diseases. Additional factors that are associated with disease development include female sex and smoking.

Grossly, the thyroid gland is symmetrically enlarged and firm, weighing up to 40 grams. Microscopically, the epithelial cells are tall and columnar and often project into the lumen of the follicles

Table 21-3
Disorders Resulting in Hyperthyroidism

Disorder	Sex	Age (years)	Etiology/ Association	Gross Pathology	Microscopic Findings	Symptoms
Graves disease	F >M	<40	Activating IgG antibodies against the TSH receptor on thyrocytes	Enlarged gland	Tall, columnar thyrocytes that project as papillae into the lumen, moth-eaten colloid, lymphocyte infiltration with occasional germinal center formation	Nervousness, emotional lability, heat intolerance, sweat profusely, increased heart rate, oligomenorrhea, proptosis
Toxic multinodular goiter	F >M	>50	Development of functional autonomy of nontoxic goiter	Multiple nodules of varying sizes in enlarged gland	Demarcated nodules consisting of large hyperplastic follicles	Symptoms less severe than Graves disease, no exophthalmos, cardiac complications may be prominent
Toxic adenoma	F >M	30s to 40s	May have somatic activating mutations in the TSH-receptor gene	Solitary enlarged nodule in a background atrophic thyroid	Demarcated nodule containing benign follicular epithelium and colloid	Symptoms of hyperthyroidism often noticeable only when nodule is >3 cm size

as papillarylike structures. The associated colloid is often depleted and appears "moth-eaten." Scattered lymphocytes and plasma cells are present in the interstitium.

Patients may present with a variety of symptoms, including nervousness, emotional lability, tremor, weight loss, tachycardia, increased sweating, and oligomenorrhea. The thyroid gland may demonstrate an audible bruit and palpable thrill on examination. The skin may demonstrate a pretibial edema termed *Graves dermopathy*. Graves disease typically demonstrates exacerbations and remissions. Treatment includes antithyroid medication, radioactive iodine, and corticosteroids.

Toxic Multinodular Goiter

Toxic multinodular goiter affects females more commonly than males and often develops after 50 years of age. The thyroid may be diffusely affected, enlarged, and demonstrate small groups of hyperplastic follicles admixed with inactive nodules of varying size or may demonstrate clearly demarcated hyperplastic nodules in a background of inactive areas of thyroid.

Clinically, patients demonstrate symptoms of hyperthyroidism, but these symptoms are less severe than those associated with Graves disease and do not involve ocular complications. Because patients with toxic multinodular goiter are often older, hyperthyroidism may lead to noticeable cardiac symptoms, including atrial fibrillation or congestive heart failure. Serum T_3 and T_4 levels are only minimally elevated. Treatment involves administration of radiolabeled iodine after a course of antithyroid therapy.

Toxic Adenoma

Toxic adenoma is a benign, solitary, hyperfunctioning tumor in a background of normal or atrophic thyroid tissue. Many lesions demonstrate somatic activating mutations of the TSH receptor. Patients, who often present in the fourth and fifth decades, generally do not have symptoms of hyperthyroidism until the tumor has grown to a large size, often greater than 3 cm. Because the adenoma can function autonomously and is not suppressed by thyroid hormone administration, treatment includes radiolabeled iodine administration or surgical excision.

Thyroiditis

Thyroiditis is a set of diseases that involve inflammation of the thyroid, which can lead to changes in thyroid function. Diseases that are associated with thyroiditis are described in Table 21-4.

Chronic Autoimmune Thyroiditis (Hashimoto Thyroiditis)

Hashimoto thyroiditis most commonly affects women in the fourth and fifth decades and is associated with the presence of autoreac-

Table 21-4
Thyroiditis

Disorder	Sex	Age (years)	Etiology/Association	Gross Pathology	Microscopic Findings	Symptoms
Hashimoto thyroiditis	F >M	30s to 40s	Antibodies against thyroid antigens that block the action of TSH	Diffuse enlarged, tan, fleshy gland with vague nodularity	Lymphocytic and plasma cell infiltrate with germinal centers, follicle destruction, Hürthle cell change	Often develop hypothyroidism, painful thyroid gland
Subacute (de Quervain) thyroiditis	F >M	30s to 40s	Often follows upper respiratory tract infection	Enlarged, firm, pale gland	Early changes include acute inflammation, later changes include chronic inflammation, multinucleated giant cells, granulomas, and fibrosis	Fever, extremely tender thyroid gland
Lymphocytic thyroiditis	F >M	<50	May occur postpartum, not associated with autoantibodies	Enlarged gland	Lymphocytic infiltrate with follicle destruction	Self-limited hypothyroidism
Riedel thyroiditis	F >M	30 to 50	Unknown	Stony hard gland with fibrosis involving surrounding soft tissues	Dense fibrous tissue and chronic inflammation replaces portions of the thyroid	Compression of the trachea or esophagus by enlarged gland, may be associated with retroperitoneal, mediastinal or orbital fibrosis

tive T cells and autoantibodies against thyroid antigens. Antibodies are most commonly directed against thyroid microsomal peroxidase, thyroglobulin, and the TSH receptor, which all lead to a blockade of TSH effects and therefore symptoms of hypothyroidism. Hashimoto thyroiditis has a familial predisposition, is often associated with other autoimmune diseases, and may occur in conjunction with high levels of iodine intake.

Grossly, the thyroid appears enlarged (up to 200 grams), tan, and fleshy, with a vaguely nodular appearance. Microscopically, the thyroid follicles are involved by a prominent lymphocytic and plasma cell infiltrate that ultimately leads to follicle destruction and atrophy. In addition, Hürthle cell change of the follicular epithelium (oxyphilic metaplasia) and interstitial fibrosis may be present.

Patients often present with a gradual development of an enlarged thyroid gland (goiter) and one-third of all patients develop hypothyroidism. Blood analysis reveals elevated TSH and the presence of circulating antithyroid antibodies. Treatment includes thyroid hormone replacement in symptomatic cases.

Subacute Thyroiditis (de Quervain or Granulomatous Thyroiditis)

Subacute thyroiditis is a self-limited disorder of the thyroid that commonly affects women between 30 and 50 years of age and often occurs following an upper respiratory tract infection.

Grossly, the thyroid appears moderately enlarged (up to 60 grams) and the cut surface is firm and pale. In the course of disease, the thyroid parenchyma is infiltrated by neutrophils and the formation of microabscesses. Later, a patchy infiltrate of lymphocytes, plasma cells, and macrophages involves the gland, leading to follicular damage. Extravasation of colloid results in a prominent granulomatous reaction with multinucleated giant cells and associated fibrosis.

Patients may present with anterior neck pain and fever, often following an upper respiratory infection. Examination of the thyroid reveals an exquisitely tender gland. Transient hyperthyroidism may occur with release of thyroid hormone following follicle destruction. This disease typically resolves within several months and treatment is predominantly symptomatic.

Lymphocytic Thyroiditis (Silent Thyroiditis, Painless Subacute Thyroiditis)

Lymphocytic thyroiditis is characterized by a painless enlargement of the thyroid gland, transient hyperthyroidism, and destruction of the thyroid gland by a lymphocytic infiltrate. This condition most commonly occurs in women, especially during the postpar-

tum period, and is not associated with the development of autoantibodies.

Grossly, the thyroid appears diffusely enlarged. Microscopically, a prominent lymphocytic infiltrate with follicle destruction
is observed. Lymphocytic thyroiditis often resolves spontaneously
within several months and treatment is symptomatic.

Riedel Thyroiditis

Riedel thyroiditis is a disease of unknown etiology that most commonly affects women during middle age and involves extensive
fibrosis of the thyroid, soft tissues of the neck, retroperitoneum,
mediastinum, and orbit. Grossly, the thyroid appears "woody"
or "stony hard," is often asymmetric, and demonstrates fibrosis
extending beyond the gland into the associated soft tissues. Microscopically, dense, hyalinized fibrous tissue and chronic inflammation replaces portions of the gland, with the unaffected portions
appearing microscopically normal.

Patients describe a painless enlargement of the thyroid and
associated local effects, including dysphagia and hoarseness. Treatment involves surgery to relieve local symptoms.

Thyroid Neoplasms

A summary of thyroid neoplasms is presented in Table 21-5.

Benign Thyroid Neoplasm: Follicular Adenoma

Follicular adenomas are benign neoplasms that more commonly
affect women and occur generally in the fourth and fifth decades.
This tumor is the most common neoplasm of the thyroid.

Grossly, follicular adenomas are encapsulated, solitary nodules that appear soft and paler than the surrounding tissue on cut
section. The nodules may also demonstrate hemorrhage and cystic
degeneration. Microscopically, the adenoma is composed of follicles of normal structure but varying size. Multiple variants of follicular adenoma exist, including variants with minimal colloid, variants with abundant colloid (colloid adenoma), and variants with
prominent Hürthle cell change (Hürthle cell adenoma). There is
no difference in clinical behavior based on morphologic subtype.

Patients generally present with a solitary nodule and normal
thyroid function. No treatment or excision is necessary.

Malignant Thyroid Neoplasms

Malignant thyroid neoplasms are uncommon overall but are one
of the most common endocrine neoplasm. The majority of cases
occur in individuals between 20 and 60 years of age.

Table 21.5

Thyroid Neoplasms

Tumor	Age	Sex	Associations	Gross Appearance	Microscopic Appearance	Treatment
Benign						
Follicular adenoma	30s to 40s	F >M	None	Solitary, circumscribed nodule often with hemorrhage or cystic change	Normal follicular structure that may have abundant colloid or Hürthle cell change	No treatment or local excision
Malignant						
Papillary thyroid carcinoma	20s to 40s	F >M	External radiation, *RET* mutations, *NTRK1* recombination	Well-demarcated, often unen capsulated, firm, tan, gritty lesions	Branching papillae with nuclear clearing, nuclear grooves, nuclear pseudoinclusions	Thyroidectomy
Follicular thyroid carcinoma	>40 years	F >M	Endemic goiter areas	Often encapsulated, pale tan, soft	Purely follicular structures with nuclear atypia and occasionally mitoses that invades capsule or shows vascular invasion	Lobectomy
Medullary thyroid carcinoma	50 years, but younger in MEN 2 patients	Slight F >M	MEN type 2, *RET* mutations	Unencapsulated, arises in upper portion of thyroid, firm and gray white	Polygonal, granular cells in a vascular stroma containing amyloid	Thyroidectomy; treatment of associated endocrine syndromes
Anaplastic thyroid carcinoma	>60 years	F >M	*p53* mutations, history of prior lower-grade thyroid carcinoma	Hard, gray-white lesion that extends to surrounding soft tissue	Sarcomalike proliferation of bizarre spindle and giant cells with abundant mitoses and necrosis	Radiation

Papillary Thyroid Carcinoma

Papillary thyroid carcinoma (PTC) accounts for as many as 90% of thyroid carcinomas in the United States. It affects women more commonly than men and often occurs between 20 and 50 years of age. A number of risk factors have been described for PTC, including the following:

- Excess iodine consumption
- External radiation, such as exposure resulting from incident at Chernobyl
- Presence of a first-degree relative with PTC
- Somatic rearrangements of the *RET* protooncogene (10q11.2)
- Recombination of the NTRK1 gene on chromosome 1

Grossly, PTC ranges from multiple microscopic foci of cancer to single large tumors. On cut section, the tumors appear pale, firm, and occasionally gritty. Less than 10% of the tumors are truly encapsulated. Microscopically, branching papillae lined by a single or stratified layer of cuboidal or columnar epithelium overlie a fibrovascular core.

An important diagnostic feature of PTC is the presence of nuclear clearing ("Orphan Annie eyes"), nuclear grooves, and the presence of salmon-colored nuclear pseudoinclusions, which represent invaginations of the cytoplasm into the nucleus. In addition, many PTCs contain lamellated calcifications, termed *psammoma bodies*. In a subset of cases, the tumor may be solely composed of small follicles that demonstrate the nuclear features of PTC and is termed *follicular variant of PTC*. Vascular invasion is uncommon in PTC, and the lesions that metastasize do so via lymphatic invasion and spread to regional lymph nodes.

Clinically, PTC may present as a painless nodule within the thyroid or may present following metastases to regional lymph nodes and therefore with lymphadenopathy. Often, a worse prognosis is associated with size of the tumor, male sex, and local invasion. Treatment involves total thyroidectomy and, if indicated, ipsilateral cervical lymph node dissection. Widespread lymphatic metastases may occur to the lungs or brain in a subset of patients.

Follicular Thyroid Carcinoma

Follicular thyroid carcinoma (FTC) affects women more commonly than men and often occurs after 40 years of age. The risk of FTC is increased in persons with marked iodine deficiency.

Grossly, FTC often occurs as a single, encapsulated nodule within the thyroid that is soft and pale tan to pink on cut section. Microscopically, FTC is formed purely of follicular structures, and the cells lining the follicles often demonstrate atypia and mitotic activity. In contrast to follicular adenoma, FTC demonstrates invasion of the surrounding capsule of the nodule and, occasionally, vascular invasion. Minimally invasive FTC is defined as a lesion that extends into the surrounding capsule, whereas invasive FTC is defined as a lesion that extends through the surrounding capsule.

FTC can metastasize via vascular channels to widespread locations such as the pelvic girdle, sternum, and skull. Patients may present with a thyroid nodule or with complications related to metastatic spread. Treatment involves thyroid lobectomy.

Medullary Thyroid Carcinoma

Medullary thyroid carcinoma (MTC) has only a slight female predominance, and most patients present between 50 and 60 years of age. MTC, which represents only 5% of all thyroid carcinomas, may be sporadic or occur in association with the MEN type 2a syndrome (pheochromocytoma, parathyroid adenoma/hyperplasia, and medullary thyroid carcinoma). MTC represents a neoplastic proliferation of the C cells of the thyroid, with associated excess calcitonin secretion and subsequent decreases in serum calcium. In many cases, sporadic forms of MTC have been associated with mutations in the RET protooncogene. Grossly, MTC commonly arises in the upper portion of the thyroid, and the nodules are not encapsulated. Sporadic forms are often solitary, whereas MTC associated with MEN type 2 is often bilateral and multicentric. On cut section, MTC is firm and gray-white. Microscopically, the tumor is formed by polygonal, granular cells within a highly vascular stroma containing amyloid, which represents the deposition of procalcitonin and stains with Congo red. Focal calcification may be present. Immunohistochemical analysis shows that the tumor cells are positive for calcitonin, neuroendocrine markers such as chromogranin and synaptophysin, and carcinoembryonic antigen (CEA).

MTC may directly invade surrounding tissues or metastasize to regional lymph nodes, lung, liver, and bone. Patients often present with symptoms associated with excess serotonin secretion (carcinoid syndrome) or ACTH secretion (Cushing syndrome). In addition, patients may present with watery diarrhea, hyperparathyroidism, and episodic hypertension. Treatment involves total thyroidectomy and treatment of associated endocrine syndromes.

Anaplastic Thyroid Carcinoma

Anaplastic thyroid carcinoma often affects women older than 60 years of age. Many patients have a history of a lower-grade thyroid carcinoma. Mutations in the *p53* tumor suppressor gene are common.

Grossly, anaplastic thyroid carcinoma presents as a large, poorly circumscribed mass in the thyroid that often extends into the surrounding soft tissues. The cut surface of the mass is hard and gray-white. Microscopically, the tumor cells appear spindled and bizarre, with giant cell formation, multinucleation, abundant mitoses, necrosis, and stromal fibrosis. Tumor thrombi may occlude surrounding vessels and lead to focal infarctions.

Patients often present with symptoms related to local extension of the cancer, including dysphagia, dyspnea, and hoarseness. Treatment involves local radiation, and only 10% of patients survive for 5 years.

Lymphoma

Lymphomas are uncommon in the thyroid but, when they occur, are predominantly B-cell lymphomas. The majority of cases occur in the setting of chronic thyroiditis, affect women, and occur after 60 years of age. Grossly, the lesions are large, soft, tan, and fleshy. Microscopically, they most commonly demonstrate features associated with diffuse large B-cell lymphoma.

THE PARATHYROID GLANDS

The parathyroid glands commonly exist as four glands located on the posterior thyroid, although the number may range from 2 to 12 and the location may range from the neck to the mediastinum. The parathyroids weigh in aggregate approximately 130 mg, although any single gland that weighs more than 50 mg is considered enlarged. The glands are composed of chief cells (secrete parathyroid hormone [PTH]), clear cells (glycogen-rich cells), and oxyphil cells. Secretion of PTH occurs in response to serum ionized calcium and magnesium levels and serves to increase serum calcium levels.

Hypoparathyroidism

Hypoparathyroidism occurs in the setting of decreased secretion of PTH from the parathyroids or end-organ insensitivity to PTH (termed *pseudohypoparathyroidism*).

Decreased Secretion of PTH

Decreased secretion of PTH may occur in a variety of settings, including the following:

- Surgical resection of the parathyroids as a complication of thyroidectomy
- Familial hypothyroidism: polyglandular syndrome that includes adrenal insufficiency and mucocutaneous candidiasis
- Familial isolated hypoparathyroidism: deficient secretion of PTH

- Idiopathic hypoparathyroidism: includes sporadic and familial forms
- Agenesis of the parathyroid glands: occurs with DiGeorge syndrome

Patients often present with signs and symptoms of hypocalcemia, including tingling in the extremities, severe muscle cramps, laryngeal stridor, convulsions, depression, paranoia, and papilledema. Treatment includes vitamin D and calcium supplementation.

Pseudohypoparathyroidism

Pseudohypoparathyroidism, or end-organ insensitivity to PTH, is a group of hereditary conditions characterized by hypocalcemia and is associated with mutations in the GNAS1 gene on chromosome 20 that results in decreased activity of G_s, which couples hormone receptors to adenylyl cyclase activity. Due to the widespread effects of G_s in the body, patients also demonstrate resistance to other cAMP-coupled hormones including TSH, glucagon, luteinizing hormone, and follicle-stimulating hormone. Patients demonstrate a characteristic phenotype (*Albright hereditary osteodystrophy*) manifested by short stature, obesity, mental retardation, subcutaneous calcification, and bone abnormalities.

Primary Hyperparathyroidism

Primary hyperparathyroidism is caused by an intrinsic disease of the parathyroids that leads to excessive secretion of PTH. The classic clinical presentation of hyperparathyroidism is described as "stones, bones, groans, and psychic overtones." Specifically, findings of hyperparathyroidism include the following:

- Skeletal system: *osteitis fibrosa cystica*, which includes bone pain, bone cysts, pathological fractures, local bone swellings (Brown cysts), and chondrocalcinosis ("bones")
- Kidney: renal "stones" often formed of calcium phosphate, renal colic, nephrocalcinosis
- Nervous system: depression, emotional lability, poor mentation, memory defects ("psychic overtones"), and hyperactive reflexes
- Gastrointestinal tract: peptic ulcer disease, chronic pancreatitis ("groans"), and constipation
- Other: hypertension, anemia

Laboratory findings in hyperparathyroidism include hypercalcemia, hyperphosphatemia, hypercalciuria, and elevated levels of PTH.

Parathyroid Adenoma

The majority of cases of primary hyperparathyroidism (85%) are caused by a solitary neoplastic mass of parathyroid tissue, termed a *parathyroid adenoma*. Parathyroid adenomas may occur sporadically or in the context of MEN type 1 and may be associated with rearrangements of the *cyclin D1* (*PRAD1*) protooncogene on chromosome 11.

Grossly, parathyroid adenomas are solitary, circumscribed, reddish-brown masses that may demonstrate hemorrhage or cystic change. Microscopically, these tumors are formed by sheets of chief cells in a vascular stroma and surrounded by a rim of normal parathyroid tissue. Often, the neoplastic cells demonstrate nuclear atypia, which is not common in either parathyroid hyperplasia or carcinoma. Immunostains show the cells are positive for PTH. The remaining three parathyroid glands are often atrophic in response to the hyperfunctioning adenoma. Treatment involves surgical resection of the adenoma.

Primary Parathyroid Hyperplasia

Primary parathyroid hyperplasia reflects hyperplasia of the chief cells and predominantly constitutes the remainder of the cases (15%) of primary hyperparathyroidism. As many as 20% of these cases are associated with MEN types 1 and 2A. The majority of the sporadic cases occur in women, and risk factors include external radiation and lithium intake.

Grossly, all four parathyroid glands are enlarged, although one gland may appear somewhat larger than the remaining glands. Microscopically, sheets, trabeculae, or follicles of uniform hyperplastic chief cells fill the glands.

Parathyroid Carcinoma

Parathyroid carcinoma accounts for only 1% of all cases of primary hyperparathyroidism, does not demonstrate a gender predominance, and often occurs between 30 and 60 years of age. Parathyroid carcinomas are often functioning tumors and demonstrate secretion of PTH. Many cases of parathyroid carcinoma show cyclin D_1 overexpression. However, in contrast to parathyroid adenomas, most parathyroid carcinomas do not stain for the retinoblastoma protein.

Grossly, parathyroid carcinomas appear as lobulated, tan, unencapsulated, firm lesions often adherent to the surrounding soft tissue. Microscopically, the cells are arranged in a trabecular pattern with mitoses, surrounding thick fibrous bands, and capsular or vascular invasion. The cells appear uniform and lack the atypia commonly present in parathyroid adenomas.

Treatment involves surgical resection. However, local recurrence is common, and metastases may occur in the regional lymph nodes, lungs, liver, and bone.

Secondary Hyperparathyroidism

Secondary hyperparathyroidism occurs primarily in the setting of chronic renal failure in which renal retention of phosphate, inadequate production of vitamin D, and chronic hypocalcemia lead to compensatory increases in PTH secretion. All four parathyroid glands are enlarged. Other causes of secondary hyperparathyroidism include vitamin D deficiency, intestinal malabsorption, Fanconi syndrome, and renal tubular acidosis. In cases of long-standing hyperplasia secondary to renal failure, the parathyroids may develop autonomous control, leading to *tertiary hypoparathyroidism*.

THE ADRENAL GLAND

Normal Anatomy and Histology

The adrenal glands are paired pyramidal organs that rest along the upper pole of each kidney and weigh approximately 4 to 6 grams. The adrenal gland is composed of the adrenal cortex and the adrenal medulla, which function as independent endocrine organs. The adrenal cortex arises from the celomic mesenchymal cells and develops into three distinct layers:

- Zona glomerulosa: outermost layer that is stimulated by angiotensin and potassium to secrete aldosterone; the cells form spherical nests and have dark-staining nuclei and moderate amounts of fat droplets in the cytoplasm
- Zona fasciculata: middle band of cortical cells that is stimulated by ACTH to secrete glucocorticoids and the weak androgen dehydroepiandrosterone; cells have a small nucleus and large, foamy cytoplasm
- Zona reticularis: innermost band of cortical cells that is stimulated by ACTH to secrete small quantities of glucocorticoids and the weak androgen dehydroepiandrosterone; cells appear as irregular anastomosing cords that have a small nucleus and lipid-poor, slightly granular cytoplasm

The adrenal medulla arises from neuroectodermal cells and forms the central portion of the gland. The chromaffin cells that constitute the medulla produce catecholamines (epinephrine and norepinephrine) and appear as nests of small polyhedral cells with pale cytoplasm and vesicular nuclei. Interspersed among the nests are postganglionic neurons and small autonomic nerve fibers.

Congenital Adrenal Hyperplasia

Synthesis of adrenal hormones (aldosterone, corticosteroids, androgens) occurs through a sequence of enzymatic conversions that modify cholesterol. Congenital adrenal hyperplasia (CAH) encompasses a variety of autosomal recessive diseases that represent enzymatic defects in the synthesis pathway of cortisol from cholesterol. The accumulated precursors are subsequently converted into alternative end products, such as androgens.

The major cause of CAH is *21-hydroxylase (P450C$_{21}$) deficiency*, which accounts for as many as 90% of all cases of CAH. 21-hydroxylase is a shared enzyme in the conversion of cholesterol to glucocorticoids and aldosterone that converts 17-hydroxyprogesterone to 11-deoxycortisol. Deficiencies in this enzyme lead to increased levels of androgens in these patients. A minor cause of CAH is *11 β-hydroxylase deficiency*, which accounts for 5% of cases of CAH. 11 β-hydroxylase regulates the final conversion step of cortisol formation.

In CAH, the adrenal glands are enlarged due to the unopposed action of ACTH on the gland caused by deficient levels of systemic cortisol. The glands may each weigh up to 30 grams and appear soft, tan, and diffusely enlarged or nodular on cut section. Microscopically, the cortex is widened between the zona glomerulosa and the medulla and this hyperplastic zone is filled by compact, granular, eosinophilic cells.

Several forms of CAH caused by 21-hydroxylase deficiency have been described as follows:

- Simple virilizing CAH: female infants exhibit pseudohermaphroditism with fused labia and an enlarged clitoris, whereas male patients show no abnormalities of the genitalia; patients of both sexes may demonstrate stunted growth and adult females may be infertile
- Salt-wasting CAH: newborns have impaired aldosterone synthesis that may manifest as hyponatremia, hyperkalemia, dehydration, hypotension, and increased renin secretion; females may demonstrate virilized external genitalia
- Late-onset CAH: virilizing symptoms may become apparent in young women at the time of puberty, whereas young men are often asymptomatic

In patients with increased levels of androgens due to *11 β-hydroxylase deficiency*, high levels of 11-deoxycortisol (a precursor) may lead to sodium retention and hypertension.

Adrenal Cortical Insufficiency

Adrenal cortical insufficiency may result from many causes including destruction of the adrenal gland, pituitary or hypothalamic dysfunction, or chronic steroid use.

Addison Disease (Primary Chronic Adrenal Insufficiency)

Addison disease is a wasting disorder resulting from complete adrenal failure with absence of glucocorticoid, mineralocorticoid, and androgen production.

The majority of cases of Addison disease have an underlying autoimmune etiology, evidenced by circulating antiadrenal antibodies, especially against 21-hydroxylase, familial history, and association with HLA-B8, HLA-DR3, and HLA-DR4 expression. In addition, patients may demonstrate *type I polyglandular autoimmune syndrome*, which manifests during childhood or adolescence with hypoparathyroidism and chronic mucocutaneous candidiasis, or *type II polyglandular autoimmune syndrome*, which occurs between 20 and 40 years of age and often demonstrates associated Hashimoto thyroiditis, Graves disease, insulin-dependent diabetes mellitus, and premature ovarian failure. Other causes of Addison disease include tuberculosis, metastatic carcinoma, amyloidosis, adrenal hemorrhage, sarcoidosis, and fungal infections.

Grossly, the adrenal gland appears pale, irregular, and shrunken, often weighing less than 3 grams. Microscopically, more than 90% of the gland has been destroyed and an intact medulla is seen surrounded by fibrous tissue containing small nests of atrophic cortical cells. Lymphoid infiltration is variable.

Patients often describe weakness, anorexia, weight loss, vomiting, diarrhea, marked personality changes, and occasionally a tan skin pigmentation caused by stimulation of skin melanocytes by proopiomelanocortin produced during ACTH processing. Lack of mineralocorticoid (aldosterone) production leads to low serum sodium and high serum potassium. Lack of glucocorticoid secretion leads to lymphocytosis and eosinophilia. The diagnosis is established by measuring corticosteroid levels after stimulation by ACTH. Treatment involves replacement of adrenal hormones by administration of glucocorticoids and mineralocorticoids.

Acute Adrenal Insufficiency

Acute adrenal insufficiency is a life-threatening condition in which a sudden loss of adrenal cortical function results in hypotension and shock. This condition may be caused by abrupt withdrawal of corticosteroid therapy following long-term administration, a sudden worsening of chronic adrenal insufficiency, or bilateral hemorrhagic infarction of the adrenal cortex caused by a meningococcal or pseudomonal septicemia (*Waterhouse-Friderichsen syndrome*). Treatment involves immediate corticosteroid administration and supportive measures.

Secondary Adrenal Insufficiency

Secondary adrenal insufficiency can occur in any setting in which secretion of hypothalamic corticotropin-releasing hormone (CRH) or pituitary ACTH is impaired. Because ACTH levels are not increased, patients typically do not demonstrate skin pigmentation. Electrolyte abnormalities are also not present in this disorder.

Adrenal Hyperfunction

Adrenal hyperfunction can lead to overproduction of corticosteroids (Cushing syndrome) or mineralocorticoids (Conn syndrome). The most common cause of adrenal hyperfunction in the United States is the chronic administration of corticosteroids.

Cushing Syndrome

Cushing syndrome is caused by excess secretion of adrenal corticosteroids. Etiologic factors include excess secretion of ACTH by pituitary corticotrope adenomas (Cushing disease), chronic administration of corticosteroids, adrenal tumors, or adrenal hyperplasia. Clinical features are generally independent of cause and include the following:

- Obesity of the face (moon facies), neck (buffalo hump), trunk, and abdomen
- Atrophic skin with loss of subcutaneous fat, purple striae, hyperpigmentation, and acanthosis nigricans
- Proximal muscle wasting, osteoporosis, and back pain
- Hypertension and congestive heart failure
- Virilization in women and erectile dysfunction and decreased libido in men
- Increased intraocular pressure
- Diabetes mellitus
- Irritability, emotional lability, depression, and paranoia

Laboratory findings include increased glucocorticoid levels, lymphopenia, low eosinophil levels, hypercalciuria, and elevated serum cholesterol and triglyceride levels. The dexamethasone suppression test is used to distinguish ACTH-dependent from ACTH-independent forms of Cushing syndrome. Dexamethasone suppresses pituitary ACTH secretion, resulting in decreased corticosteroid levels in ACTH-dependent forms, whereas it has no effect on ACTH-independent forms, such as adrenal tumors or ectopic ACTH production.

ACTH-dependent Cushing Syndrome

Causes of ACTH-dependent Cushing syndrome include the following:

- Ectopic ACTH production by a nonpituitary tumor: most commonly caused by small cell carcinoma of the lung
- Hypersecretion of ACTH by the pituitary (Cushing disease):

most commonly occurs in women between 25 and 45 years of age, often from a corticotrope microadenoma
- Inappropriate secretion of CRH by the hypothalamus

The adrenal glands appear diffusely and bilaterally enlarged, with each gland weighing up to 20 grams. *Diffuse adrenal hyperplasia* describes a grossly broadened cortex composed of an inner brown layer and a yellow, lipid-rich cap that is represented microscopically by a prominent zona fasciculata with large clear cells filled with lipid. *Nodular adrenal hyperplasia* refers to adrenal glands containing nodules measuring at least 2.5 cm in diameter that compress the overlying cortex.

ACTH-independent Cushing Syndrome

Causes of ACTH-independent Cushing syndrome include adrenal adenoma, adrenal carcinoma, bilateral micronodular hyperplasia of the adrenal cortex, and chronic administration of corticosteroids.

Adrenal Adenoma

Adrenal adenomas most commonly occur after 50 years of age and often demonstrate a female predominance. Grossly, these lesions appear as encapsulated, firm, yellow, slightly lobulated masses that measure approximately 4 cm in diameter. The cut surface is mottled yellow and brown, and may appear black due to the deposition of lipofuscin. Necrosis and calcification may be present. Microscopically, clear, lipid-laden cells are present in sheets or nests with scattered compact, eosinophilic cells. The remainder of the adrenal gland is often atrophic. Functional versus nonfunctional adenomas cannot be distinguished on the basis of morphology.

Adrenal Carcinoma

Adrenal carcinomas more commonly affect women and often occur around 40 years of age; however, this tumor may also occur in children. The majority of adrenal carcinomas are functional. Grossly, adrenal carcinomas are large (often greater than 100 grams), soft, encapsulated, and lobulated. On cut section, the tumors appear pink, brown, or yellow; irregular; and often with necrosis or cystic change. Microscopically, a mixture of clear and compact cells is present with varying degrees of nuclear polymorphism, mitoses, and vascular invasion. This tumor is highly aggressive and local extension and micrometastases are often present at the time of surgery. Most patients survive only 1 to 3 years.

Other ACTH-independent Diseases

Bilateral micronodular hyperplasia of the adrenal cortex (*Carney complex* or *primary pigmented nodular adrenocortical disease*) is disease of children or young adults. Approximately 50% of all cases are caused by an autosomal dominant form of the disease that also manifests with pigmented lesions on the body, myxomas, testicular tumors, and somatotrope adenomas of the pituitary. A subset of patients contain a mutation in a regulatory subunit of protein kinase A. Grossly, the adrenal glands contain small brown or black nodules that consist of large eosinophilic cells filled with lipofuscin granules.

Conn Syndrome

Conn syndrome is the inappropriate secretion of aldosterone caused by an adrenal adenoma or hyperplastic adrenal glands. Approximately 75% of cases are caused by a solitary adrenal adenoma (aldosteronoma). The remainder is caused by bilateral adrenal hyperplasia.

Aldosteronomas are more common in women and occur between 30 and 50 years of age. Grossly, these tumors are solitary, small, and yellow. Microscopically, they have clear, lipid-rich cells arranged in cords or alveolar structures. Because aldosterone does not inhibit ACTH secretion, the background adrenal gland is not atrophic.

Bilateral adrenal hyperplasia is characterized by multiple cortical nodules, measuring less than 2 cm in diameter, that are formed by clear cells.

Excess aldosterone secretion is manifested clinically hypertension, hypokalemia, and metabolic alkalosis. Treatment involves surgical resection of aldosteronomas and dietary sodium restriction and spironolactone administration for hyperplasia.

Other Adrenal Lesions

A variety of other lesions may occur in the adrenal glands and include the following:

- Adrenal myelolipoma: mixture of mature adipose tissue and hematopoietic marrow
- Adrenal cysts: most likely represent pseudocysts formed by cystic degeneration of benign adrenal tumors
- Metastatic cancer: often include metastatic lung and breast cancer and malignant melanoma

Adrenal Medullary Tumors

A summary of adrenal medullary tumors, derived from neural crest cells, is shown in Figure 21-2.

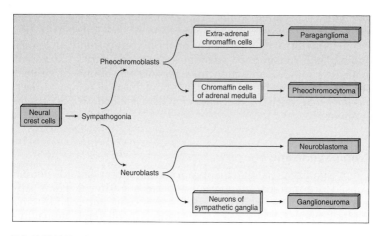

FIGURE   21-2
Histogenesis of tumors of the adrenal medulla and extraadrenal sympathetic nervous system. (From Rubin E, Gorstein F, Rubin R, et al. Rubin's Pathology, 4th ed. Philadelphia: Lippincott Williams & Wilkins, 2005, p. 1164.)

Pheochromocytoma

Pheochromocytomas are tumors of the chromaffin cells of the adrenal medulla that secrete catecholamines. These tumors occur slightly more often in women and may occur at any age, although are often more common in adults with rare presentation after 60 years of age. Pheochromocytomas follow the "ten-percent rule": 10% of pheochromocytomas are malignant, extraadrenal in location (termed *paragangliomas*), multiple, occur in childhood, and are associated with other conditions.

Pheochromocytomas are often sporadic, although a subset may occur in association with the following heritable syndromes:

- MEN type 2A (Sipple syndrome): also associated with medullary thyroid carcinoma and parathyroid carcinoma/hyperplasia and is caused by *RET* protooncogene mutations
- MEN type 2B: associated with medullary thyroid carcinoma, ganglioneuromas of the conjunctiva, oral cavity, larynx, and gastrointestinal tract (mucosal neuroma syndrome), is associated with *RET* protooncogene mutations, and occurs 10 years earlier than MEN type 2A syndrome
- Familial medullary thyroid carcinoma: at least four family members are affected and no other signs of MEN type 2A are identified
- Von Hippel-Lindau disease

- Neurofibromatosis type 1
- McCune-Albright syndrome

Grossly, pheochromocytomas are variably sized, encapsulated, spongy, reddish masses with central scars, hemorrhage, and cystic degeneration. Microscopically, nests of cells (zellballen) are present in a highly vascular stroma. The cells are polyhedral, with a granular cytoplasm often containing eosinophilic globules and vesicular nuclei. Nuclear pleomorphism, mitoses, necrosis, and invasion of the capsule or blood vessels may be present. There are no reliable histologic findings suggestive of malignancy, and only metastases (often to regional lymph nodes, bone, lung, or liver) demonstrate the aggressive nature of some lesions. The tumor cells stain with neuroendocrine markers, including chromogranin and synaptophysin.

A proposed precursor of pheochromocytomas, *adrenal medullary hyperplasia*, demonstrates an expanded medulla with nests of enlarged chromaffin cells.

Patients with pheochromocytomas often present with symptoms of episodic catecholamine release, including hypertension, paroxysms of convulsions, anxiety, hyperventilation, palpitations, headaches, sweating, abdominal pain, or vomiting. The release of catecholamines may be severe enough to lead to myocardial infarction or aortic dissection in some instances. The majority of patients demonstrate hypertension, which may be resistant to therapy. Episodic catecholamine release may be triggered by meals rich in tyramine (beer, wine, cheese), exercise, bending, or lifting.

Diagnosis is established by elevated urine catecholamine metabolites, such as metanephrine, vanillylmandelic acid, and unconjugated catecholamines. Treatment involves surgical resection of the tumor and adjunct treatment of symptoms with α-adrenergic blocking agents and β-adrenergic receptor antagonists.

Paraganglioma

Paragangliomas occur within paraganglia throughout the body, including the retroperitoneum, bladder, and head and neck region. Generally, paragangliomas of the head and neck are benign, whereas paragangliomas of the retroperitoneum are malignant. One of the more common paragangliomas is the *carotid body tumor*, which arises at the carotid bifurcation and often forms a palpable mass. These tumors occur most frequently in young adults and may be multicentric. Microscopically, these lesions are similar to pheochromocytomas.

Neuroblastoma

Neuroblastoma is a malignant tumor of neural crest origin that originates in the adrenal medulla or sympathetic ganglia and most commonly occurs within the first 3 years of life, accounting for 10% of all childhood cancers. Neuroblastomas are most commonly sporadic and are often characterized by chromosome 1 deletions, unbalanced 17q translocations, extrachromosomal double minutes, and homogeneously staining regions on chromosome 2 that represent *N-myc* amplification. Up to one third of neuroblastomas occur in the adrenal gland, whereas the majority of the remaining tumors occur in the abdomen or posterior mediastinum.

Grossly, neuroblastomas vary in size and appear as round, irregularly lobulated masses with a soft, friable, maroon cut surface. Necrosis, hemorrhage, cystic change, and calcification are common. Microscopically, these tumors are composed of sheets of small, round to fusiform cells with hyperchromatic nuclei and scant cytoplasm that are morphologically similar to lymphocytes (i.e., small round blue cell tumor). Mitotic figures are common. Tumor cells may form rosettes (circular structures with central fibrillary material) or pseudorosettes (cells palisading around blood vessels). Neuroblastomas often infiltrate locally and metastasize to regional lymph nodes, the liver, lung, bones, orbit, and other sites.

The clinical manifestations of neuroblastomas are variable and include an enlarging abdomen, a firm, nontender abdominal mass, ascites from hepatic metastases, respiratory distress from large masses in the thorax, and irritability. Diagnosis includes the presence of urinary catecholamines and their metabolites and imaging studies. Localized tumors are treated by surgical excision, whereas disseminated tumors are treated by chemotherapy and sometimes radiation. Favorable prognostic indices include the following:

- Age less than 2 years
- Extra-adrenal tumors
- Stage I tumors (confined to the organ of origin) or stage IVS tumors (absence of chromosomal abnormalities and often undergo spontaneous remissions)
- Low-grade tumors
- Vanillylmandelic acid: homovanillic acid ratio of 1 or greater
- Absence of *N-myc* amplification

Ganglioneuroma

Ganglioneuromas are benign tumors that originate from neural crest cells and occur most commonly in older children and young adults. These tumors arise in sympathetic ganglia, commonly in the posterior mediastinum and adrenal medulla. Chromosomal abnormalities are absent.

Grossly, ganglioneuromas are well encapsulated and display a myxoid, glistening, cut surface. Microscopically, the tumor cells are well-differentiated, mature ganglion cells and associated spindle cells in a loose, abundant fibrillar stroma. A subset of ganglioneuromas may represent differentiated neuroblastomas.

THE PINEAL GLAND

Normal Anatomy and Histology

The pineal gland is situated below the posterior edge of the corpus callosum, between the superior colliculi, and measures only 5 to 7 mm in size. It is composed of cords and clusters of large epitheliallike cells (pinealocytes) and cells that appear similar to astrocytes. The pineal gland produces melatonin, serotonin, and several peptides.

Neoplasms of the Pineal Gland

Pineal gland neoplasms are rare and include the following:

- Germ cell tumors (germinomas, dysgerminomas): most common pineal tumor, derived from misplaced stem cells, and are identical to those found in other sites
- Pineocytoma: benign, well-circumscribed tumor formed by nests of small tumor cells with round nuclei and eosinophilic cytoplasm
- Pinealoblastoma: highly malignant tumor of young adults composed of small oval cells with dark nuclei, scant cytoplasm, numerous mitoses, and often hemorrhage and necrosis

Pineal gland neoplasms often present with signs and symptoms related to compression of surrounding structures and include headaches, visual disturbances, and changes in behavior. Precocious puberty may occur in boys.

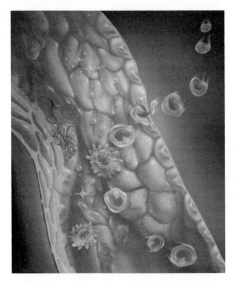

Diabetes Mellitus

Chapter Outline

Regulation of Blood Glucose

Classification of Diabetes Mellitus
    Type I Diabetes Mellitus
    Type II Diabetes Mellitus

Complications of Diabetes Mellitus
    Atherosclerosis, Diabetic Nephropathy, and Diabetic Retinopathy
    Diabetic Neuropathy
    Infections
    Pregnancy Complications

The pancreas functions as both an endocrine and exocrine organ. The most common disorders of the endocrine pancreas include diabetes mellitus and tumor formation. Neoplasia of the endocrine pancreas is discussed in Chapter 13.

Regulation of Blood Glucose

Under normal conditions, ingestion of a carbohydrate-rich meal results in increased blood glucose levels, which induces the secretion of insulin from pancreatic β cells. Insulin functions to reduce blood glucose levels by the following mechanisms:

- Increasing glucose uptake by skeletal muscle and adipose tissue
- Inhibiting gluconeogenesis in the liver
- Promoting glycogen synthesis in the liver
- Inhibiting the release of glucagon from the pancreas

The insulin receptor—present on skeletal muscle, liver, and adipose cells—is a heterotetrameric glycoprotein containing two extracellular α subunits and two transmembrane β subunits. When bound to insulin, the β subunits function as a tyrosine kinase to activate downstream signaling molecules. Ultimately, glucose transport and metabolic proteins are activated to reduce levels of circulating glucose.

Abnormalities in any of these pathways may lead to diabetes mellitus, which is characterized by increased blood glucose levels (hyperglycemia), excretion of excess sugar in the urine (glucosuria) with secondary increased urine volume (polyuria), and thirst (polydipsia).

Classification of Diabetes Mellitus

Diabetes may be a primary disease or occur secondary to a variety of conditions including pancreatic disease, endocrine abnormalities, pregnancy, or pharmaceutical drug use.

Forms of diabetes mellitus include the following:

- Type I diabetes: less than 10% of all diabetic patients; juvenile onset; autoimmune destruction of pancreatic β cells
- Type II diabetes: majority of diabetic patients; more commonly demonstrates an adult onset; associated with obesity; combination of impaired insulin secretion and peripheral insulin resistance
- Gestational diabetes: β-cell defect and insulin resistance of pregnancy
- Glucocorticoid-induced diabetes: occurs with Cushing syndrome and corticosteroid administration

Type I Diabetes Mellitus

Type I diabetes (also known as insulin-dependent diabetes mellitus [IDDM]) is caused by the autoimmune destruction of pancreatic β cells. Decreased insulin production causes sustained, elevated levels of blood glucose with loss of glucose into the urine, metabolism of body fat resulting in the production of ketone bodies (acetoacetic acid and β-hydroxybutyric acid), and continued production of glucose by the liver (Fig. 22-1).

Type I diabetes is most common among persons of northern European ancestry. Peak onset usually occurs at the time of puberty

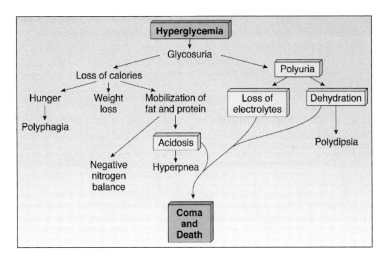

FIGURE 22-1
Symptoms and signs of uncontrolled hyperglycemia in diabetes mellitus. (From Rubin E, Gorstein F, Rubin R, et al. Rubin's Pathology, 4th ed. Philadelphia: Lippincott Williams & Wilkins, 2005 p. 1175.)

and most patients are younger than 20 years of age at onset of disease. Factors that have been proposed to promote the development of type I diabetes include the following:

- Expression of the major histocompatibility complex types HLA-DR3 or HLA-DR4: occurs in 95% of patients
- Autoimmune, cell-mediated β cell destruction: CD8+ (cytotoxic) T lymphocytes infiltrate and damage pancreatic islets, termed insulinitis; may recur in a transplanted donor pancreas due to immune-memory; 10% of patients have a second autoimmune disease such as Graves disease or pernicious anemia
- Viral infection: mumps, group B coxsackie viruses; possibly due to shared antigen epitopes between β cells and viral proteins (molecular mimicry)
- Chemical exposure

Patients with type I diabetes present with polyuria, polyphagia, and polydipsia, hyperglycemia, and reduced serum insulin levels due to a severe reduction in pancreatic β cells and insulin production. Some cases may be heralded by the development of ketoacidosis in which the patient demonstrates severe acidosis due to increased ketone production. Due to the lack of insulin production, these patients require exogenous insulin.

Microscopically, the pancreatic findings in type I diabetes are variable. Early disease demonstrates a lymphocytic infiltrate in the pancreatic islets (insulinitis). More advanced disease demonstrates variably sized, ribbonlike islets due to loss of the β-cell population. The associated exocrine pancreas often contains interlobular and interacinar fibrosis.

Type II Diabetes Mellitus

Type II diabetes mellitus (also known as noninsulin-dependent diabetes mellitus [NIDDM]) is characterized by reduced tissue sensitivity to insulin (insulin resistance) and reduced glucose-stimulated insulin secretion. Type II disease is most common in adults and often affects elderly and obese persons, although there is an increasing incidence of type 2 diabetes in young patients; ethnic minority groups are most frequently affected in the United States. A comparison of type I and type II diabetes mellitus is provided in Table 22-1. Proposed factors that may promote the development of type II diabetes include the following:

Table 22-1

Comparison of Type I and Type II Diabetes Mellitus

Feature	Type I	Type II
Age at onset	Usually before age 20	Usually after age 20
Type of onset	Abrupt; often severe with ketoacidosis	Gradual; usually subtle, asymptomatic
Usual body weight	Normal	Overweight
Genetics (parents/ siblings with diabetes)	<20%	>60%
Monozygotic twins	50% concordant	90% concordant
HLA association	HLA-DR3, HLA-DR4	None
Islet cell antibodies	Secondary to injury	None
Islet lesions	Early inflammation; late atrophy and fibrosis	Fibrosis, amyloid
β cells	Markedly reduced	Normal or slight reduced
Blood insulin	Markedly reduced	Elevated or normal
Management	Insulin required	Diet, exercise, oral medication, insulin

- Multigenic inheritance: 60% of patients have a parent or sibling with NIDDM; both monozygotic twins are usually affected
- Obesity, especially visceral-abdominal obesity: adipose cells release free fatty acids and cytokines (tumor necrosis factor-α/TNF-α and adiponectin) that reduce peripheral insulin sensitivity, leading to insulin resistance
- Hypertension, reduced levels of exercise, dyslipidemia: cardiovascular risk factors that lead to insulin resistance and compensatory hyperinsulinemia, termed *metabolic syndrome*
- African-American race
- Increased age

Patients often present with polyuria, polydipsia, and polyphagia. Ketoacidosis is typically not a classic presentation in patients with type II diabetes mellitus. In cases of severe blood glucose elevation in the setting of dehydration, patients may experience *nonketotic hyperosmolar coma.*

Microscopically, a variable reduction in pancreatic β cells is identified and the islets of Langerhans contain an accumulation of fibrous tissue and amyloid. Type II diabetes can be treated initially with diet and exercise; however, more severe cases are treated with oral antihyperglycemics and insulin, when necessary.

Complications of Diabetes Mellitus

Chronic elevation of blood glucose is the major factor in the development of diabetic complications (including retinopathy, nephropathy, and neuropathy), which frequently affect small vessels (microvascular changes). Macrovascular complications (such as atherosclerosis) occur in older patients with diabetes mellitus, although the pathophysiology of these changes in relation to hyperglycemia is unclear.

Multiple pathophysiologic mechanisms lead to the pathologic changes evident in diabetes:

- Protein glycosylation: glucose binds nonenzymatically to many proteins including hemoglobin; elevation of serum hemoglobin A_{1c} reflects poor glucose control during preceding 6 to 8 weeks; crosslinking of glycosylated proteins leads to thickened basement membranes of vessels
- Aldose reductase pathway: excess glucose in tissues is metabolized by aldose reductase leading to the formation of sorbitol, which may be toxic to cells
- Protein kinase C (PKC) activation: diacylglycerol synthesized from glycolytic intermediates activates PKC; promotes increased cytokine production, microvascular contractility and permeability, and proliferation of endothelial and smooth muscle cells
- Excessive reactive oxygen species: promotes mitochondrial oxidative phosphorylation

Atherosclerosis, Diabetic Nephropathy, and Diabetic Retinopathy

Hyperglycemia affects blood vessels of all caliber by increasing the rate of atherosclerosis. Atherosclerotic heart disease and ischemic stroke are major causes of death in adults with diabetes. Peripheral vascular disease is also common in this population, leading to distal ulcers and gangrene, which accounts for approximately 40% of nontraumatic limb amputations in the United States. Small vessel disease—caused by hyaline arteriolosclerosis, capillary basement membrane thickening, and increased platelet aggregation—causes renal failure and blindness.

Diabetic nephropathy accounts for 20% to 40% of all cases of renal failure, and kidney disease secondary to diabetes is the most common reason for renal transplantation in adults. The pathogenesis of diabetic nephropathy begins with glomerular hypertension and renal hyperperfusion, which results in a cascade of protein deposition in the mesangium, glomerulosclerosis, and renal failure. In addition, thickening of the glomerular basement membrane due to glycosylation products occurs. The major pathologic finding in the kidneys of patients with diabetes is nodular glomerulosclerosis (Kimmelstiel-Wilson disease), which demonstrates basement membranelike material deposited as lobules or diffusely throughout the glomerulus (see Chapter 16).

Worsening renal function is heralded by albuminuria and increasing glomerular filtration rate, serum creatinine, and serum urea nitrogen. The primary route of prevention of diabetic nephropathy is strict control of blood glucose and the addition of antihypertensive medication, especially angiotensin-converting enzyme (ACE) inhibitors, when necessary.

Diabetic retinopathy leads to blindness in a significant proportion of patients with diabetes and the prevalence of diabetic retinopathy is related to the duration and severity of hyperglycemia. Microscopic changes in diabetic retinopathy are discussed in Chapter 29.

Diabetic Neuropathy

A common complication of diabetes, diabetic neuropathy affects primarily the autonomic and peripheral sensory nervous systems. Alterations have been identified in the axons, myelin sheath, Schwann cells, and small blood vessels surrounding the nerves. Peripheral neuropathy initially causes pain and abnormal sensations in the distal extremities. Ultimately, it leads to loss of touch, pain sensation, and proprioception, often in a "stocking-and-glove" distribution. Loss of distal extremity sensation often makes patients unaware of injurious stimuli on the foot and ankle, leading to ulcer formation. Autonomic dysfunction contributes to postural hypotension, diarrhea, erectile dysfunction, and hypotonic urinary bladder.

Infections

Patients with poorly controlled hyperglycemia are at increased risk for bacterial and fungal infection due to decreased leukocyte function. The most commonly seen infections are urinary tract infections, in which the glucose-rich urine provides a medium for organism growth.

Pregnancy Complications

Poor glycemic control during pregnancy leads to large birth-weight infants (macrosomia), occasionally necessitating a cesarean section. During fetal gestation, increased circulating glucose levels cause pancreatic β-cell hyperplasia in the infant, often leading to hypoglycemic episodes during the neonatal period. An additional complication of hyperglycemia during pregnancy includes major developmental abnormalities, such as heart and great vessel anomalies and neural tube defects such as spina bifida and anencephaly.

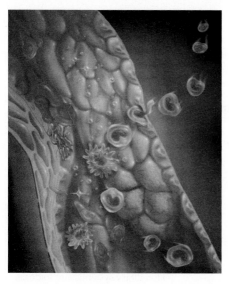

Amyloidoses

Chapter Outline

Amyloid
Common Amyloidoses
Clinical Features of Amyloidoses

Amyloid

Amyloidosis describes an extracellular deposition of characteristic proteins that may occur in a localized or systemic manner with several disease processes. Amyloid itself is composed of a disease-specific fibrillogenic protein and a common set of components, which includes the amyloid P component (AP) derived from serum amyloid P, basement membrane components (laminin, collagen type IV, and perlecan), and apolipoprotein E.

With routine stains (H&E), amyloid appears amorphous, pale pink, and glassy. Special stains may be used to highlight the presence of amyloid protein, the most common of which is the Congo red stain. Amyloid stained with Congo red demonstrates a red-apple green birefringence under polarized light. Additional stains that highlight amyloid include thioflavin T (viewed under ultraviolet light), alcian blue, and immunohistochemical stains against disease-specific proteins.

The various amyloids share a similar ultrastructural appearance. By electron microscopy, amyloid has groups of fibers ar-

Table 23-1

Classification of Amyloids

Amyloid Protein	Protein Precursor	Clinical Setting

AA
AL
	apoSAA
	κ or λ light chain
		Persistent acute inflammation
		Multiple myeloma, plasma
		  cell dyscrasias, and primary
		  amyloid

AH
ATTR
	γ chain
	Transthyretin
		Waldenstrom macroglobulinemia
		Familial amyloidotic
		  polyneuropathy, normal TTR
		  in senile systemic amyloid

AGel ACys ALys	Gelsolin Cystatin C Lysozyme	Famial amyloidosis, Finnish HCHWA, Icelandic Hereditary systemic amyloidosis, Ostertag-type
AFib Aβ	Fibrinogen β-protein precursor	Hereditary renal amyloidosis Alzheimer disease Down syndrome, HCHWA Dutch
APrP ACal	Prion protein (Pro)calcitonin	CJD, scrapie, BSE, GSS, Kuru Medullary carcinoma of the thyroid
AANF AIAPP	Atrial naturetic factor Islet amyloid polypeptide	Isolated atrial amyloid Type 2 diabetes, insulinomas

CJD, Creutzfeldt-Jakob disease; BSE, bovine spongiform encephalopathy; GSS, Gerstmann-Staussler-Sheinker syndrome; HCHWA, hereditary cerebral hemorrhage with amyloid; TTR, transthyretin.
Modified from Rubin E, Gorstein F, Rubin R, et al. Rubin's Pathology, 4th ed. Philadelphia: Lippincott Williams & Wilkins, 2005, p. 1190.

ranged in parallel arrays, with each group having a different orientation; this configuration contributes to the property of birefringence under polarized light. The individual protein subunits are primarily organized as β-pleated sheets. The specific protein subunits, that are disease specific and an integral part of the amyloid structure, are listed in Table 23-1.

Common Amyloidoses

Amyloidoses have been previously categorized as primary (no known underlying disease), secondary to a known disease process, or familial. This classification scheme has been changed to reflect the disease-specific protein involved in amyloid formation. Some of the more common diseases that feature amyloid deposition include the following:

- *Familial Mediterranean fever*: autosomal recessive disease; mapped to short arm of chromosome 16; characterized by polymorphonuclear leukocyte dysfunction and recurrent episodes of serositis
- *Alzheimer disease*: deposition of the Aβ peptide derived from proteolytic cleavage of the amyloid precursor protein (APP) by secretases; localized deposition in the brain; see chapter 28
- *Diabetes*: islet amyloid polypeptide cleavage results in amyloid deposition in the pancreas
- *AL amyloidosis*: derived from the κ or λ light chain of antibodies; produced by neoplastic cells and therefore varies in sequence between patients; may occur in primary amyloidosis, multiple myeloma, B-cell lymphomas, or other plasma cell dyscrasias
- *AA amyloidosis*: derived from normal serum amyloid A protein; occurs with persistent inflammatory, neoplastic, and hereditary conditions; AA sequence is the same between patients

Clinical Features of Amyloidoses

The clinical features vary depending on the location of predominant amyloid deposition. Multiple organs and structures may be involved, including the following:

- Kidneys: may result in the nephrotic syndrome and renal failure
- Vessels: amyloid is often present in the walls of blood vessels and may lead to hemorrhagic complications, especially in the brains of elderly patients
- Heart: myocardial deposition may lead to cardiomegaly, congestive heart failure, arrhythmias if the conduction system is affected, and restrictive cardiomyopathy
- Gastrointestinal tract: most commonly affects ganglia, smooth muscle vasculature, and submucosa leading to constipation or diarrhea
- Peripheral nerves

Most commonly, amyloid deposits within the stroma of affected organs and may lead to organ enlargement with a pale, waxy appearance on cut section or to organ atrophy due to impairment of circulation. Ultimately, the diagnosis of amyloidosis is dependent on the demonstration of this material histologically.

In systemic forms of amyloidosis, the disease is progressive and may lead to death within a short period of time. For example, patients with AL amyloidosis usually die within 1 to 2 years from complications of amyloidosis or the underlying disease process itself. Treatment of amyloidosis involves regulation of the underlying disease process, inhibition of nidus formation in amyloid (i.e., colchicine treatment of familial Mediterranean fever), and acceleration of amyloid removal (i.e., treatment of AL amyloidosis patients with an iodinated analogue of doxorubicin). Other potential treatment modalities include reduction in the amyloid precursor concentration and inhibition of molecular interactions.

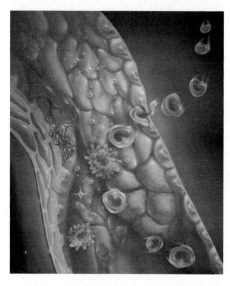

CHAPTER *24*

The Skin

Chapter Outline

Systemic Lupus Erythematosus
Lichen Planus

Blistering Diseases
Pemphigus Vulgaris
Bullous Pemphigoid
Dermatitis Herpetiformis
Epidermolysis Bullosa

Granulomatous Inflammation
Sarcoidosis
Granuloma Annulare

Acne Vulgaris

Disease of the Dermal Connective Tissue: Scleroderma

Leukocytoclastic Vasculitis

Inflammatory Disorders of the Panniculus
Erythema Nodosum
Erythema Induratum

Melanocytic Lesions
Freckle
Lentigo
Acquired Melanocytic Nevus
Dysplastic (Atypical) Nevus
Malignant Melanoma

Epidermal Lesions
Benign Epidermal Lesions
Premalignant and Malignant Epidermal Lesions

Adnexal Tumors

Fibrohistiocytic Lesions
Dermatofibroma
Dermatofibrosarcoma Protuberans
Atypical Fibroxanthoma

Mycosis Fungoides

Kaposi Sarcoma

Normal Anatomy and Histology

The skin performs multiple physiologic functions, including the formation of a protective barrier against organisms, the regulation of body temperature, immunoregulatory modulation, and sensation. The skin is formed of the epidermis, dermis, hair follicles, and sweat glands.

Epidermis

The epidermis is formed by stratified squamous epithelium that rests on a basement membrane (Fig. 24-1). Free nerve endings extend into the epidermis and provide sensory information. The four layers of the epidermis are as follows:

- Stratum basalis: mitotically active single layer of cuboidal cells ("basal cells") that rest on the basement membrane and appear slightly basophilic
- Stratum spinosum (prickle cell layer): multiple layers of keratinocytes with short processes between the cells
- Stratum granulosum (granular cell layer): flattened keratinocytes that contain numerous keratohyaline granules
- Stratum corneum: anucleated keratinocytes that form a protective barrier on the surface of the skin (keratin)

Numerous cell types are found within the epidermis and include the following:

- Keratinocytes: produce keratin and function as the primary water barrier of the skin; contain tonofibrils that terminate on cell–cell adhesion junctions called desmosomes

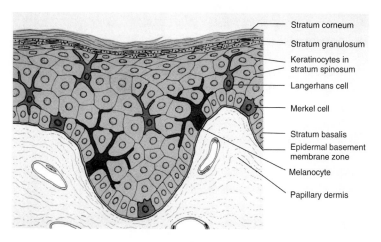

FIGURE 24-1

Normal epidermis. Keratinocytes form the multilayered epidermis, protecting against water loss and bacterial invasion. Melanocytes provide color as well as protection against ultraviolet radiation. Langerhans cells function in immunological regulation. Merkel cells provide tactile sensation. (From Rubin E, Gorstein F, Rubin R, et al. Rubin's Pathology, 4th ed. Philadelphia: Lippincott Williams & Wilkins, 2005, p. 1204.)

- Melanocytes: derived from the neural crest and produce melanin, which is transferred to adjacent keratinocytes to provide skin color
- Langerhans cells: HLA-DR containing cells that recognize and process antigens and are immunopositive for CD1a and S-100. Birbeck granules (tennis racket–shaped vesicles) are identified by electron microscopy
- Merkel cells: modified epidermal cells in the lips, oral cavity, hair follicles, and palmar skin of the digits that serve as mechanoreceptors

Basement Membrane Zone

The basement membrane zone (BMZ) rests between the epidermis and dermis and is responsible for epithelial cell polarity. The BMZ contains multiple layers containing types IV and VII collagen, among other components (Fig. 24-2). A number of disease conditions affect the BMZ, including bullous pemphigoid.

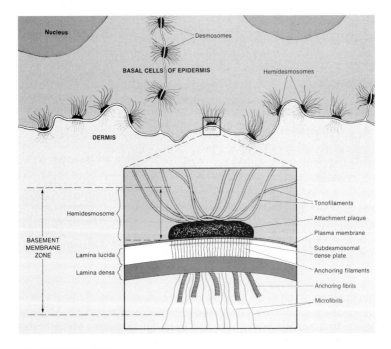

FIGURE   24-2
The dermal-epidermal interface and the basement membrane zone. (From Rubin E, Gorstein F, Rubin R, et al. Rubin's Pathology, 4th ed. Philadelphia: Lippincott Williams & Wilkins, 2005, p. 1209.)

Dermis

The dermis rests deep to the BMZ and contains predominantly collagen embedded in a hyaluronic acid matrix, with interspersed myelinated nerve endings (including Meissner's corpuscles and Pacinian corpuscles) and cutaneous vasculature. The two main divisions of the dermis are as follows:

- Papillary dermis: immediately deep to the BMZ and is formed of delicate collagen fibrils
- Reticular dermis: deep to the papillary dermis and contains bundles of collagen and elastic fibers

The dermal papillae contain capillary beds, which help regulate body temperature and can allow egress of inflammatory cells. Lymphatic channels are present near the epidermis, which may be involved in the metastases of cutaneous neoplasms.

Hair Follicles

Hair follicles are formed by an invagination of the epidermis and contain bulbs composed of epithelial and mesenchymal tissue. Hair, formed of hard keratin, grows in a cyclical phase, with the majority of hair undergoing active growth (anagen phase of hair growth). Hair follicles are associated with arrector pili muscles that regulate hair position and "goosebumps." *Alopecia* (baldness) is a loss of hair commonly caused by the cessation of mitosis of the growing hair.

Sweat Glands

The three types of glands found in the skin are as follows:

- Sebaceous glands: produce the oily substance sebum that coats the skin
- Eccrine sweat glands: located throughout the skin and can help regulate body temperature
- Apocrine sweat glands: located in the axilla, genitoanal region, and around the areola and produces a protein-rich secretion that may be acted on by bacteria to produce an odor

Terminology of Skin Disease

Specific terms used to describe the clinical findings in skin disease include the following:

- Macule: flat lesion that appears as a different color from the surrounding skin
- Patch: a large macule
- Papule: elevated lesion less than 5 mm in diameter

- Nodule: a large papule
- Vesicle: small, fluid-filled blister
- Bulla: large, fluid-filled vesicle
- Pustule: pus-filled vesicle
- Scale: exfoliated epidermis that appears as flakes
- Lichenification: thickened skin with prominent skin markings

Microscopic findings that may be common to various skin diseases include the following:

- Hyperkeratosis: increased keratin with thickening of the stratum corneum
- Parakeratosis: nuclei within the cells of the stratum corneum
- Erosion: partial loss of the epidermis
- Ulceration: full-thickness loss of the epidermis
- Spongiosis: edema between the cells of the epidermis
- Acantholysis: loss of cell-cell adhesion in the epidermis
- Papillomatous hyperplasia: elongation of the papillary dermis

Infectious Skin Diseases

Impetigo

Impetigo is a superficial bacterial infection of the skin often caused by staphylococci or streptococci. This disease most commonly affects children, who are infected by minor breaks in the skin. Grossly, the hands, extremities, and face demonstrate honey-colored crusted erosions or ulcers that often have an area of central healing. Eventually, vesicles or bullae may form and rupture, resulting in a thin, seropurulent discharge that dries on the surface. Microscopically, abundant neutrophils are present below the stratum corneum and the epidermis shows reactive changes including spongiosis and elongation of the rete ridges.

Superficial Fungal Infections

Superficial fungal infections of nonviable keratinized epithelium are caused by dermatophytes, which ingest keratin, and are termed *dermatophytosis, tinea,* or *ringworm*. Infection often occurs secondary to an altered microenvironment, often caused by corticosteroid use or excessive sweating. The most common causal organism is *Trichophyton rubrum*; however, *Candida* species and *Malassezia furfur* may also produce infection. Special stains such as Periodic acid–Schiff (PAS) may demonstrate the organisms. Clinically, the dermatophytoses are named by site of infection (e.g., *tinea capitis* for infection of the scalp; *tinea cruris* for infection of the pubic area). Hyperkeratosis, epidermal hyperplasia, and chronic perivascular inflammation in the dermis are often present.

Deep Fungal Infections

Deep fungal infections often occur secondary to pulmonary infection, especially following inhalation of aerosols containing *Histoplasma* or *Blastomyces*. Special stains for fungus, such as PAS, can demonstrate the organism. Grossly, these lesions appear as nodules or ulcers and may be bilateral. Introduction of organisms may also occur locally and can demonstrate a chancrelike appearance. Microscopically, there may be epidermal hyperplasia, intraepidermal microabscesses, and suppurative granulomatous inflammation of the dermis.

Viral Infections

Many types of viruses can lead to skin infection. Examples include the following:

- *Molluscum contagiosum* is an infection that occurs in children and young adults and is spread by direct contact. Grossly, lesions are firm, dome-shaped, smooth-surfaced papules with a central umbilication on the face, trunk, and anogenital area. The lesions are often self-limited. Microscopically, epidermal cells contain large, eosinophilic cytoplasmic viral inclusions (molluscum bodies) in a background of papillomatous epidermal hyperplasia.
- Human papillomavirus (HPV) infection may result in warty growth of the epidermis (see Benign Epidermal Lesions, Verrucae).

Arthropod Infestations

Arthropod infestations are often pruritic, and tissue reactions are produced in response to arthropod products. Such infections include the following:

- *Scabies*: caused by the mite *Sarcoptes scabei*, which burrows beneath the stratum corneum of the fingers, wrists, trunk, and genital skin and results in a lymphocytic and eosinophilic infiltration
- *Pediculosis*: produced by lice present along hair shafts

Biting insects form small, pruritic papules to large, weeping nodules on the skin.

Inherited Abnormalities of Keratinization

Ichthyoses

The ichthyoses are composed of a heterogeneous group of heritable diseases that share a marked thickening of the stratum corneum.

These diseases have their onset in infancy or childhood, and affected patients demonstrate coarse, fishlike scales. Four major types of ichthyoses have been described as follows:

- Ichthyosis vulgaris
- X-linked ichthyosis
- Lamellar ichthyosis
- Epidermolytic hyperkeratosis

Ichthyoses are generally characterized by increased cohesiveness of the stratum corneum, abnormal keratinization, and increased basal cell proliferation.

Darier Disease

Darier disease is an autosomal dominant disorder involving the *ATP2A2* gene that is characterized by multifocal keratoses. Patients present during childhood or adolescence with skin-colored papules on the chest, nasolabial folds, back, scalp, forehead, ears, and groin that eventually develop crusts.

Dermatoses and Inflammatory Conditions of the Skin

A subset of conditions that cause dermatoses is listed in Table 24-1.

Urticaria and Angioedema

Urticaria and angioedema are type I hypersensitivity reactions that are mediated by immunoglobulin E. They both result in degranulation of mast cells to specific antigens and exaggerated permeability of the venules.

Urticaria (hives) is characterized by raised, erythematous, well-demarcated pruritic lesions associated with edema in the upper portion of the dermis, which are termed *wheals*. These lesions appear following antigen exposure and resolve within several hours. However, in the chronic form, the lesions may recur for several weeks.

Angioedema is a more pronounced, intensely pruritic reaction in which the wheals are larger and edema extends into the subcutis. The lesions are characterized by interstitial edema and dilated cutaneous vessels.

Allergic Contact Dermatitis

Allergic contact dermatitis is a type IV hypersensitivity reaction (cell-mediated) that follows antigen exposure. Common offending agents include members of the plant genus *Rhus*, such as poison ivy and poison oak. The plants contain antigens called *haptens* that

Table 24-1
Conditions Associated with Dermatoses

Disease	Anatomic Location	Pathologic Findings
Urticaria (hives)	Variable	Raised, erythematous, well-demarcated pruritic lesions; degranulation of mast cells and dermal edema
Allergic contact dermatitis	Region of contact	Intensely pruritic, erythematous, small vesicles that crust without scarring; epidermal edema (spongiotic dermatitis), vesicles, lymphocytes, and macrophages that surround the superficial venular bed; eosinophils after 24 hours
Erythema multiforme	Scattered patches; may be widespread; may also involve mucous membranes	Target lesions with central red region surrounded by pale rim and additional erythematous rim; lymphocytic infiltration of the dermal–epidermal junction and upper dermis; keratinocyte apoptosis; occasional subepidermal blisters
Psoriasis	Dorsal extensor surfaces or areas exposed to trauma	Large, well-defined erythematous scaly plaques with silver hue; hyperplastic epidermis with thinning over papillae, hyperkeratosis, parakeratosis, neutrophilic infiltration in epidermis with Munro abscess formation
Systemic lupus erythematosus (SLE)	Often face (malar rash), skin, chest, back, extensor surfaces	Maculopapular rash; vacuolization of the basal cells, altered epithelial thickness, hyperkeratosis, plugging of hair follicles, and dense lymphocytic infiltrate involving basal cells, basement membrane, and dermis
Lichen planus	Often flexor surfaces of wrists	Violaceous, flat-topped papules; hyperkeratosis, hypergranulosis, band-like infiltrate of lymphocytes at dermal–epidermal junction, sawtoothlike appearance of epithelium

couple with carrier molecules, after which the complex is processed by Langerhans cells; this results in the formation of memory T cells. Patients demonstrate lesions 5 to 7 days following reexposure to the hapten. Grossly, these lesions appear as intensely pruritic, erythematous, small vesicles that last approximately 3 weeks. Eventually, the lesions crust and healing occurs without scarring. Microscopically, these lesions demonstrate prominent epidermal edema, termed *spongiotic dermatitis*, with lymphocytes and macrophages surrounding the superficial venular bed and the vesicles. After 24 hours, eosinophils infiltrate the epidermis and dermis.

Erythema Multiforme

Erythema multiforme is an acute, self-limited disorder that is most common during late adolescence and early adulthood. It is often induced by an infectious agent (herpesvirus, *Mycoplasma*) or drug reaction. The disorder ranges in severity from scattered erythematous macules and blisters to widespread ulceration of the skin and mucous membranes that is often fatal (Stevens-Johnson reaction).

Grossly, the lesions have a "target" appearance, with a central dark red zone and occasional blister formation, surrounded by a paler region that is further surrounded by an erythematous rim. Microscopically, the dermal-epidermal junction and the upper dermis have a lymphocytic infiltrate. The epidermis has apoptosis of keratinocytes and occasionally subepidermal blister formation with the roof of the blister formed by necrotic epidermis.

Psoriasis

This common chronic skin condition affects as much as 2% of the population and often occurs in late adolescence or young adulthood. It is characterized by large, well-defined, erythematous, scaly plaques with a silvery hue that are found most often on the dorsal extensor surfaces or areas exposed to trauma.

The underlying pathophysiology involves a variety of factors, including the following:

- Genetic factors: strong association with HLA-Cw6 expression
- Environmental factors: may be incited by infection, drugs, photosensitivity
- Abnormal cellular proliferation
- Microcirculatory changes: capillary loops of the dermal papillae develop increased basal lamina material and neutrophilic infiltration
- Immunological factors: T lymphocytes have been proposed to play a central role in lesion development

Microscopically, the epidermis is hyperplastic, with elongated rete ridges and thinning over the papillae, and demonstrates hyperkeratosis and parakeratosis. The dermal papillae become clubbed

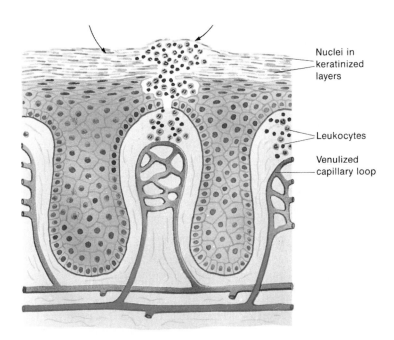

Nuclei in keratinized layers

Leukocytes

Venulized capillary loop

FIGURE 24-3
Psoriasis. Neutrophils emerge from the tips of the venulized capillary loop and involve the epidermis. (From Rubin E, Gorstein F, Rubin R, et al. Rubin's Pathology, 4th ed. Philadelphia: Lippincott Williams & Wilkins, 2005, p. 1216.)

and contain tortuous dilated venules that allow an efflux of neutrophils into the epidermis. Within the epidermis, neutrophils can form small abscesses in the upper stratum spinosum and stratum corneum, termed *Munro abscesses*. The superficial vascular plexus of the dermis is surrounded by variable numbers of lymphocytes (Fig. 24-3).

Clinically, patients demonstrate lesions of varying severity. Disruption of the overlying scale results in pinpoint foci of bleeding from the markedly dilated capillaries in the dermal papillae. As many as 7% of patients may develop an associated seronegative arthritis, which is most common in patients who have an HLA-B27 haplotype. The disease is often intermittent and treatment options include corticosteroids, methotrexate, phototherapy, and vitamin A and D derivatives.

Systemic Lupus Erythematosus

Systemic lupus erythematosus (SLE) is an autoimmune disease that commonly affects young to middle-aged adults.

The epidermal injury that occurs in SLE is often triggered by exogenous agents. The disease process involves deposition of immune-complexes along the epidermal basement membrane, vacuolization of basal keratinocytes, and release of DNA into the circulation.

There appears to be an inverse relationship between the level of cutaneous disease and systemic manifestations. The manifestations of SLE vary with the type of disease, as shown in the following:

- Chronic cutaneous (discoid) lupus erythematosus: commonly affects only the face, ears, and scalp and may result in scar formation; characterized by altered epithelial thickness, hyperkeratosis, plugging of hair follicles, and a dense lymphocytic infiltrate involving the basal cells, basement membrane, and dermis
- Subacute cutaneous lupus erythematosus: may be accompanied by involvement of the musculoskeletal system and kidneys and demonstrates a milder lymphocytic infiltrate involving the basement membrane and prominent vacuolar degeneration of the basal keratinocytes; commonly affects the upper chest, upper back, and extensor surfaces of the arms
- Acute SLE: occurs in association with disease of the kidneys and joints and is manifested by a malar rash and a maculopapular eruption of the chest; characterized by edema of the papillary dermis

Lichen Planus

Lichen planus is a disease of unknown etiology. The disease may occur alone or in association with SLE, myasthenia gravis, drug administration, or external agents. Grossly, lichen planus presents with violaceous, flat-topped papules, often on the flexor surfaces of the wrists. Microscopically, the epidermis demonstrates hyperkeratosis (without parakeratosis) and a wedge-shaped thickening and hypergranulosis of the stratum granulosum. A bandlike infiltrate of lymphocytes and macrophages obscures the dermal–epidermal junction (Fig. 24-4). The epidermis projects into the underlying inflammatory infiltrate with a pointed, sawtoothlike, appearance. Eosinophilic, globular, fibrillary bodies (which represent apoptotic keratinocytes) are present in the inflammatory infiltrate.

Blistering Diseases

Pemphigus Vulgaris

Pemphigus vulgaris (PV) is an autoimmune disease that occurs most commonly between 40 and 60 years of age.

PV is caused by antibodies directed against a keratinocyte anti-

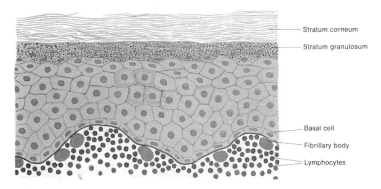

FIGURE   24-4
Lichen planus. The epidermis shows hyperkeratosis, hypergranulosis, epidermal hyperplasia, and a bandlike infiltrate of lymphocytes at the dermal-epidermal junction, and the formation of fibrillary bodies. (From Rubin E, Gorstein F, Rubin R, et al. Rubin's Pathology, 4th ed. Philadelphia: Lippincott Williams & Wilkins, 2005, p. 1232.)

gen called desmoglein 3, which resides at the desmosome. Desmoglein 3 is located in the lower epidermis and binding of antibodies to this antigen results in dyshesion of the keratinocytes, with separation between the basal layer and the remaining epidermis and subsequent bulla formation.

Four variants of PV include the following:

- Pemphigus foliaceus: antibodies directed against desmoglein 1 in the outer spinous and granular epidermal layers
- Pemphigus erythematosus: milder version of pemphigus foliaceus often involving a malar distribution
- Pemphigus vegetans: healing in intertriginous areas is characterized by complex papillary epidermal hyperplasia
- Drug-induced pemphigus: most commonly associated with penicillamine and captopril

Grossly, these lesions appear as large, easily ruptured blisters that form denuded or crusted areas and are most common on the scalp, mucous membranes, and periumbilical and intertriginous areas. Lateral pressure on these lesions results in the epidermis appearing to slide off the affected area. Microscopically, a distinct separation is present between the basal cell layer and the upper layers of the epidermis. The resulting bulla contains a mixture of inflammatory cells and rounded, acantholytic keratinocytes. Immunofluorescence reveals immunoglobulin (Ig) G antibodies in the epidermis that appear as a lacelike pattern outlining the keratinocytes. Treatment involves corticosteroids or immunosuppressive agent administration.

Bullous Pemphigoid

Bullous pemphigoid is an autoimmune disease that often presents in the elderly with large bullae on the trunk, extremities, and intertriginous areas. The condition is caused by antibodies directed against the basement membrane proteins BPAG1 and BPAG2 and demonstrates a clinical presentation similar to pemphigus vulgaris.

Grossly, the bullae of bullous pemphigoid are subepidermal, with the base of the lesion formed by the lamina densa and roof formed by the epidermis. These bullae contain abundant eosinophils, as well as lymphocytes, neutrophils, and fibrin. Immunofluorescence reveals a linear deposition of C3 and IgG along the epidermal basement membrane. The disease is treated by systemic corticosteroids.

Dermatitis Herpetiformis

Dermatitis herpetiformis (DH) is characterized by intensely pruritic, grouped vesicles ("herpeslike") over the extensor surfaces of the body, especially the elbows, knees, and buttocks. The condition often affects young to middle-aged males and is often associated with the haplotypes HLA-DR3, HLA-B8, and HLA-DQw2. DH is caused by gluten sensitivity. Ingestion of gluten in wheat, barley, rye, or oats results in the formation and deposition of IgA at the dermal-epidermal junction and at the tips of the dermal papillae. IgA immune complexes ultimately result in the recruitment of neutrophils to dermal-epidermal junction during the following 12 hours (Fig. 24-5). Subepidermal bullae filled with neutrophils and eosinophils may subsequently develop. Immunofluorescence reveals deposition of IgA in the dermal papillae. Lesions often heal with scarring. Treatment includes a gluten-free diet, dapsone, or sulfapyridine.

Epidermolysis Bullosa

Epidermolysis bullosa (EB) is a group of heritable diseases characterized by blisters that form at sites of minor trauma and which are often noted shortly after birth. Three major categories of EB include the following:

- Epidermolytic EB: autosomal dominant disease in which cytolysis of the basal cells results in a blister within the epidermis that heals without scarring

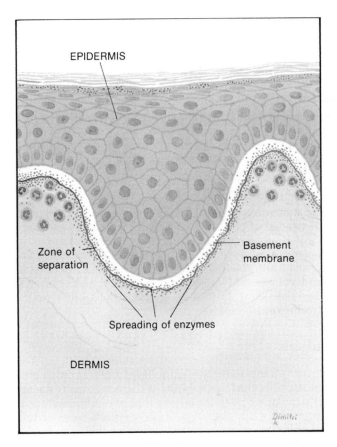

F I G U R E   24-5
Dermatitis herpetiformis. Deposition of immunoglobulin A complexes at the tips of the dermal papillae and the dermal-epidermal junction lead to the formation of subepidermal bullae filled with neutrophils and eosinophils. In addition, neutrophils accumulate at the tips of the dermal papillae. (From Rubin E, Gorstein F, Rubin R, et al. Rubin's Pathology, 4th ed. Philadelphia: Lippincott Williams & Wilkins, 2005, p. 1227.)

- Junctional EB: autosomal recessive disease caused by mutations in type VII collagen in which blisters form within the lamina lucida of the basement membrane zone and may be fatal within the first 2 years of life
- Dermolytic EB: autosomal dominant or recessive disease in which mutations in collagen type VII leads to blisters that heal by scarring and abnormalities of the nails and teeth

Granulomatous Inflammation

Granulomatous inflammation may be idiopathic or occur in association with a foreign antigen or infectious agent.

Sarcoidosis

Sarcoidosis is a systemic disease that primarily affects the lungs, but may also involve the skin. Grossly, asymptomatic papules, plaques, and nodules may be present. Microscopically, epithelioid granulomas lacking caseous necrosis are identified.

Granuloma Annulare

Granuloma annulare is a benign, self-limited disorder of unknown etiology that often affects children and young adults, especially women. Grossly, asymptomatic, skin-colored, or erythematous annular plaques are present on the dorsal surface of the hands and feet. Microscopically, the lesions contain a central area of acellular degenerated collage and mucin in the superficial dermis surrounded by palisading histiocytes. These lesions often resolve without treatment.

Acne Vulgaris

Acne vulgaris is a disease of the hair follicles and sebaceous units that commonly affects adolescents and is characterized by the formation of papular or pustular lesions that may ultimately scar. The pathogenesis of this disease most likely reflects the activity of *Propionibacterium acnes* on sebaceous secretions that may lead to the subsequent influx of neutrophils. Noninflammatory acne is characterized by closed and open comedones, which are accumulations of lipids, keratin, and bacteria that form a central plug, and it results in follicular dilation. Inflammatory acne is characterized by progressive follicular distention and rupture, and leads to the presence of erythematous skin lesions.

Disease of the Dermal Connective Tissue: Scleroderma

Scleroderma most commonly affects women between 30 and 50 years of age and is characterized by progressive fibrosis of the skin, kidneys, lungs, heart, esophagus, and small intestine. *Morphea* is a similar, but more limited, disease that only affects patchy areas of the skin.

Early in the course of the disease, patients demonstrate Raynaud phenomenon and nonpitting edema of the hands or fingers. Enlarged collagen bundles that run parallel to the epidermis fill the dermis and a patchy lymphocytic infiltrate is present. Over time, the face develops a masklike appearance, and the skin becomes hard and tense. Hair follicles become obliterated, and the sweat ducts become entrapped by the collagen.

Leukocytoclastic Vasculitis

Leukocytoclastic vasculitis, also termed *cutaneous necrotizing vasculitis*, is an immune-complex mediated disease that can occur in association with a variety of disease conditions, including autoimmune disease and infection. In this disease, immune complexes are deposited along vascular walls, which lead to subsequent C5a complement activation and neutrophil infiltration. Neutrophil activity results in endothelial damage and fibrin deposition.

Grossly, these lesions appear as red, palpable lesions that do not blanch under pressure and are termed *purpuric papules*. Often, these lesions present in crops on the lower extremities or at sites of pressure. Microscopically, the dermal vessels demonstrate a neutrophilic infiltrate that results in vascular damage with extravasation of red blood cells, fibrin deposits in the vessel, and breakdown of neutrophil nuclei ("leukocytoclasia") with the formation of dustlike nuclear remnants.

Lesions generally resolve after a month, but may result in residual hyperpigmentation or scarring.

Inflammatory Disorders of the Panniculus

Inflammation of the subcutis is termed *panniculitis* and may be caused by a variety of factors, including drugs and microorganisms. Septal panniculitis refers to inflammation of the septa, and lobular inflammation refers to inflammation of the fat lobules.

Erythema Nodosum

Erythema nodosum is a self-limited disease that often affects patients between 20 and 30 years of age. It is characterized by the acute onset of erythematous, tender nodules on the extensor surfaces of the lower extremities. Erythema nodosum is associated with infection, drugs, and various systemic conditions and has been proposed to represent an immunologic response to foreign antigens.

Early in the course of disease, the subcutaneous fibrous septa demonstrate neutrophilic infiltration and extravasation of erythrocytes (septal panniculitis). Late in the course of disease, the septa become widened and contain giant cells and lymphocytes. In general, lesions usually resolve within 6 weeks without scarring.

Erythema Induratum

Erythema induratum describes chronic, recurrent subcutaneous nodules or plaques on the legs that may be associated with DNA of *Mycobacterium tuberculosis*. Patients demonstrate recurrent, tender, erythematous nodules on the legs, especially the calf. The subcutaneous fat demonstrates marked lymphocytic infiltrates (lobular panniculitis) that may form granulomas or cause coagulative necrosis. A prominent vasculitis caused by lymphocytic infiltrate in the wall of the vessel can lead to ischemic fat necrosis. These lesions tend to ulcerate and resolution may occur over several years and lead to scarring.

Melanocytic Lesions

Freckle

A freckle, or *ephelidis*, is a small, brown macule that occurs on sun-exposed skin and is common in persons with fair skin. Pigmentation varies with sun exposure and most freckles appear by age 5 years. These lesions demonstrate an increased number of melanocytes and increased pigmentation of the basal keratinocytes.

Lentigo

A lentigo is a brown macule that appears at any age and the pigmentation does not vary with sun exposure. These lesions demonstrate elongated rete ridges, increased numbers of melanocytes, and increased melanin pigment in the melanocytes and basal keratinocytes.

Acquired Melanocytic Nevus

An acquired melanocytic nevus, or *mole*, most commonly develops between the time of birth and 20 years of age and is dependent on exposure to ultraviolet light. Over time, nevi may flatten or ultimately disappear. Persons who develop >100 nevi are at an increased risk of melanoma.

Grossly, nevi appear as well-demarcated, flat or slightly elevated, brown lesions with a regular peripheral outline. Microscopically, nevi demonstrate increased numbers of monomorphic melanocytes in the basal epidermis, dermal–epidermal junction, or dermis that may form nests. In general, nevi demonstrate maturation (i.e., smaller cell size) with depth in the dermis, a symmetrical distribution of cells, and an absence of mitoses. Nevi may be subdivided based on the location of cells:

- Junctional nevus: melanocytes form nests at the tips of the rete ridges

- Compound nevus: nests involve the dermal–epidermal junction and the dermis
- Dermal nevus: nests are present only in the dermis

Congenital Melanocytic Nevus

Congenital melanocytic nevi are present at birth and represent an increased number of intraepidermal and dermal melanocytes. Some lesions achieve a large size (giant hairy nevus or garment nevus) and are at increased risk of melanoma.

Spitz Nevus

Spitz nevi occur in children and adolescents and appears grossly as an elevated, pink, round nodule, often on the head and neck. The lesion typically grows rapidly to a size of 3 to 5 mm and demonstrates hyperkeratosis, parakeratosis, and nests of spindled and epithelioid melanocytes in the dermis and at the dermal–epidermal junction.

Blue Nevus

A blue nevus is a dark blue, gray, or black nevus on the dorsum of the hand or feet, buttocks, scalp, or face. The dermis contains melanin-containing melanocytes with long dendritic processes.

Dysplastic (Atypical) Nevus

In some instances, nevi may demonstrate persistent melanocytic growth and appear grossly as larger and more irregular lesions. The irregular portion of the lesion grows asymmetrically away from the parent nevus and often measure greater than 5 mm in diameter. Microscopically, these lesions often demonstrate melanocytes with large, atypical nuclei that appear to bridge between the rete ridges. In addition, lamellar fibroplasias (surrounding eosinophilic connective tissue) and a lymphocytic infiltrate may be present.

Malignant Melanoma

Malignant melanoma occurs most commonly on regions that have been intermittently exposed to the sun, especially in areas of sunburn. Melanomas may commonly undergo initial radial growth and spread upward in the epidermis and along the superficial dermis; lesions in this phase of growth rarely metastasize. Lesions that enter the vertical growth phase extend into the dermis, demonstrate increased mitotic activity, and may contain minimal pigment; lesions in the vertical phase are more likely to undergo metastatic spread via lymphatic or hematogenous routes and most commonly affect regional lymph nodes.

Grossly, malignant melanoma can be described using the "ABCD" rule: **A**symmetry, **B**order irregularity, **C**olor variation, and **D**iameter greater than 6 mm. Later stages of melanoma growth may also demonstrate itching, bleeding, or oozing. Microscopically, the malignant cells are large epithelioid melanocytes that demonstrate decreased maturation with depth and mitotic activity.

The prognosis of malignant melanoma may be evaluated using the following factors:

- Tumor thickness: thickness is measured from the superficial aspect of the stratum granulosum to the point of deepest invasion and is associated with a worse prognosis
- Dermal mitotic rate: associated with a worse prognosis
- Lymphocytic response: tumor-infiltrating lymphocytes can disrupt the tumor and form rosettes around melanoma cells; correlates with better prognosis
- Location: lesions on the head, neck, trunk, or sole of the foot do more poorly
- Sex: females commonly have a better prognosis

Grossly, lesions appear blue-white and demonstrate a widened papillary dermis. Lentigo maligna melanoma is a large, pigmented, macular form of malignant melanoma that occurs most commonly in elderly, fair-skinned persons and affects sun-exposed skin, especially the face and dorsal hands. Microscopically, atypical melanocytes form nearly contiguous row of cells within the basal layer of the epidermis, although later lesions may undergo vertical growth.

Epidermal Lesions

Benign Epidermal Lesions

A variety of benign conditions affect the epidermis, many of which represent benign neoplastic proliferations that demonstrate little to no risk of metastatic spread.

Verrucae

Verrucae are circumscribed, elevated, or flat epidermal proliferations that demonstrate a tan appearance and occur in the setting of human papilloma virus (HPV) infection. Several types of verrucae exist and include the following:

- Verruca vulgaris (common warts): most common on the dorsal surface of the hands or on the face and display hyperkeratosis, epidermal hyperplasia and koilocytosis (viral change that demonstrates raisinlike nucleus with a perinuclear halo)
- Plantar warts: painful, hyperkeratotic nodules on the soles of the feet that display endophytic or exophytic epithelial proliferation and abundant cytoplasmic inclusions

- Verruca plana: small, flat papules on the face that display an elongation of the rete ridges (acanthosis), hypergranulosis, and koilocytosis
- Condyloma acuminatum: genital warts that display papillary epidermal proliferation and koilocytosis

Seborrheic Keratosis

Seborrheic keratosis is a disease of unknown etiology that most commonly affects the trunk of elderly persons. Grossly, these lesions appear as tan-brown, scaly, elevated papules or plaques, with scales that can be easily rubbed off. Microscopically, seborrheic keratosis demonstrates hyperkeratosis and broad anastomosing cords of mature stratified squamous epithelium often associated with small cysts of keratin. The appearance of numerous seborrheic keratoses has been associated with internal malignancies (Leser-Trélat sign).

Keratoacanthoma

Keratoacanthomas develop on sun-exposed skin, often the hands or face, of middle-aged or elderly persons. These lesions grow rapidly over a period of 3 to 6 weeks and appear as flesh-colored nodules with central keratin. Keratoacanthomas are endophytic, papillary proliferations of keratinocytes, with a central, cup-shaped crater of keratin. The base of this crater is lined by large, glassy keratinocytes. In some instances, associated inflammation or dermal fibroplasias may be present.

Fibroepithelial Polyp

Fibroepithelial polyps, also termed *skin tags* or *acrochordons*, are common lesions that occur in middle-aged to elderly persons and often affect the face, neck, trunk, or axillary regions. Grossly, these lesions appear as flesh-colored, polypoid protrusions that are lined by benign squamous epithelium and contain a central fibrovascular core.

Epithelial Cysts

Several types of benign epithelial cysts occur, including the following:

- Epithelial inclusion cyst: cyst that often occurs on the head, neck, and trunk and is lined by keratin-producing stratified squamous epithelium without associated appendages
- Dermoid cyst: cyst that often occurs on the head and around the eyes, which is lined by keratin-producing stratified squamous epithelium and contains associated dermal appendages
- Trichilemmal (pilar) cyst: often occurs on scalp and is lined by stratified squamous epithelium that lacks a granular cell layer,

leading to abrupt keratinization and contents consisting of "wet keratin"

Premalignant and Malignant Epidermal Lesions

Actinic Keratosis

Actinic keratosis is a premalignant proliferation of keratinocytes that typically affects middle-aged to elderly persons and preferentially affects sun-exposed areas. Light-skinned, fair-haired persons are at greater risk for these lesions. Actinic keratosis appears as patches or plaques demonstrating hyperkeratosis, dense parakeratosis, and marked epidermal atypia most prominent in deeper layers of the epidermis. These lesions demonstrate a risk of transformation to squamous cell carcinoma.

Squamous Cell Carcinoma

Squamous cell carcinoma (SCC) may be caused by exposure to ultraviolet light, ionizing radiation, chemical carcinogens, HPV infection, or chronic scarring processes, such as sinus tracts and burns (termed a Marjolin's ulcer). SCC most commonly affects middle-aged to elderly persons, especially those with fair skin and light hair. Mutations in *p53* have been described in a large majority of SCCs. Less than 2% to 5% of these lesions undergo metastatic spread by the time of diagnosis.

Grossly, these lesions range in appearance from small, scaly, erythematous papules to large, ulcerating lesions. Microscopically, the tumors mimic the appearance of the cells of the stratum spinosum (in well- to moderately differentiated) lesions and demonstrate invasion into the dermis. The tumor cells demonstrate nuclear enlargement, hyperchromasia, variable mitotic activity, and, occasionally, perineural invasion.

Basal Cell Carcinoma

Basal cell carcinoma (BCC) is one of the most common epidermal malignancies and most often affects sun-exposed skin of elderly persons, especially those with pale skin. BCC may also occur in conjunction with the *nevoid BCC syndrome*, in which patients develop multiple BCCs (often on skin that has not been exposed to sun) in conjunction with dyskeratoses on the palms and soles, mandibular cysts, hypertelorism, and occasionally medulloblastoma. Mutations in *PTCH* have been described in heritable and sporadic forms of BCCs.

Grossly, BCC demonstrates a pearly white, nodular appearance with fine branching vessels (telangiectasias) and occasional pigmentation or central ulceration (rodent ulcer). Microscopically, these lesions demonstrate nests of basaloid cells at the dermal-epidermal junction or in the dermis with peripheral palisading and an overall basophilic appearance at low magnification. These lesions may demonstrate increased mitotic activity and apoptosis. These tumors rarely metastasize.

Merkel Cell Carcinoma

Merkel cell carcinoma is an aggressive tumor that occurs most commonly on the head and neck of elderly patients and is derived from neural-crest cells. Grossly, these lesions appear as solitary, dome-shaped, red-to-purple nodules. Microscopically, these tumors have a small cell appearance, with evenly disbursed granular chromatin, frequent mitotic figures, and apoptotic debris. Merkel cell carcinoma stains for the neuroendocrine markers chromogranin and synaptophysin.

Adnexal Tumors

Adnexal tumors often appear at the time of puberty and are typically benign lesions that differentiate toward various skin appendages (although malignant variants may occur). These lesions appear grossly as nodular elevations of the skin. A summary of adnexal tumors is presented in Table 24-2.

Fibrohistiocytic Lesions

Dermatofibroma

Dermatofibromas are benign tumors that often occur on the extremities of middle-aged persons. Grossly, these lesions appear as dome-shaped, firm, rubbery nodules with ill-defined borders and a yellow-white cut surface. Microscopically, these lesions demonstrate a dermal infiltrate of bland spindled cells (neoplastic fibroblasts) admixed with macrophages that may blend with the surrounding tissue. Typically, mitotic activity is not present. The overlying epidermis is hyperplastic and often hyperpigmented.

Dermatofibrosarcoma Protuberans

Dermatofibrosarcoma protuberans (DFSP) is a slow-growing tumor that often appears on the trunk of young adults. Microscopically, DFSP demonstrates a poorly defined, infiltrative lesion in the dermis or subcutis composed of a storiform (pinwheellike) arrangement of spindled cells that may demonstrate prominent mitotic activity. These lesions are immunopositive for CD34, which helps to distinguish them from dermatofibromas. These lesions may recur after excision.

Table 24-2

Adnexal Tumors

Tumor	Common Location(s)	Gross Appearance	Microscopic Appearance
Cylindroma	Scalp	Solitary or multiple nodules	Sharply circumscribed nests of deeply basophilic cells surrounded by a hyalinized, thickened basement membrane
Syringoma	Eyelid and upper cheek	Small, elevated, flesh-colored papules	Small, elongated, comma-shaped nests of epithelium in the upper dermis that form ductlike structures containing eosinophilic material and which are surrounded by a fibrotic stroma
Poroma	Sole or sides of the foot, hands, or fingers	Solitary, rubbery nodules	Broad sheets of monomorphic cuboidal cells that extend into the dermis and may form cystic spaces
Trichoepithelioma	Face, scalp, neck and upper trunk	Solitary or multiple flesh-colored nodules	Symmetric lesion composed of nodular aggregates of basaloid cells that may demonstrate follicular differentiation in a cellular stroma. Cysts containing keratin are often present.
Trichilemmoma	Nose, cheek, and upper lip	Solitary flesh-colored lesions	Circumscribed proliferation of cells with clear cytoplasm, resembling the outer root sheath of a hair follicle, surrounded by a thick basement membrane
Spiradenoma	Trunk and extremities	Solitary, often painful, nodules	Solid component containing large and small cells with admixed lymphocytes and cystic component that resembles dilated ducts containing globules of basement membranelike material

Atypical Fibroxanthoma

Atypical fibroxanthoma is a dome-shaped lesion that often occurs on the sun-exposed skin of elderly persons. These lesions demonstrate atypical, pleomorphic spindled and epithelioid cells with occasional atypical mitotic figures and multinucleated giant cells that involve the dermis. Local recurrence is common following excision.

Mycosis Fungoides

Mycosis fungoides is a cutaneous T-cell lymphoma that preferentially affects the elderly population and demonstrates progressive skin involvement. Early in the disease, scaly erythematous macules and plaques appear on the lower abdomen, buttocks, and upper thighs that are characterized microscopically by psoriaform changes of the epithelium. Over time, increased infiltration by atypical T-lymphocytes leads to epidermal infiltration (epidermotropism), aggregation of atypical lymphocytes in the epidermis (Pautrier abscesses), and nodular and bandlike dermal infiltrates. The characteristic appearance of the atypical lymphocyte in this disorder is termed a *Sézary-Lutzner cell*, which contains a large, cerebriform nucleus. Systemic involvement by mycosis fungoides is termed Sézary syndrome.

Kaposi Sarcoma

Kaposi sarcoma is a malignant tumor of endothelial cells that most commonly arises in the setting of HIV infection. The lesions of Kaposi sarcoma progress through patch, plaque, and nodular stages. Microscopically, slitlike vascular channels are lined by a single layer of atypical endothelial cells. These vessels are surrounded by fascicles of spindled cells in a background of extravasated red blood cells, hemosiderin deposition, and a sparse inflammatory infiltrate of lymphocytes and plasma cells.

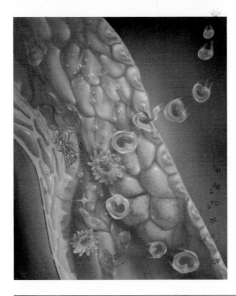

CHAPTER 25

The Head and Neck

Chapter Outline

THE ORAL CAVITY

Normal Anatomy and Histology

The oral cavity includes the hard and soft palates, lower labial (inner lip) mucosa, buccal (inner cheek) mucosa, the floor of the

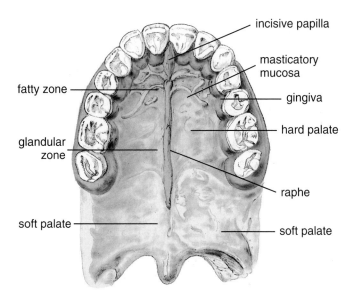

F I G U R E   25-1
Diagram of the roof of the oral cavity. (From Ross MH, Kaye PI, and Pawlina W. Histology: A Text and Atlas, 4th ed. Philadelphia: Lippincott Williams & Wilkins, 2003, p. 436.)

mouth, the tongue, the teeth, the gingiva, and the tonsillar pillars (Fig. 25-1). The oral cavity is covered by stratified squamous epithelium that is nonkeratinized or only lightly keratinized.

The dorsum of the tongue contains specialized gustatory mucosa, which appears as irregular elevations termed lingual papillae. The lingual papillae include filiform papillae (which have a mechanical function) and fungiform, circumvallate, and foliate papillae (which contain taste buds).

The oral cavity serves as host for a variety of commensal organisms that may cause disease under certain conditions.

Developmental Anomalies

A variety of developmental anomalies involve or originate from the oral cavity. Some of these anomalies arise from residual developmental structures, including branchial arches or the thyroid gland, which originates from the base of the tongue and descends into the neck. These anomalies include the following:

- *Cleft upper lip* (harelip): may occur in association with a cleft palate

- *Lingual thyroid nodule*: heterotopic functioning thyroid tissue often located at the foramen cecum of the tongue
- *Thyroglossal duct cyst*: cystic structure containing thyroid tissue that occurs at the midline neck along the path of thyroid descent
- *Branchial cleft cyst*: arises from branchial arch remnants and is located on the lateral anterior neck or parotid gland; lined by squamous or respiratory epithelium and contains watery or gelatinous fluid

Infections

Localized inflammation of the oral cavity may involve the lips (*cheilitis*), gums (*gingivitis*), tongue (*glossitis*), or oral mucosa (*stomatitis*). Bacteria, fungi, and spirochetes frequently cause oral infections and are described in Table 25-1. Viruses, especially herpes simplex virus type 1 (HSV1), also infect the oral cavity and generally are manifested as vesicular or ulcerative lesions, as described in Table 25-2.

Benign Tumors and Tumorlike Conditions
of the Oral Cavity

Lesions that occur in the oral cavity include nevi, fibromas, hemangiomas, lymphangiomas, and squamous papillomas, which occur at other sites of the body as well.

A specific lesion of the oral cavity is *giant cell reparative granuloma* (peripheral giant cell granuloma), which is a proliferative reaction to local injury that appears as a mass on the gingival or the alveolar process, often in young or middle-aged adults. The lesion is extraosseous and is proposed to arise from the deeper soft tissues of the oral cavity. Grossly, the lesion appears as a brown-to-black mass covered with mucosa, which may be ulcerated. Microscopically, the lesion is nonencapsulated and vascular, with numerous multinucleated giant cells, a fibrous stroma, chronic inflammation, and hemosiderin-laden macrophages.

Leukoplakia is a clinical term that denotes the appearance of an asymptomatic white lesion on the mucosal surface. Several factors may result in the appearance of leukoplakia, ranging from a benign hyperkeratosis to the malignant squamous carcinoma in situ. Lesions are often fairly well demarcated and often occur on the buccal mucosa, tongue, and floor of the mouth. Microscopic analysis is necessary to determine the cause of leukoplakia.

Erythroplakia refers to the presence of a red lesion on the mucosa. In contrast to leukoplakia, erythroplakia is less well demarcated and more frequently reflects an underlying premalignant or malignant condition, such as squamous carcinoma.

Table 25-1

Infectious Disease of the Oral Cavity

Infection	Organism(s)	Predisposing Factors	Gross and Microscopic Appearance
Scarlet fever	β-Hemolytic streptococcus (*Streptococcus pyogenes*)	Often occurs in children	Strawberry tongue (white coating with hyperemic papillae), rash
Aphthous stomatitis (canker sores)	Unknown	None	Painful, recurrent, solitary or multiple small ulcers of the oral mucosa covered by a fibrinopurulent exudate
Pyogenic granuloma	Nonspecific organisms	Minor trauma	Elevated red/purple mass covered by a lobulated, ulcerated surface; often on gingiva
Acute necrotizing ulcerative gingivitis	Fusiform bacillus, *Borrelia vincentii* (spirochete)	Immunodeficiency, inadequate nutrition, poor oral hygiene	Punched-out erosions of the interdental papillae that may spread across gingiva; covered by a necrotic pseudomembrane
Noma (cancrum oris)	Form of acute necrotizing ulcerative gingivitis	Immunocompromised children	Rapidly spreading gangrene of the oral and facial tissues
Ludwig angina	Oral flora	Chronic illness, dental extraction, trauma	Rapidly spreading cellulitis that originates in the submaxillary or sublingual space
Diphtheria	*Corynebacterium diphtheriae*	Often occurs in children and adolescents	Patchy pseudomembrane that begins on the tonsils and pharynx
Syphilis	*Treponema pallidum*	Infection primary to oral cavity or secondary/tertiary disease	Chancre (primary), multiple gray-white patches over ulcerated surface (secondary), gummas (tertiary)
Actinomycosis	*Actinomyces bovis*, *Actinomyces israelii*	Immunocompromise	Chronic granulomatous inflammation and abscesses
Candidiasis (thrush)	*Candida albicans*	Immunocompromise	White, slightly elevated soft patches containing fungi

Table 25-2

Viral Infections of the Oral Cavity

Virus	Gross Appearance	Microscopic Appearance	Additional Findings
Herpes simplex virus 1 (HSV1)	Painful mucosal inflammation followed by vesicles that rupture to form shallow, painful ulcers (herpes labialis/cold sores and herpetic stomatitis)	The edge of the mucosal ulcer contains large, multinucleated giant cells with "ground glass" nuclei and ballooning degeneration of epithelial cells	Transmitted by contact with infected saliva; the virus can remain latent in the trigeminal ganglion and be reactivated following exposure to certain stressors
Cytomegalovirus (CMV)	Vesicular lesions that can ulcerate	Endothelial cells are most commonly infected and contain large, eosinophilic inclusions in the nucleus and cytoplasm	Often occurs in the setting of immunocompromise
Epstein-Barr virus (EBV)	Ulceration of the posterior oral mucosa. Patients with HIV may have oral hairy leukoplakia, which presents with shaggy, white lesions on the oral mucosa, especially the lateral tongue	In oral hairy leukoplakia, the mucosa shows parakeratosis and edema. The infected cells have vacuolated cytoplasm and eosinophilic inclusions	Patients with HIV are prone to the development of the more severe form of the disease, oral hairy leukoplakia

Squamous Cell Carcinoma

Squamous cell carcinoma (SCC) is the most common malignant lesion of the oral cavity. The lesion has a male predominance and occurs, with descending frequency, on the floor of the mouth, the alveolar mucosa, the palate and the buccal mucosa. Multiple separate carcinomas may be identified within the oral cavity, termed field cancerization. Risk factors for SCC include the following:

- Tobacco use
- Alcohol use
- Iron deficiency (Plummer-Vinson syndrome)
- Physical and chemical irritants
- Betel nuts
- Poor oral hygiene
- Possibly human papillomavirus infection

Microscopically, the lesions in SCC range from well- to poorly differentiated. Often, adjacent regions of squamous carcinoma in situ may be identified. Oral SCC metastasizes to the submandibular, superficial, and deep cervical lymph nodes; hematogenous spread to the lungs, liver, and bones may occur.

Benign Diseases of the Lips

The lips may be affected by systemic or localized disorders.

Solar cheilitis is analogous to solar keratosis of the skin and presents in the vermilion border of the lower lip. This lesion is caused by sun exposure and microscopically demonstrates hyperkeratosis, epithelial hyperplasia, and a band of damaged collagen under the epithelium.

A *mucocele* occurs secondary to trauma and is most likely caused by the escape of mucus from minor salivary glands. The lesion is cystic, lined by granulation tissue, and is filled with mucus and numerous macrophages.

Diseases of the Tongue

Macroglossia refers to an enlargement of the tongue that may occur with a variety of systemic and localized processes. Macroglossia present at birth may occur with a diffuse lymphangioma or hemangioma. An enlarged, protruding tongue may occur in association with congenital hypothyroidism, Hurler syndrome, and Down syndrome, among other diseases. Acquired macroglossia can occur in amyloidosis, acromegaly, and lymphatic obstruction by tumors.

Glossitis is an inflammation of the tongue caused by a variety of factors including microorganisms, pernicious anemia, pellagra, riboflavin deficiency, and physical and chemical agents.

Diseases of the Teeth and Associated Soft Tissues

A diagram of the tooth and associated tissue is presented in Figure 25-2.

Dental Caries (Tooth Decay) and Associated Lesions

Dental caries is a common, chronic infectious disease of the enamel, dentin, and cementum of the teeth. The development of dental caries is the result of numerous factors, including the following:

- Bacteria: oral flora initially coalesce into a soft mass (dental plaque) that leaches mineral in the dental tissues; process is often initiated by *Streptococcus mutans*
- Saliva: helps prevent caries by neutralizing microbially produced acids and acting as a bacteriostatic factor
- Dietary factors: diets high in carbohydrates promote caries formation, whereas diets with roughage help prevent caries
- Fluoride: present in the drinking water; is incorporated into the enamel to protect teeth

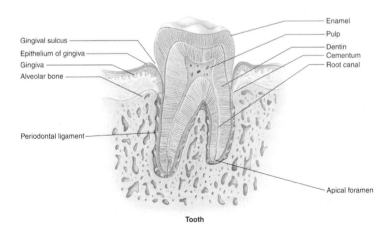

Tooth

FIGURE   25-2

The tooth, composed of a crown and root, is suspended in its bony socket, the alveolus, by a dense, collagenous connective tissue called the periodontal ligament. The crown of the tooth consists of two calcified tissues, dentin and enamel, whereas the root is composed of dentin and cementum. The blood vessels, lymphatics, nerve fibers, and odontoblasts (which maintain and repair dentin) are contained in the pulp. (From Gartner LP, Hiatt JL. Color Atlas of Histology, 3rd ed. Philadelphia: Lippincott Williams & Wilkins, 2000, p. 256.)

The development of caries proceeds in a stepwise fashion and includes the disintegration of the enamel by bacterial action, the formation of a small pit that ultimately extends to the dentinoenamel junction, lateral spread of the lesion along the dentin, and ultimately invasion of the dental pulp, which produces pain.

Several lesions of the dental pulp and periapical tissues may complicate dental caries as described in the following list:

- *Pulpitis*: inflammation of the pulp by bacteria in dental caries that is associated with pain and may be accompanied by abscesses
- *Apical* (or periapical) *granuloma*: most common sequel of pulpitis; composed of chronically inflamed periapical granulation tissue surrounded by a fibrous capsule that is attached to the root
- *Radicular cyst* (apical periodontal cyst): proliferation of the squamous epithelium of an apical granuloma to form a cyst lined by stratified squamous epithelium
- *Periapical abscess*: abscess around the root of a tooth
- *Osteomyelitis*: uncommon, but may develop by extension of a periapical abscess into the adjacent bone

Periodontal Disease

Periodontal disease refers to acute and chronic disorders of the soft tissues surrounding the teeth, which eventually lead to the loss of supporting bone. The periodontium is composed of the gingiva (gum) and the periodontal ligament. Periodontal disease may occur in persons with poor oral hygiene or in association with a strong family history of the disease. The disease begins with the accumulation of bacteria, often including *Bacteroides gingivalis*, under the gingiva in the periodontal pocket. As this dental plaque ages, it mineralizes to form tartar. Chronic inflammation associated with this process results in destruction of the periodontium, resulting in loosening and loss of teeth.

Periodontal disease may also occur secondary to hematological disorders (agranulocytosis), infectious mononucleosis, acute and chronic leukemias (often acute monocytic leukemia), and scurvy.

Odontogenic Cysts and Tumors

A variety of cysts and tumors arise in the jawbone and surrounding soft tissues. Odontogenic cysts include inflammatory and developmental cysts.

Radicular (also termed *apical* or *periodontal*) *cysts*, the most common odontogenic cysts, involve the apex of an erupted tooth. Radicular cysts often occur following infection of the dental pulp and are lined by stratified squamous epithelium.

Dentigerous cysts are associated with the crown of an impacted, embedded, or unerupted tooth, often the mandibular and maxillary third molars. This cyst forms when fluid accumulates between the crown and the overlying epithelium. Dentigerous cysts are unilocular and lined by stratified squamous epithelium. Complications of dentigerous cysts include adjacent bone resorption due to pressure, recurrence after incomplete removal, development of an ameloblastoma, and progression to squamous cell carcinoma.

Ameloblastomas arise from the odontogenic epithelium and are slow-growing, locally invasive tumors. The majority of ameloblastomas arise in the mandible and may be subdivided into the conventional solid or multicystic type (85%), the unicystic type (14%), and the peripheral/extraosseous type (1%). Radiologically, these lesions have a cystlike appearance with a smooth periphery accompanied by expansion of the bone and thinning of the cortex. Microscopically, ameloblastomas resemble developing enamel with peripheral columnar cells oriented perpendicularly to the basement membrane and central, loosely organized, polyhedral cells. Occasionally, microcysts may be present.

THE SALIVARY GLANDS

Normal Anatomy and Histology

Salivary glands are separated into major salivary glands that are often paired organs (parotid, submandibular, and sublingual glands) and minor salivary glands that are widespread in the mucosa of the lips, cheeks, palate, and tongue. Salivary glands produce serous, mucous, or mixed serous and mucous saliva.

A variety of clinical terms are used to describe conditions of altered salivary gland function:

- *Xerostomia*: chronic dryness of the mouth from the lack of saliva due to many causes (e.g., sarcoidosis, Sjögren syndrome, drugs)
- *Sialorrhea*: increased salivary flow due to many causes (e.g., rabies, Parkinson disease, pregnancy)
- Enlargement: unilateral enlargement often caused by inflammation, cysts, or neoplasms, whereas bilateral enlargement often caused by inflammation or diffuse neoplastic involvement
- *Sialolithiasis*: calcified stones that often affect the submandibular gland and may lead to duct obstruction

Inflammatory Diseases of the Salivary Glands

Sjögren Syndrome

Sjögren syndrome is a chronic inflammatory disease of the salivary and lacrimal glands that leads to dry mouth (xerostomia) and dry eyes (keratoconjunctivitis sicca). Sjögren syndrome may occur in isolation or in conjunction with a systemic collagen vascular disease.

The parotid gland and occasionally the submandibular gland will be unilaterally or bilaterally enlarged. A periductal infiltrate of lymphocytes and plasma cells surrounds, then infiltrates, the glands. Myoepithelial cells proliferate around the damaged ducts, resulting in the formation of epimyoepithelial islands. Over time, the affected glands become atrophic and demonstrate fibrosis and fatty replacement.

Acute Suppurative Parotitis

Acute suppurative parotitis is caused by ascent of bacteria, often *Streptococcus aureus*, from the oral cavity. This condition often occurs in the setting of reduced salivary flow.

Mumps

Mumps (epidemic parotitis) is a viral disease that spreads via infected saliva and may be accompanied by pancreatitis and orchitis. This disease is described in greater detail in Chapter 9.

Tumors of the Salivary Glands

The salivary glands are affected by a variety of benign and malignant lesions. Approximately 75% of lesions occur in the parotid gland, 10% in the submandibular glands, and 15% in the minor salivary glands. Table 25-3 presents the more common tumors of the salivary glands.

Benign Tumors
Pleomorphic Adenoma (Benign Mixed Tumor)

Pleomorphic adenoma is the most common tumor of the salivary glands and occurs most often in middle-aged adults, with a female predominance. The lesion most commonly arises within the parotid gland, especially in the superficial lobe. Pleomorphic adenomas have a fibrous capsule and appear clinically as a painless, mobile, firm, slow-growing nodule.

Microscopically, the lesion contains epithelial (ductal and myoepithelial) and stromal components and may have a variety of appearances. An inner ductal and outer myoepithelial cells may form tubules or cystic structures that contain clear fluid or eosinophilic periodic acid-Schiff (PAS)-positive material. The myoepithelial cells may appear spindled or plasmacytoid. The stroma is myxoid or mucous and can demonstrate regions of cartilage and bone formation.

Table 25-3
Tumors of the Salivary Glands

Tumor	Average Age	Common Location	Microscopic Appearance
Benign			
Pleomorphic adenoma (benign mixed tumor)	Middle aged	Parotid	Epithelial (ductal and myoepithelial) components may be tubular, trabecular or cystic; stroma is myxoid of mucous and may contain cartilage or bone; fibrous capsule
Warthin tumor	>50 years	Parotid	Well-delineated lesion; cystic space lined by eosinophilic epithelium with underlying lymphoid stroma containing germinal centers
Oncocytoma	50–60 years	Parotid	Encapsulated; solid or trabecular pattern; cells with pink granular cytoplasm and small, round nuclei
Basal cell adenoma	Elderly	Parotid	Uniform basal cells form solid trabecular structures with peripheral palisading; prominent basement membrane material separates nests
Malignant			
Carcinoma ex pleomorphic adenoma	Middle aged to elderly	Parotid	Arises out of preexistent pleomorphic adenoma; demonstrates identifiable carcinoma that is often poorly differentiated
Mucoepidermoid carcinoma	40–50 years	Parotid, minor salivary glands	Mixture of neoplastic squamous cells, mucus-secreting cells, and epithelial cells of an intermediate type; may form solid, ductlike, or cystic spaces
Adenoid cystic carcinoma	40–60 years	Parotid, minor salivary glands	Often cribriform or tubular pattern of small cells with scant cytoplasm; tubules are filled with blue-tinged basement membrane material; perineural invasion
Acinic cell carcinoma	40–50 years	Parotid	Tumor cells resemble serous salivary gland cells with finely granular cytoplasm or clear cells

If a pleomorphic adenoma is incompletely excised or if implants are formed at the time of surgery, the lesion may recur as multiple foci with local growth.

Warthin Tumor

Warthin tumor is a benign tumor of the parotid gland, which may be bilateral in 15% of cases. This tumor is the only salivary gland neoplasm that has a male predominance. In the majority of cases, patients are older than 50 years of age. The well-delineated lesion is composed of cystic spaces lined by eosinophilic (oncocytic) epithelial cells with underlying stroma composed of lymphoid tissue with follicle formation. It has been proposed that these lesions arise from salivary gland inclusions within intraparotid lymph nodes.

Oncocytoma

Oncocytomas are benign lesions that often occur in the parotid gland in patients aged 50 to 60 years. These lesions are often encapsulated. Microscopically, nests or trabecular arrangements of eosinophilic, granular cells with abundant pink, granular cytoplasm and small, round nuclei are identified.

Basal Cell Adenoma

Basal cell adenoma is a benign tumor that most commonly occurs in the parotid gland of elderly patients. Microscopically, this lesion contains uniform basal cells that form solid trabecular structures with peripheral palisading. Prominent basement membrane material separates the nests of cells.

Malignant Tumors

Carcinoma ex Pleomorphic Adenoma

Carcinoma ex pleomorphic adenoma results from malignant transformation of a pleomorphic adenoma, which is evidenced clinically by rapid growth or pain of an existing pleomorphic adenoma of the parotid gland. This occurs in middle-aged to elderly adults. The carcinoma is readily identified and may appear as a poorly differentiated carcinoma or as virtually any type of salivary gland neoplasm.

Mucoepidermoid Carcinoma

Mucoepidermoid carcinoma is a malignant neoplasm that affects adults of an average age of 40 to 50 years. The lesion arises from the salivary gland ducts and commonly affects adult women. This carcinoma accounts for 5% to 10% of major salivary gland tumors (most commonly the parotid) and 10% of minor salivary gland tumors. This tumor is typically slow growing.

Clinically, these lesions present as a painless, firm mass, often in the parotid or on the palate. Microscopically, mucoepidermoid carcinoma is composed of a mixture of neoplastic squamous cells, mucus-secreting cells, and epithelial cells of an intermediate type. Histologic patterns may appear irregularly solid, cystic, or ductlike. Poorly differentiated carcinomas demonstrate a marked pleomorphic cell population.

Mucoepidermoid carcinoma can metastasize. The 5-year survival for low-grade carcinomas in greater than 90%, whereas poorly differentiated carcinoma have a 5-year survival of 20% to 40%.

Adenoid Cystic Carcinoma (Cylindroma)

Adenoid cystic carcinoma is the most common malignant neoplasm of the salivary glands. It is slow growing and most commonly presents between 40 to 60 years of age. This lesion constitutes 5% of all major salivary gland tumors and 20% of minor salivary gland tumors. In addition, these lesions may occur at other sites, including the lacrimal glands, nasopharynx, nasal cavity, and lower respiratory tract.

Microscopically, adenoid cystic carcinoma demonstrates varying patterns, including solid sheets, groups, strands, or columns or small cells with scant cytoplasm. The tumor cells often connect to form cystic spaces that may be tubular or cribriform. The cystic cavity is filled with blue-tinged basement membrane material. These lesions often infiltrate the perineural space and are therefore painful. Adenoid cystic carcinomas often invade locally and recur after surgery, resulting in an overall poor prognosis for this lesion. In addition, hematogenous spread to the lungs may occur.

Acinic Cell Carcinoma

Acinic cell carcinoma is an uncommon, aggressive neoplasm that arises most commonly in the parotid gland. This tumor occurs most commonly between the ages of 40 to 50 years. Microscopically, the tumor cells resemble serous salivary glands and demonstrate finely granular cytoplasm or clear cells. This lesion may recur locally following resection or develop regional and distant metastases.

THE NOSE AND PARANASAL SINUSES

Normal Anatomy and Histology

The nose serves both a respiratory and olfactory function. Air flows into the nose via the anterior nares (nostrils) to the nasal vestibule, which is a space lined by skin containing hairs and sebaceous glands. The nasal fossae, situated behind the vestibules, consist of

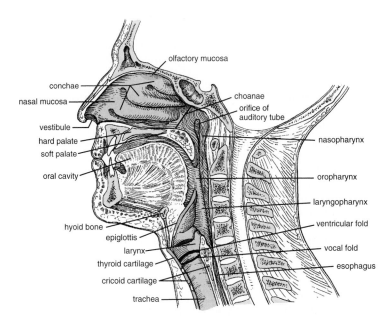

FIGURE 25-3
Diagram of the relationship of the pharynx to the respiratory and digestive systems. (From Ross MH, Kaye GI, and Pawlina W. Histology: A Text and Atlas, 4th ed. Philadelphia: Lippincott Williams & Wilkins, 2003 p. 570.)

respiratory and olfactory regions; the nasal fossae are separated by the nasal septum. The lateral wall is composed of the superior, middle, and inferior nasal conchae, or turbinates. The nasal mucosa is lined by ciliated, columnar epithelium with scattered goblet cells. The sinuses are composed of the maxillary, ethmoid, frontal, and sphenoid sinuses (Fig. 25-3).

Diseases of the External Nose and Nasal Vestibule

The skin that covers the nose is subject to virtually all diseases of the skin, and is commonly affected by solar damage, basal cell carcinoma, squamous cell carcinoma, and malignant melanoma. Additional diseases of the external nose and vestibule include the following:

- Rhinophyma: protuberant bulbous mass on the nose caused by marked hyperplasia of the sebaceous glands and chronic inflammation

- Pyogenic granuloma: exuberant granulation tissue secondary to trauma
- Epistaxis (nosebleed): caused by trauma, inflammation, and neoplasms and often originates in the anterior nasal septum

Diseases of the Nasal Cavity and Paranasal Sinuses

Inflammation

Rhinitis is an inflammation of the mucous membranes of the nasal cavity and sinuses and may be viral or allergic in nature.

Viral rhinitis is the most common cause of acute rhinitis. On infection, the virus replicates in the epithelium, causing shedding of the epithelium, edema, and infiltration by neutrophils and leukocytes. Abundant mucus production leads to rhinorrhea. A few days after initial infection, secondary infection by normal pathogens occurs, causing a mucopurulent discharge. The disease usually resolves in a few days to a week.

Allergic rhinitis (hay fever) occurs when allergens are deposited on the nasal mucosa and may be seasonal (acute) or chronic. Mast cells in the mucosa bind to allergens by immunoglobulin (Ig) E receptors and subsequently secrete histamine, heparin, and leukotrienes. These mediators are responsible for the sneezing and rhinorrhea associated with allergic rhinitis. Microscopically, the nasal mucosa demonstrates edema and numerous eosinophils.

Chronic rhinitis is caused by repeated episodes of acute rhinitis and is characterized by a thickening of the nasal mucosa secondary to hyperplasia of the mucous glands and infiltration by lymphocytes and plasma cells.

Nasal Polyps

Sinonasal inflammatory polyps are reactive lesions that may be single or multiple, unilateral or multilateral, and often arise from the lateral nasal wall or the ethmoid recess. Patients may be asymptomatic or produce nasal obstruction, rhinorrhea, and headaches. Microscopically, the polyps are lined by respiratory epithelium and contain mucous glands within a loose mucoid stroma that is infiltrated by plasma cells, lymphocytes, and eosinophils. Often, there is basement membrane thickening and goblet cell hyperplasia. These polyps may occur secondary to allergy, cystic fibrosis, infections, or diabetes mellitus.

Sinusitis

Sinusitis is an inflammation of the mucous membranes of the paranasal sinuses that often occurs in conditions that interfere with the normal drainage of the sinus. *Acute sinusitis* lasts less than 3 weeks and is often caused by extension of pathogens, such as *Haemophilus influenzae* and *Branhamella catarrhalis*, from the nasal mucosa. Maxillary sinusitis may be caused by odontogenic infections. Chronic sinusitis occurs following incomplete resolution of acute sinusitis or recurrent acute sinusitis and often contains anaerobic bacteria. A variety of complications may occur following sinusitis, including the following:

- Mucocele: accumulation of mucous secretions in a nasal sinus that develops slowly and may result in bone resorption
- Osteomyelitis: occurs rarely when a suppurative infection of the frontal sinus extends to the bone; can cause overlying cellulitis or abscess formation
- Septic thrombophlebitis: infection may penetrate the bone and spread into the frontal and diploe venous systems
- Intracranial infections: includes epidural, subdural, and cerebral abscesses and purulent leptomeningitis

Leprosy

Leprosy is the result of infection with *Mycobacterium leprae*, which spreads by infected nasal secretions. Nasal involvement is usually the first symptom of leprosy. The skin surrounding the nares and anterior nasal mucosa shows nodules, ulceration, or perforation. Microscopically, chronic granulomatous inflammation is present.

Rhinoscleroma

Rhinoscleroma is a chronic inflammatory process that usually remains localized to the nose and is most common in Mediterranean countries and in parts of Asia, Africa, and Latin America. Risk factors include poor domestic and personal hygiene and close personal contact with an infected person. The infectious agent is *Klebsiella rhinoscleromatis*. Infected tissue appears firm, thickened, irregularly nodular, and ulcerated. Microscopically, plasma cells, lymphocytes, foamy histiocytes with phagocytosed bacteria, and granulation tissue is present. This condition is treatable with antibiotics.

Fungal Infections

Sinonasal fungal infections occur in immunocompromised patients, including patients with immunodeficiency, diabetes, and patients undergoing chemotherapy. Fungal infections may be invasive or noninvasive. Noninvasive fungal sinusitis demonstrates surface colonization of the nasal mucosa by fungi and may produce symptoms of nasal obstruction. Invasive fungal sinusitis is an emergent medical condition in which fungi invade the nasal mucosa and may spread to the venous sinuses, meninges, or brain. Fungal infections may be caused by a variety of organisms including the following:

- *Candida albicans*: white plaques on the oral and pharyngeal mucosa (thrush) and nasal infections
- *Aspergillus*: often involves the paranasal sinuses and may be invasive or noninvasive; noninvasive fungal sinusitis may produce fungal balls called aspergilloma that cause nasal obstruction
- *Rhinosporidium seeberi* (rhinosporidiosis): common in India, South America, and Central America; forms vascular polypoid masses in the nose, upper respiratory tract, ear, and skin; presence of spherical sporangia may induce giant cell reaction
- Zygomycetes: mucormycosis, *Rhizopus*; often invasive

Allergic fungal sinusitis is a hypersensitivity to fungal antigens that commonly occurs in younger patients and presents with allergic symptoms.

Leishmaniasis

The initial lesion in patients affected with *Leishmania braziliensis* is a cutaneous nasal sore that heals in a few months. After many months to years, mucocutaneous lesions develop in the nose or upper lip. The infected mucosa exhibits polypoid lesions and superficial ulcers, with parasite-containing macrophages early in the disease and a granulomatous reaction late in the disease. The anterior cartilaginous septum may collapse due to soft tissue destruction.

Wegener Granulomatosis

Wegener granulomatosis involves the lungs, kidneys, and small arteries of the body, but may be localized. Ischemic-type necrosis, vasculitis, mixed chronic inflammatory cell infiltrate, scattered multinucleated giant cells, poorly formed granulomas, and microabscess formation may be noted. The disease often manifests as septal perforation and mucosal ulceration. Often patients also describe constitutional symptoms such as weight loss, fever, and malaise. Over time, nasal involvement may lead to destruction of the nose and paranasal sinuses, which form a "saddle nose deformity." Clinical tests show increased serum anti neutrophil cytoplasmic antibodies (ANCA).

Benign Tumors of the Nasal Cavity

Benign tumors of the nose include the papillomas, such as the following:

- *Squamous papilloma*: most frequent benign tumor of the nasal cavity; occurs most often in the nasal vestibule; appear morphologically similar to a wart (verruca vulgaris)
- An *inverted papilloma:* involves the lateral nasal wall with occasional spread to the paranasal sinuses; occurs in middle-aged persons; appear as involutions of the surface squamous epithelium into the underlying stroma. Most commonly, human papillomaviruses types 6 and 11 are associated with these lesions. In a small number of cases, inverted papillomas may give rise to squamous carcinoma.

Malignant Tumors of the Nasal Cavity

Of the carcinomas that arise in the nose, approximately 50% arise in the antrum of the maxillary sinus, 30% in the nasal cavity, 10% in the ethmoid sinus, and 1% in the frontal and sphenoid sinuses. The vast majority are squamous cell carcinomas, with the remainder consisting of adenocarcinomas, transitional cell carcinomas, or undifferentiated carcinomas. Risk factors for the development of nasal carcinoma include exposure to nickel, chromium, and aromatic hydrocarbons. Nasal carcinomas are very locally aggressive but often do not give rise to metastases.

Olfactory Neuroblastoma

Olfactory neuroblastoma (esthesioneuroblastoma) occurs at any age and most likely arises from the neural crest cells. This lesion most often arises from the superior third of the nasal septum, the cribriform plate, and the superior turbinate. It appears polypoid, is highly vascular, and contains small round blue cells with hyperchromatic nuclei and a background pink stroma. The cells form pseudorosettes around blood vessels or form true neural rosettes with orientation around a fibrillary center. These lesions invade locally and may demonstrate lymphatic metastases to regional and distant lymph nodes. The 5-year survival rate is only 50%.

Nasal-type Angiocentric T-cell/Natural Killer-cell Lymphoma

T-cell/natural killer (T/NK)-cell lymphoma is a necrotizing, ulcerating mucosal lesion of the upper respiratory tract that often affects the midline of the nose (hence the prior name, *lethal midline granuloma*) and is Epstein-Barr virus (EBV)-related. T/NK-cell lymphoma demonstrates an insidious onset with symptoms of nonspecific sinusitis or rhinitis that progresses to an ulceration of the nasal mucosa with ulcers covered by a black crust. Microscopically, this disease shows a malignant infiltrate of atypical lymphocytes surrounding small- to medium-sized blood vessels. Vascular invasion and vessel occlusion may occur. If untreated, lesions ultimately erode the underlying cartilage and bone, and often the skin of the midface is involved. Half of all patients will develop disseminated disease. Death often ensues secondary to bacterial infection, aspiration pneumonia, or hemorrhage.

THE NASOPHARYNX

Continuous with the nasal cavities, the nasopharynx is lined early in life by pseudostratified columnar epithelium that is replaced over time by nonkeratinizing squamous epithelium. Waldeyer ring is a band of lymphoid tissue located at the opening of the oropharynx into the respiratory and digestive tracts and contains the adenoids (covered by respiratory epithelium) and the palatine tonsils (covered by squamous mucosa). Waldeyer ring is well developed in children and demonstrates prominent lymphoid follicles with germinal centers; with advancing age, Waldeyer ring gradually involutes.

Diseases Involving Lymphoid Tissue

- *Bruton X-linked agammaglobulinemia:* congenital absence of lymphoid tissue; demonstrates minimal to no lymphoid tissue in the tonsils, pharynx, and intestines of affected males, although these patients often have a normal thymus. Atrophy of pharyngeal lymphoid tissue may also occur in AIDS, chronic immunosuppression, and local radiation therapy.
- *Hyperplasia of the pharyngeal lymphoid tissue:* occurs following infections or chronic irritation of the pharynx

Inflammation of the Nasopharynx

Inflammation of the nasopharynx may occur from a variety of infectious causes and is termed *pharyngitis* and *tonsillitis*. These conditions are most common in childhood through early adulthood. Infections may be bacterial or viral in nature, with the most common viral pathogens consisting of influenza, parainfluenza, adenovirus, respiratory syncytial virus, and rhinovirus. Infectious mononucleosis is a viral disease accompanied by sore throat and producing exudative pharyngitis. *Streptococcus pyogenes* is an important cause of pharyngitis and tonsillitis because of the serious suppurative and nonsuppurative sequelae.

Other inflammatory diseases include the following:

- Acute tonsillitis: caused by bacterial infection, often *S. pyogenes*, and causes follicular tonsillitis with pinpoint exudates that can be extruded from the crypts

- Pseudomembranous tonsillitis: occurs in diphtheria or in Vincent angina and is represented by a necrotic mucosa covered by a coat of exudate
- Recurrent tonsillitis: may occur following repeated bouts of acute tonsillitis and cause obstructive enlargement of the tonsils
- Peritonsillar abscess: usually occurs following incompletely treated acute bacterial tonsillitis and may lead to extension into the pyriform sinus, parapharyngeal space, wall of the carotid artery, mediastinum, or cranial cavity

Tumors of the Nasopharynx

Several types of tumor of the nasopharynx are discussed in this section. Additional malignant tumors that arise in this region include lymphomas (often diffuse B-cell lymphomas), plasmacytoma, and chordoma.

Juvenile Nasopharyngeal Angiofibroma

Juvenile nasopharyngeal angiofibroma is an uncommon, highly vascular neoplasm of the nasopharynx that occurs in adolescent boys. The lesion appears rounded and has a sessile or pedunculated attachment to the posterior or lateral nasopharyngeal wall. This lesion is locally aggressive and may grow into adjacent structures and is associated with bony destruction. Microscopically, the vascular component contains vessels that vary in size and shape and the vessel wall is characterized by the absence of a smooth muscle layer or by irregularly arranged smooth muscle. These vessels form a slitlike appearance in a collagenous background stromal component. These abnormal vessels are less likely to undergo vasoconstriction following trauma and are therefore more likely to bleed; biopsies are often contraindicated. Management includes surgical excision or radiation.

Squamous Cell Carcinoma

Squamous cell carcinomas occur in the nasopharynx and are often more aggressive than those in the anterior oral cavity and frequently metastasize to the superior deep jugular and submandibular lymph nodes.

Nasopharyngeal Carcinoma

Nasopharyngeal carcinoma (NPC) is a carcinoma of the nasopharynx that is classified into keratinizing or nonkeratinizing subtypes.

Nonkeratinizing NPC

Nonkeratinizing NPC is associated with EBV infection and presence in tumor cells and B lymphocytes. It is divided into two types: differentiated or undifferentiated:

- Differentiated nonkeratinizing NPC has a stratified appearance with distinct cell margins.
- Undifferentiated nonkeratinizing NPC appears as clusters of poorly differentiated cells with a syncytial appearance, scant cytoplasm, and oval nuclei in a background of lymphoid infiltration. Cytokeratin stains are often necessary to distinguish this variant from malignant lymphoma. The undifferentiated form of nonkeratinizing NPC is common in Asia and Africa and may have both genetic and environmental causes.

Keratinizing NPC

Keratinizing NPC (squamous cell) occurs in older individuals and does not have an EBV association. NPCs are asymptomatic for a long time due to their location and often first present with a palpable cervical lymph node metastasis. These tumors are highly radiosensitive and localized disease may be effectively treated in many cases.

THE EAR

Normal Anatomy and Histology

The ear is formed by external, middle, and inner components. The external ear is formed by elastic cartilage of the auricle and external ear canal that is covered by skin. The external ear ends at the tympanic membrane (eardrum), which is covered on the outer surface by squamous epithelium and the inner surface by cuboidal epithelium. The middle ear (tympanic cavity) is an oblong space in the temporal bone that is lined by a mucous membrane. The middle ear contains the opening of the eustachian tube and the auditory ossicles (malleus, incus, and stapes). The middle ear opens posteriorly into the mastoid antrum. The inner ear is formed by the cochlea and vestibular labyrinth, which are housed in the petrous portion of the temporal bone. The cochlea contains the organ of Corti, which contains numerous hair cells and is the end organ of hearing. The vestibular labyrinth aids in equilibrium and is formed by the utricle, saccule, and semicircular canals.

The External Ear

The external ear may demonstrate a variety of lesions, including the following:

- *Keloids*: thick, hyalinized bundles of collagen in the deep dermis that occur following piercing or trauma
- *Cauliflower ears*: organized subperichondrial hematomas that deform the ears following repeated trauma
- *Relapsing polychondritis*: rare, chronic disease that causes intermittent inflammation and destroys the cartilaginous structures in the ears, nose, larynx, tracheobronchial tree, ribs, and joints
- *Malignant otitis externa*: infection by *Pseudomonas aeruginosa* that may spread through skin and cartilage and may result in death; often in patients with diabetes or blood dyscrasias
- *Aural polyps*: benign polyps formed by granulation tissue

The Middle Ear

Otitis media is common inflammatory condition of the middle ear that usually results from an upper respiratory tract infection that extends from the nasopharynx, but may occur following obstruction of the eustachian tube. Various forms of otitis media include the following:

- *Acute serous otitis media*: obstruction of the eustachian tube by sudden changes in atmospheric pressure that may or may not have superimposed bacterial infection
- *Chronic serous otitis media*: recurrent or chronic serous effusions caused by obstructions of the eustachian tube; goblet cell metaplasia may occur on the mucosal lining of the middle ear; may form cholesterol granulomas
- *Acute suppurative otitis media*: caused by virulent pyogenic bacteria that invade the middle ear, especially *Streptococcus pneumoniae* and *H. influenzae*; accumulation of purulent material in the middle ear with possible eardrum rupture
- *Acute mastoiditis*: caused by spread of inadequately treated acute otitis media
- *Chronic suppurative otitis media and mastoiditis*: repeated infections of the middle ear lead to chronic inflammation of the mucosa or destruction of the periosteum covering the ossicles; eardrum is always perforated and there is often hearing loss and discharge; cholesteatoma may form. *Cholesteatoma* is a mass of accumulated keratin and squamous mucosa that results from the growth of squamous epithelium from the external ear canal through the perforated eardrum into the middle ear.

Complications of acute and chronic otitis media, if inadequately treated, include meningitis, cerebral abscess formation, and petrositis.

Jugulotympanic paraganglioma is the most frequent benign tumor of the middle ear and arises from the middle ear paraganglia.

These lesions grow slowly but may cause destruction of the middle ear. Microscopically, paragangliomas demonstrate nests of cells embedded in a richly vascular stroma. These lesions stain for catecholamines such as epinephrine and norepinephrine.

The Inner Ear

Otosclerosis

Otosclerosis is the formation of new spongy bone around the stapes and oval window, which results in progressive deafness. This disease is inherited in an autosomal dominant manner and is the most common cause of conductive hearing loss in young and middle-aged adults. The disease tends to be bilateral. Microscopically, the early lesion shows resorption of bone with the formation of highly cellular fibrous tissue with wide vascular spaces and osteoclasts. Over time, the lesion undergoes repeated remodeling.

Ménière Disease

Ménière disease is the triad of vertigo, sensorineural hearing loss, and tinnitus that occurs in the fourth and fifth decades and is bilateral in 15% of cases. The cause of Ménière disease is unknown. The disease is intermittent at first, but over time may become more frequent and result in permanent hearing loss. Microscopically, early lesions show a dilation of the cochlear duct and saccule. As the disease progresses, the entire endolymphatic system becomes dilated and the membranous wall frequently tears. Treatment involves a low-salt diet and diuretic administration to improve symptoms.

Labyrinthine Toxicity

A variety of drugs can cause transient or permanent sensorineural hearing loss. The most common agents that induce permanent hearing loss are the aminoglycoside antibiotics.

Viral Labyrinthitis

Congenital deafness may result from prenatal infection with cytomegalovirus or rubella. Mumps is the most common cause of deafness associated with postnatal viral infections.

Acoustic Trauma

Noise-induced hearing loss is a significant source of morbidity in industrialized countries and is caused by damage to the organ of Corti.

Tumors

The most common tumors of the inner ear include *schwannomas*, which arise from the vestibular nerve and may be associated with neurofibromatosis type 2, and meningiomas that arise in the cerebellopontine angle. These lesions are discussed in further detail in Chapter 28.

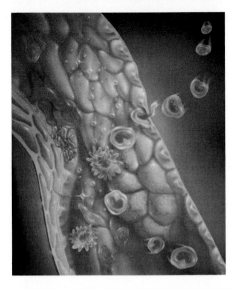

CHAPTER 26

Bones, Joints, and Soft Tissues

Chapter Outline

BONE AND CARTILAGE

Normal Anatomy and Histology

Bone is a specialized form of connective tissue that performs numerous important functions in the body, including mechanical support, protection of internal organs, mineral storage, and hematopoiesis. Bones are the principal reservoir of calcium in the body, and they also store phosphate, sodium, and magnesium.

Bones can be macroscopically subdivided into compact (cortical) bone and spongy (cancellous) bone. *Compact bone* is dense bone that makes up 80% of the skeleton and forms the outside layer of bones. *Spongy* (cancellous) *bone* is found at the ends of long bones within the medullary canal and demonstrates a high surface-to-volume ratio. The bridging spicules of bone that make up spongy bone are called *trabeculae* and the spaces between the trabeculae are often filled with bone marrow and blood vessels. The bone marrow is present within the medullary canal and consists of red marrow (containing hematopoietic elements and located in the axial skeleton in adults) and yellow marrow (containing fat and located in the bones of the limbs).

Changes in the rate of bone turnover are primarily manifested in the cancellous bone.

The blood supply of the long bones occurs via two main artery types and associated canals:

- *Nutrient arteries*: supply marrow space and internal one-third of the cortex; enter bone via nutrient foramen
- *Perforating arteries*: small straight vessels that extend inward from the periosteal arteries; anastomose with nutrient arteries in the cortex
- *Haversian canals*: spaces that course parallel to the long axis of the bone; each canal contains vessels, lymphatics, and nerves
- *Volkmann canals*: spaces within the cortex that run perpendicular to the long axis of the bone; connect haversian canals; contain blood vessels

Bone is formed of cells (10% of total tissue), an organic matrix (30% of total tissue) and inorganic matrix (60% of total tissue). The *inorganic,* or mineralized, *matrix* is predominantly formed by poorly crystalline hydroxyapatite. The *organic matrix* is primarily formed of type I collagen, as well as lipids, glycosaminoglycans, osteocalcin (formed by osteoblasts), and osteopontin (helps anchor cells to bone matrix).

Four cell types are present in bone:

- *Osteoprogenitor cell*: derived from a primitive stem cell; can differentiate into osteoblasts and osteoclasts, as well as other cell types; small stellate or spindle cell difficult to recognize by light microscopy

- *Osteoblast*: protein synthesizing cells that produce and mineralize bone tissue; derived from precursor cells by CBFA-1; large mononuclear and polygonal cells that are arrayed in a line along the bone surface; produces eosinophilic organic bone matrix termed *osteoid*; produces growth factors
- *Osteocyte*: an osteoblast completely embedded in the bone matrix within a lacuna; loses capacity for protein synthesis; numerous processes extend through canaliculi to contact other osteocytes
- *Osteoclast*: bone-resorptive cell; multinucleated cell rich in lysosomes and hydrolytic enzymes; attaches to bone along its ruffled membrane and reduces pH of surrounding bone to 4.5 via a proton pump; acts only on mineralized bone

The periosteum is a specialized connective tissue that covers all bones of the body and is composed of an inner, loosely arranged layer and an outer dense, fibrous layer that contains blood vessels.

Throughout life, bone is a dynamic structure that undergoes constant remodeling to maintain the skeleton. Bone may be microscopically divided into lamellar or woven bone. Unmineralized bone is termed *osteoid*.

- *Lamellar bone* is produced slowly, is highly organized, and forms the adult skeleton. Lamellar bone is defined by a parallel arrangement of type I collagen fibers, few osteocytes, and uniform osteocytes in lacunae parallel to the long axis of the collagen fibers.
- *Woven bone* is deposited more rapidly than lamellar bone, demonstrates low tensile strength, and is haphazardly arranged. Woven bone is found primarily in the developing fetus, in areas surrounding tumor or infection, and as part of a healing fracture, and is therefore not a normal finding in adults. Woven bone is characterized by an irregular arrangement of type I collagen fibers, numerous osteocytes, and variation in the size and shape of osteocytes.

Cartilage is formed of both an organic and an inorganic matrix, but unlike bone, it does not contain blood vessels, nerves, or lymphatics. Cartilage provides resilience and lubrication to the articular surfaces of joints. The inorganic matrix of cartilage is predominantly formed of calcium hydroxyapatite crystals, similar to bone. However, the organic matrix is composed of 80% water, with the remaining 20% predominantly composed of type II collagen and proteoglycans. These proteoglycans are attached to long side arms of polysaccharides called glycosaminoglycans, which are composed of chondroitin-4-sulfate, chondroitin-6-sulfate, and keratan sulfate.

The three types of cartilage are as follows:

- Hyaline cartilage: articular surface of joints, trachea, growth plates

- Fibrocartilage: hyaline cartilage that contains numerous type I collagen fibers for tensile and structural strength; annulus fibrosus of the intervertebral disk, symphysis pubis
- Elastic cartilage: epiglottis, arytenoids cartilage of the larynx, external ear

Chondrocytes are derived from primitive mesenchymal cells that are similar to the precursors of bone cells.

The *transverse cartilage plate* is present in the growing child at the ends of long bones and defines the epiphysis, metaphysis, and diaphysis (Fig. 26-1).

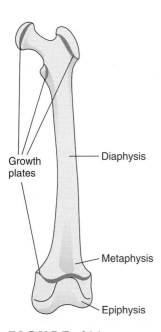

FIGURE   26-1
Structure of a typical long bone. The diaphysis (shaft) of a long bone contains a large marrow cavity surrounded by a thick-walled tube of compact bone. The proximal and distal ends, or epiphyses, of the long bone consist chiefly of spongy bone with a thin outer shell of compact bone. The expanded or flared part of the diaphysis nearest the epiphysis is referred to as the metaphysis. Except for the articular surfaces that are covered by hyaline (articular) cartilage, the outer surface of the bone is covered by a fibrous layer of connective tissue called the periosteum. (From Rubin E, Gorstein F, Rubin R, et al. Rubin's Pathology, 4th ed. Philadelphia: Lippincott Williams & Wilkins, 2005, p. 1308.)

- *Epiphysis:* forms the ends of the long bones and, in articulating joints, is covered by articular cartilage.
- *Metaphysis:* forms the flared portion of the long bone adjacent to the epiphysis. During development, the epiphysis and the metaphysis are situated on opposite ends of the growth plate.
- *Diaphysis:* corresponds to the body or shaft of the bone.

Bone Formation and Growth

Bone formation may occur via *endochondral ossification* (bone tissue replaces cartilage) or *intramembranous ossification* (bone tissue replaces fibrous tissue laid down by the periosteum). Most of the skeleton develops from cartilage anlagen present during fetal development, except for the clavicles and calvaria. Bone is therefore first represented by tissue cartilage, which undergoes resorption followed by bone replacement, termed *endochondral ossification.*

Primary Ossification

This process directs the formation of bone along a temporal sequence that includes the formation of cartilage at the site of future bone, deposition of woven bone on the surface of the cartilage core (termed *primary center of ossification*), calcification and removal of the central cartilage (termed *cylinderization*), and invasion of vessels into the cartilage core.

Secondary Ossification

This process occurs at the cartilaginous ends of the future bone. The secondary center of ossification is formed at the ends of the bone when cartilage is resorbed. Ultimately, a zone of cartilage is trapped between the end of the bone and the diaphysis, which then forms the growth plate. The growth plate controls the longitudinal growth of the bones and ultimately determines adult height. Within the growth plate, chondrocytes are arranged in vertical rows. The growth plate is divided into several zones, as is diagrammed in Figure 26-2. In general, the growth plate is obliterated at a specific age for each bone, and closure of the growth plate is induced by sex hormones and occurs earlier in girls. Eventually, the entire growth plate is replaced by bone.

Congenital and Inherited Disorders of Bone

A variety of inherited and congenital disorders affect bone formation and growth, as are summarized in Table 26-1.

Cretinism

Cretinism is caused by maternal iodine deficiency and results in impaired linear growth of the skeleton, resulting in dwarfism with

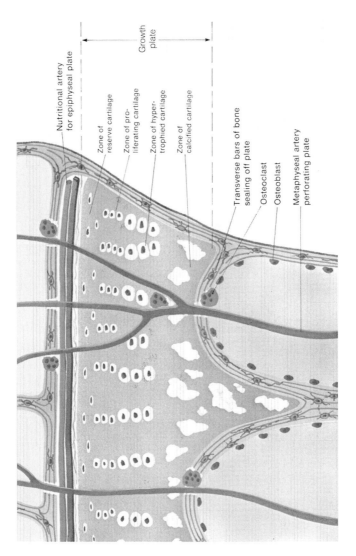

FIGURE 26-2

Normal structure of the growth plate. During closure, the epiphyseal cartilage ceases to grow, and metaphyseal vessels penetrate the cartilage plate. Transverse bars of bone separate the growth plate from the metaphysis. (From Rubin E, Gorstein F, Rubin R, et al. Rubin's Pathology, 4th ed. Philadelphia: Lippincott Williams & Wilkins, 2005, p. 1315.)

Table 26-1
Congenital and Inherited Disorders of Bone Formation and Growth

Disease	Pathophysiology	Microscopic Findings	Clinical Findings
Cretinism	Maternal iodine deficiency	Narrow zone of proliferative cartilage; retarded maturation of the hypertrophic zone	Short-limbed dwarfism, unusually large head, delayed shedding of deciduous teeth
Morquio syndrome	Mucopolysaccharidosis type IV	Chondrocytes filled with mucopolysaccharides; disordered growth plate; transverse bar of bone	Dwarfism, corneal clouding, hearing defects; mental retardation, keratan sulfituria
Achondroplasia	Activating mutation of FGF-3 receptor	Greatly thinned growth plate; near absent zone of proliferative cartilage; transverse bar of bone	Dwarfism with short, thick limbs, normal mentation, average life span
Osteopetrosis	Defects in osteoclast activity	Overgrowth and sclerosis of bone	Brittle bones that readily fracture, occasionally impaired hematopoiesis
Osteogenesis imperfecta	Defects in type I collagen synthesis	Osteopenia with cortical thinning	High risk of fractures; type II is fatal in the perinatal period

disproportionately short limbs and an unusually large head. In addition, there is delayed shedding of deciduous teeth and eruption of permanent teeth. Maturation of the hypertrophic zone of the growth plate is delayed and endochondral ossification does not occur.

Achondroplasia

Achondroplasia is the most common genetic form of dwarfism (1: 15,000 live births) and represents a failure of normal epiphyseal cartilage formation. Achondroplasia is inherited as an autosomal dominant trait and is caused by an activating mutation in the FGF-3 receptor on chromosome 4 (4p16.3). This mutation arrests chondrocyte proliferation and differentiation and results in a greatly thinned growth plate with a severely attenuated zone of proliferative cartilage. In addition, a transverse bar of bone seals off the growth plate. However, intramembranous ossification is undisturbed, resulting in short, thick bones and a large head. Patients demonstrate dwarfism with short limbs and macrocephaly but have normal mentation and a normal life span. Occasionally, severe kyphoscoliosis may be a complication.

Osteopetrosis

Osteopetrosis encompasses a group of rare, inherited disorders in which failed osteoclastic bone resorption underlies the clinical findings. Osteopetrosis is characterized pathologically by the retention of the primary spongiosum with its cartilage cores, lack of funnelization of the metaphysis, and a thickened cortex. Bones are short, blocklike, radiodense, and extremely radiopaque, and they weigh as much as three times more than normal bone. Although bones are thick, improper development due to faulty remodeling leads to disorganized bones that can easily fracture.

Examination of the bones from patients with osteopetrosis reveals bones that are widened at the metaphysis and diaphysis, resulting in an Erlenmeyer flasklike appearance. Almost all bones contain a residual cartilage core. In some cases, suppression of hematopoiesis may occur due to replacement by sheets of abnormal osteoclasts or extensive fibrosis, which leads to the development of extramedullary hematopoiesis.

The most frequent type of osteopetrosis is *autosomal dominant osteopetrosis* (ADO) *type II*, which is caused by a mutation of chromosome 1p21 and results in frequent fracture. A severe autosomal recessive form occurs in infants and children, and may result in death secondary to marked anemia, cranial nerve entrapment, hydrocephalus, and infections.

Osteogenesis Imperfecta

Osteogenesis imperfecta (OI) encompasses a group of autosomal dominant disorders caused by mutations in the genes for collagen type I, which affect the skeleton, joints, ears, ligaments, teeth, sclera, and skin. Mutations in the *COL1A1* gene on chromosome 17 occur in all types of OI, whereas mutations in the *COL1A2* gene on chromosome 7 occur in types II, III, and IV. These genes encode the proalpha1 and proalpha2 chains of type I procollagen. Four types of OI have been described as follows:

- Type I: mildest form; multiple fractures when child begins walking and sitting, blue sclera (thin sclera with underlying choroids), hearing abnormalities (fusion of ossicles), extremely thin and curved bones, misshapen and bluish yellow teeth
- Type II: lethal, perinatal disease; blue sclera; infants are stillborn or die within days from crush injury in birth canal
- Type III: progressive, most severely deforming type of OI; many bone fractures, growth retardation, severe skeletal deformities; fractures present at birth, blue sclera only at birth, teeth abnormalities
- Type IV: similar to type I; white sclera; bone cortex may mature during adolescence or afterwards

Enchondromatosis

Enchondromatosis (*Ollier disease*) is characterized by the development of numerous cartilaginous masses that lead to bony deformities. Residual anlage or growth plate cartilage does not undergo endochondral ossification but remains in the bone, often at the metaphysis. With growth of the child, these lesions ultimately settle in the diaphysis of the bone. Microscopically, these lesions appear as multiple, tumorlike masses of abnormally arranged hyaline cartilage with zones of proliferation and hypertrophied cartilage, and they have a tendency to undergo malignant transformation into chondrosarcomas in adult life.

The disorder known as *Maffucci syndrome* is characterized by multiple enchondromas and cavernous hemangiomas that manifest in childhood, leading to skeletal deformities. Approximately half of patients develop chondrosarcomas and other malignant tumors. In contrast, *solitary enchondroma* primarily affects the tubular bones of the hands and feet and only rarely undergoes malignant transformation.

Reactive Bone Formation

Reactive bone formation occurs in response to stress on bones or soft tissues, and may occur in regions of tumor, infection, or trauma. Reactive bone is derived from the periosteum or the endosteal tissue of the marrow, and may consist of woven or lamellar bone. Woven bone typically occurs in rapidly expanding processes and lamellar bone typically occurs in indolent processes. Formation of reactive bone by the periosteum may appear as a sunburst or onionskin pattern (with progressive layering of the periosteum). Endosteal bone formation occurs on the marrow surface and may appear as a thickened cortex radiographically with denser cancellous bone. Heterotopic calcification is the deposition of acellular mineral in soft tissue, and may consist of woven or lamellar bone. In contrast to reactive bone formation, which often has a spicular or trabeculated pattern, heterotopic calcification demonstrates an irregular, splotchy, amorphous appearance radiographically. Heterotopic calcification often occurs in areas of soft tissue necrosis.

Myositis Ossificans

Fracture

Fractures represent the most common bone lesion, and are defined as a discontinuity of the bone. Fractures demonstrate not only injury to the bone, but also extensive muscle necrosis, hemorrhage, tearing of ligaments and tendons, and occasionally nerve damage. Different forces on the bones can produce specific types of fractures, including the following:

- Transverse fracture: force applied perpendicular to the long bone
- Compression fracture: force applied in the long axis of the bone
- Spiral fracture: torsional force applied to a long bone

Fracture Healing

Fractures undergo healing to ultimately reform normal cortical bone. Healing occurs through a progression of stages, including the inflammatory, reparative, and remodeling phases, and the length of each phase is dependent on the patient's age, site of fracture, and the patient's overall health. Figure 26-3 illustrates the phases of fracture healing.

The *inflammatory phase* begins immediately following fracture and lasts for approximately 1 week. During this phase, extensive necrosis of bone (characterized by the absence of osteocytes and empty osteocyte lacunae) and hemorrhage occurs within the first several days. By 2 to 5 days, the hemorrhage forms a large clot, which undergoes neovascularization beginning at the periphery. By 7 days, woven bone begins to form, which corresponds to the "scar" of bone. The granulation tissue containing bone or cartilage is termed a *callus*.

The *reparative phase* begins following the first week after the fracture and continues for months. This process involves the differentiation of fibroblasts and osteoblasts from pluripotential cells, the resorption of the blood clot, and the construction of the bone callus. Osteoclasts tunnel towards the site of the fracture by the

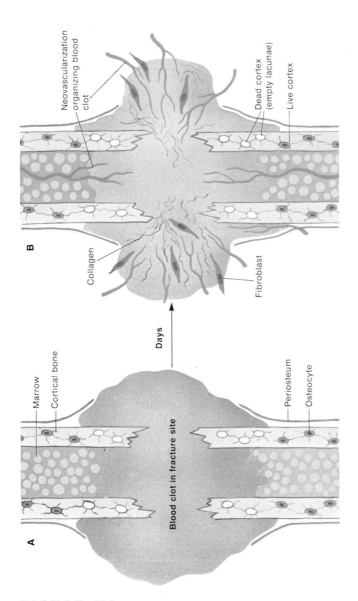

FIGURE 26-3

Healing of a fracture. A: Soon after a fracture is sustained, an extensive blood clot forms in the subperiosteal and soft tissue, as well as in the marrow cavity. The bone at the fracture site is jagged. B: The inflammatory phase of fracture healing is characterized by neovascularization and beginning organization of the blood clot. Because the osteocytes in the fracture site are dead, the lacunae are empty. (*continues*)

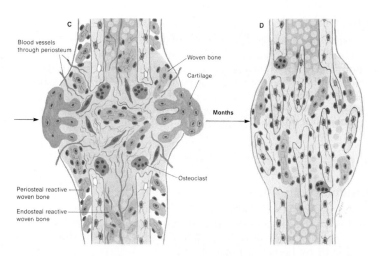

FIGURE   26-3

(*continued*) C: The reparative phase of fracture healing is characterized by the formation of a callus of cartilage and woven bone near
the fracture site. The jagged edges of the original cortex have been
remodeled and eroded by osteoclasts. The marrow space has been
revascularized and contains reactive woven bone, as does the periosteal area. D: In the remodeling phase, during which the cortex is
revitalized, the reactive bone may be lamellar or woven. The new
bone is organized along stress lines and mechanical forces. Extensive
osteoclastic and osteoblastic cellular activity is maintained. (From
Rubin E, Gorstein F, Rubin R, et al. Rubin's Pathology, 4th ed. Philadelphia: Lippincott Williams & Wilkins, 2005, p. 1323.)

formation of cutting cones, and are accompanied by new vessel
ingrowth. In addition, an external callus arising from the periosteum and an internal callus arising from the medullary cavity
grows toward the fracture site.

The *remodeling phase* begins several weeks after the fracture,
when the ingrowth of callus has sealed the ends of the fractured
bone. During this phase, bone is reorganized to restore the original
cortex. Remodeling can continue for several years.

In certain instances, fractures may not follow the above sequence of healing events. In cases of *primary healing*, the fracture
does not result in bone displacement and therefore no soft tissue
reaction or callus formation occurs. In *nonunion*, the fracture site
does not heal due to excessive motion, interposition of soft tissues,
infection or poor blood supply. Continued movement at the un-
healed fracture site results in pseudoarthrosis, a condition in which
jointlike tissue is formed, which must be removed surgically for
proper healing to occur.

Stress Fracture

A stress fracture refers to an accumulation of stress-induced microfractures, which eventually result in a true fracture through the bone cortex. Stress fractures result from repeated mechanical injury that results in the formation of periosteal and endosteal calluses that strengthen the bone while active remodeling takes place. Stress fractures produce pain and swelling over the bone, with more severe pain at the time of fracture.

Infections

Osteomyelitis

Osteomyelitis is an inflammation of the bone and the bone marrow, and is most commonly used in the context of bacterial infections.

Organisms are introduced into the bone either by direct penetration or by hematogenous spread.

Direct penetration occurs in the context of penetrating wounds, fractures, or surgery, and often involves infection by staphylococci and streptococci. In cases of postoperative infection, up to 25% of infections are caused by anaerobic organisms.

Hematogenous spread originates reaches the bone from a primary source outside of the skeletal system and most commonly affects the metaphyses of the long bones, such as the knee, ankle, and hip (Fig. 26-4). In adults, osteomyelitis frequently involves the vertebral bodies (*vertebral osteomyelitis*) and spread often occurs between adjacent vertebrae via the intervertebral disk. Approximately half of all cases are caused by *Staphylococcus aureus*, although enteric organisms such as *Escherichia coli* have also been identified as causative agents. Predisposing factors include intravenous drug abuse, upper urinary tract infections, and hematogenous spread of organisms from other sites.

Several specific lesions may occur in osteomyelitis:

- Cloaca: hole formed in the bone during formation of a draining sinus
- Sequestrum: fragment of necrotic bone embedded in pus
- Brodie abscess: reactive periosteal and endosteal bone that surrounds and contains the infection
- Involucrum: periosteal new bone forms a sheath around the sequestrum

Symptoms of osteomyelitis include pain, swelling, erythema, and tenderness over the involved bone. In addition, patients may demonstrate a low-grade fever and increased sedimentation rate. Some patients may experience vertebral collapse and associated epidural abscesses if the vertebral column is involved. Leukocytosis is common.

A

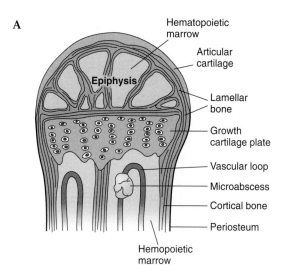

Hematopoietic marrow

Articular cartilage

Epiphysis

Lamellar bone

Growth cartilage plate

Vascular loop

Microabscess

Cortical bone

Periosteum

Hemopoietic marrow

B

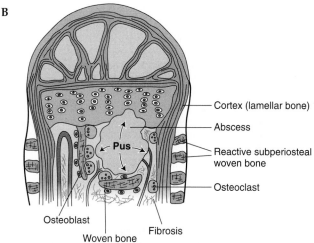

Cortex (lamellar bone)

Abscess

Pus

Reactive subperiosteal woven bone

Osteoclast

Osteoblast

Woven bone

Fibrosis

FIGURE 26-4

Pathogenesis of hematogenous osteomyelitis. A: The epiphysis, metaphysis, and growth plate are normal. A small, septic microabscess is forming at the capillary loop. B: Expansion of the septic focus stimulates resorption of adjacent bony trabeculae. The abscess expands into the cartilage and stimulates reactive bone formation by the periosteum. (*continues*)

C

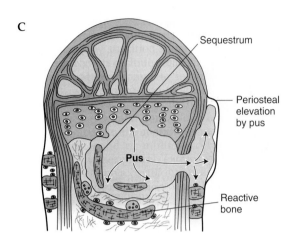

Sequestrum

Periosteal
elevation
by pus

Pus

Reactive
bone

D

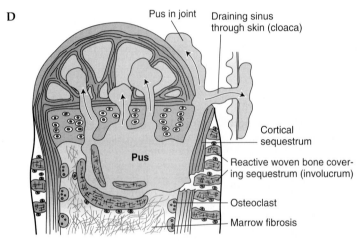

Pus in joint

Draining sinus
through skin (cloaca)

Cortical
sequestrum

Reactive woven bone covering sequestrum (involucrum)

Osteoclast

Marrow fibrosis

Pus

F I G U R E   26-4

(*continued*) C: The abscess, which continues to expand through the cortex into the subperiosteal tissues, shears off the perforating arteries that supply the cortex with blood, thereby leading to necrosis of the cortex. D: The extension of this process into the joint space, the epiphysis, and the skin produces a draining sinus. The necrotic bone is called a *sequestrum*. The viable bone surrounding a sequestrum is termed the *involucrum*. (From Rubin E, Gorstein F, Rubin R, et al. Rubin's Pathology, 4th ed. Philadelphia: Lippincott Williams & Wilkins, 2005, p. 1329.)

Complications of osteomyelitis include the following:

- Septicemia: dissemination of organisms in the bloodstream
- Acute bacterial arthritis: joint infection resulting in digestion of articular cartilage; medical emergency
- Pathological fractures
- Squamous cell carcinoma: occurs in bone or sinus tract of long-standing chronic osteomyelitis
- Amyloidosis: rare; more common in preantibiotic era
- Chronic osteomyelitis: difficult to treat, as necrotic tissue is avascular and antibiotics are therefore ineffective

Early osteomyelitis can be treated with intravenous antibiotics for 6 or more weeks. Abscesses are managed by surgical intervention.

Tuberculosis of Bone

Tuberculosis of bone often originates from the lung or lymph nodes, and reaches the bone by hematogenous spread. Infection of the spine, termed *tuberculous spondylitis* (Pott disease) is a complication of childhood tuberculosis and affects the bodies of the vertebrae, with sparing of the lamina and adjacent vertebrae. The thoracic vertebrae are most commonly affected. Tuberculosis causes disease by the formation of caseating granulomas within the marrow, which leads to slow reabsorption of bone and little to no reactive bone formation. Collapse of the vertebrae may occur, leading to kyphosis and scoliosis. If the infection ruptures into the soft tissue anteriorly, pus and necrotic debris reach the spinal ligaments to form a cold abscess (containing an absence of acute inflammatory elements).

Tuberculosis may also result in arthritis, with destruction of articular cartilage, or osteomyelitis of the long bones. With current antibiotic treatment, tuberculosis of the bone is rare.

Syphilis

Syphilis of bone is a rare disease and is characterized by a slowly progressive, chronic, inflammatory disease of bone.

Syphilis may be acquired either by transplacental spread or via sexual contact. Involvement of the bone by congenital syphilis may occur as early as the fifth month of gestation. Spirochetes are present in the epiphysis and periosteum, where they produce inflammation. Occasionally, the epiphysis may become dislocated. The knee is most often affected by congenital syphilis, and the growth plate is widened and displays a yellow discoloration. Microscopically, granulomas, necrosis, and marked reactive bone formation are present. Lymphocytes, plasma cells, and spirochetes are present in the marrow space.

Acquired syphilis produces bony lesions primarily of the tibia, nose, palate and skull, during the tertiary phase approximately 2 to 5 years after infection. Periostitis is the predominant finding. Tibial lesions may result in new bone deposition along the medial and anterior aspects, termed *saber shin deformity*. Ultimately, the affected bones become short and deformed with growth. Lysis and collapse of the nasal and palatal bones results in saddle nose deformity.

Osteonecrosis (Avascular Necrosis, Aseptic Necrosis)

Osteonecrosis refers to death of bone in the absence of infection. A variety of conditions may predispose to osteonecrosis—including trauma, emboli, and radiation—and are summarized in Table 26-2.

Coarse cancellous bone and cortex undergo different mechanisms of repair. Necrotic coarse cancellous bone heals by creeping substitution, in which the necrotic marrow is replaced by invading neovascular tissue, thus providing the pluripotential cells necessary for bone repair. Ultimately, the necrotic bone becomes sandwiched between surrounding viable bone and is remodeled by osteoclastic activity.

Legg-Calvé-Perthes disease refers to osteonecrosis in the femoral head of children. Idiopathic *osteonecrosis* refers to osteonecrosis in the femoral head of adults. Both diseases can result in collapse of the femoral head and subsequent severe arthritis. Radiographi-

Table 26-2
Causes of Osteonecrosis Trauma

Surgery
Emboli
Systemic diseases
   Polycythemia
   Lupus erythematosus
   Sickle cell disease
Radiation
Corticosteroid administration
Osteochondritis dissecans (condition of unknown etiology in which a
   piece of articular cartilage and subchondral bone breaks off into a joint)
Autografts and allografts
Thrombosis of local vessels
Idiopathic factors
   Alcoholism

Modified from Rubin E, Gorstein F, Rubin R, et al. Rubin's Pathology, 4th ed. Philadelphia: Lippincott Williams & Wilkins, 2005, p. 1326.

cally, the necrotic region in avascular necrosis may appear radio-dense due to relative osteoporosis in the surrounding bone, addition of new bone by creeping substitution, formation of calcium soaps from marrow fat necrosis, and compaction of the preexisting dead bone. Often the necrotic zone appears wedge-shaped.

Metabolic Bone Disease

Metabolic disorders result in secondary, systemic structural defects of the skeleton, including diminished bone mass caused by decreased synthesis or increased destruction, reduced bone mineralization, or both. Figure 26-5 summarizes the bone findings associated with metabolic bone disease.

Osteomalacia and Rickets

Osteomalacia is an adult disease of soft bones, which is characterized by inadequate mineralization of newly formed bone matrix. Rickets is a similar childhood disease and it characterized by inadequate mineralization of bone and the cartilaginous matrix of the open growth plate. Osteomalacia and rickets may be caused by abnormal vitamin D metabolism, phosphate deficiency, and mineralization defects. The metabolic pathway leading to synthesis of vitamin D is described in Figure 26-6.

Decreased levels of vitamin D result from the following:

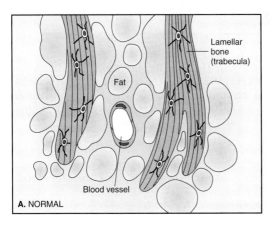

FIGURE 26-5
Metabolic bone diseases. A: Normal trabecular bone and fatty marrow. The trabecular bone is lamellar and contains evenly distributed osteocytes. (*continues*)

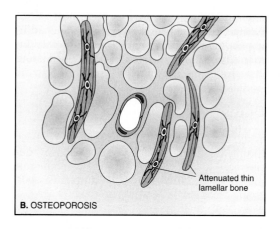

Attenuated thin
lamellar bone

B. OSTEOPOROSIS

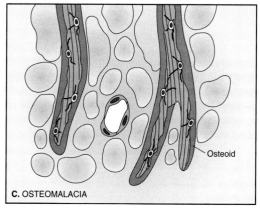

Osteoid

C. OSTEOMALACIA

F I G U R E   26-5
(*continued*) B: Osteoporosis. The lamellar bone exhibits discontin-
uous, thin trabeculae. C: Osteomalacia. The trabeculae of the lamellar
bone have abnormal amounts of nonmineralized bone (osteoid).
These osteoid seams are thickened and cover a larger than normal
area of the trabecular bone surface. (*continues*)

- Inadequate dietary intake: to prevent this, milk and other foods
  are fortified with vitamin D in developed countries; still occurs
  in developing countries
- Inadequate exposure to sunlight
- Defective intestinal absorption: diseases of the small intestine
  (celiac disease, Crohn disease), liver disease (reduced hydroxylation of vitamin D), biliary obstruction (bile salts help absorb vitamin D), chronic pancreatic insufficiency

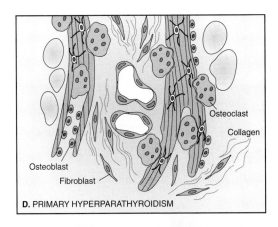

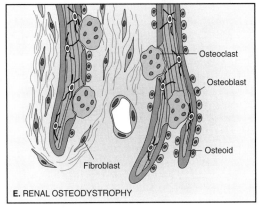

FIGURE 26-5

(*continued*) D: Primary hyperparathyroidism. The lamellar bone trabeculae are actively resorbed by numerous osteoclasts that bore into
each trabecula. Osteoblastic activity also is pronounced. The marrow
is replaced by fibrous tissue adjacent to the trabeculae. E: Renal
osteodystrophy. The morphological appearance is similar to that of
primary hyperparathyroidism, except that prominent osteoid covers
the trabeculae. (From Rubin E, Gorstein F, Rubin R, et al. Rubin's
Pathology, 4th ed. Philadelphia: Lippincott Williams & Wilkins,
2005, p. 1335.)

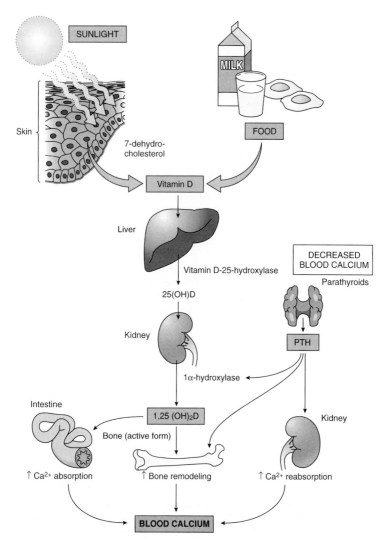

F I G U R E   26-6
Metabolism of vitamin D and the regulation of blood calcium. (From
Rubin E, Gorstein F, Rubin R, et al. Rubin's Pathology, 4th ed. Phila-
delphia: Lippincott Williams & Wilkins, 2005, p. 1339.)

Heritable syndromes that disturb vitamin D metabolism include:

- *Vitamin D-dependent rickets type I*: autosomal recessive; deficiency of 1α-hydroxylase activity; elevated levels of serum PTH and alkaline phosphatase; treated by $1,25(OH)_2D$ administration
- *Vitamin D-dependent rickets type II*: autosomal recessive; mutations of the vitamin D receptor; elevated levels of serum $1,25(OH)_2D$; treated by repeated intravenous calcium administration

Acquired alterations in vitamin D metabolism include defective renal 1α-hydroxylation and end-organ insensitivity.

Impaired reabsorption of phosphate by the proximal renal tubules may also result in both rickets and osteomalacia. Syndromes that lead to impaired phosphate reabsorption include the following:

- *X-linked hypophosphatemia*: autosomal dominant; most common type of hereditary rickets; mutations in *PHEX* gene on Xp22; impaired transport of phosphate across the luminal membrane of proximal renal tubular cells; patients have wide osteoid seams and hypomineralized areas surrounded by osteocytes, termed "halos"; treated with lifelong phosphate and $1,25(OH)_2D$
- *Fanconi syndromes*: includes Wilson disease, glycogen-storage diseases, tyrosinemia, among others; disease of proximal renal tubule that causes wasting of phosphate, glucose, bicarbonate, and amino acids
- *Tumor-associated osteomalacia*: phosphate-wasting syndrome associated with benign and malignant tumors of soft tissue and bone

Finally, rickets and osteomalacia can occur with *defective mineralization* of bone. *Hypophosphatasia* is a rare autosomal recessive disease associated with low activity of alkaline phosphatase in the bones and blood, leading to defective mineralization. In addition, bisphosphonates and high dose fluoride may interfere with bone mineralization.

Osteomalacia demonstrates an osteopenic radiographic pattern and can result in vertebral compression fractures due to decreased bone thickness, similar to osteoporosis. In patients with rickets, the growth plate becomes conspicuously thickened, irregular, and lobulated because of the lack of osteoclastic activity. The zones of proliferating cartilage are distorted, and disordered chondrocytes are separated by small amounts of matrix. The epiphysis becomes flared and cup-shaped.

Adult patients with osteomalacia may have nonspecific complaints, including muscle weakness or diffuse aches and pains. Occasionally, patients present with an acute fracture of the femoral neck, pubic ramus, spine, or ribs.

Children with rickets are apathetic, irritable, and have a short attention span. Flattening of the skull (frontal bossing), delayed dentition, an outward curvature of the sternum ("pigeon breast"), beading of the costochondral junction, weak muscles, and bowing of the arms are present. Potbelly may be present due to weak abdominal musculature. Frequent fractures may occur.

Osteoporosis

Osteoporosis is characterized by a decreased mass of normally mineralized bone to a point that it no longer provides adequate mechanical support. Osteoporosis may be due to a number of causes, but demonstrates the similar outcome of loss of skeletal mass with eventual fracture. Although reduced in volume, the remaining bone contains a normal ratio of mineralized to nonmineralized (osteoid) matrix.

Under normal conditions, bone mass peaks between the ages of 25 and 35 years and declines thereafter. African Americans have a reduced risk of osteoporosis due to higher peak bone mass, whereas women are more prone to osteoporosis due to both menopause and aging. Fractures most commonly affect the neck and intertrochanteric region of the femur (hip fracture), the vertebral bodies, and the distal radius (Colles fracture). By 80 years of age, 15% of Americans have experienced a hip fracture due to osteoporosis.

Regardless of the cause, osteoporosis reflects enhanced bone resorption relative to formation. Throughout life, bone is constantly remodeled via a cycle of osteoclast resorption and osteoblast bone synthesis. Within aging, less bone is replaced following resorption, leading to a net deficit over time. Osteoporosis may be described as primary (idiopathic) or secondary (due to identified underlying disorders).

Changes are most conspicuous in the spine, where loss of cancellous bone leads to vertebral deformation and compression fractures. Following each compression fracture, the spine becomes shorter and the patient develops kyphosis (Dowager's hump). Microscopically, osteoporosis demonstrates decreased thickness of the cortex and reduction in the number and size of trabeculae of the coarse cancellous bone. Senile osteoporosis contains reduced trabecular thickness, whereas postmenopausal osteoporosis contains disrupted connections between trabeculae.

Prevention of osteoporosis may be achieved by estrogen therapy following menopause, although this harbors an increased risk of breast and endometrial cancer development. Bisphosphonates have also been recently used to prevent osteoporosis.

Primary Osteoporosis

Primary osteoporosis is the most common form of osteoporosis and occurs in postmenopausal women (type 1) and elderly persons of both sexes (type 2). Figure 26-7 illustrates the pathogenesis of this form of osteoporosis.

Type 1 primary osteoporosis is due to an absolute increase in osteoclast activity, principally affects postmenopausal women, and is a direct result of estrogen withdrawal. Estrogen has been proposed to mediate osteoclast activity through the actions of cytokines produced by the marrow stroma. Typically, postmenopausal osteoporosis becomes recognizable within 10 years following menopause.

Type 2 primary osteoporosis (*senile osteoporosis*) occurs in patients older than 70 years of age, affects both sexes, and is caused by attenuated osteoblast function. Causes of type 2 primary osteoporosis include the following:

- Genetic factors: related to the formation of peak bone mass
- Calcium intake: controversial; recommended daily intake is 800 mg/day

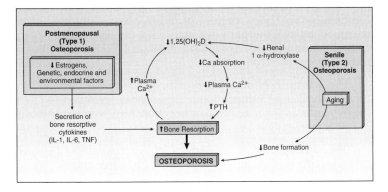

F I G U R E   26-7
Pathogenesis of primary osteoporosis. (From Rubin E, Gorstein F, Rubin R, et al. Rubin's Pathology, 4th ed. Philadelphia: Lippincott Williams & Wilkins, 2005, p. 1337.)

- Calcium absorption and vitamin D: the active form of vitamin D, $1,25(OH)_2D$, promotes calcium absorption in the intestine; reduced levels of active vitamin D is caused by decreased activity of 1α-hydroxylase in the kidney due to reduced PTH actions; see Figure 26-7
- Exercise: physical activity maintains bone mass
- Environmental factors: smoking in women increases osteoporosis

Secondary Osteoporosis

Secondary osteoporosis occurs in association with a variety of etiologic factors, including:

- Endocrine conditions: excess corticosteroids (inhibit osteoblastic activity), estrogen deficiency
- Hyperparathyroidism: increased osteoclastic activity
- Hyperthyroidism: accelerated bone turnover and increased osteoclastic activity
- Hypogonadism: deficiency in estrogen or anabolic androgens; Klinefelter syndrome, Turner syndrome
- Hematological malignancies: multiple myeloma may secrete osteoclast-activating factor
- Malabsorption: gastrointestinal and hepatic disease; loss of calcium, phosphate, and vitamin D from gastrointestinal tract
- Alcoholism: direct inhibitor of osteoblasts; may inhibit calcium absorption

Primary Hyperparathyroidism

Primary hyperparathyroidism results in generalized bone resorption due to inappropriate secretion of PTH, which is relatively uncommon today. Ninety percent of primary hyperparathyroidism is caused by parathyroid adenomas, and the remaining 10% is caused by parathyroid hyperplasia. Elevated PTH has multiple effects, including the following:

- Osteoclastic bone resorption
- Renal calcium reabsorption and phosphate excretion
- Enhances intestinal calcium absorption by increasing synthesis of active vitamin D

The histological changes of primary hyperparathyroidism are called osteitis fibrosa and are represented by three stages:

- Early stage: osteoclasts advance into the cortex; collagen deposited adjacent to trabeculae
- Osteitis fibrosa: trabecular bone resorbed; marrow replaced by loose fibrosis, hemosiderin-laden macrophages, areas of hemorrhage, and reactive woven bone

- Osteitis fibrosa cystica: cystic degeneration; presence of many giant cells

Skeletal radiographs of most patients with primary hyperparathyroidism are normal. However, some radiographs reveal mottled bone cortices, with an irregular frayed surface of the skull, tufts of the terminal digits, and shafts of the metacarpals. Multiple localized lytic lesions, which represent hemorrhagic cysts or masses of fibrous tissue ("brown tumor"), may be present. Resorption around tooth sockets may occur.

The clinical picture is represented by "stones" (kidney stones), "bones" (skeletal changes), "moans" (psychiatric depression), and "groans" (gastrointestinal irregularities). Low serum phosphate and high serum calcium levels are characteristic. Treatment of primary hyperparathyroidism involves surgical resection of one or more parathyroid glands.

Renal Osteodystrophy

Renal osteodystrophy occurs in the context of chronic renal failure in patients on long-term dialysis. The pathophysiology involves secondary hyperparathyroidism with osteoclastic resorption of bone. Ultimately, reduced glomerular filtration, active vitamin D deficiency, and decreased intestinal calcium absorption in part cause hyperphosphatemia and hypocalcemia.

Renal osteodystrophy is characterized by varying degrees of osteomalacia, osteitis fibrosa, osteomalacia, osteosclerosis, and adynamic bone disease. Hyperphosphatemic patients may develop metastatic calcification at various sites in the body.

Paget Disease of Bone

Paget disease is a chronic condition that is characterized by disorganized remodeling of bone. Paget disease affects men and women older than 60 years of age and may affect as much as 3% of the population.

Although the etiology of Paget disease is unclear, a slow virus has been hypothesized to serve an etiologic role in that the marrow of these patients contains paramyxovirus nucleocapsid transcripts and osteoclasts demonstrate nuclear inclusions. A familial form of Paget disease has been linked to chromosome 18q21–22.

Paget disease may involve one or many bones and commonly affects the axial skeleton, including the spine, skull, and pelvis. Initially, excessive bone resorption results in lytic lesions, which is followed by disorganized and excessive bone formation. The lesions of Paget disease evolve through three stages, although various lesions may be at different stages at a given point in time:

- "Hot" or osteoclastic resorptive stage: sharply defined, flame- or wedge-shaped lytic lesion of the cortex; widespread osteolysis with marrow fibrosis and dilation of the marrow sinusoids
- Mixed stage of osteoblastic and osteoclastic activity: radiographically, bones appear larger than normal (only seen otherwise in fibrous dysplasia); cortex thickened; cancellous bone accentuated; "picture-frame" appearance of vertebrae
- "Cold" or burnt-out stage: radiologically thickened and disordered bones; little cellular activity; mosaic pattern of bone

In general, the osteoclast functions abnormally in Paget disease and appears to be hyperresponsive to vitamin D and the growth factor RANK-L. The nuclei of osteoclasts may contain nuclear inclusions. Osteoclasts may have more than 100 nuclei (as compared to approximately 12 in the normal osteoclast).

The histology of Paget disease is severe osteitis fibrosa, with peritrabecular marrow fibrosis, irregular trabeculae, woven bone collagen, numerous osteoclasts, and large active osteoblasts. Over time, lesions burn out and appear histologically as islands of irregular bone separated by prominent cement lines, which resembles a jigsaw puzzle.

Patients with Paget disease may have a number of findings, including the following:

- Pain over affected bone possibly due to microfractures, stimulation of free nerve endings
- Skull alterations: lysis of the frontal and parietal bones; thickening of the frontal and occipital bones; hearing loss due to ossicle involvement; misshapen jaws; loss of teeth
- Pagetic steal: blood shunted from brain to bones resulting in light-headedness
- High-output cardiac failure: due to blood shunting
- Bone fractures and secondary osteoarthritis
- Sarcomatous transformation: less than 1% of cases; usually in femur, humerus, or pelvis
- Giant cell tumor: increased osteoclastic response with associated fibroblastic response; radiation therapy curative

In addition, they have markedly elevated serum alkaline phosphatase levels but normal serum calcium and phosphorus levels.

Nonneoplastic Lesions of Bone

Nonneoplastic lesions of bone are outlined in Table 26-3.

Fibrous Dysplasia

Fibrous dysplasia is a developmental abnormality of the skeleton characterized by a disorganized mixture of fibrous and osseous

Table 26-3
Nonneoplastic Lesions of Bone

Tumor	Age (years)	Location	Radiology	Histology
Nonossifying fibroma	4–10	Metaphysis of femur, tibia	Central lucency with surrounding scalloped margin	Bland spindle cells in a whorled pattern with giant cells
Solitary bone cyst	<20	Metaphysis of proximal humerus and femur	Thin, well-marginated, lucent	Lined by giant cells, hemosiderin-laden macrophages, reactive bone
Aneurysmal bone cyst	10–20	Long bones, vertebrae	Fluid-fluid levels	Granulation tissue containing multinucleated giant cells, osteoid trabeculae

elements in the interior of affected bones. Cases may be involve a single bone (monostotic), multiple bones (polyostotic), or be associated with skin pigmentation and endocrine dysfunction (McCune-Albright syndrome). Fibrous dysplasia is caused by activating mutations in the α-subunit of the stimulatory guanine nucleotide-binding protein ($G_s\alpha$), which leads to activation of adenylyl cyclase and increased levels of cyclic AMP.

The three types of fibrous dysplasia are as follows:

- *Monostotic fibrous dysplasia*: most common form; second and third decades; most common in proximal femur, tibia, ribs, and facial bones
- *Polyostotic fibrous dysplasia*: usually occurs in childhood; female predominance; often associated with fractures, limb deformities, limb-length discrepancies
- *McCune-Albright syndrome*: usually occurs in females during childhood; characterized by endocrine dysfunction (acromegaly, Cushing syndrome, hyperthyroidism) and pigmented café-au-lait spots that do not cross the midline; may cause short stature and precocious puberty

The radiographic lesions consist of a lucent ground-glass appearance with well-marginated borders and a thin cortex. Involved bones may be ballooned, deformed, or enlarged. Microscopically, benign fibroblastic tissue is arranged in a loose, whorled pattern. Irregularly arranged spicules of woven bone that lack osteoblastic rims are embedded in this fibroblastic tissue and are termed "Chinese figures." In 10% of cases, islands of hyaline cartilage may be present. In less than 1% of cases, malignant degeneration to an osteosarcoma, chondrosarcoma, or fibrosarcoma may occur, although these cases have been associated with prior radiation exposure.

Treatment involves curettage, fracture repair, and prevention of deformities.

Nonossifying Fibroma

Nonossifying fibroma is common and affects as many as 25% of all children between 4 and 10 years of age, after which it regresses. The lesion is solitary and occurs in the metaphysis of a long bone, most commonly the tibia or femur. Radiologically, nonossifying fibromas demonstrate a cortical, eccentric position and well-demarcated, central lucent zones surrounded by scalloped, sclerotic margins. On gross examination, the lesion appears granular and dark red to brown. Microscopically, bland spindle cells are arranged in an interlacing, whorled pattern with multinucleated giant cells and macrophages. Rarely, these lesions may cause pain or fracture.

Solitary (Unicameral) Bone Cyst

Solitary bone cysts are fluid-filled, unilocular lesions with a male predilection. These lesions classically occur in the proximal humerus or femur, often within the metaphysis. They grow via slow expansion of the fluid cavity, which results in the resorption of bone via osteoclasts. Radiologically, solitary bone cysts appear as thin, well-marginated, radiolucent bone lesions, which are never greater in diameter than the growth plate. These lesions are prone to fracture. Microscopically, cysts are lined by fibrous tissue, scattered giant cells, hemosiderin-laden macrophages, chronic inflammatory cells, and reactive bone. The cysts are filled with amorphous proteinaceous material.

Aneurysmal Bone Cyst

Aneurysmal bone cyst (ABC) is a rapidly growing, expansive, hyperemic lesion that occurs in children and young adults and is most frequent in the long bones and vertebral column. By magnetic resonance imaging (MRI), ABCs demonstrate fluid-fluid levels between red blood cells and plasma contained within the lesion. The periosteum surrounding an ABC is ballooned, but intact. On cut section, ABCs are spongy and contain blood and blood clots. The walls of the lesion are formed by granulation tissue containing multinucleated giant cells and occasional osteoid trabeculae. Patients often have pain and swelling overlying the lesion. Occasionally, ABCs may rupture and result in local hemorrhage. Treatment involves extraperiosteal excision and curettage.

Bone Tumors

Benign bone tumors are uncommon (Table 26-2). The majority of benign lesions occur at the metaphysis, and 80% of lesions occur sat the distal femur or the proximal tibia. Figure 26-8 illustrates the common locations of several benign and malignant bone tumors.

Benign Tumors of Bone

Benign tumors of bone are outlined in Table 26-4.

Osteoid Osteoma

Osteoid osteoma is a small, painful lesion composed of central osseous tissue (the nidus), often in the diaphysis of the tubular bones of the lower extremity, and surrounded by a halo of reactive bone. This lesion occurs more commonly in boys and occurs between the ages of 5 and 25 years. Grossly, osteoid osteoma is a spherical, hyperemic lesion up to 1 cm in diameter, which is softer than the surrounding bone. Microscopically, this lesion contains

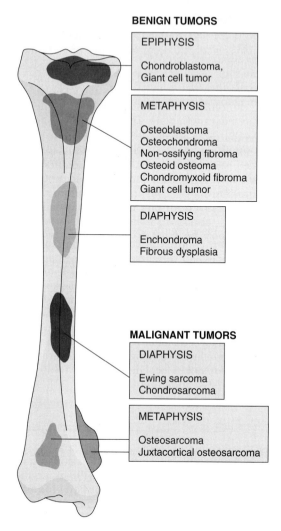

BENIGN TUMORS

EPIPHYSIS

Chondroblastoma,
Giant cell tumor

METAPHYSIS

Osteoblastoma
Osteochondroma
Non-ossifying fibroma
Osteoid osteoma
Chondromyxoid fibroma
Giant cell tumor

DIAPHYSIS

Enchondroma
Fibrous dysplasia

MALIGNANT TUMORS

DIAPHYSIS

Ewing sarcoma
Chondrosarcoma

METAPHYSIS

Osteosarcoma
Juxtacortical osteosarcoma

FIGURE 26-8
Location of primary bone tumors in long tubular bones. (From Rubin
E, Gorstein F, Rubin R, et al. Rubin's Pathology, 4th ed. Philadelphia:
Lippincott Williams & Wilkins, 2005, p. 1351.)

Table 26-4

Benign Tumors of Bone

Tumor	Age (years)	Location	Radiology	Histology
Osteochondroma	<30	Metaphysis of knee	Mushroom shaped stalk with cartilaginous cap and under lying cortical bone	Disorganized cartilage; medullary cavity of lesion and native bone communicate
Osteoid osteoma	5–25	Diaphysis of long tubular bones of the lower leg	Radiolucent with surrounding reactive/sclerotic bone	Spherical lesion; central nidus of trabecular bone with surrounding osteoblasts and vascular stroma
Osteoblastoma	10–35	Spine and long bones	Purely radiolucent lesion	Similar to osteoid osteoma
Chondroma	Any age	Metacarpals and phalanges of the hand	Well-delineated radiolucent area, +/– stippled calcifications	Well-differentiated cartilage with sparse (enchondroma) chondrocytes
Chondroblastoma	5–25	Upper femur, tibia, humerus; often para-articular	Eccentric, radiolucent appearance with sharp borders-	Sheets of round-to-polygonal chondrocytes in a primitive matrix
Chondromyxoid fibroma	<30	Femur or tibia	Eccentric, radiolucent appearance with scalloped border of sclerotic bone	Sparsely cellular lobules with spindle and stellate cells and multinucleated giant cells in chondroid or myxoid matrix
Giant cell tumor of bone (may rarely be malignant)	20–40	Junction of metaphysis and epiphysis; knee region; sacrum	Multilocular radiolucent "soap bubble" appearance	Giant cells in a background of mononuclear "stromal" cells and vascularized stroma

thin, irregular, trabeculae within a cellular granulation tissue containing osteoblasts and osteoclasts. The trabeculae are more mature in the center. Patients classically report nocturnal pain that is exacerbated by alcohol and relieved by aspirin, mediated by prostaglandins produced by the tumor. These lesions are readily enucleated.

Osteoblastoma

Osteoblastoma is similar to osteoid osteoma histologically but is larger and not accompanied by nocturnal pain. This lesion occurs in people between 10 and 35 years of age, has no sex predilection, and mainly affects the spine and long bones. Radiographically, this lesion is purely radiolucent with only a shell of surrounding bone. These lesions are cured by curettage or resection, depending on the size.

Chondromas

Chondromas are slow-growing tumors composed of well-differentiated hyaline cartilage. Chondromas may be single or multiple, with multiple lesions associated with enchondromatosis or Maffucci syndrome. When these lesions occur within bone, they are termed *enchrondromas*. Chondromas typically affect the metacarpals and phalanges of the hand, with some lesions affecting any of the other tubular bones. Radiologically, the lesion appears as a small, well-delimited radiolucent area with occasional stippled calcifications. Grossly, the lesion appears semitranslucent with or without a few calcified areas. Microscopically, it is composed of well-differentiated cartilage with sparse chondrocytes. Most cases are asymptomatic; painful lesions are treated with curettage and bone grafting.

Chondroblastoma

Chondroblastoma is a slow-growing lesion that occurs in people between 5 and 25 years of age; has a male predilection; and often affects the upper femur, tibia, and humerus. Radiologically, chondroblastoma demonstrates an eccentric, radiolucent appearance with sharply delimited borders. Chondroblastoma typically occurs in a para-articular area. Grossly, the tumor is soft with scattered gray or hemorrhagic areas. Microscopically, primitive chondroblasts form sheets of round-to-polyhedral cells with well-defined cytoplasmic borders and large, ovoid nuclei that often have nuclear grooves. Variable amounts of calcification occur. Osteoclasts often participate in bone resorption. Patients often present with joint symptoms, including pain, mild swelling, and functional limitation of joint movement. Treatment involves curettage. A small number of lesions may recur.

Chondromyxoid Fibroma

Chondromyxoid fibroma is a cartilagelike tumor of bone that occurs in the femur or tibia of children and young adults. Radiologically, this lesion appears as an eccentric, radiolucent defect with a thin scalloped border of sclerotic bone. Grossly, the tumor is firm, lobulated, gray-white or gray-yellow and appears to replace and thin the cortex. Microscopically, the lobules are sparsely cellular and show spindle and stellate cells and multinucleated giant cells embedded within a chondroid or myxoid matrix. Bands of plump, round, mononuclear cells and multinucleated cells separate the lobules. These lesions are best treated by surgical excision, due to their high propensity for recurrence following curettage.

Giant Cell Tumor of Bone

Giant cell tumor of bone is a locally aggressive neoplasm that most commonly affects the junction of the metaphysis and epiphysis surrounding the knee (distal femur and proximal tibia) and may affect the radius, humerus, sacrum, and fibula. The disorder most frequently affects people between the third to fourth decades and may occasionally occur in the elderly secondary to radiation.

This slow-growing, lytic lesion elicits a surrounding periosteal reaction and thin rim of bone. Radiologically, these lesions are radiolucent and have a multiloculated, or "soap bubble" appearance. Grossly, the lesion is circumscribed, light brown, soft, lacks calcification, and appears like a sponge filled with blood. Cystic and necrotic areas may be present. Occasionally, the lesion may penetrate the cortex. Microscopically, multinucleated, osteoclastic giant cells are present in a background of plump mononuclear ("stromal") cells with large nuclei and rich vasculature. Diffuse interstitial hemorrhage is common.

Giant cell tumor presents with pain involving the joint adjacent to the lesion. Microfractures and pathologic fractures may occur. Giant cell tumor of bone rarely metastasizes, but when this occurs (usually after curettage), it may be secondary to surgical dislodgement. Metastatic lesions, often to the lungs, may be readily resected. Rarely, sarcomatous transformation may occur. The lifespan of patients with giant cell tumor of bone is normal.

Malignant Tumors of Bone

The most common tumors of bone are metastatic lesions that reach the skeleton often by hematogenous spread (Table 26-5). These lesions may be osteolytic (bone destruction) or osteoblastic (bone forming), although the majority of metastases have features of both elements. Primary malignant bone tumors are less common.

Table 26-5
Malignant Tumors of Bone

Tumor	Age (years)	Location	Radiology	Histology
Osteosarcoma	10–20	Knee and proximal humerus	Codman triangle (incomplete rim of reactive bone)	Malignant osteoblast-like cells producing haphazard woven bone; +/− pleomorphic giant cells
Chondrosarcoma Central	Middle age	Medullary cavity of pelvis, ribs and long bones	Poorly defined borders, thickened shaft, perforated cortex	Intertrabecular spaces filled by neoplastic cartilage
Peripheral	>20	Cartilaginous cap of an osteochondroma	Radiopacities representing ossification or calcification	Large bosselated mass that surrounds the base of an osteochondroma and invades bone
Juxtacortical	Middle age	Outer surface of cortex on metaphysis of long bones	Translucent or focally calcified	Malignant cells in various stages of maturity; zones of calcification
Ewing sarcoma	<20	Midshaft or metaphysis of humerus, tibia, or femur	Lytic lesion with indistinct border between tumor and bone	Sheets of closely packed, round cells with little cytoplasm
Multiple myeloma	Elderly	Skull, ribs, pelvis, and femur	Punched-out lytic lesions	Sheets of plasma cells in varying stages of maturation; +/− amyloid

Osteosarcoma

Osteosarcoma, or osteogenic sarcoma, is the most common primary malignant bone tumor (20% of all bone tumors) and is characterized by the formation of bone by the malignant cells.

This tumor occurs most commonly between the ages of 10 and 20 years, demonstrates a male predilection, and more commonly affects tall persons. If osteosarcoma arises in older patients, it is often a result of Paget disease or radiation exposure. Two thirds of cases have mutations in the retinoblastoma (Rb) gene, and many also harbor lesions of the p53 gene.

The most common locations of osteosarcoma are the knee (lower femur, upper tibia, or fibula) or the proximal humerus. Radiologically, "Codman's triangle" may be evident, which appears as a shell of bone intersecting the cortex at one end and open at the other end and is caused by a lifting of the periosteum from the cortical surface by the tumor. Surrounding this site, the periosteal reaction may form a sunburst pattern on imaging.

Grossly, the tumor may appear hemorrhagic, cystic, soft, or bony. Microscopically, highly malignant cells with osteoblastic differentiation produce haphazardly arranged woven bone. Foci of malignant cartilage or pleomorphic giant cells may be present.

Patients often present with mild or intermittent pain around the involved area, which may become swollen. The serum alkaline phosphatase is increased in 50% of patients. Hematogenous spread to the lungs results in rapid clinical deterioration and death. Treatment involves chemotherapy and limb-sparing surgery.

A rare variant of osteosarcoma is *juxtacortical osteosarcoma*, which occurs on the periosteal surface of the bone, affects patients older than 25 years, and is more common in women. These lesions have a favorable prognosis and are treated by surgical excision.

Chondrosarcoma

Chondrosarcoma is a malignant tumor that arises from cartilage cells and produces cartilage throughout its evolution, usually occurs in the fourth to sixth decades, and is more common in men. Chondrosarcoma is the second most common primary malignant bone tumor. Although most patients have no preexisting lesions, a subset have enchondromas, solitary osteochondroma, or hereditary multiple osteochondromas.

Chondrosarcoma may be described as the following:

- Central chondrosarcoma: middle-aged men; medullary cavity of pelvic bones, ribs, and long bones; radiologically has poorly defined borders, thickened shaft, and perforated cortex; stippled radiopacities (calcifications); neoplastic cartilage compressed within bone with hemorrhage, necrosis, and cystic change; causes deep pain

- Peripheral chondrosarcoma: people older than 20 years of age; outside the bone in the pelvis, femur, vertebrae, sacrum, humerus, and other long bones; radiologically has radiopacities of calcification; appears as a large bosselated mass that surrounds the base of an osteochondroma and invades the bone; causes pain and local symptoms
- Juxtacortical chondrosarcoma: middle-aged men; outer surface of the cortex in the metaphysis of long bones; radiologically translucent or with focal calcification; malignant cartilage cells in various stages of maturation; zones of calcification; association of histologic grade with prognosis

  - ➤ Trisomy 7: chondrosarcoma
  - ➤ Rearrangement of short arm of chromosome 17: high-grade chondrosarcoma
  - ➤ 12q13 Alterations: myxoid features
  - ➤ Translocation (9;22)(q31;q12): extraskeletal myxoid chondrosarcoma

  Wide excision is the usual treatment.

Ewing Sarcoma

Ewing sarcoma (EWS) is a disease of young persons; two thirds of patients presenting are under the age of 20 years. EWS affects the midshaft or metaphysis of long bones, especially the humerus, tibia, and femur, and its distribution tends to parallel the distribution of red marrow.

It has been suggested that EWS arises from immature mesenchymal elements or primitive marrow elements. The underlying genetic defect is a reciprocal translocation between chromosomes 11 and 22, t(11;22)p(13;q12), which results in the formation of a transcription factor formed by the fusion of the *EWS* gene to the *FLI-1* gene.

The radiologic appearance is variable but generally demonstrates a lytic lesion with an indistinct border between the tumor and the surrounding bone. Grossly, these tumors are soft, gray-white, and demonstrate regions of hemorrhage and necrosis. Microscopically, sheets of closely packed small cells with scant cytoplasm infiltrate the cortical bone in a diffuse or nodular pattern. Fibrous bands separate the cells into nests. Occasionally, rosettes may be identified. Mitotic figures are infrequent. The tumor cells contain intracytoplasmic glycogen, which may be identified by PAS stain.

Patients often present with mild pain and swelling of the affected area. Fever and leukocytosis may be present. Treatment involves a combination of chemotherapy, radiation, and surgery.

Multiple Myeloma

Multiple myeloma is a malignant disease of plasma cells that affects elderly persons, more commonly men. Bone lesions in multiple myeloma (the diffuse form of the disease) or in plasmacytoma (the localized form of the disease) appear as punched-out, lytic lesions that often involve the skull, spine, ribs, pelvis, and femur. Microscopically, sheets of plasma cells in varying stages of maturity are present. Some cases may contain associated amyloid produced by the neoplastic cells. Plasmacytoma has a 60% 5-year survival, whereas multiple myeloma has a median survival of only 32 months despite radiation and chemotherapy.

Langerhans Cell Histiocytosis (LCH)

LCH encompasses three diseases that are characterized by the clonal proliferation of Langerhans cells (tissue macrophages) in various tissues.

Bone lesions in LCH appear as punched-out lytic defects with little to no reactive bone formation. These lesions often occur in the metaphysis or diaphysis of long bones, or in flat bones such as the skull. These lesions may lead to fractures or periosteal callus formation. LCH is characterized by collections of large, phagocytic cells with pale, eosinophilic, foamy cytoplasm and convoluted nuclei.

JOINTS

Normal Anatomy and Histology

A joint (articulation) is a union between two or more bones, whose construction varies with the function of the joint. Synovial (diarthrodial) joints are movable joints lined by synovial membrane. A synarthrosis is a joint that demonstrates minimal movement.

Synarthroses are subclassified as follows:

- Symphysis: articulation joined by fibrocartilage and firm ligaments (symphysis pubis)
- Synchondrosis: at the ends of bones; contains articular cartilage but no synovium or significant joint cavity (sternal manubrial joint)
- Syndesmosis: articulation joined by fibrous tissue without cartilage (cranial sutures)
- Synostosis: pathological bony bridge between bones (ankylosing spondylitis)

Synovial joints are subclassified as uniaxial, biaxial, polyaxial, and plane joints based on the type of movement they permit.

Joints are buffered by the surrounding muscles, joint deformation, and synovial fluid. Synovial joints are lined by synovium, which rests directly on the subsynovial tissue without an intervening basement membrane. The synovium regulates diffusion in and out of the joint, ingestion of debris, secretion of hyaluronate, and lubrication of the joints by secretion of glycoproteins. The synovial fluid serves as the main source of nourishment for chondrocytes of the articular cartilage.

The articular cartilage is hyaline cartilage that covers the ends of the bones. Grossly, articular cartilage appears glistening, smooth, white, and semirigid. A notable feature of the articular cartilage is the tidemark, which separates mineralized and unmineralized cartilage, and appears as an undulating blue line. Cartilage cells are renewed at the tidemark, and recently formed chondrocytes migrate upwards from the tidemark to the joint surface.

Inflammatory Joint Diseases

Osteoarthritis

Osteoarthritis (OA; degenerative joint disease) is a slowly progressive destruction of the articular cartilage of weight-bearing joints and fingers of elderly persons, as well as younger persons subjected to trauma. OA is the most common form of joint disease. The prevalence of primary OA increases with age, and as many as 85% of persons 75 years of age or older show evidence of this disease. Following 55 years of age, women are more commonly affected.

OA may be primary (due to an intrinsic defect in the joint cartilage) or secondary (due to a known underlying cause). A variety of factors underlie its pathogenesis, including abnormal force on the cartilage, biochemical abnormalities, and rarely mutations in the type II collagen gene in familial variants.

The progressive destruction of articular cartilage in OA results in joint narrowing, subchondral bone thickening, and ultimately a nonfunctioning, painful joint. The most commonly affected bones in OA include the proximal and distal interphalangeal joints of the upper extremity, knees and hips, and the cervical and lumbar segments of the spine. Radiologically, OA is manifested by the following:

- Narrowing of the joint space: loss of articular cartilage
- Increased thickness of the subchondral bone
- Subchondral bone cyst: cracking of the eroded bone surface allowing synovial fluid to enter the subchondral bone marrow
- Osteophytes: large peripheral growths of bone and cartilage

Grossly, joints with OA demonstrate thick, shiny, smooth exposed areas of eroded cartilage with exposed subchondral bone (termed eburnation). Microscopically, the cartilage may appear frayed and the tidemark thickened.

Patients experience various symptoms, including enlarged, tender, boggy joints with crepitus, deep, achy joint pain relieved by rest, or short periods of stiffness in the morning or after periods of minimal activity. Treatment involves exercise, weight loss, anti-inflammatory medications, and joint replacement if the disease is debilitating.

Rheumatoid Arthritis

Rheumatoid arthritis (RA) is a systemic, chronic inflammatory disease that manifests with symmetric, bilateral chronic polyarthritis that is often punctuated by remissions and exacerbations. The onset is usually in the third or fourth decades, and the prevalence increases with age. The regions most commonly affected include the proximal interphalangeal and metacarpophalangeal joints of the hands, elbows, knees, ankles, and spine. The prevalence is higher in women.

A variety of factors may contribute to the pathogenesis of RA, including the following:

- Association with HLA-DR allele expression (DR4, DR1, DE10, DR14) that shares a common epitope with the hypervariable segment of the *HLA-DRB1* gene
- Humoral immunity: production of rheumatoid factor in 80% of patients, which represents primarily immunoglobulin (Ig) M antibodies directed against the Fc fragment of IgG (associated with a worse prognosis); lymphocytes and plasma cells within the synovium
- Cellular immunity: T lymphocytes in the synovium produce cytokines
- Infectious agents: most patients develop antibodies against a nuclear antigen in EBV-infected B cells termed the *RANA antigen*
- Local factors: decreased synovial cell response to glucocorticoids

The early pathological changes of RA consist of synovial edema, increased vascularity fibrin exudate in the joint space (rice bodies), and an infiltrate of plasma cells, lymphocytes, and macrophages in the subsynovial tissue. Rheumatoid nodules may be present in extraarticular locations and consist of a core of fibrinoid necrosis surrounded by palisading macrophages, which are then surrounded by lymphocytes. Rheumatoid nodules are not specific for RA and may be found in lupus and rheumatic fever.

Over time, the synovium undergoes hyperplasia to form a three- to eight-cell layer thick lining thrown into numerous villi and frondlike folds that fill the peripheral recesses of the joint. This synovium creeps over the surface of the articular cartilage and is termed a *pannus*. The pannus erodes the articular cartilage and adjacent bone, probably through the action of secreted collagenase. The characteristic bone loss is juxtaarticular, immediately adjacent to both sides of the joint. Over time, the joint may be destroyed and undergo fibrous fusion, termed *ankylosis*. The synovial fluid demonstrates a massive increase in volume, increased turbidity, decreased viscosity, and increased inflammatory cells.

The clinical diagnosis of RA is complicated and is based on a number of criteria. The onset of RA may be acute, slowly progressing, or insidious. Most patients describe slowly developing fatigue, weight loss, weakness, and vague musculoskeletal discomfort that eventually localizes to the involved joints. Diseased joints are warm, swollen, and painful, which is worsened by motion and most severe after times of disuse. Over time, patients may develop joint deformities, such as ulnar deviation of the fingers and a characteristic "swan-neck" appearance of the extended fingers, and an increased risk of infection.

Spondyloarthropathies

Spondyloarthropathies encompass a variety of disorders, including ankylosing spondylitis, Reiter syndrome, psoriatic arthritis, and arthritis associated with inflammatory bowel disease. These conditions share a number of features, including the following:

- Seronegativity for rheumatoid factor
- Association with MHC class I antigens, especially HLA-B27
- Sacroiliac and vertebral involvement
- Asymmetric involvement of only few peripheral joints
- Tendency to inflammation of periarticular tendons and fascia
- Systemic involvement of other organs, especially uveitis, carditis, and aortitis
- Preferential onset in young men

Ankylosing Spondylitis

Ankylosing spondylitis begins at the sacroiliac joints bilaterally and then ascends the spinal column, with ultimate destruction of these joints after which the spine becomes fused. Approximately 30% of patients have an asymmetric peripheral arthritis and systemic manifestations. Rarely, AA amyloidosis, uremia, and cardiac disease may occur. The classic patient is a male about age 20, and over 90% of patients are positive for HLA-B27.

Reiter Syndrome

Reiter syndrome is a triad of seronegative polyarthritis, conjunctivitis, and nonspecific urethritis. This disorder occurs almost entirely in men, follows a venereal exposure or bacillary dysentery, and has a strong HLA-B27 association. Half of all patients develop mucocutaneous lesions on the palms, soles, and trunk. In the majority of cases, the disease resolves, although 20% of patients develop progressive arthritis, including ankylosing spondylitis.

Juvenile Arthritis (Still Disease)

Juvenile arthritis (Still disease) refers to a number of different chronic arthritic conditions in children, who may eventually develop ankylosing spondylitis, psoriatic arthritis, and other connective tissue diseases.

Gout

Gout is caused by an increased serum uric acid level (hyperuricemia) and, in a subset of patients, deposition of urate crystals in the joints and kidneys. Gout can be primary (idiopathic) or secondary (leukemia, lymphoma). The majority of cases affect men and demonstrate an onset in the fifth decade.

Uric acid, which is fairly insoluble, is normally derived from the diet or synthesized de novo and is converted to the soluble allantoin by urate oxidase (Fig. 26-9). Uric acid is eliminated only in the urine. Increased uric acid levels are a result of the following:

- Overproduction of purines
- Augmented catabolism of nucleic acids caused by increased cell turnover (leukemia, lymphoma, chemotherapy)
- Decreased salvage of free purine bases
- Decreased urinary excretion of uric acid

The majority of primary gout is caused by impaired excretion of uric acid by the kidneys, although the underlying disorder is unknown. Many cases of secondary gout result from leukemia, lymphoma, dehydration, diuretics, and chemotherapy. In addition, a correlation exists between hyperuricemia and weight, protein intake, alcohol consumption, and social status. Often, gouty attacks may be precipitated by ethanol or meat ingestion.

The development of pathologic findings in gout reflects the precipitation of sodium urate crystals from supersaturated body fluids, including synovial fluid, which then absorbs fibronectin, complement, and other proteins. Neutrophils that have ingested urate crystals release activated oxygen species and lysosomal enzymes that mediate tissue injury and promote inflammation.

Microscopically, long, needle-shaped crystals are present, which are negatively birefringent under polarized light. Deposition of these crystals in soft tissue leads to the development of a tophus, which is a deposit of urate crystals surrounded by foreign-body giant cells and associated mononuclear cells. Tophi may also occur in cartilage or the subchondral bone marrow adjacent to joints. Tophi appear grossly as chalky white deposits on the surfaces of intraarticular structures, including the articular cartilage. Radiologically, these regions appear as punched-out, juxtaarticular, lytic ("rat bite") lesions with only minimal reactive bone. In addition, urate renal stones may occur in a subset of patients.

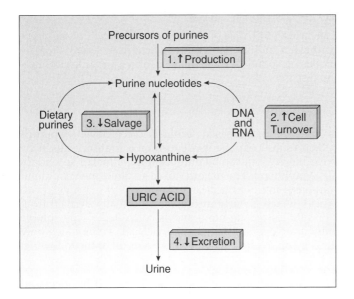

FIGURE 26-9

**Pathogenesis of hyperuricemia and gout. Purine nucleotides are syn-
thesized de novo from nonpurine precursors or derived from preformed purines in the diet. Purine nucleotides are catabolized to
hypoxanthine or incorporated into nucleic acids. The degradation
of nucleic acids and dietary purines also produces hypoxanthine.
Hypoxanthine is converted to uric acid, which in turn is excreted
into the urine. Hyperuricemia and gout result from (a) increased
de novo purine synthesis, (b) increased cell turnover, (c) decreased
salvage of dietary purines and hypoxanthine, and (d) decreased uric
acid excretion by the kidneys. (From Rubin E, Gorstein F, Rubin R,
et al. Rubin's Pathology, 4th ed. Philadelphia: Lippincott Williams &
Wilkins, 2005, p. 1372.)**

Clinically, patients may progress through a series of clinical
syndromes due to hyperuricemia, including the following:

- *Asymptomatic hyperuricemia*
- *Acute gouty arthritis*: usually involves a painful and red first
  metatarsophalangeal joint (great toe), termed podagra; often
  begins at night and is exquisitely painful
- *Intercritical period*: asymptomatic interval between initial attack
  and subsequent episodes
- *Tophaceous gout*: tophi in cartilage, synovial membranes, tendons, and soft tissue

Approximately 10% of patients die from renal failure.

The treatment of gout is to reduce serum urate levels to prevent future attacks, to promote the dissolution of urate deposits, and to alkalinize the urine. Interruption of the inflammatory process may be accomplished by nonsteroidal anti-inflammatory drugs. Colchicine is used to prevent the leukocyte response to urate crystals. Allopurinol is a competitive inhibitor of xanthine oxidase, which converts xanthine and hypoxanthine to uric acid, and is used to treat chronic attacks.

Another disease that results in enhanced purine synthesis is *Lesch-Nyhan syndrome*, which is an X-linked (Xq26–q27) deficiency of HPRT that leads to accumulation of PP-ribose-P. Children are normal at birth but exhibit delays in development and neurological dysfunction in the first year. Most are mentally retarded and exhibit self-mutilation. In addition, these patients may develop obstructive nephropathy, gouty arthritis, and hematological disorders.

Calcium Pyrophosphate Dihydrate-deposition Disease

Calcium pyrophosphate dihydrate-deposition disease (CPPD) is caused by the accumulation of this compound in synovial membranes (*pseudogout*), joint cartilage (*chondrocalcinosis*), ligaments, and tendons. The majority of patients are older than 85 years of age, and many of them demonstrate preexistent joint damage. CPPD may be idiopathic or occur following trauma or with metabolic disorders.

The major predisposing factor is an excessive level of inorganic pyrophosphate in the synovial fluid, which derives from the hydrolysis of nucleoside triphosphates in the chondrocytes of the joint. CPPD deposition may also occur in the joints following trauma or after surgical removal of the meniscus. Additional causes of CPPD include hyperparathyroidism, hypothyroidism, hemochromatosis, and hypophosphatemia (inherited deficiency of alkaline phosphatase that hydrolyzes pyrophosphate).

Radiologically, asymptomatic cases may demonstrate punctate or linear calcifications in fibrocartilage or hyaline cartilage surfaces. Grossly, CPPD deposits appear as chalky white areas on the cartilaginous surfaces. In contrast to gout, crystals in CPPD are short and rhomboid ("coffin-shaped") in appearance, birefringent under polarized light, and do not dissolve in water. Only few mononuclear cells and macrophages surround these crystals.

Pseudogout refers to self-limited attacks of acute arthritis lasting from 1 day to 4 weeks and involving one or two joints. Patients often have inflammation and swelling of the knees, ankles, wrists, hips, or shoulders with sparing of the metatarsophalangeal joints, which are classically affected by gout.

Other Causes of Joint Disease

Hemophilia may have extensive bleeding into the joints (hemarthrosis), especially the knees, elbows, ankles, shoulders, and hips. Half of all patients with *hemochromatosis* may demonstrate arthritis. *Ochronosis* is a rare, autosomal recessive disease caused by a defect in homogentisic acid oxidase, which leads to the deposition of ochronotic pigment in the cartilage of the joints including the intravertebral disks, eventually causing them to become brittle and degenerate.

Tumors and Tumorlike Lesions of Joints

True neoplasms arising in the joint are rare and most tumors that involve the synovium are metastatic carcinomas or lymphoproliferative disorders.

Ganglion Cysts

A ganglion cyst is a thin-walled, simple cyst containing clear mucinous fluid, which most commonly occurs on the extensor surfaces of the hands and feet, especially the wrist. The cyst arises from the synovium or from areas of myxoid change in the connective tissue. The lesion is painful and can readily be removed surgically.

Baker's Cyst

A Baker's cyst is a herniation of the synovium of the knee joint into the popliteal space. It is often seen with arthritis.

Synovial Chondromatosis

Synovial chondromatosis is a benign, self-limited disease in which hyaline cartilage nodules that form in the synovium detach and float in the synovial fluid. These nodules produce chronic irritation, which stimulates the synovium to secrete large amounts of synovial fluid and also causes bleeding. Synovial chondromatosis involves the large synovial joints of young and middle-aged men, especially the knees. Symptoms include pain, stiffness, and locking of the joint.

Because the cartilage nodules are formed de novo in the synovium, microscopically, no tidemark is evident. These nodules may occasionally undergo calcification; this is termed *synovial osteochondromatosis*. Treatment involves joint evacuation and partial synovectomy.

Pigmented Villonodular Synovitis

Pigmented villonodular synovitis is a benign neoplasm of the synovial lining characterized by an exuberant proliferation of synovial lining cells with extension in to the subsynovial tissue. These lesions may sometimes insinuate through joint capsules and encompass nerves and arteries. This disease usually involves a single joint, most commonly the knee, and occurs in young adults.

Grossly, enlarged synovial folds and excrescences may be noticeable. Microscopically, bland mononuclear cells with scattered multinucleated giant cells containing peripheral nuclei are present. Hemosiderin-laden macrophages reflect prior hemorrhage.

Localized nodular synovitis is a similar condition of the knee that involves only one portion of the synovium and present with pain, joint locking, and joint effusions. *Localized nodular tenosynovitis* (giant cell tumor of the tendon sheath) involves the tendon sheath of the hands and feet and is the most common soft tissue tumor of the hand. This lesion occurs almost exclusively in young and middle-aged women and involves the flexor surface of the middle or index finger.

Treatment of these lesions involves surgery.

SOFT TISSUE

Soft Tissue Tumors and Tumorlike Conditions

These tumors occur in the skeletal muscle, fat, fibrous tissue, blood vessels, and lymphatics and include peripheral nerve tumors. These tumors are rare, accounting for less than 1% of all cancers, and are most commonly benign. Conditions associated with the development of soft tissue tumors include neurofibromatosis type 1, tuberous sclerosis, Osler-Weber-Rendu disease, and mesenteric fibromatosis in Gardner syndrome. In addition, radiation injury has been incited as a causative agent in some cases. General principles involving these lesions include the following:

- Superficial tumors tend to be benign
- Deep lesions are often malignant
- Large tumors are more often malignant
- Rapidly growing tumors are more likely malignant
- Calcification may occur in both benign and malignant lesions
- Most malignant tumors are hypervascular
- Some tumors are classified on the basis of molecular findings

Fibrous Lesions
Nodular Fasciitis

Nodular fasciitis is a rapidly growing reactive lesion that commonly affects the superficial tissues of the forearm, trunk, and back. Because of its rapid growth, it may be mistaken for a malignant lesion. Most cases occur in adults. Microscopically, the lesion is hypercellular with abundant mitoses and numerous, pleomorphic, spindle shaped cells. The lesion is self-limited and cured by surgical excision.

Fibromatosis

Fibromatosis is a locally invasive, slow-growing lesion that occurs almost anywhere in the body and often arises from muscular fascia. Grossly, these lesions are large, firm, and whitish with poorly demarcated borders and a whorled, cut surface. Microscopically, sheets and interdigitating fascicles of benign-appearing spindle cells (fibroblasts) extend between preexisting structures, making these lesions difficult to fully excise surgically. An aggressive form of fibromatosis that involves abdominal and extra-abdominal sites is termed a desmoid tumor. Minimal mitotic activity is evident. Three specific types of fibromatosis are identified:

- *Palmar fibromatosis* (*Dupuytren contracture*): most common form of fibromatosis; fibrous nodules and cordlike bands in the palmar fascia lead to flexion contractures of the fingers
- *Plantar fibromatosis*: similar to palmar fibromatosis but occurs in the plantar aponeurosis
- *Penile fibromatosis* (*Peyronie disease*): least common form; induration or mass in the shaft of the penis, causing it to curve to the affected side (penile strabismus); leads to urethral obstruction and pain on erection

Fibrosarcoma

Fibrosarcomas are malignant tumors of fibroblasts that arise in connective tissue, such as fascia, scar tissue, periosteum, and tendons. Most fibrosarcomas arise in adults and most commonly involve the thigh, especially around the knee. Congenital fibrosarcoma (CFS) occurs in infancy and is characterized by the translocation t(12;15)(p13;q26) encoding an ETV6-NTRK3 fusion gene; this lesion has a poor prognosis.

Grossly, fibrosarcomas appear well demarcated with necrosis and hemorrhage. Microscopically, pleomorphic fibroblasts form interlacing bundles and fascicles, termed a *herringbone pattern*. Patients with more poorly differentiated fibrosarcomas have a worse prognosis; however, the 5-year survival rate for all fibrosarcomas is only 40%.

Malignant Fibrous Histiocytoma

Malignant fibrous histiocytoma (MFH) commonly occurs in older adults and often arises in the deep fascia or within a skeletal muscle. This lesion has been associated with prior radiation therapy, surgical scars, and foreign bodies.

Microscopically, a highly variable morphologic pattern is present, with areas of benign-appearing spindle-shaped tumor cells arrayed in an irregular whorled (storiform) pattern adjacent to pleomorphic sheets of cells. Occasionally, plump cells, abundant mitoses, xanthomatous cells, chronic inflammation, giant cells, and myxoid areas may be present. The extent of collagen deposition varies. The karyotype demonstrates numerous chromosomal aberrations.

The prognosis depends on the degree of cytological atypia, mitotic activity, and degree of necrosis. Metastatic disease may occur, especially to the lungs.

Adipose Tissue

Lipoma

Lipoma is composed of well-differentiated adipocytes and represents the most common soft tissue mass. These lesions are benign, circumscribed, and may occur in any region containing fat, especially on the trunk and neck. These lesions occur predominantly in adults and appear grossly as encapsulated, soft, yellow lesions that vary in size. Deeper tumors may be less well circumscribed. Microscopically, these lesions are indistinguishable from normal fat.

Angiolipomas are small, well-circumscribed subcutaneous lipomas that have extensive vascular proliferation, affect mainly adolescents, and may be multiple and painful.

Liposarcoma

Liposarcomas are the second most common sarcoma in adults and usually occur after 50 years of age. These lesions are malignant, slow-growing, and most commonly affect the deep thigh and retroperitoneum. Most cases demonstrate a characteristic translocation t(12;16)(q13;p11), which results in a fusion between the TLS/FUS and CHOP genes that results in a novel RNA-binding protein.

Grossly, these lesions average 5 to 10 cm in diameter and the cut surface varies based on the proportions of adipose, mucinous, and fibrous tissue. Well-differentiated lesions may be confused with lipomas both grossly and microscopically, and have a 5-year survival of over 70%.

Poorly differentiated lesions may demonstrate necrosis, hemorrhage, and cystic degeneration. The most common microscopic pattern is one of variably differentiated "signet-ring" lipoblasts embedded in a vascularized myxoid stroma. Other poorly differentiated forms may have uniform round cells with vesicular nuclei. The 5-year survival for poorly differentiated liposarcomas is less than 20%.

Rhabdomyosarcoma

Rhabdomyosarcoma is the most frequent soft tissue sarcoma of children and young adults and is characterized by striated muscle differentiation. Four types of rhabdomyosarcomas occur:

- *Embryonal rhabdomyosarcoma*: 3 to 12 years of age; involves the head and neck, genitourinary tract, and retroperitoneum; variable histology from well-differentiated with rhabdomyoblasts (cells with large eosinophilic cytoplasm and cross-striations) to poorly differentiated
- *Botryoid embryonal rhabdomyosarcoma* (sarcoma botryoides): polypoid, grapelike tumor masses; involve hollow visceral organs, including the vagina and bladder; malignant cells scattered in an abundant myxoid stroma
- *Alveolar rhabdomyosarcoma*: 10 to 25 years of age; rarely elderly patients; upper and lower extremities affected; club-shaped tumor cells arranged in clumps that are outlined by fibrous septa; cells with intense eosinophilia and occasional multinucleated giant cells; t(2;13)(q35;q14) encoding PAX3-FKHR fusion or t(1;13)(p36;q14) encoding PAX7-FKHR fusion
- *Pleomorphic rhabdomyosarcoma*: least common; older persons; skeletal muscle, especially the thigh; pleomorphism of irregularly arranged cells; cells with large, granular, eosinophilic cytoplasm; no cross-striations

Smooth Muscle Tumors

Leiomyoma

Leiomyomas are benign nodules that arise in the subcutaneous tissue or the walls of blood vessels. These lesions are painful and appear grossly as firm, yellow, circumscribed nodules. Microscopically, intersecting fascicles of regular smooth cells with minimal mitotic activity are evident.

Leiomyosarcoma

Leiomyosarcoma is a malignant neoplasm that often arises in the wall of blood vessels in the extremities of adults. Grossly, these lesions are well circumscribed, but are larger than leiomyomas and demonstrate necrosis, hemorrhage, and cystic degeneration. The tumor cells are arranged in fascicles, often with palisaded nuclei. The atypia is variable, but often cells have a high mitotic rate. Most lesions eventually metastasize, although metastases may occur as late as 15 years following the primary resection.

Vascular Tumors

Vascular tumors include benign hemangiomas and malignant angiosarcomas. These lesions are discussed in Chapter 10.

Synovial Sarcoma

Synovial sarcoma is a highly malignant lesion that arises in the region of a joint, often in association with a tendon sheath, bursa, or joint capsule. These lesions occur in adolescents and young adults and manifests as a painful mass, often in the vicinity of a large joint, especially the knee. Less than 10% of these lesions are intra-articular. Although the lesion bears a microscopic resemblance to synovium, it is unclear whether this is the cell of origin. Synovial sarcomas demonstrate a balanced translocation t(x; 18)(p11.2;q11.2) that results in fusion of the SYT and SSX genes.

Grossly, these lesions are usually circumscribed, round or multilobular masses attached to tendons, tendon sheaths, or the exterior wall of the joint capsule. They are surrounded by a glistening pseudocapsule and may be cystic. Microscopically, these lesions have a biphasic appearance with fluid-filled glandular spaces lined by epitheliumlike tumor cells in a background of sarcomatous spindle cells. These lesions often express cytokeratin or epithelial membrane antigen.

The recurrence rate of these lesions is high and metastases occur in over 60% of cases. The 5-year survival rate is 50%.

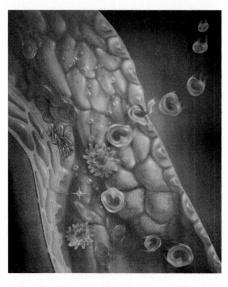

CHAPTER 27

Skeletal Muscle

Chapter Outline

Normal Anatomy and Histology

Muscle is composed of fascicles (groups of muscle fibers) that are separated from one another by connective tissue termed perimysium. Each muscle fiber, in turn, is surrounded by an endomysium and is formed of numerous myofibrils. Scattered satellite cells are present within the muscle, which serve as progenitor cells during muscle regeneration. Each muscle fiber is innervated by a single axon, although a given nerve may innervate multiple fibers. The lower motor neuron and its associated innervated fibers are termed a motor unit. Muscle fibers respond to neuronal transmission by signaling through nicotinic acetylcholine receptors clustered at the motor endplate.

Muscle fibers are subdivided into type I and type II fibers, the phenotype of which may be influenced by signaling from the lower motor neuron.

- Type I fibers (also called red or slow-twitch fibers) have increased oxygen-storage capacity and increased numbers of mitochondria. Activation of these fibers results in a slow, prolonged contraction that is highly resistant to fatigue.
- Type II fibers (also called white or fast-twitch fibers) use the Embden-Myerhof pathway for anaerobic glycolysis. Activation of these fibers results in faster, shorter, and more powerful contraction than type I fibers. These fibers stain prominently with myosin ATPase.

The majority of human muscle is formed of a combination of type I and type II fibers, although the proportion of these fibers varies by location.

Survey of muscle disease is performed by muscle biopsy, with the quadriceps femoris and the biceps brachii serving as common biopsy sites. In patients with peripheral neuropathy, the gastrocnemius muscle and sural nerve are often sampled.

General Pathological Reactions

In a variety of myopathies, muscle fibers undergo a cycle of necrosis and regeneration. Injury to the muscle fiber results in a focal (segmental) necrosis of the fiber, which leaves a residual basement membrane and nerve supply. Macrophage infiltration and activation of satellite cells, which form regenerating myoblasts, result in the restoration of the muscle fiber. In general, the regenerating muscle fiber is smaller in diameter than the parent fiber; large, centrally located, vesicular nuclei with prominent nucleoli are located within the fiber. Return of function can occur within several weeks following injury.

Muscular Dystrophy

Muscular dystrophy refers to a group of disorders characterized by a progressive weakness of the voluntary muscles caused by a primary muscle disorder. In general, muscular dystrophy is a progressive disease that is characterized by muscle fiber necrosis and regeneration resulting in progressive muscle fibrosis and replacement of muscle tissue by fatty tissue. These disorders are not associated with a prominent inflammatory component.

Duchenne Muscular Dystrophy

Duchenne muscular dystrophy is an X-linked disorder that manifests with progressive degeneration of muscle fibers, often involving the pelvic and shoulder girdles. Mutations and deletions of *dystrophin* (Xp21) results in greatly reduced to absent levels of this protein on the inner surface of the sarcolemma. Diagnosis can be established by polymerase chain reaction (PCR) of genomic DNA derived from leukocytes or by muscle biopsy, which shows little to no dystrophin protein by immunostaining or immunoblot. Serum creatine kinase activity is greatly increased.

Boys affected by Duchenne muscular dystrophy often demonstrate weakness by 3 to 4 years of age, especially in the shoulder and pelvic girdles. Pseudohypertrophy of the calf muscles is common and is caused by replacement of muscle by fibroadipose tissue. Many patients often demonstrate variable degrees of mental retardation. Patients are often wheelchair-bound by 10 years of age, and death often occurs secondary to respiratory complications or cardiac arrhythmia.

Becker Muscular Dystrophy

Becker muscular dystrophy is a milder form of Duchenne muscular dystrophy in which a truncated dystrophin protein is present on the muscle fibers. The disorder manifests during childhood. Serum creatine kinase activity is also greatly increased.

Myotonic Dystrophy

Myotonic dystrophy is an autosomal dominant disorder characterized by slowed muscle relaxation (myotonia) and progressive muscle weakness and wasting. The disorder commonly presents during adulthood, although the age of onset is highly variable. Myotonic dystrophy is caused by a mutation chromosome 19 (19q13.3), which encodes a novel serine-threonine protein kinase and results in the expansion of a triplet CTG repeat. Affected patients often demonstrate greater than 50 repeats of this sequence. A congenital form of this disorder occurs in offspring of women who have symptomatic myotonic dystrophy.

Most patients demonstrate atrophy of type I muscle fibers and hypertrophy of type II muscle fibers. The ATPase reaction shows numerous ring fibers, which refer to a circumferential concentration of heavily stained sarcoplasm. In contrast to Duchenne muscular dystrophy, necrosis and regeneration are not prominent features of this disease.

Patients frequently present with slowly progressive muscle weakness and stiffness, often of the distal limbs, face, and jaw. Multiple systems may be affected and additional findings include testicular atrophy, personality alterations, and cataracts.

Congenital Myopathies

Congenital myopathies often manifest in the newborn period with generalized hypotonia (Table 27-1). In general, the persistent hypotonia does not progress and does not appear to affect life span. In contrast, several forms of "malignant" myopathy (Pompe disease, Werdnig-Hoffman disease) have a rapidly progressive course that results in death within the first year of life. Congenital myopathies—including central core disease, nemaline myopathy, and central nuclear myopathy—have a number of the same features. Patients often demonstrate congenital hypotonia, decreased deep tendon reflexes, decreased muscle bulk, and delayed motor milestones. Muscle biopsy shows an abnormal predominance of type I fibers, but myofiber necrosis and fibrosis are not present. The serum creatine kinase level is normal.

Inflammatory Myopathies

Inflammatory myopathies represent an uncommon group of acquired disorders, which feature symmetric proximal muscle weakness, increased serum levels of muscle-derived enzymes, and non-suppurative inflammation of skeletal muscle (Table 27-2). These conditions, which include dermatomyositis, polymyositis, and inclusion body myositis, have been proposed to represent autoimmune processes, although specific antigens have not been identified.

Patients with inflammatory myopathy often demonstrate progressive symmetric proximal muscle weakness, leading to difficulties in climbing steps or combing the hair. Patients also demonstrate increased serum creatine kinase levels, as well as the presence of antinuclear and anticytoplasmic antibodies. Inflammatory myopathies are characterized by a mononuclear inflammatory infiltrate, necrosis and phagocytosis of muscle fibers, a mixture of regenerating and atrophic fibers, and muscle fibrosis.

Myasthenia Gravis

Myasthenia gravis is an acquired autoimmune disease caused by circulating polyclonal antibodies against the acetylcholine receptor

Table 27-1

Congenital Myopathies

Myopathy	Mode of Inheritance	Genetic Defect	Muscle Findings	Associated Findings
Central core disease	Autosomal dominant	Ryanodine receptor (19q13.1)	Predominance of type I fibers that show a central zone of degeneration	Most patients become ambulatory. Rare association with malignant hyperthermia.
Rod (nemaline) myopathy	Autosomal dominant or autosomal recessive	Multiple genes, including slow α-tropomyosin, skeletal muscle α-actin, α-tropomyosin among others	Predominance of type I fibers that show aggregates of rod-shaped structures in the cytoplasm	May have severe involvement of the face, pharynx and neck. Kyphoscoliosis may be present.
Central nuclear myopathy	Autosomal dominant, autosomal recessive, X-linked forms	X-linked form caused by mutation in a tyrosine phosphatase	Predominance of type I fibers showing small, round fibers with a central nucleus	X-linked forms may be fatal in the neonatal period, whereas autosomal dominant forms have a later onset

Table 27-2
Inflammatory Myopathies

Myopathy	Age of Onset	Etiology	Muscle Findings	Associated Finding
Polymyositis	After age 20 years	Affected muscles express MHC-I antigen, which may lead to CD8$^+$ T cell response	Endomysial inflammation and mononuclear infiltration of healthy-appearing muscle fibers	Some patients may have interstitial lung disease, Raynaud phenomenon, nonerosive arthritis
Dermatomyositis	Children and adults	Immune complexes in blood vessel walls results in a microangiopathy and loss of myofibers; may be partially mediated by CD4$^+$ T cells	Intramuscular blood vessels show endothelial hyperplasia, fibrin thrombi, obliteration and the myofibers show peripheral atrophy (perifascicular atrophy)	Rash on the upper eyelids, face, trunk. May occur in association with other autoimmune diseases or with lung carcinoma
Inclusion body myositis	Adulthood	Involvement of the endomysium by cytotoxic T cells	Single fiber necrosis and regeneration. Myofibers contain slitlike vacuoles and eosinophilic cytoplasmic inclusions (intracellular amyloid)	

at the motor endplates of muscle fibers. The binding of the antibodies results in increased endocytosis of the acetylcholine receptor, leading to muscle weakness and easy fatigability. This condition most commonly affects young adults, with a female predominance.

Patients with myasthenia gravis often demonstrate waxing and waning muscle weakness and fatigability, which may often affect the muscles of the eye, leading to ptosis and diplopia. Muscles of the trunk and extremities may also be affected, and a subset of patients develops respiratory insufficiency due to involvement of the respiratory muscles. Muscle biopsy shows minimal findings, such as atrophy of type II muscle fibers and focal collections of lymphocytes within muscle fascicles. A large number of patients have either an associated thymoma or thymic hyperplasia, and surgical removal of the thymoma may be curative. Treatment includes corticosteroids, anticholinesterase drugs, or plasmapheresis.

Lambert-Eaton Syndrome

Lambert-Eaton syndrome is a paraneoplastic syndrome often associated with small cell carcinoma of the lung, as well as other malignancies, which manifests with muscular weakness and wasting of the proximal muscles.

Inherited Metabolic Diseases

A variety of hereditary abnormalities affect the skeletal muscle, including glycogen-storage diseases, lipid myopathies, mitochondrial disease, as well as other enzyme deficiencies (Table 27-3).

Rhabdomyolysis

Rhabdomyolysis is the noninflammatory necrosis of muscle fibers that may result in release of large amounts of myoglobin from the cells and possibly acute renal failure secondary to myoglobinemia. Rhabdomyolysis may be acute, subacute, or chronic, and it may be induced by influenza, exercise, heat stroke, or malignant hyperthermia. Acute rhabdomyolysis is characterized by swollen, tender, and weak muscles. Scattered necrosis of muscle fibers with focal regeneration and clusters of macrophages is identified.

Denervation

Damage to the lower motor neuron results in axonal degeneration and subsequent irregularly scattered, angular atrophy of type I and type II muscle fibers. In cases of severe denervation, clusters of angular atrophic fibers appear, which immunostain intensely for

Table 27-3

Inherited Metabolic Diseases Involving Skeletal Muscle

Disease	Mode of Inheritance	Molecular Defect	Microscopic Findings	Associated Findings
Glycogen-storage diseases				
Type II glycogenosis (acid maltase deficiency, Pompe disease)	Autosomal recessive	Altered acid maltase activity (reduced breakdown of glycogen and accumulation within lysosomes)	Muscle contains massive accumulations of membrane-bound glycogen	Hypotonia. Most severe form is Pompe disease in which infants may die secondary to cardiac failure
Type III glycogenosis	Autosomal recessive	Debranching enzyme deficiency (reduced hydrolysis of glycogen)	Electron microscopy reveals large aggregates of glycogen granules in the sarcoplasm	Hepatomegaly, growth retardation
Type V glycogenosis (McArdle disease, myophosphorylase deficiency)	Autosomal recessive	Myophosphorylase deficiency (reduced cleavage of glycogen)	Subtle accumulation of glycogen granules in the sarcoplasm	Prominent myofiber necrosis may occur in association with prolonged exercise

Lipid myopathies

Carnitine deficiency	Autosomal recessive	Carnitine deficiency (reduced transport of long-chain fatty acids into the mitochondria)	Massive accumulation of lipid droplets in the sarcoplasm	Exercise intolerance, progressive proximal muscle weakness

Mitochondrial disease

Mitochondrial encepahalomyopathies	Maternal transmission	Often, impaired activity of cytochrome oxidase	Accumulation of mitochondria that appear as reddish granular material in the sarcoplasm (ragged red fibers)	Kearns-Sayre syndrome (ophthalmoplegia, retinal pigmentary degeneration, cardiac arrhythmias); MELAS syndrome (myopathy, encephalopathy, lactic acidosis, strokelike episodes)
Familial periodic paralysis	Autosomal dominant	Abnormalities of sodium and potassium fluxes in and out of muscle cells	Later in the course of disease, muscle fibers show sarcoplasmic vacuolization	Episodes of muscular weakness or paralysis, followed by a rapid recovery

nonspecific esterase and NADH-TR (in contrast to atrophy caused by disuse or wasting). As surviving neurons sprout new terminals, reinnervated muscle fibers become type I or type II fibers, depending on signal from the innervating axon. Over time, larger motor units appear that demonstrate large clusters of type I fibers adjacent to large clusters of type II fibers (termed *type grouping*). Patients with type grouping manifest muscle cramping in addition to muscle weakness. In cases in which reinnervation does not occur, muscle fibers progressively atrophy and are ultimately replaced by fibroadipose tissue, resulting in muscle weakness.

Spinal Muscular Atrophy

Spinal muscular atrophy (SMA) is a group of autosomal recessive disorders caused by abnormalities in 5q11.2-13.3, which demonstrates degeneration of the anterior horn cells of the spinal cord. Subtypes of SMA include the following:

- Werdnig-Hoffmann disease (type I or infantile SMA): progressive and severe weakness in infancy, with death often occurring in the first year; microscopically demonstrates groups of minute, rounded, atrophic fibers that are still identifiable as type I or II fibers by ATPase staining in association with hypertrophied type I fibers
- Kugelberg-Welander disease (type III or juvenile SMA): later-onset form of SMA that may not progress; microscopically demonstrates type grouping

Type II Fiber Atrophy

Type II fiber atrophy often occurs secondary to other conditions and reflects a selective angular atrophy of type II fibers as demonstrated by ATPase stain. Steroid myopathy is a form of type II fiber atrophy that manifests with muscle weakness and occurs following prolonged corticosteroid administration.

Critical Illness Myopathy

Patients who receive high-dose steroids in conjunction with neuromuscular blocking agents may demonstrate critical illness myopathy, manifested by a loss of thick myosin filaments as documented by electron microscopy. These filaments often reconstitute following withdrawal of corticosteroids.

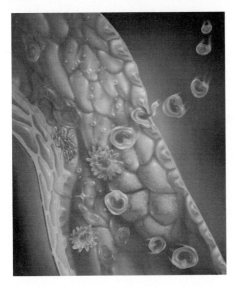

CHAPTER *28*

The Nervous System

Chapter Outline

The nervous system is subdivided into the central and peripheral nervous systems. Although both systems function to rapidly transmit information, the basic components are slightly varied.

THE CENTRAL NERVOUS SYSTEM

Normal Anatomy and Histology

The central nervous system (CNS) is composed of five major components, which include neurons, astrocytes, oligodendroglia, ependymal cells, and microglia.

Neurons

Neurons relay information along intricate and plastic neuronal networks. Signals originate in the cell body, which are then transmitted along axons to the dendrites of neighboring neurons. Myelination of neurons by oligodendroglia allows a rapid transmission of signals along the length of the axon. The number of neurons present in the CNS decreases with age, and only a small number of neurons are created during adult life.

Neurons are large cells with a centrally located round nucleus and a prominent nucleolus. The cytoplasm is abundant and demonstrates prominent basophilic granules, termed *Nissl bodies*, which represent ribosome-laden endoplasmic reticulum. Neurons of the substantia nigra and locus ceruleus contain neuromelanin and therefore demonstrate a brown appearance.

Neurons are extremely sensitive to injury, with a limited ability to regenerate axons following injury and an extremely limited ability to recover following demyelination. Neuronal injury may manifest in the following ways:

- Chromatolysis: reversible process that involves neuronal swelling, cytoplasmic expansion, and eccentric positioning of the nucleus

- Atrophy: reduction in brain volume or weight evidenced microscopically by hyperchromatic neurons and a reduction in neuronal size
- Neuronophagia: phagocytosis of neuronal debris by brain macrophages or microglia
- Intraneuronal inclusions: cytoplasmic and nuclear inclusions that occurs in certain infectious or neurodegenerative diseases

Astrocytes

Astrocytes are glial cells that serve a supportive and signaling role in the CNS, as well as function in the CNS response to injury. Astrocytes have a star-shaped appearance with a round nucleus with homogenous chromatin. Some astrocytes terminate their foot processes on blood vessels and may assist in the maintenance of the blood-brain barrier. Astrocytes stain for glial fibrillary acidic protein (GFAP). Following injury, astrocytes proliferate locally, which leads to the formation of a scar; this process is termed *gliosis*. Astrocytes are also responsible for the formation of amorphous, basophilic, rounded structures called corpora amylacea, which are aggregates of carbohydrates and proteins accumulated with normal aging. Finally, astrocytes may undergo neoplastic transformation.

Oligodendroglia

Oligodendroglia are glial cells responsible for the formation of myelin surrounding axons. These cells have a small, dark, round nucleus and a thin rim of cytoplasm, and are situated as satellites around neurons in the gray matter and longitudinally between myelinated fibers in the white matter. These cells can undergo neoplastic transformation or demyelination.

Ependymal Cells

Ependymal cells regulate the fluid transfer between the cerebrospinal fluid (CSF) and the CNS. These cells line the ventricular system, including the ventricular chambers, aqueduct of Sylvius, the central canal of the spinal cord, and the filum terminale, as a single layer of cuboidal or flat cells. Ependymal cells can undergo malignant transformation.

Microglia

Microglia are the phagocytic cells of the CNS. These cells contain hyperchromatic, elongated nuclei and a thin rim of cytoplasm elaborated into fine processes. Following injury, the proliferation of microglia results in the formation of microglial nodules (aggregates of microglia and astrocytes) or diffuse microgliosis. The accumulation of cellular debris and lipids by microglia lead to the formation of gitter cells.

Congenital Malformations of the CNS

Specific congenital malformations may often have multiple potential causes, and the identical insult may result in various malformations depending on the developmental stage of the fetus. The pathogenesis and clinical findings of congenital malformations involving the neural tube and spinal cord are presented in Table 28-1.

Epilepsy may occur in association with underlying congenital abnormalities or in association with a variety of other CNS disorders such as intracranial tumors or arteriovenous malformations. Epilepsy is defined as paroxysmal, transient disturbances in brain function, which are termed *seizures*. Epilepsy has a prevalence of 6 per 1,000 and the majority of cases are idiopathic. Microscopically, the brains of patients with epilepsy often demonstrate gliosis (glial scarring), although it is unclear whether this represents a cause or effect of the seizure activity.

CNS Trauma

Trauma may result in intracranial hemorrhage (epidural, subdural, and subarachnoid hematomas, direct damage (penetrating trauma), or paralysis (spinal cord injuries). Table 28-2 compares the different types of intracranial hemorrhages.

Concussion

A *concussion* is a transient loss of consciousness due to trauma that causes a rapid torque on the brainstem, leading to a paralysis of neurons of the reticular formation.

Epidural Hematoma

Trauma to the temporal bone may result in transection of the middle meningeal artery, which is situated between the calvaria and dura. Damage to this artery causes a progressive accumulation of blood within the epidural space, termed an *epidural hematoma* (Fig. 28-1). Within the first 4 to 8 hours, patients are often asymptomatic; however, when a critical volume of 30 to 50 mL collects within the epidural space, patients demonstrate symptoms of a space-occupying lesion.

Table 28-1

Congenital Malformations of the Central Nervous System

Malformation	Pathogenesis	Findings
Neural tube defects		
Spina bifida	Failure of dorsal neural tube closure, hypervitaminosis A or folic acid deficiency	Most common congenital malformation and most frequently affects the dorsal lumbosacral region of the vertebral column. Severe forms of spina bifida may show sensory loss, lower limb paralysis, and incontinence.
Spina bifida occulta		Vertebral arch defect with external dimple or tuft of hair
Meningocele		Protrusion of meninges as fluid-filled sac; apical ulceration
Meningomyelocele		Exposed spinal canal; nerve roots trapped in scar tissue
Rachischisis		Spinal column appears as gaping canal often without recognizable spinal cord
Anencephaly	Possible failure of anterior neuropore closure or abnormal angiogenesis	Congenital absence of all or part of the brain and cranial vault; cerebrum is a highly vascularized, poorly differentiated structure; hypoplastic upper spinal cord
Spinal cord malformations		
Hydromyelia		Dilation of the central canal of the spinal cord
Syringomyelia	Occasionally trauma, ischemia, tumors	Tubular cavitation extends along the length of the spinal cord; may not communicate with central canal; filled with clear fluid; may cause sensory/motor deficits

(*continues*)

Table 28-1

(continued)

Malformation	Pathogenesis	Findings
Arnold-Chiari malformation	Increased intracranial pressure or possible tethering of cord by meningomyelocele	Caudal aspect of cerebellar vermis herniates through wide foramen magnum to level C3 to C5; beaking of quadrigeminal plate, inferior colliculus; caudally displaced brainstem; hydrocephalus
Congenital hydrocephalus	Congenital atresia of the aqueduct of Sylvius; viruses; many others	Ventricular enlargement
Cerebral gyri disorders		
Polymicrogyria		Small and excessive gyri; MR
Pachygyria		Reduced number of gyri; very broad gyri; MR
Lissencephaly	Neuronal migration defect	Smooth cortical surface; MR
Heterotopias	Neuronal migration defect	Ectopic nerve and glia, often in white matter, MR
Chromosomal abnormalities		
Down syndrome	Trisomy 21	MR, distinctive facial features, reduced brain weight; slender superior temporal gyri
Trisomy 13–15	Trisomy 13–15	Holoprosencephaly (absent interhemispheric fissure), arrhinencephaly (absence of olfactory tracts), absence of corpus callosum; cyclopia, cleft palate, polydactyly, "rocker bottom" feet

MR, mental retardation.

Table 28-2

Comparison of Intracranial Hemorrhages

	Epidural	Subdural	Subarachnoid
Vessel	Middle meningeal artery	Bridging vein	Arterial aneurysm
Injury	Temporal	Frontal/occipital	Variable/none
Time course	Rapid	Moderate/slow	Rapid
Bilateral	Rare	Common	Rare
Blood in CSF	No	No	Yes
Early symptom	None	Headache	Severe headache

As the hematoma enlarges, the large venous sinuses are compressed, leading to global cerebral hypoxia, ischemia, and confusion. In response to such injury, patients may demonstrate a *Cushing reflex*, which is attempts to increase cerebral blood flow and oxygen delivery by slowing the heart rate (increased ventricular filling), increasing myocardial contraction, and increasing blood pressure. If epidural hematomas are left untreated, they can cause transtentorial herniation, as evidenced by a fixed and dilated pupil

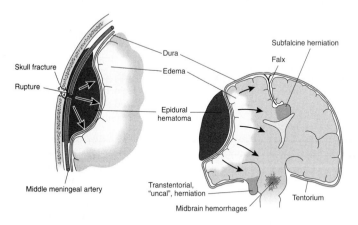

FIGURE   28-1

Development of an epidural hematoma. Transection of a branch of the middle meningeal artery by the sharp fracture initiates bleeding under arterial pressure that dissects the dura from the calvaria and produces an expanding hematoma. After an asymptomatic interval of several hours, transtentorial herniation becomes life-threatening. (From Rubin E, Gorstein F, Rubin R, et al. Rubin's Pathology, 4th ed. Philadelphia: Lippincott Williams & Wilkins, 2005, p. 1426.)

on the side of the lesion and unconsciousness, as well as midbrain ischemia and necrosis. Within 24 to 48 hours, an epidural hematoma may be fatal if untreated.

Subdural Hematoma

Subdural hematomas occur in the context of trauma to the frontal or occipital regions of the head that causes a rapid displacement of the cerebral hemispheres against the inner aspect of the skull, such as in falls, assaults, or car accidents. This trauma causes a shearing effect on the bridging veins within the subdural space, leading to the formation of a subdural hematoma (Fig. 28-2). Most commonly, blood accumulates to a volume of 25 to 50 mL, which then results in a tamponade effect on the ruptured bridging vein. However, in some cases, venous thrombosis and ischemia may develop in the bridging veins. Subdural hematomas may be bilateral due to the nature of the injury.

Patients with subdural hematomas may demonstrate headaches, contralateral weakness, or seizures. Bilateral hematomas may result in impaired cognitive function.

The outcome of subdural hematomas is variable. During the first several weeks, subdural hematomas develop overlying granulation tissue secondary to irritation between the hematoma and dura. Over time, the hematoma may resolve, remain static, or enlarge. Lesions that resolve contain only foci of hemosiderin-laden macrophages microscopically. Lesions that remain static demonstrate blood clot and occasionally calcification. Lesions that expand do so sporadically, often within 6 months of initial injury.

Subarachnoid Hemorrhage

Subarachnoid hemorrhage may occur following trauma or rupture of a berry aneurysm in the Circle of Willis, as well as in instances of vasculitis and tumors (Fig. 28-3). Subarachnoid hemorrhage produces a sudden severe headache and photophobia due to meningeal irritation that may be followed by coma. Often, patients experience a progressive decline in consciousness if they survive the initial hemorrhage. A subarachnoid bleed may be diagnosed by the presence of blood within the CSF when performing a lumbar puncture.

Cerebral Contusion

Contusions also occur when a rapid anteroposterior displacement of the brain occurs. A *coup* injury occurs at the site of impact, whereas a *contrecoup* injury is contralateral to the site of initial injury. A contusion describes damage to the cortex in the form of a bruise or laceration, which may be associated with hemorrhage. The velocity of the acceleration and the abruptness of the deceleration of the head mediate the severity of a contusion. Mild contusions result in cortical bruising, whereas severe contusions may

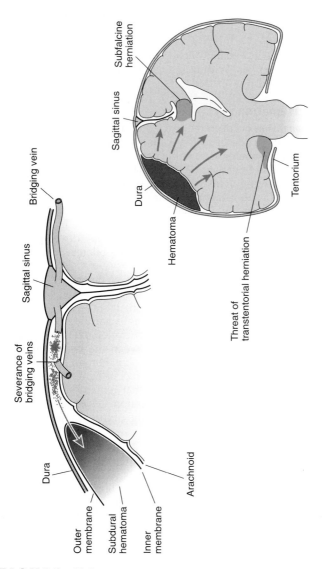

Bridging vein

Sagittal sinus

Severance of
bridging veins

Sagittal sinus

Subfalcine
herniation

Dura

Dura

Hematoma

Tentorium

Threat of
transtentorial herniation

Arachnoid

Outer
membrane

Subdural
hematoma

Inner
membrane

F I G U R E 28-2
Development of a subdural hematoma. With head trauma, the dura
moves with the skull, and the arachnoid moves with the cerebrum.
As a result, the bridging veins are sheared as they cross between the
dura and the arachnoid. Venous bleeding creates a hematoma in the
expansile subdural space. Subsequent transtentorial herniation is
life-threatening. (From Rubin E, Gorstein F, Rubin R, et al. Rubin's
Pathology, 4th ed. Philadelphia: Lippincott Williams & Wilkins,
2005, p. 1429.)

Cross section of the brain

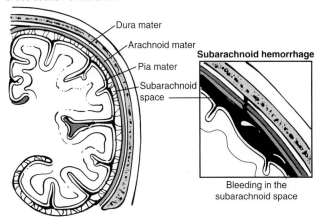

F I G U R E   28-3
Development of a subarachnoid hemorrhage. Subarachnoid hemor-rhages may occur in the setting of an arterial aneurysm rupture, arte-riovenous malformation, infection, or neoplasm. Blood spreads below the subarachnoid membrane to cover the cerebral hemisphere.

result in deep cavitary lesions within the brain that extend into the white matter and cause a mass effect. Contusions may be life-threatening if complicated by edema and hemorrhage, which pre-dispose to transtentorial herniation.

The foci of necrotic brain tissue formed by a contusion is phagocytosed by macrophages and replaced by scar formed by reactive astrocytes. In addition, diffuse axonal shearing injuries, which occur in the context of a contusion, are identified microscopi-cally by axonal spheroids (ends of severed axons which retract) and multiple small hemorrhages.

Penetrating Wounds

Penetrating wounds may be caused by objects such as bullets and knives, which result in direct injury to brain parenchyma, as well as associated hemorrhage. The immediate concern is the develop-ment of extensive hemorrhage, which produces a space-occupying lesion and a risk of transtentorial herniation. Seizures may occur 6 to 12 months following a penetrating brain injury and arises from the region of scar formation.

Spinal Cord Injuries

The spinal cord may be injured by penetrating wounds, fractures of the vertebrae, hyperextension, or hyperflexion. Injury of the spinal cord often extends to levels above and below the point of original injury.

- *Hyperextension injury*: rapid posterior displacement of the head tears the anterior spinal ligament, damaging the posterior spinal cord against the posterior process of the vertebral body.
- *Hyperflexion injury*: the head is driven forcefully forward and downward, resulting in a fracture of the underlying vertebral body and injury of the anterior spinal cord.

Injury to the spinal cord may result in a concussion of the spinal cord, contusion of the spinal cord, or transection of the spinal cord, which can lead to paraplegia or quadriplegia.

Circulatory Disorders of the CNS

Vascular Malformations

Vascular malformations vary in location and histology. Clinically, vascular malformations may be asymptomatic or present with a variety of symptoms, including seizures. Specific malformations include the following:

- *Arteriovenous malformation*: most common congenital malformation composed of anastomosing, abnormal thick walled arteries and veins that can enlarge over time; arteriovenous malformations increase the risk of seizures and intracranial hemorrhage
- *Cavernous angioma*: large, irregular, thin-walled vascular channels that are often asymptomatic
- *Telangiectasia*: focal aggregate of uniformly small vessels that may cause seizures
- *Venous angioma*: focus of a few enlarged veins that is often asymptomatic

Cerebral Aneurysms

Cerebral aneurysms may be caused by developmental defects of the arterial wall, hypertension, atherosclerosis, bacterial infection, or trauma.

Berry Aneurysms

Berry (saccular) aneurysms are most likely caused by a developmental defect in the arterial muscle at points of bifurcation, resulting in an arterial wall composed of only endothelium, an internal elastic lamina and adventitia. Intravascular pressure at this site leads to expansion and potential rupture of the aneurysm. The most common sites of berry aneurysms are demonstrated in Figure 28-4. In 20% of cases, multiple berry aneurysms occur.

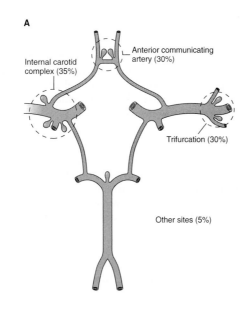

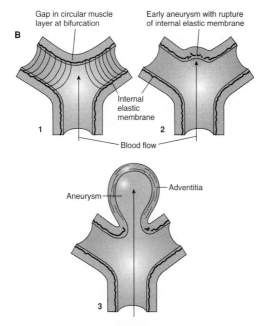

FIGURE 28-4
Berry aneurysm. A: The incidence of saccular aneurysms (berry aneurysms), which preferentially involve the carotid tributaries, is shown. B: The lesion evolves as a result of blood acting on an early embryonic defect. (From Rubin E, Gorstein F, Rubin R, et al. Rubin's Pathology, 4th ed. Philadelphia: Lippincott Williams & Wilkins, 2005, p. 1436.)

Rupture of a berry aneurysm results in life-threatening subarachnoid hemorrhage and often intracerebral or intraventricular hemorrhage as well. Patients who survive the initial event may develop a progressive decline in consciousness secondary to arterial spasm and ischemia or aneurysmal rebleeding.

Atherosclerotic Aneurysms

Atherosclerotic aneurysms are situated primarily in large cerebral arteries (basilar, internal carotid, and vertebral) and are caused by fibrous replacement of the media and destruction of the internal elastic membrane of the arterial wall. These aneurysms most commonly result in thrombosis rather than rupture.

Mycotic Aneurysms

Mycotic aneurysms result from septic emboli that originate in infected cardiac valves and can cause arterial rupture, cerebral abscess, or meningitis.

Cerebral Hemorrhage

Spontaneous cerebral hemorrhages generally occur as a consequence of long-standing hypertension. With persistent hypertension, the arteriolar walls undergo lipid and hyaline deposition (lipohyalinosis), which weakens the wall, leading to Charcot-Bouchard aneurysms. Formation and rupture of these aneurysms occurs most commonly along the trunk of the vessel, rather than at points of bifurcation, and most commonly affects the following:

- Basal ganglia-thalamus (65%)
- Pons (15%)
- Cerebellum (8%)

Rupture of a Charcot-Bouchard aneurysm leads to cerebral hemorrhage (hemorrhagic stroke) that can cause progressive neurological symptoms, especially weakness and possibly death if untreated. Occasionally, hemorrhage may extend into the ventricular system, which may lead to distention of the fourth ventricle and compression of the medulla. *Pontine hemorrhage* may damage the reticular system, leading to loss of consciousness. *Cerebellar hemorrhage* may produce abrupt ataxia, occipital headache, and vomiting; an expanding hemorrhage may encroach on the medulla or produce cerebellar herniation through the foramen magnum by mass effect.

Cerebral Ischemia and Infarction

Globally decreased oxygenation of the brain caused by hypoxia (near-drowning, carbon monoxide poisoning, suffocation) or generalized decreased blood flow (cardiac arrest, external hemorrhage) may lead to diffuse (global) ischemia of the brain. By contrast, regional ischemia results from occlusive cerebrovascular disease (cerebral artery thrombosis), which is localized to a specific vascular distribution.

Global Ischemia

Global ischemia most prominently affects regions of the brain that are most sensitive to diminished blood flow. One of these regions is the territories between the anterior, middle, and posterior cerebral arteries, in which there are no anastomoses between vessels. Decreased blood flow or hypoxia to these regions results in *watershed infarcts*. Another region affected by global ischemia is the deeper layers of the neocortex (cortical layers V and VI) where short penetrator vessels that originate from pial vessels enter the gray matter; global ischemia results in *laminar necrosis* of this region of the cortex. Finally, certain neuronal types are more sensitive to decreased oxygen and include the Purkinje neurons of the cerebellum and the pyramidal neurons of the Sommer sector of the hippocampus. Figure 28-5 summarizes neuronal regions most sensitive to global ischemia.

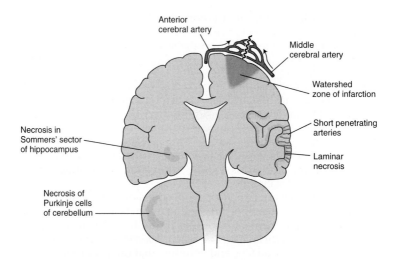

F I G U R E   28-5
Consequences of global ischemia. A global insult induces lesions that reflect the vascular architecture (watershed infarcts, laminar necrosis) and the sensitivity of individual neuronal systems (pyramidal cells of Sommer sector, Purkinje cells). (From Rubin E, Gorstein F, Rubin R, et al. Rubin's Pathology, 4th ed. Philadelphia: Lippincott Williams & Wilkins, 2005, p. 1439.)

Regional Ischemia

Regional ischemia, which affects a single vascular distribution, often results from arterial thrombosis or embolism secondary to atherosclerosis. Whereas thrombotic disease progresses slowly over time and deprives downstream vessels of blood flow, embolic disease occurs suddenly and often causes downstream vascular necrosis and subsequent hemorrhage.

The clinical findings associated with regional ischemia reflect the underlying function of the region of the brain affected. For example, damage to the internal capsule results in hemiparesis or hemiplegia, whereas ischemia of the parietal cortex produces motor and sensory defects.

Regional ischemia produces three distinct clinical syndromes:

- *Transient ischemic attacks* (TIAs): lasts for a few minutes to less than 24 hours and is followed by complete neurological recovery; due to transient vascular occlusion
- *Stroke in evolution*: progression of neurological symptoms while patient is observed; usually caused by a propagation of a thrombus or embolus through a vessel
- *Completed stroke*: stable neurological deficit caused by an infarction

In addition to the subdivision of ischemic events by clinical syndromes, regional occlusive cerebrovascular disease may be subdivided into subtypes based on the size and nature of the vessel involved:

- Large extracranial and intracranial vessel occlusion (carotid, vertebral and basilar arteries): carotid arteries commonly affected by atherosclerosis; carotid artery occlusion may present with ipsilateral hemisphere impairment or often middle cerebral artery damage
- Circle of Willis vessel occlusion: often the middle cerebral artery by atherosclerosis and the trifurcation of the middle cerebral artery by emboli
- Parenchymal artery and arteriole occlusion: often damaged by hypertension resulting in lacunar infarcts that are typically small; impairment of cognition by multiple lacunar infarcts is termed *multiple infarct dementia; hypertensive encephalopathy* manifests as headache and vomiting that can progress to coma and death
- Capillary bed occlusion: small emboli consisting of fat (following long bone trauma) or air (following rapid ascent from deepsea diving, *Caisson disease*) often cause multiple white matter infarcts and petechiae
- Cerebral vein occlusion: secondary to systemic dehydration, phlebitis, neoplastic obstruction, or sickle cell disease; abrupt

thrombosis may cause bilateral frontal lobe hemorrhage due to blood stagnation in the sagittal sinus

Microscopically, an acute infarction initially and primarily consists of necrotic brain tissue that subsequently undergoes phagocytosis by macrophages and revascularization by capillary ingrowth. After many months, an infarct appears as a gliosis-lined cystic cavity. If the infracted region was large, the cavity may be bridged by atretic cobwebs of blood vessels.

Cerebrospinal Fluid and Hydrocephalus

Cerebrospinal fluid (CSF) is produced by the choroid plexus, which is located in the third ventricle, the oramina of Monro, and the lateral ventricles. Following production, the CSF circulates throughout the ventricular system and is ultimately absorbed by the arachnoid villi. An adult has approximately 150 mL of CSF that serves to transport nutrients to cells of the nervous system, remove metabolic waste, and cushion structures. *Hydrocephalus* reflects a dilation of the ventricular system due to increased CSF volume behind a region of obstruction and is often accompanied by neurological symptoms. In general, the sulci of the brain are compressed and the white matter is reduced in volume.

During infancy, hydrocephalus results in expansion of the cranium (due to open suture lines) and may present with seizures, optic atrophy, weakness, or spasticity, although cognition is often spared. In adults, increased intracranial pressure results in headache, vomiting, papilledema and, if advanced, mental deterioration. The obstruction may be relieved by surgical CSF drainage or shunting.

Noncommunicating hydrocephalus occurs when an obstruction to CSF flow resides within the ventricular system. Noncommunicating hydrocephalus may occur with congenital malformations (aqueduct of Sylvius malformations), neoplasms (ependymomas), inflammation (viral ependymitis), or hemorrhage.

Communicating hydrocephalus occurs when CSF cannot be reabsorbed by the arachnoid villi and may occur with subarachnoid hemorrhage, meningitis, and tumor spread.

Infectious Diseases of the CNS

The CNS is prone to infection by bacteria, viruses, parasites, and prion diseases. The specific clinical findings associated with each infection are often distinct. Inflammation of the meninges is termed *meningitis*, inflammation of the cortex is termed *encephalitis*, and inflammation of the spinal cord is termed *myelitis*.

Meningitides

Selected forms of meningitis are described in Table 28-3.

Bacterial Meningitis

Bacterial meningitis occurs when bacteria reach the meninges via bloodborne spread. Bacterial meningitis may affect the pia and arachnoid meninges (*leptomeningitis*) or the dura (*pachymeningitis*). Leptomeningitis involves infection of the CSF, which is a rich culture medium for many organisms. In contrast, pachymeningitis commonly occurs with extension of chronic sinusitis or mastoiditis into the external layer of the dura, often without additional spread within the CNS.

The most common bacteria that cause meningitis include the following:

- *Escherichia coli*: affects newborns in whom a lack of transplacental maternal immunoglobulin (Ig) M protection against gram-negative bacteria leads to disease; associated with a high mortality rate
- *Haemophilus influenzae*: gram-negative organism that affects infants between 3 months and 3 years
- *Streptococcus pneumoniae*: occurs in adulthood and has high incidence following basilar skull fracture
- *Neisseria meningitidis*: affects persons in crowded places, such as schools or barracks; resides in nasopharynx; early symptoms include fever, malaise, petechial rash and may result in adrenal hemorrhages (*Waterhouse-Friderichsen syndrome*) or acute fulminant meningitis

Macroscopic examination of the brain in patients that have succumbed to bacterial meningitis reveals an opacification of the meninges caused by a purulent exudate that is most evident over the cerebral hemispheres and base of the brain. Occasionally, infection may spread to subarachnoid spaces. Although the pia is a strong barrier to spread of infection, cerebral abscesses may occur in rare instances.

Findings may be similar irrespective of infectious organism. Most patients present with headache, vomiting, and fever. Children may also have convulsions. Classic findings include cervical rigidity, inability to straighten knee following hip flexion due to pain (Kernig sign), and knee and hip flexion following neck flexion due to pain (Brudzinski sign). Lumbar puncture often reveals polymorphonuclear leukocytes (neutrophils), increased protein, and decreased glucose levels.

Tuberculous Meningitis

Tuberculous meningitis often occurs following hematogenous spread of mycobacteria to the leptomeninges and presents with

Table 28-3
Forms of Meningitis

Disease	Organism(s)	Pathologic Findings	Lumbar Puncture Findings
Bacterial meningitis	*Escherichia coli, Haemophilus influenzae, Streptococcus pneumoniae, Neisseria meningitidis*	Opacified meninges; purulent exudates	Neutrophils, ↓ glucose, ↑ protein, organism by stain
Tuberculous meningitis	*Mycobacterium tuberculosis*	Meningeal granulomas; organisms by AFB stain	Lymphocytes, ↓ glucose, ↑ protein, organism by AFB stain
Viral meningitis	Enterovirus (e.g., echovirus)	Often no findings	Lymphocytes, normal glucose, slight ↑ protein
Cryptococcal meningitis	*Cryptococcus neoformans*	1-mm white nodules containing organisms; minimal inflammation	Spheres with a halo by India ink; lymphocytes
Syphilitic meningitis	*Treponema pallidum*	Meningeal and perivascular lymphocytic infiltrate; +/− spirochetes	↑ lymphocytes, elevated protein, normal glucose

symptoms similar to those of bacterial meningitis. Organisms are present on the leptomeninges and in the CSF, and are identified by special stains for acid-fast bacilli. The meninges demonstrate granulomas composed of epithelioid histiocytes, Langerhans giant cells, and lymphocytes that surround regions of caseous necrosis. Lumbar puncture often demonstrates increased numbers of lymphocytes in the CSF. If not properly treated, tuberculous meningitis may result in meningeal fibrosis, communicating hydrocephalus, and arteritis that may result in infarcts. Untreated tuberculous meningitis may be fatal in 4 to 6 weeks. *Potts disease* refers to tuberculous infection of the spine in which an epidural granulomatous mass destroys the spine and causes spinal cord compression.

Viral Meningitis

Viral meningitis affects children and young adults and is often caused by infection with enterovirus (coxsackie B virus, echovirus). Symptoms include a sudden fever and severe headache. Lumbar puncture demonstrates lymphocytes and increased protein, but normal glucose. Most cases resolve without sequelae.

Cryptococcal Meningitis

Cryptococcus neoformans causes meningitis primarily in immunocompromised hosts and infection is often initiated by inhalation of contaminated bird excreta. Lumbar puncture reveals large (5 to 15 μm) encapsulated spherical organisms that demonstrate a halo (capsule) when mixed with India ink. The latex cryptococcal antigen test may be used to confirm the diagnosis on CSF. Macroscopically, 1-mm white nodules are widely disseminated on the meninges, ependyma, and choroid plexus. Microscopically, organisms may be identified, although the surrounding inflammation may be minimal with rare multinucleated giant cells and lymphocytes.

Amebic Meningoencephalitis

Amebic meningoencephalitis is commonly caused by the amoeba *Naegleria* and *Acanthamoeba*.. Infection with *Acanthamoeba* produces a more protracted meningitis, as well as parenchymal abscesses and a granulomatous reaction. Infection with *Naegleria*, which occurs during swimming in infested waters, results in fulminant, often fatal, meningitis. *Naegleria* and *Acanthamoeba* can penetrate the cribriform plate and enter the cranial compartment by way of the olfactory nerves. Microscopically, these amoebae appear similar to macrophages.

Syphilitic Meningitis

The spirochete *Treponema pallidum* may affect the CNS following hematogenous spread. Often, the organisms are rapidly cleared from the meninges, and only a minor inflammatory reaction involving lymphocytes and plasma cells is present. However, three severe manifestations of tertiary syphilis may occur:

- Meningovascular syphilis: thickened meninges caused by a fibroblastic response and obliterative endarteritis resulting in multiple small infarcts; microscopically shows plasma cells surrounding cortical arterioles
- Tabes dorsalis: transient infection around the dorsal nerve roots of the spinal cord causes wallerian degeneration of axons that extends to the posterior fasciculi and causes loss of position sense in lower extremities
- Dementia paralytica (luetic dementia): occurs many years after infection and results in dementia accompanied by focal loss of cortical neurons with "windblown" appearance, astrogliosis, rod cell formation of microglia, and ependymal granulations

Cerebral Abscess

Cerebral abscesses originate when bloodborne microorganisms lodge within the capillary network of the cortex. These organisms incite an acute inflammatory reaction (cerebritis) with neutrophil influx, edema, and liquefactive necrosis. Expansion of the abscess may result in compression of blood vessels leading to ischemia or mass effect leading to transtentorial herniation or rupture into a ventricle. Resolution of an abscess involves the formation of a fibroblastic capsule surrounding the abscess and astrocytic repair of the cortex.

Viral Encephalomyelitides

Viruses that infect the CNS typically localize to specific sites within the brain and spinal cord and therefore demonstrate distinct clinicopathologic findings. Typically, the onset of encephalitis is abrupt, but the duration of disease may vary from weeks to years. Commonly, viral infections demonstrate perivascular lymphocytes surrounding arteries and arterioles, and many viruses will demonstrate nuclear or cytoplasmic inclusions. Additional microscopic findings include glial nodules (aggregates of microglia and lymphocytes) and neuronophagia (ingestion of dying neurons by macrophages). The most common viruses that affect the CNS are listed in Table 28-4.

Poliomyelitis

Poliomyelitis is caused by a nonenveloped, single-stranded RNA enterovirus that preferentially infects the anterior horn cells and bulbar motor nuclei of the spinal cord. Transmission occurs via the fecal-oral route and the disease may spread rapidly among children

Table 28-4
Viral Encephalomyelitis

Disease	Virus Type	Location of Infection	Viral Inclusions	Clinical Features
Poliomyelitis	Nonenveloped, SS RNA (enterovirus)	Anterior horn cells and bulbar motor nuclei of spinal cord	None	Fever, malaise followed by meningitis and paralysis
Rabies	Enveloped, SS RNA (rhabdovirus)	Brainstem and cerebellum; originally, peripheral nerve	Eosinophilic Negri body in cytoplasm	Throat spasm, difficulty with swallowing, encephalopathy
HSV-1	DS DNA	Temporal lobes; hemorrhagic necrotic parenchyma,	Small, eosinophilic intranuclear inclusion	Often children and young adults; changes in mood, behavior, memory
HSV-2	DS DNA	Cerebrum and cerebellum of newborns; obtained from birth canal	Small, eosinophilic intranuclear inclusion	Neonates; may cause severe, hemorrhagic, necrotizing encephalomyelitis
VZV	DS DNA	Severe meningitis	Glia and neurons	Often immunocompromised patients; well-delineated lesions with demyelination and necrosis
Cytomegalovirus	DS DNA	Transplacental spread to periventricular areas in utero; immunocompromised hosts	Large cytoplasmic and nuclear inclusions in neurons and astrocytes	Severe hemorrhagic, necrotic encephalomyelitis
Arthropod-borne	Togavirus, Bunyavirus	Mild meningitis to diffuse encephalitis	None	Flulike symptoms to severe meningoencephalitis
SSPE	Measles virus (SS RNA)	Gray and white matter of cortex	Prominent basophilic nuclear inclusions with halo	Cognitive and behavioral deficits; motor/sensory deficits
PML	JC virus (DS DNA)	White matter of cortex; widespread demyelination	Nuclear ground-glass oligodendroglial inclusions	Dementia, weakness, visual loss, ataxia, death within 6 months

in close quarters, although the development of effective vaccines has dramatically decreased the incidence of this disease. Poliovirus binds to and enters motor neurons. Following infection, neurons undergo chromatolysis and subsequent ingestion by macrophages (neuronophagia). Microscopically, lymphocytes surround blood vessels in the spinal cord and brainstem and inflammation may spread to the meninges. The cortex may demonstrate glial nodules; viral inclusions are not present. Patients with poliomyelitis initially experience fever, headaches, and malaise, followed by meningitis and variable paralysis. Death can result from respiratory failure following paralysis of the respiratory muscles.

Rabies

Rabies is caused by an enveloped, single-stranded RNA rhabdovirus. Rabies is transmitted by contaminated saliva from animal bites (dogs, wolves, foxes, skunks, etc.) that serve as a reservoir for the virus. The virus infects peripheral nerves at the site of a bite and is transported to the spinal cord and brain by retrograde axoplasmic flow. Infection with the rabies virus demonstrates a specific cytoplasmic inclusion termed a *Negri body*. The onset of disease varies from 10 days to 3 months following infection. Patients initially demonstrate painful throat spasms, difficulty swallowing, and a tendency to aspirate fluids early in the course of disease. Ultimately, a generalized encephalopathy characterized by irritability, agitation, seizures, and delirium ensues and death may occur within weeks unless a postexposure vaccination is administered.

Herpes Simplex Virus

- Herpes simplex virus type 1 (HSV-1) causes the cold sore on the lips and can retrogradely infect the gasserian ganglion via the mandibular nerve trunk. Infection of the CNS primarily affects the temporal lobes and results in swollen, hemorrhagic, necrotic brain parenchyma with perivascular lymphocytic cuffing. Infected neurons contain small, eosinophilic nuclear inclusions that can be specifically identified by immunostains for HSV-1.
- Herpes simplex virus type 2 (HSV-2) is a sexually transmitted disease that causes vesicular lesions of the vagina and penis. Transmission of HSV-2 to newborns during passage through the birth canal results in severe neonatal encephalitis with liquefactive necrosis of the cerebrum and cerebellum.

Arboviruses

Arboviruses (togavirus, Bunyavirus) are transmitted to humans by the bite of infected mosquito or ticks. Patients may demonstrate a range of presentations, from flulike symptoms to meningoencephalitis associated with severe inflammation of the gray matter, necrosis, and vessel thrombosis. In severe cases, patients may die within days. The insect-borne viral encephalitides includes St. Louis encephalitis, Western equine encephalitis, and tickborne encephalitis, among others.

Subacute Sclerosing Panencephalitis

Subacute sclerosing panencephalitis (SSPE) is caused by infection with the measles virus, which persists in the CNS for years and results in a chronic neurodegenerative process. Viral infection primarily affects the cortex, with marked gliosis in the gray and white matter, patchy loss of myelin, ubiquitous perivascular lymphocytes and macrophages, prominent basophilic nuclear inclusions rimmed by a prominent halo, and occasionally neurofibrillary tangles. Over time, SSPE causes behavioral changes, cognitive defects, and motor and sensory impairments, and seizures.

Progressive Multifocal Leukoencephalopathy

Progressive multifocal leukoencephalopathy (PML) is caused by infection with the polyomavirus JC virus, which primarily affects the white matter of the brain. PML infection demonstrates multiple discrete foci of demyelination near the gray-white junction in the cerebral hemispheres and brainstem. Typically, lesions measure several millimeters in diameter, demonstrate a central area devoid of myelin with residual axons and few oligodendrocytes, and macrophage infiltration. The oligodendrocytes within the lesion appear enlarged and contain hyperchromatic intranuclear inclusions with a ground-glass appearance. Astrocytes appear pleomorphic with multiple irregular nuclei and dense chromatin. Typically, PML affects immunocompromised patients and manifests with dementia, weakness, visual loss, and ataxia. Death often occurs within 6 months.

AIDS Encephalopathy

AIDS encephalopathy occurs as a direct affect of macrophage and microglial infection by the HIV-1 retrovirus. Macroscopically, the brains of these patients demonstrate mild cerebral atrophy. Microscopically, diffuse demyelination, astrogliosis, neuronal loss, microglial nodules and multinucleated giant cells are present. Patients classically present with encephalopathy (AIDS dementia complex), which includes mild to severe cognitive impairment, paralysis, and loss of sensory function.

Prion Diseases

Prion diseases, the spongiform encephalopathies, are a group of disorders that involve conformational changes of the human prion protein and are characterized clinically by slowly progressive ataxia and dementia. Prion diseases may be autosomal dominant (fatal familial insomnia) or infectious (kuru, corneal transplants). The human prion gene (*PRNP*) is located on the short arm of chromosome 20 and encodes a constitutively expressed cell-surface glycoprotein of unknown function. Both normal prion protein (PrP^c) and diseased prion protein (PrP^{sc}) have identical protein sequences but exist as different three-dimensional configurations. The conformation of PrP^{sc} makes this molecule resistant to protein degradation and allows it to self-propagate by converting normal prion protein to abnormal protein in an autocatalytic, exponentially expanding manner.

Lesions often occur in the cortical gray matter, but may involve the deeper nuclei of the basal ganglia, hypothalamus, and cerebellum. Microscopically, these lesions are characterized by vacuolization and microcystic change (spongiform degeneration), neuronal degeneration and loss, gliosis, and accumulations of insoluble prions with properties of amyloid. Specific forms of prion diseases are listed in Table 28-5 and include the following:

Table 28-5

Prion Diseases

Human
Creutzfeldt-Jakob disease (CJD)
  Sporadic (85% of all CJD cases; incidence 1 per million worldwide)
  Inherited mutation of the prion gene, autosomal dominant transmission
    (15% of all CJD cases)
  Iatrogenic
    Hormone injection
    Human growth hormone
    Human pituitary gonadotropin
  Tissue grafts
  Medical devices (inadequate sterilization)
    Depth electrodes
    Surgical instruments (not definitely proven)
  New variant
Gerstmann-Staussler-Scheinker disease (GSS; inherited prion gene mutation, autosomal dominant transmission)
Fetal familial insomnia (FFI; inherited prion gene mutation, autosomal dominant transmission)
Kuru (confined to the Fore people of Papua New Guinea, formerly transmitted by cannibalistic ritual)

Animal
Scrapie (sheep and goats)
Bovine spongiform encephalopathy (BSE: "mad cow disease")
Chronic wasting disease of deer or elk
Experimental transmission to many species, including primates and transgenic mice

From Rubin E, Gorstein F, Rubin R, et al. Rubin's Pathology, 4th ed. Philadelphia: Lippincott Williams & Wilkins, 2005, p. 1459.

- Sporadic Creutzfeldt-Jakob disease (CJD): 75% of cases of CJD; median age of onset 65 years; triad of dementia, myoclonus, and periodic spike-wave EEG complexes; death within 4 to 12 months
- Inherited CJD: 15% of cases of CJD; several different mutations of the *PNRP* gene; autosomal dominant
- Iatrogenic CJD: human pituitary-derived growth hormone, tissue grafts, medical devices
- New variant CJD (vCJD): median age of onset 26 years; most likely associated with BSE; behavioral and sensory changes in addition to ataxia
- Fatal familial insomnia: profound sleep-wake cycle disturbances, abnormal endocrine function, signs of pyramidal and cerebellar dysfunction; often cognitive function remains intact
- Kuru: first identified transmissible prion disease, related to cannibalistic practices of human brain ingestion, and results in severe ataxia of limbs and trunk due to severe cerebellar involvement

Demyelinating Diseases of the CNS

Demyelinating diseases refer to disorders in which a selective loss of myelin occurs.

Leukodystrophy

Leukodystrophies refer to inherited disorders of myelin formation and preservation.

Metachromatic Leukodystrophy

The most common leukodystrophy, metachromatic leukodystrophy (MLD), is an autosomal recessive disease caused by a deficiency in the activity of arylsulfatase A. It is frequently manifested in infancy. Arylsulfatase A is a lysosomal enzyme involved in the degradation of myelin sulfatides; deficiencies result in an accumulation of sulfatides in Schwann cells and oligodendrocytes (white matter). The brain demonstrates diffuse myelin loss and accumulation of 15 to 20 μm cytoplasmic granules that stain metachromatically with cresyl violet and toluidine blue.

Krabbe Disease

Krabbe disease, or *globoid cell leukodystrophy*, is an autosomal recessive disorder caused by a deficiency of galactocerebroside β-galactosidase. The disease is manifested in early infancy with severe motor, sensory, and cognitive deficits; it progresses to death within 1 to 2 years. The brain is small, with regions of partial and total demyelination and prominent astrogliosis, and there is almost a complete loss of oligodendroglia and myelin. A characteristic feature is the presence of perivascular, large (50 μm) mononuclear and multinucleated "globoid cells," which are macrophages that contain undigested galactocerebroside.

Adrenoleukodystrophy

Adrenoleukodystrophy (ALD) manifests between the ages of 3 and 10 years. This X-linked (Xq28) inherited disorder involves dysfunction of the adrenal cortex and demyelination of the nervous system, and is associated with high levels of saturated very-long-chain fatty acids (VLFCAs). Defects in the peroxisomal membrane prevent degradation of VLFCAs and increased levels and accumulation of these fatty acids results in loss of myelinated axons and oligodendroglia. The brain demonstrates confluent, bilaterally symmetrical demyelination, especially of the subcortical white matter of the parietooccipital region. The adrenals are atrophic and electron microscopy reveals membrane-bound curvilinear inclusions of VLFCAs in the adrenal, Schwann cells, and CNS macrophages. Patients demonstrate neurologic symptoms that progress to a vegetative state prior to death.

Alexander Disease

Alexander disease is caused by mutations in the gene encoding glial fibrillary acidic protein (GFAP), which leads to aggregates of extracellular Rosenthal fibers consisting of GFAP aggregates bound to protein chaperones. The Rosenthal fibers are deposited in the subpial regions of the brain and spinal cord and in the perivascular region of white matter. This disease is accompanied by a loss of oligodendrocytes and myelin in the brain. Alexander disease presents during infancy or early childhood with psychomotor retardation, progressive dementia, and paralysis, leading ultimately to death.

Multiple Sclerosis

Multiple sclerosis (MS) is a chronic demyelinating disease that most commonly affects young adults with a 2:1 female to male predominance and a prevalence of 1 in 1,000. MS is commonly characterized by a relapsing-remitting disease course over many years.

A number of mechanisms have been proposed to play a role in the pathogenesis of MS:

- Genetic factors: 25% concordance for MS in monozygotic twins, familial aggregation, and linkage to a number of MHC alleles
- Immune factors: injection of myelin basic protein may induce a similar disease in mice; identification of oligoclonal T cells

in the CSF and perivascular lymphocyte and macrophage accumulation
- Infectious agents: disease of temperate climates, and risk varies with age of relocation to various climates

The classic pathologic feature of MS is the demyelinated plaque, which is a discrete region of demyelination usually less than 2 cm in diameter. These plaques occur in the white matter and occasionally the gray-white junction. The plaques are most common in the optic nerves, optic chiasm, and periventricular white matter. Microscopically, active plaques are well-demarcated and demonstrate prominent macrophage infiltration and selective loss of myelin in a region of axonal preservation. In addition, lymphocytes often surround small veins and arteries, and edema may be prominent. The neuronal cell body is unaffected by the disease process, whereas the axon may undergo degeneration. Inactive MS plaques demonstrate gliosis and minimal to no inflammation.

The classical clinical feature associated with MS is the accumulation of lesions in different regions of the brain at different periods (lesions separated in time and space). This feature underlies the common relapsing-remitting course of MS, although some patients may demonstrate a relentless, progressive course of the disease. Early symptoms include loss of vision in one eye, blurred vision, vertigo, and weakness or numbness of one or both legs. These symptoms may resolve, but development of additional lesions results in permanent defects.

Over time, the degree of functional impairment varies from minor to severe, with many patients developing paralysis, dysarthria, severe visual defects, incontinence, and dementia. Most patients survive 20 to 30 years following the onset of disease and may ultimately die of respiratory failure or urinary tract infection. Some patients benefit from treatment with interferon-β.

Postinfectious and Postvaccinal Encephalomyelitis

- Postinfectious encephalomyelitis: occurs days to weeks following a viral rash; often presents with the sudden onset of headache, vomiting, fever, and meningeal signs. Microscopically, focal perivascular demyelination and mononuclear cell infiltrates around small- to medium-sized venules in the white matter are apparent.
- Postvaccinal encephalomyelitis: a similar disease process; occurs following vaccination with agents containing cross-reacting antigens

Central Pontine Myelinolysis

Central pontine myelinolysis occurs following rapid correction of hyponatremia in which demyelination of the pons occurs. This results in a variety of lesions, from small asymptomatic foci to large lesions presenting with quadriparesis, pseudobulbar palsy, or depression of consciousness.

Neuronal Storage Diseases

This group of inherited diseases is caused by enzyme deficiencies that result in the accumulation of normal metabolic products in lysosomes. These disorders are discussed in detail in Chapter 6 and are briefly described here.

- Tay-Sachs disease: a lethal autosomal recessive disorder that manifests by 6 months of age and is caused by a deficiency in hexosaminidase A, which leads to the accumulation of gangliosides in CNS neurons. Infants develop a delay in motor development with subsequent flaccid paralysis, weakness, blindness, mental impairment and death. Nerve cells of the CNS and peripheral nervous system are distended and contain cytoplasmic lipid droplets. By electron microscopy, lysosomes are filed with lipids and termed "myelin figures." A characteristic cherry red spot is present in the macula with retinal involvement.
- Hurler syndrome: an autosomal recessive disorder that results from deficient glycosaminoglycan metabolism, leading to intraneuronal accumulation of mucopolysaccharides. Involvement of the CNS is variable.
- Gaucher disease: an autosomal recessive disorder caused by a deficiency in glucocerebrosidase and accumulation of glucocerebroside in macrophages. The CNS is most severely involved in the infantile, or type II, form of the disease. Infants demonstrate severe neuronal loss and failure to thrive, with death at an early age.
- Niemann-Pick disease: an autosomal recessive disorder caused by a deficiency of sphingomyelinase that results in intraneuronal storage of sphingomyelin. Patients demonstrate a failure to thrive. Retinal degeneration is common and a cherry-red spot may also be present in the macula. The brains of patients with Niemann Pick disease are atrophic with marked astrogliosis.

Metabolic Neuronal Diseases

Various metabolic neuronal diseases contribute to neuronal dysfunction.

Phenylketonuriais an autosomal recessive disorder caused by a deficiency in phenylalanine hydroxylase, which converts phenylalanine to tyrosine. The disease presents within the first several months of life with mental retardation, seizures, and impaired physical development. Early institution of a phenylalanine-free diet can prevent neurological impairment. Cretinism (severe infantile hypothyroidism) results in stunted growth and cognitive impairments, but is reversible early in the disease by administration of thyroxine.

Wilson disease is an autosomal recessive disorder caused by mutations in the *WD* gene that lead to defective copper metabolism. Defective biliary copper excretion results in deposition in the brain and the development of athetoid movements and insidious cirrhosis. In addition, the limbus of the cornea demonstrates a visible golden-brown band termed the Kayser-Fleischer ring. Grossly, the lenticular nuclei of the brain show a light golden discoloration, and often small cysts or clefts are present in the putamen or deep layers of the neocortex. Microscopically, mild neuron loss and gliosis are present.

Metabolic Disorders

Alcoholism

Disorders caused by chronic alcohol use reflect direct toxic injury to neurons as well as injury occurring secondary to nutritional deficits. CNS lesions that occur with alcoholism include the following:

- *Wernicke syndrome*: due to thiamine (vitamin B_1) deficiency; rapid onset of thermal regulatory disturbances, altered consciousness, ophthalmoplegia and nystagmus; lesions in hypothalamus, mamillary bodies, periaqueductal region of the midbrain, pons; rapidly reversed by thiamine administration
- *Korsakoff syndrome*: disordered recent memory compensated for by confabulation reflected in the degeneration of neurons in the medial-dorsal nucleus of the thalamus
- Cerebral atrophy
- Atrophy of the superior aspect of the vermis of the cerebellum: atrophy of Purkinje and granular cells resulting in truncal ataxia
- Central pontine myelinolysis: demyelination of the pons caused by rapid correction of hyponatremia

Hepatic Encephalopathy

Hepatic encephalopathy occurs with liver failure and manifests as delirium, seizures, and coma. The only CNS findings are altered astroglia in the thalamus (Alzheimer type II astrocytes), which demonstrate enlarged nuclei and marginated chromatin.

Subacute Combined Degeneration of the Spinal Cord

This disease is a result of vitamin B_{12} deficiency, and it may occur in pernicious anemia, extensive gastric resection, malabsorption syndromes, or in strict vegetarians. Initially, the posterolateral columns of the spinal cord demonstrate symmetric myelin and axonal loss at the thoracic level. Often, burning sensations on the soles of the feet or other paresthesias are the earliest signs. Over time, gliosis and atrophy of the posterolateral columns occurs and results in weakness, defective postural sensation, and ataxia. This disease is rapidly progressive and poorly reversible.

Neurodegenerative Diseases

Neurodegenerative diseases are a heterogeneous group of disorders that share several features in common, including familial and sporadic forms, an autosomal dominant pattern of inheritance of heritable forms, and the formation of filamentous amyloid lesions either intracellularly or extracellularly. Selected neurodegenerative diseases are presented in Table 28-6.

Parkinson Disease

Parkinson disease (PD) occurs in the sixth to eighth decades and affects 2% of the population of North America. The majority of cases are sporadic, but rare cases of early onset, autosomal dominant, familial PD occurs. The disease has also been reported to occur following viral encephalitis and intake of the drug MPTP.

Macroscopically, PD is characterized by a loss of pigmented, dopaminergic neurons in the substantia nigra and locus ceruleus. Microscopically, Lewy bodies (spherical, eosinophilic cytoplasmic inclusions) are present throughout the brain and represent aggregates of α-synuclein (a synaptic protein of unknown function). Lewy bodies have been hypothesized to arise following oxidative stress produced by the autooxidation of catecholamines during melanin formation by neurons in the substantia nigra and locus ceruleus. Damage to the extrapyramidal system results in the classic symptoms of PD, which include a slowness of voluntary movements, muscular rigidity through the entire range of movement, and a coarse tremor of the distal extremities present at rest that disappears with voluntary movement. Additional findings include an expressionless (masklike) facies and a reduced rate of swallowing, which leads to drooling. Late stages may be characterized by depression and dementia.

Treatment of PD includes levodopa administration, which becomes ineffective following several years. Newer treatments may include deep-brain stimulation and possibly dopaminergic cell transplants.

Two diseases that are clinically very similar to PD are striatonigral degeneration and progressive supranuclear palsy.

Table 28-6
Neurodegenerative Diseases

Disease	Lesion	Components	Location	Symptoms
Parkinson disease	Lewy bodies	α-Synuclein	Intracytoplasmic	Resting tremors, muscular rigidity, expressionless face, lability
Dementia with Lewy bodies	Lewy bodies	α-Synuclein	Intracytoplasmic	Dementia, Parkinsonian symptoms
Amyotrophic lateral sclerosis (ALS)	Spheroids	Neurofilament subunits/superoxide dismutase (SOD-1)	Intracytoplasmic	Early hand weakness; late limb weakness, respiratory muscle weakness, unintelligible speech
Trinucleotide repeat diseases: Huntington disease	Inclusions	Polyglutamine tracts	Intracellular	Choreoathetoid movements, emotional and cognitive disturbances
Alzheimer disease	Senile plaques/neurofibrillary tangles	Amyloid-β, tau	Extracellular, intracytoplasmic	Progressive memory loss, cognitive decline, eventual dementia
Pick disease	Neurofibrillary tangles	tau	Intracytoplasmic (Pick bodies)	Similar to Alzheimer disease
Striatonigral degeneration	Glial inclusions	tau	Intracytoplasmic	PD, Shy-Drager disease, and olivopontocerebellar atrophy
Prion diseases	Prion deposits	Prions	Extracellular	Slowly progressive ataxia and dementia

Modified from Rubin E, Gorstein F, Rubin R, et al. Rubin's Pathology, 4th ed. Philadelphia: Lippincott Williams & Wilkins, 2005, p. 1468.

- *Striatonigral degeneration*: clinically identical to PD; atrophy of the corpus striatum and less atrophy of substantia nigra and locus ceruleus; may be component of multiple system atrophy (in addition to Shy-Drager disease and olivopontocerebellar atrophy); α-synuclein inclusions
- *Progressive supranuclear palsy*: clinically similar to PD with additional progressive paralysis of vertical eye movements; more widespread neuronal loss, including globus pallidus and dentate nuclei; neurofibrillary tangles

Amyotrophic Lateral Sclerosis

Amyotrophic lateral sclerosis (ALS) most commonly occurs in the fifth decade and demonstrates a male predominance. Approximately 5% of cases show autosomal dominant inheritance and are caused by a mutation in the superoxide dismutase 1 (*SOD1*) gene on chromosome 21q.

ALS is characterized pathologically by a loss of motor neurons in the brain and spinal cord, specifically the anterior horn cells of the spinal cord, the motor nuclei of the brainstem (especially the hypoglossal nuclei), and the upper motor neurons of the cerebral cortex. Loss of neurons is accompanied by a mild gliosis and often aggregations of neurofilaments within the axons to form spheroids. Myelin stains demonstrate a striking pallor of the lateral corticospinal tracts of the spinal cord. The muscles innervated by injured spinal areas become atrophic.

ALS begins as weakness and wasting of the muscles of the hand, often accompanied by painful cramps of the arm. Fasciculations (irregular rapid contractions of the muscles that do not result in limb movements) are characteristic. ALS is progressive and results in weakness of the limbs leading to total disability, unintelligible speech, and respiratory weakness. Dementia is uncommon in ALS. Patients often succumb within 10 years.

Trinucleotide Repeat Expansion Syndromes

A large number of diseases can be classified under triplet repeat expansion syndromes. Triplet repeats are normal components of many genes and represent three nucleotides that repeat in sequence. The expansion of triplet repeats to certain critical amounts can lead to disease states. Triplet repeat diseases may be inherited in an X-linked, autosomal dominant, or autosomal recessive manner. An increase in triplet repeat length with each subsequent generation can lead to an earlier onset of disease, termed anticipation. Triplet repeats may occur within a coding region of a gene, leading to abnormal protein formation, or in a noncoding region of a gene, leading to transcriptional interference.

Huntington Disease

Huntington disease (HD) is a triplet-repeat disease caused by expansion of CAG repeats in the coding region of the *HD* gene on chromosome 4p16.3. The *HD* gene product huntingtin is expressed widely throughout the body, including in neurons and glia, although the function is unknown; expansion of triplet repeats in this gene most likely leads to a gain of toxic function. HD demonstrates an autosomal dominant inheritance pattern, although sporadic forms have been identified. This disease commonly affects whites of northwestern European ancestry and has an incidence of 1 in 20,000. The average age of onset is 40 years, and patients present initially with cognitive and emotional disturbances followed in several years by the development of choreoathetoid movements.

Patients ultimately develop severe intellectual deterioration, often accompanied by paranoia and delusions, as well as severe, debilitating movement disorder. Death occurs at an average of 15 years after HD as been diagnosed. At autopsy, the frontal cortex is symmetrically and moderately atrophied. In addition, the caudate nuclei undergo symmetric atrophy with an expansion of the lateral ventricles. Microscopically, loss of small neurons with associated microgliosis is identified. Accumulation of abnormal huntingtin protein occurs in neuronal nuclei and processes, although its role in pathogenesis is unclear.

Inherited Spinocerebellar Ataxias

The inherited spinocerebellar ataxias include a heterogeneous group of disorders that share features of a broad, but system-based, topography, a genetic contribution, and a precocious loss of neurons in the cerebellum, brainstem, and spinal cord. A subset of these diseases demonstrates expanded trinucleotide repeats. The most common inherited spinocerebellar ataxia is *Friedreich ataxia (FA)*, which in inherited in an autosomal recessive manner and demonstrates a prevalence in European populations of 1 in 50,000. FA may also occur sporadically. Onset of disease typically occurs before 25 years of age and progresses until death, which occurs approximately 30 years following diagnosis. FA is caused by expansion of a GAA repeat in the *frataxin* gene located at 9q13.3–21.1, which functions in iron transport into the mitochondria. Frataxin is most highly expressed in the heart and spinal cord, and disease occurs by loss of function of the frataxin protein. Patients demonstrate a combined ataxia of the upper and lower limbs, and frequently dysarthria, lower-limb areflexia, extensor plantar reflexes, and sensory loss. In addition, many patients also demonstrate skeletal deformities, hypertrophic cardiomyopathy, and diabetes mellitus. At autopsy, degeneration of the posterior columns (sensory loss), distal corticospinal tracts, and spinocerebellar tracts (ataxia) is evident.

Alzheimer Disease

Alzheimer disease (AD) is the most common cause of dementia in the elderly and demonstrates an increasing prevalence with age, with 10% of persons older than 85 years of age demonstrating features of the disease. The majority of AD cases are sporadic, although a familial form is recognized.

A variety of genetic factors appear to contribute to the development of AD, including the following:

- Apolipoprotein E: chromosome 19q13.2; ε4 allele associated with increased risk ad earlier onset of AD
- Presenilin-1: chromosome 14; mutations associated with early-onset familial AD
- Presenilin-2: chromosome 1; mutations associated with Volga German familial AD

AD is characterized by the formation of senile (neuritic) plaques and neurofibrillary tangles (NFTs). Senile plaques are spherical aggregates of Aβ up to several hundred micrometers in diameter. Aβ is formed by altered cleavage of the amyloid precursor protein (APP), which is a transmembrane protein located on neurons and glia and found on chromosome 21. Normal degradation of APP results in proteolytic cleavage in the center of the Aβ region, located on the extracellular aspect of APP. In contrast, abnormal cleavage at either end of the Aβ portion of the molecule (in patients with mutated APP) results in the production of a 42–amino-acid, highly amyloidogenic, nonsoluble Aβ peptide that accumulates in senile plaques. Extensive senile plaque formation and early AD onset is characteristic of patients with Down syndrome, who have an extra copy of chromosome 21, thereby supporting the role of the Aβ peptide in the development of dementia. In contrast, many cognitively intact elderly persons may have extensive plaque formation without clinical cognitive impairment.

Neurofibrillary tangles (NFTs) are a second prominent pathologic feature of AD. NFTs are formed by an abnormal form of a microtubule-associated protein (MAP) termed *tau*. In AD, tau undergoes aberrant phosphorylation, which results in dissociation of the protein from microtubules and aggregation of paired helical filaments within the neuronal cytoplasm. Neuronal transport is therefore interrupted and contributes to the compromised neuronal function.

On gross examination, the brain of patients with AD appears atrophic, evidenced by an average weight loss of 200 grams, narrow gyri and widened sulci. The atrophy is symmetrical and predominantly in the frontal and hippocampal cortex. Microscopically, neuronal loss, gliosis, and the formation of senile plaques and NFTs are identified. Senile plaques are immunopositive for Aβ at the core and periphery, and are also positive for Congo red, thioflavin

S, and argentophilic. NFTs appear as irregular bundles of fibrils in the neuronal cytoplasm that are immunoreactive for tau.

Patients with AD present clinically with a gradual loss of memory and cognitive function, difficulty with language, and behavioral changes. The disease progresses, with development to full-blown dementia within 5 to 10 years. Most patients die as a result of bronchopneumonia.

Pick disease appears clinically similar to AD, although the cortical atrophy is initially unilateral and localized to the frontotemporal lobe, but ultimately becomes bilateral. Many neurons contain tau immunoreactive cytoplasmic inclusions termed *Pick bodies*. Pick disease is commonly a sporadic disease that often presents in mid adult life and progresses to death in 3 to 10 years.

Tumors of the CNS

The majority of neoplasms within the CNS are actually metastatic lesions, although a variety of primary neoplasms may occur. Primary CNS neoplasms may be classified according to cell of origin, including the following:

- Neuroectoderm: gliomas (astrocytomas, oligodendrogliomas, ependymomas) and neuronal tumors (medulloblastoma)
- Mesenchymal structures: meningiomas, schwannomas
- Ectopic tissues: craniopharyngiomas, dermoid cysts, lipomas, dysgerminomas
- Retained embryonic structures: paraphyseal cysts
- Metastases

Approximately 60% of primary CNS neoplasms are gliomas, 20% are meningiomas, and the remainder is composed of various other neoplasms. Neuronal tumors are uncommon. When they occur in childhood, they are often primitive, rapidly growing lesions that involve the cerebellum (medulloblastomas). Typically, the behavior of CNS neoplasms cannot be readily categorized into benign versus malignant, because many lesions may demonstrate indolent growth and cause mortality only many years following diagnosis. In addition, the vast majority of CNS neoplasms do not metastasize outside of the CNS.

The majority of CNS neoplasms also demonstrate specific intracranial locations and relatively well-defined age of onsets. Classical locations of CNS neoplasms are presented in Figure 28-6.

Intracranial tumors may demonstrate similar symptoms that are primarily caused by local infiltration and mass effect. Infiltration may result in motor or sensory deficits, with general sparing of cognitive function. Irritation of neuronal regions may result in the development of seizures. Mass effect may be caused directly by the tumor or by surrounding edema, and increases the risk of

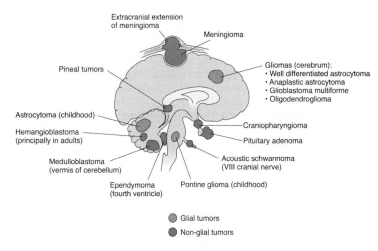

FIGURE 28-6

The distribution of common intracranial tumors. (From Rubin E, Gorstein F, Rubin R, et al. Rubin's Pathology, 4th ed. Philadelphia: Lippincott Williams & Wilkins, 2005, p. 1481.)

hydrocephalus and herniation. Various types of herniation include the following:

- Transtentorial herniation: medial aspect of the hippocampus herniates through the tentorium; may result in third nerve palsy, midbrain necrosis
- Foramen magnum herniation: cerebellar tonsils herniated into the foramen magnum; compression of the cardiac and respiratory centers in the brainstem
- Subfalcine herniation: cingulate gyrus herniates beneath the falx

Gliomas

Astrocytomas

ocytomas range greatly in levels of differentiation, with malignancy often correlating with increased age of the patient. Generally, astrocytomas demonstrate expression of GFAP, reflecting their origin from glial astrocytes, although poorly differentiated lesions may demonstrate some loss of this molecule. Astrocytomas are subclassified into four types, based on the pathological findings.

Grade I Astrocytomas

Grade I astrocytomas often occur in children and young adults and demonstrate the most favorable prognosis of all astrocytomas.

Pilocytic astrocytomas represent a grade I astrocytoma, and often occur in the posterior fossa, although the third ventricle, hypothalamus, and thalamus may be involved. Outcome is dependent on the extent of resection, with completely resected tumors having nearly 100% 10-year survival. Pilocytic astrocytomas are often microcystic and demonstrate regions of parallel bundles of fibrillar ("piloid" or "hairlike") processes that are positive for GFAP. In addition, Rosenthal fibers, which are highly eosinophilic irregular aggregations within glial processes, and eosinophilic intracellular or extracellular protein droplets (eosinophilic granular bodies) may be identified.

Grade II Astrocytomas

Grade II astrocytomas (diffuse astrocytomas) account for approximately 20% of all CNS neoplasms and affect the spinal cord, optic nerve, third ventricle, midbrain, pons, and cerebellum in young adults, and the cerebral hemispheres in adults. The average age of onset is between 20 to 40 years of age. These lesions are often poorly demarcated and are composed of a hypercellular cortex containing infiltrating, small, hyperchromatic single glial cells demonstrating pleomorphic nuclei and rare to no mitotic figures. Patients with grade II astrocytomas demonstrate an average life expectancy of 5 years, and transformation to a higher grade astrocytoma may occur.

Grade III Astrocytomas

Grade III astrocytomas (anaplastic astrocytomas) often occur in patients between the ages of 30 to 40 years and most commonly affect the cerebral hemispheres. Microscopically, these tumors are characterized by pleomorphic cells, greater cellularity, and modest mitotic activity. The rapid growth of this lesion results in an average life expectancy of 2 to 3 years.

Grade IV Astrocytomas

Grade IV astrocytomas (glioblastoma multiforme) account for 40% of all primary CNS neoplasms and most commonly occurs in patients over the age of 40 years. These lesions may affect any region of the brain and can cross the midline of the brain via the corpus callosum to give a butterflylike effect on radiographic imaging. Microscopically, this lesion is characterized by markedly pleomorphic cells, mitoses, palisading necrosis, and glomeruloid vascular proliferation (endothelial proliferation within the vascular lumen). These lesions are highly aggressive and life expectancy is only 18 months.

Oligodendroglioma

Oligodendrogliomas represent approximately 15% of all gliomas and most commonly occur in adults. These lesions are typically located in the white matter of the cerebral hemispheres. Grossly, oligodendrogliomas appear gelatinous or soft and often obscure the gray-white junction of the cortex. Microscopically, these lesions are composed of cells with small round nuclei with a perinuclear halo (clearing) caused by fixation ("fried egg cells"). These cells often surround large cortical neurons, a process termed *satellitosis*. Mitotic figures and necrosis are typically absent, although they may occur in higher grade lesions. The neoplastic cells are often surrounded by delicate small vessels. Oligodendrogliomas infiltrate the surrounding the surrounding brain and are positive for GFAP. Loss of heterozygosity for 1p and 19q tend to occur in these lesions and serves as a useful molecular test. In some instances, oligodendrogliomas may undergo anaplastic transformation. The average life expectancy following diagnosis is 5 to 10 years.

Ependymoma

Ependymomas most commonly occur during the first two decades of life and are often located in the fourth ventricle. Growth within the fourth ventricle may give rise to hydrocephalus. In contrast to other gliomas, ependymomas demonstrate a more discrete border with the surrounding brain, and appear grossly as soft, fleshy lesions. A common microscopic feature of ependymomas is the formation of true rosettes and pseudorosettes. True rosettes appear similar to tire spokes, in which a circular arrangement of cells rims central fibrillar processes. When these structures surround blood vessels, they are termed pseudorosettes. Ependymomas stain positively for GFAP and may be subdivided into a number of types based on morphology. Outcome is related to the extent of surgical resection.

Neuronal Tumors

Gangliocytoma

Gangliocytomas are formed of large neurons that have the morphologic appearance of ganglion cells. When admixed with neoplastic glial cells, these lesions are termed *gangliogliomas*. These tumors are most common in children and young adults and preferentially affect the temporal lobes, although any site of the brain may be affected. Radiographically and macroscopically, these lesions are well-circumscribed and most commonly demonstrate a cystic structure containing a mural nodule. Microscopically, gangliocytomas are formed of large, disordered neurons in a background of fibrillary stroma (neuronal processes) with little to no intervening brain tissue. Additional microscopic findings include cytoplasmic eosinophilic granular bodies, microcalcification, and perivascular lymphocytic infiltrates. Patients often present with seizures.

Central neurocytoma

Central neurocytomas often occur in young adults and appear grossly and radiographically as well-circumscribed, intraventricular lesions. These tumors occur within the ventricular system near the foramen of Monro and therefore may present with obstruction of CSF flow and manifestations of hydrocephalus. Microscopically, these lesions are formed by uniform, small, round neurons with finely speckled chromatin in a background fibrillar stroma formed by neuronal processes.

Medulloblastoma

Medulloblastomas occur within the first two decades of life and represent the most common neuroblastic tumor in the CNS. In addition to sporadic forms, these tumors may arise in association with Turcot or Gorlin syndromes. These lesions most likely arise from the external granular layer of the cerebellum, which may explain why these tumors are located almost exclusively in the cerebellum. Microscopically, these tumors contain hyperchromatic, round to oval nuclei, and scant cytoplasm, typical of "small cell" neoplasms. The cells often crowd together and overlap, although rosette formation may be present. Immunostains for neurofilament protein and synaptophysin are often positive. Multiple underlying molecular abnormalities have been identified, including c-*myc* amplication, isochromosome 17q formation, and loss of 17p heterozygosity. Patients often present with ataxia and signs of hydrocephalus. These lesions are highly sensitive to radiotherapy, but the 10-year survival rate is only 50% because of the highly infiltrative behavior of this neoplasm and its ability to disseminate within the CSF.

Meningioma

Meningiomas arise from the meningothelium and often occur in the fourth or fifth decades, although young adults may also be affected. Meningiomas account for 20% of all primary CNS neoplasms and most commonly occur in the parasagittal regions of the cerebral hemispheres, olfactory groove, and lateral sphenoid wing. These lesions most commonly occur sporadically, although prior radiation treatment or association with a genetic disorder such as neurofibromatosis type 2 (NF2) may predispose to these lesions.

Meningiomas grow as well-demarcated, firm, bosselated lesions attached to the meninges and often cause symptoms, such as seizures, by compression of adjacent brain parenchyma. Involvement of the meninges, which are innervated, may also cause headaches. The cut surface of meningiomas is gray and often demonstrates a homogeneous appearance. Microscopically, these lesions are classically characterized by whorled patterns of meningothelial cells associated with psammoma bodies (laminated, spherical calcium deposits). Various morphological forms may occur, some of which appear to be more aggressive. Due to their position, meningiomas may occasionally invade the skull, although this is not associated with a worsened prognosis. In contrast, local brain invasion portends a poorer outcome. Meningiomas are positive for epithelial membrane antigen and negative for GFAP and cytokeratin.

Choroid Plexus Papilloma

Choroid plexus papillomas are uncommon and often occur during the first decade of life, commonly in the lateral ventricles. Hydrocephalus may be a presenting feature. Grossly, choroid plexus papillomas appear as papillary excrescences within the ventricle. Microscopically, these lesions are composed of well-differentiated columnar epithelium resting on a fibrovascular stroma, similar to normal-appearing choroid plexus. These lesions are commonly immunopositive for cytokeratin and S-100, and only rarely for GFAP. These lesions are typically benign, although transformation into *choroid plexus carcinoma* may occur.

Craniopharyngioma

Craniopharyngiomas arise above the sella turcica during the first two decades of life. Grossly, these lesions may demonstrate a solid and cystic component. Craniopharyngiomas originate from the epithelium of Rathke's pouch and may be lined by squamous or adamantinous epithelium and produce keratin at different stages of maturation. These lesions may present with visual deficits, headaches, or pituitary failure.

Tumors of Germ Cell Origin

Germinomas arise in the CNS as a result of misplaced germ cells during embryogenesis and often occur in the midline of the CNS of young adult men, especially in the pineal gland and suprasellar region. Germinomas appear microscopically as nests or sheets of large neoplastic cells admixed with lymphocytes and prominent collagenous stroma. The large neoplastic cells are typically immunopositive for placental alkaline phosphatase (PLAP) and c-kit.

Other types of germ cell tumors that may arise in the CNS include teratoma, endodermal sinus tumor, embryonal carcinoma, and choriocarcinoma.

Hemangioblastoma

Hemangioblastomas often present as an expanding cerebellar mass in people between 20 and 40 years of age, and more commonly affect men. Grossly, these lesions are solid or demonstrate a cystic structure containing a mural nodule. Microscopically, hemangioblastomas are highly vascularized and feature endothelium-lined canals admixed with interstitial (or "stromal") cells. In 20% of cases, these cells secrete erythropoietin and cause polycythemia. *Lindau syndrome* refers to the hereditary occurrence of cerebellar hemangioblastoma without additional lesions, whereas *von Hippel-Lindau syndrome* refers to VHL gene mutations demonstrating cerebellar hemangioblastoma associated with retinal hemangiomas and other tumors.

Colloid Cyst

Colloid cysts occur along the anterior, midline portion of the tegmental portion of the third ventricle. At this location, they can occlude the foramen of Monro, elevate and compress the fornix, and compress the lateral wall of the third ventricle. Grossly, colloid cysts are discrete masses that appear translucent and are filled with mucinous material. Microscopically, these cysts are lined by ciliated cuboidal epithelium. Patients present with hydrocephalus, alterations in personality, weakness of the lower legs, and loss of bladder control.

CNS Lymphoma

Lymphomas that involve the brain often occur secondary to systemic disease, although primary CNS lymphoma can occur and is usually represents a B-cell lesion. CNS lymphomas often affect immunosuppressed patients. Primary CNS lymphomas often involve the bilateral periventricular regions and comprise a mixture of small and large cells.

Schwannoma

Schwannomas are derived from Schwann cells, which produce both collagen and myelin. These lesions may occur at many locations, including spinal nerve roots and along the eighth cranial nerve, termed an acoustic neuroma. *Acoustic neuromas* arise at the oligodendroglial-Schwann cell junction and may cause tinnitus and deafness, as well as additional nerve compression if it has extended into the cerebellopontine angle. Microscopically, these lesions demonstrate interwoven fascicles of spindled cells, some of which form a parallel array termed a Verocay body. These lesions may occur in conjunction with *NF2* gene deletion. Excision is usually curative.

Metastatic Lesions

Metastases to the CNS occur by hematogenous spread and make up the majority of overall CNS neoplasms. Determination of the site of neoplastic origin is based on a combination of clinical features, radiologic findings and immunostaining.

Hereditary Intracranial Neoplasms

A variety of hereditary syndromes may be associated with the development of various CNS neoplasms. A listing of these disorders and associated genetic defects is presented in Table 28-7.

PERIPHERAL NERVOUS SYSTEM

Normal Anatomy and Histology

The peripheral nervous system (PNS) is external to the brain and spinal cord and is composed of cranial nerves, dorsal and ventral spinal roots, spinal nerves, and ganglia. Somatic motor and preganglionic autonomic fibers arise from nerve cell bodies in the CNS, whereas somatic sensory and postganglionic autonomic fibers arise from cell bodies situated within ganglia. Peripheral nerves are ensheathed by an endoneurium, perineurium, and epineurium. The epineurium binds together nerve fascicles and contains nutrient arteries that supply the nerves. Peripheral nerve fibers may be myelinated or unmyelinated; although Schwann cells ensheathe both forms of nerve fibers, the axons that are destined to become myelinated fibers direct Schwann cell myelination. The axon diameter is proportional to the conduction velocity, myelin thickness, and distance between the nodes of Ranvier.

Peripheral Nerve Injury

In contrast to nerves in the CNS, peripheral nerves may undergo regeneration and remyelination in certain instances. Peripheral nerve degeneration occurs following injury to the neuronal cell body or the axon. Three types of *axonal degeneration* can occur:

- Distal axonal degeneration: distal ends of larger, longer fibers; often cause stocking-and-glove distal neuropathies; may regenerate if the proximal axon and cell body are not affected
- Neuronopathy: due to damage or death of the neuronal cell body; little potential for recovery of function
- Wallerian degeneration: axonal degeneration occurs distal to a crush injury or transection; may regenerate in some instances

Loss of myelin from a portion of the neuron is termed *segmental demyelination* and may occur with Schwann cell dysfunction (primary demyelination) or axonal abnormalities (secondary demyelination). Following injury, macrophages clear the myelin debris, which is then followed by Schwann cell proliferation, remyelination, and recovery of function. Repeated episodes of myelin injury result in multiple rounds of remyelination, with resultant supernu-

Table 28-7

Hereditary Syndromes Associated with Intracranial Tumors

Disease	Chromosome Locus	Gene (Protein)	Nervous System Tumor(s)
Neurofibromatosis 1	17q11	*NF1* (neurofibromin)	Neurofibroma Malignant peripheral nerve sheath tumor Juvenile pilocytic astrocytoma of the optic nerves ("optic glioma")
Neurofibromatosis 2	22q12	*NF2* (schwannomin/merlin)	Schwannoma Meningioma Ependymoma (spinal cord) Bilateral acoustic neuromas
Tuberous sclerosis	9q34 16p13.3	*TSC1* (hamartin) TSC2 (tuberin)	Subependymal giant cell tumor Astrocytoma
von Hippel-Lindau syndrome	3p25	*VHL*	Hemangioblastoma

From Rubin E, Gorstein F, Rubin R, et al. Rubin's Pathology, 4th ed. Philadelphia: Lippincott Williams & Wilkins, 2005, p. 1490.

merary Schwann cells around axons (onion-skinning) and nerve enlargement (hypertrophic neuropathy).

Peripheral Neuropathies

Peripheral neuropathies may affect any age group and may be hereditary or acquired. Peripheral neuropathies may be subclassified into those that demonstrate primarily axonal degeneration (axonal neuropathy) or those that demonstrate primarily segmental demyelination (demyelinating neuropathy). A defining characteristic of demyelinating neuropathies is decreased nerve conduction velocity demonstrated by electrophysiological studies, which is in contrast to the normal nerve velocity of axonal neuropathies.

Clinically, patients with peripheral neuropathies may have muscle weakness, muscle atrophy, altered sensation, and autonomic dysfunction. Sensory abnormalities may include involvement of large caliber fibers (position and vibration sense) or small caliber fibers (pain and temperature). The disease may be acute, subacute, or chronic and affect one nerve (mononeuropathy), several nerves (mononeuropathy multiplex), or diffuse nerves in a symmetrical pattern (polyneuropathy). The most common causes of peripheral neuropathy include diabetes, renal failure, alcoholism, neurotoxic drugs, autoimmune diseases, and HIV infection.

Diabetic Neuropathy

Diabetic neuropathy is the most common peripheral neuropathy and can manifest with distal sensory or sensorimotor polyneuropathy (a stocking-and-glove distribution), autonomic neuropathy, mononeuropathy, or mononeuropathy multiplex. Distal sensory polyneuropathy is the most common finding. Nerve ischemia has been postulated to play a pathophysiological role in the development of nerve disease. Diabetic neuropathy is characterized pathologically by a predominance of axonal degeneration, with some degree of segmental demyelination. Both large and small caliber nerve fibers may be involved.

Acute Inflammatory Demyelinating Polyneuropathy (Guillain-Barré Syndrome)

Acute inflammatory demyelinating polyneuropathy (AIDP) is an immune-mediated neuropathy that often follows immunization or infection by a variety of agents, including *Campylobacter jejuni*. AIDP is the most common cause of acute polyneuropathy in children and adults. Patients usually demonstrate predominantly motor dysfunction. Severe complications may include compromise of respiratory function, cardiac arrhythmias, or hypotension. Most patients improve within several weeks, and beneficial effects have been demonstrated with plasmapheresis and intravenously administered gamma globulin. Microscopically, AIDP demonstrates endoneurial lymphocyte and macrophage infiltrates, segmental demyelination, and relative sparing of axons.

Dorsal Root Ganglionitis (Sensory Neuronopathy)

Dorsal root ganglionitis (sensory neuronopathy) is a subacute or chronic sensory polyneuropathy associated with sensory ataxia. This disorder may be idiopathic or occur in conjunction with paraneoplastic syndromes in which anti-Hu antibodies (antineuronal autoantibodies) occur.

Monoclonal Gammopathy-associated Neuropathies

Monoclonal gammopathy-associated neuropathies are caused by amyloid neuropathy, a cryoglobulinemia-associated vasculitic neuropathy, a chronic axonal polyneuropathy, or a chronic demyelinating polyneuropathy. This disease may occur with monoclonal gammopathy of undetermined significance (MGUS) or plasma cell neoplasms. In many cases, the paraprotein binds to myelin-associated glycoprotein, which may lead to ultimate neuronal dysfunction.

Amyloid Neuropathy

Amyloid neuropathy leads to prominent autonomic dysfunction and often occurs in association with light-chain (AL) amyloidosis associated with primary systemic amyloidosis or multiple myeloma. Certain dominantly inherited, familial amyloid polyneuropathies are caused by a point mutation in the transthyretin (prealbumin) gene. Microscopically, amyloid depositions are identified in peripheral nerves, dorsal root ganglia, autonomic ganglia, and often walls of blood vessels. Loss of both myelinated and unmyelinated fibers occurs. An additional complication is carpal tunnel syndrome, which can result from amyloid infiltration of the flexor retinaculum.

Charcot-Marie-Tooth Disease

Hereditary neuropathies are the most common form of chronic neuropathy in children. One of the most common hereditary neuropathies is Charcot-Marie-Tooth disease (CMT), which encompasses a variety of disorders that demonstrate slowly progressive distal sensorimotor polyneuropathies in childhood and early adulthood. *CMT1* is the most common type of CMT, has autosomal dominant inheritance, and demonstrates a chronic demyelinating polyneuropathy with onion skinning and axonal loss. *CMT2* is also an autosomal dominant disease, but demonstrates dying-back neuropathy. A summary of hereditary neuropathies is presented in Table 28-8.

Table 28-8

Charcot-Marie-Tooth Disease (CMT) and Related Hereditary Motor and Sensory Neuropathies

Disease	Inheritance	Linkage	Candidate Gene	Pathology
CMT1A (HMSN IA)	Dominant	Chromosome 17	Peripheral myelin protein-22 (PMP22)	Chronic demyelinating polyneuropathy with numerous onion bulbs and nerve hypertrophy; distal axonal degeneration also is present
CMT1B (HMSN IB)	Dominant	Chromosome 1	Myelin protein zero (P_0) (a protein of PNS myelin)	Same as CMT1A
CMTX1	Dominant	Chromosome X	Connexin-32 (a gap junction protein)	Same as CMT1A
	Dominant	Chromosome 1	Unknown	Distal axonal degeneration
	Recessive or dominant	Chromosome 1 or 17	PMP22 or P_0	Same as CMT1A
	Dominant	Chromosome 17	PMP22	Chronic demyelinating polyneuropathy with focally thickened myelin sheaths (tomacula) and axonal degeneration

From Rubin E, Gorstein F, Rubin R, et al. Rubin's Pathology, 4th ed. Philadelphia: Lippincott Williams & Wilkins, 2005, p. 1498.

Peripheral Nerve Trauma

Nerve injury may occur via crush or transection of the nerve.

- *Traumatic neuromas:* form at the end of the proximal stump of a transected nerve. Within 1 week of injury, neuronal sprouts arise from the distal ends of the intact axons in the proximal nerve stump. If the apposing nerve end is not approximated, these nerve sprouts grow haphazardly into the scar tissue at the end of the proximal stump to form a painful swelling termed a traumatic neuroma.
- *Plantar interdigital neuromas:* painful, sausage-shaped swellings of the plantar digital nerve between the second and third or third and fourth metatarsal bones that often occur in women who wear high heels. These lesions most likely are caused by repeated nerve compression and are composed of fibrosis of the nerve sheath.

Tumors of the Peripheral Nervous System

PNS tumors arise from neurons or the nerve sheath.

Schwannoma

Schwannomas are benign, slow growing, encapsulated neoplasms of Schwann cells that can occur in the cranial nerves, spinal roots, or peripheral nerves. These lesions may occur along the eighth cranial nerve (acoustic neuromas) and within the spinal canal. Schwannomas occur in adults and may vary in size from several millimeters to several centimeters. The cut surface is tan to gray and firm, and it often shows focal hemorrhage, necrosis, and cystic degeneration.

Microscopically, a biphasic pattern comprising Antoni A and Antoni B regions is present. Antoni A regions are characterized by interwoven fascicles of spindled cells with elongated nuclei, eosinophilic cytoplasm, and indistinct cytoplasmic borders. Parallel, palisaded cells may form Verocay bodies. Antoni B regions are characterized by spindled or oval cells with indistinct cytoplasm in a loose vacuolated background.

Neurofibroma

Neurofibromas are benign, slowly growing neoplasm composed of Schwann cells, perineuriallike cells and fibroblasts. Neurofibromas may be solitary or multiple and may occur in both children and adults. Commonly, neurofibromas may involve skin, major nerve plexuses, large deep nerve trunks, the retroperitoneum, and the gastrointestinal tract. Solitary cutaneous neurofibromas are commonly benign, sporadic lesions. Multiple neurofibromas or plexiform neurofibromas may be associated with *neurofibromatosis 1* (NF1), which demonstrates an increased risk of sarcomatous transformation to a malignant peripheral nerve sheath tumor.

Grossly, neurofibromas appear as poorly circumscribed, fusiform nerve enlargements; on occasion, the fascicles may be so enlarged that they appear as cords (plexiform neurofibroma). These lesions may involve extensive tracts of nerves, therefore making surgical excision impossible. The cut surface is soft and light gray. Microscopically, an endoneurial proliferation of spindled cells with elongated nuclei, eosinophilic cytoplasm and indistinct cell borders is present. The spindled cells are present within an extracellular myxoid matrix, wavy bands of collage and residual nerve fibers. Increased cellularity and mitotic figures indicates malignant transformation.

Malignant Peripheral Nerve Sheath Tumor

Malignant peripheral nerve sheath tumor (MPNST) is a poorly differentiated, spindle-cell sarcoma of the peripheral nerve. These lesions may occur de novo or arise from a neurofibroma. Approximately half of these lesions occur in patients with neurofibromatosis. MPNST appears grossly as an unencapsulated, fusiform enlargement of a nerve. Microscopically, the appearance is similar to that of a fibrosarcoma. This lesion can demonstrate blood-borne metastases and local recurrence.

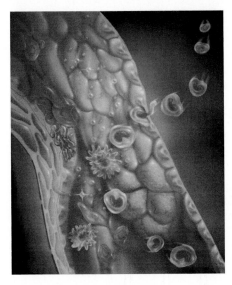

CHAPTER 29

The Eye

Chapter Outline

Normal Anatomy and Histology

The eye is a complex structure. It comprises multiple layers and is protected by the eyelids and surrounding bony socket (Fig. 29-1).

- Outermost layer is composed of the cornea and the sclera; central layer is composed of the uvea (ciliary body, ciliary processes, iris, and choroid); innermost layer is composed of the retina and retinal pigment epithelium.
- Eye chambers include the anterior chamber (between cornea and iris), the posterior chamber (between the iris and the lens), and the vitreous chamber (between the lens and the retina). The aqueous humor refers to the fluid in the anterior and posterior chambers and the vitreous humor is the gel-like material that fills the vitreous chamber.
- Iris is the contractile diaphragm that covers the anterior surface of the lens and contains pigment within the stroma.
- Pupil is the central circular opening of the eye that changes diameter to regulate the amount of light passing through the lens.
- Lens is a biconvex, crystalline structure that is situated between the ciliary bodies and stretched by adherent fibers to allow for accommodation to occur.
- Blood vessels: the central retinal artery and vein regulate blood flow to the eye and these enter through the center of the optic nerve at the back of the eye.

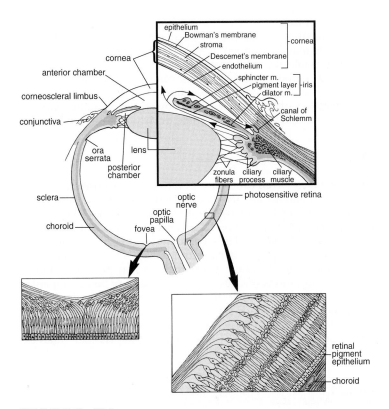

FIGURE 29-1

The structure of the eye. This drawing shows a horizontal section of the eyeball. (Upper inset) Enlargement of the anterior and posterior chambers shown in more detail. Note the direction of the flow of aqeous humor (*arrows*), which is drained by the scleral venous sinus (canal of Schlemm) at the iridocorneal angle. (Lower insets) Typical organization of the cells and nerve fibers of the fovea centralis (*left*) and the retina (*right*). (From Ross MH, Kaye G, Pawlina W. Histology: A Text and Atlas, 4th ed. Philadelphia: Lippincott Williams & Wilkins, 2003, p. 795.)

Physical and Chemical Injuries of the Eye

A variety of manifestations of ocular injury may occur:

- Black eye: result of ecchymosis of the vascular eyelids caused by physical trauma
- Superficial disruptions of the corneal epithelium: result of traumatic abrasion, contact lens wear, foreign bodies, ultraviolet light, caustic chemicals

- Blowout fracture: fracture of the bones of the orbital floor into the maxillary sinus caused by blunt trauma; inferior rectus muscle may be trapped in the fracture leading to a sinking of the eye into the orbit (*enophthalmos*)
- Injury caused by foreign bodies: can result in acute inflammation, granulomatous inflammation, retinal degeneration, discoloration of the ocular tissues by iron-containing particles (*siderosis bulbi*), cataracts, retinal detachment, glaucoma

Orbit

An abnormal forward protrusion of the eyeball is termed *exophthalmos* when bilateral and *proptosis* when unilateral. A variety of causes, including thyroid disease, orbital dermoid cysts, hemangiomas, inflammation, lymphomas, and neoplasms, result in forward protrusion of the eyeball. The most common cause of exophthalmos is Graves disease, a form of hyperthyroidism that most commonly affects middle-aged women. Exophthalmos may precede or follow other manifestations of Graves disease and may be accompanied by retraction of the upper eyelid (due to increased sympathetic tone) and a characteristic stare appearance. Ocular complications of this disease include corneal exposure with ulceration and optic nerve compression, both of which may lead to eventual blindness if uncorrected.

Eyelids

The eyelids are composed of a dense tarsal plate with overlying muscle, glands, and skin. The glands of the eyelid include eccrine sweat glands, meibomian glands (produce oily layer to prevent tear evaporation), and sebaceous glands/glands of Zeis (empty into the follicles of the eyelashes), among others. Various conditions that affect the eyelids include:

- *Blepharitis*: inflammation of the eyelids that produces an acute, red, tender mass
- *Hordeolum (sty)*: acute, inflammatory, focal lesion of the eyelids that may involve the meibomian or sebaceous glands
- *Chalazion*: granulomatous inflammation centered around the meibomian or sebaceous glands; probable reaction to extruded lipid secretions; results in a painless swelling of the eyelid
- *Inflammatory pseudotumor of the orbit*: idiopathic chronic inflammatory condition associated with variable fibrosis; may cause proptosis and partial immobility of the eyeball
- *Xanthelasma*: yellow plaque of lipid-containing macrophages often on the nasal aspect of the eyelid; affects older persons and persons with elevated lipids

Conjunctiva

The conjunctiva is a transparent membrane that extends from the lateral margin of the cornea across the sclera (bulbar conjunctiva) and the internal surface of the eyelids (palpebral conjunctiva). It may undergo *hemorrhage* following blunt trauma, anoxia, severe bouts of coughing, or spontaneously on first arising after sleep.

Inflammation of the conjunctiva is termed *conjunctivitis*, which may occur secondary to allergy or infection. Infectious conjunctivitis occurs as a result of microorganisms on the surface of the eye, hematogenous spread of microorganisms to the eye from another site, or iatrogenic introduction of organisms by infected eyedrops. Conjunctivitis may be accompanied by *keratitis* (corneal inflammation) or corneal ulceration.

Pink Eye

Pink eye refers to a common infectious form of conjunctivitis characterized by hyperemic conjunctival blood vessels and an inflammatory exudate that commonly crusts, causing the eyelids to stick together in the morning. The inflammatory exudates may be purulent, fibrinous, serous, or hemorrhagic and contain inflammatory cells that vary with the etiological agent.

Trachoma

Trachoma is a conjunctivitis caused by serotypes A, B, and C of *Chlamydia trachomatis*. This infection is the most common cause of blindness in the world and is especially prevalent in Asia, the Middle East, and parts of Africa. Trachoma is not highly contagious, but may spread from person to person in conditions of overcrowding or poor hygiene. Trachoma commonly heals spontaneously in children, but may progress in adults. The disease is almost always bilateral and more extensively involves the upper half of the conjunctiva and the corneal epithelium. The cellular infiltrate is composed of lymphocytes, with the formation of lymph follicles and necrotic germinal centers. Eventually, lymphocytes and blood vessels invade the superior portion of the cornea (trachomatous pannus) that ultimately results in scarring of the conjunctiva and eyelids and distortion of the eyelids. Microscopically, the conjunctival epithelium contains glycogen-rich intracytoplasmic inclusions and associated large macrophages contain nuclear fragments (Leber cells). This disease may be complicated by secondary bacterial infection.

Other Conjunctival Infections

- Chlamydial infections: inclusion blennorrhea, a purulent conjunctivitis, or inclusion conjunctivitis, a chronic follicular conjunctivitis with focal lymphoid hyperplasia (inclusion conjunctivitis). In contrast to trachoma, inclusion conjunctivitis usually involves the lower tarsal conjunctiva and does not result in scarring, necrosis, or keratitis.

- Ophthalmia neonatorum: a severe, acute conjunctivitis accompanied by a copious purulent exudate in the newborn; caused by *Neisseria gonorrhoeae*. The infection is acquired during passage through the birth canal of an infected mother and may result in corneal ulceration, perforation, and scarring of the eye. Treatment includes erythromycin, tetracyclines, or silver nitrate.
- Pinguecula: yellowish conjunctival lump that is usually located nasal to the corneoscleral limbus; consists of sun-damaged connective tissue.
- Pterygium: often associated with pinguecula; represents a fold of vascularized conjunctiva that grows horizontally onto the cornea in the shape of an insect wing.

Cornea

The cornea is transparent, is situated on the anterior aspect of the eye, and consists of multiple layers that include, from anterior to posterior:

- The corneal epithelium: nonkeratinized stratified squamous epithelium; continuous with the bulbar conjunctiva; may regenerate from basal cells following minor injury
- Bowman's membrane: anterior basement membrane; prevents spread of infections into the eyeball; damage to this membrane is associated with recurrent corneal erosions
- Corneal stroma: thickest portion of cornea
- Descemet's membrane
- Corneal endothelium: single layer of squamous epithelium that allows for transfer of nutrients between the cornea and the aqueous humor

Some corneal disorders are described below.
Herpesvirus (HSV) includes type 1 and type 2 disease.

- *HSV type 1* has a predilection for the corneal epithelium and may cause localized ocular lesions in childhood, which are accompanied by regional lymphadenopathy, systemic infection and fever. The majority of ocular lesions are asymptomatic plaques, although an acute unilateral follicular conjunctivitis and corneal ulcers may occur. HSV becomes latent in the trigeminal ganglion and can reactivate following trauma, exposure to ultraviolet light or sunlight, vaccination, or menstruation. Reactivation of HSV results in multiple, minute discrete, intraepithelial corneal ulcers (*superficial punctate keratopathy*). These lesions enlarge and coalesce to form a branching pattern with intervening epithelial desquamation, resulting in irregular geographic ulcers. Infected epithelial cells are multinucleated and have eosinophilic, intranuclear inclusion bodies (Lipschütz bodies). In addition, corneal stromal lesions may occur, including the development of a central disc-shaped corneal opacity below the epithelium (*disciform keratitis*).

- *HSV type 2* may infect newborns during passage through the birth canal of an infected mother and can cause widespread lesions of the cornea and retina.

Onchocerciasis is caused by the nematode *Onchocerca volvulus*, which is transmitted by bites of infected blackflies after which microfilaria released from fertilized adult female worms migrate into ocular tissues. When the microfilaria die, an inflammatory response causes corneal opacification and visual impairment (river blindness). This disease is the most prevalent in Africa and Latin America.

Arcus lipoides (*arcus senilis*) occurs in patients with certain disorders of lipid metabolism, which appears as a white arc caused by lipid deposition in the peripheral cornea.

Band keratopathy is an opaque horizontal band across the superficial central cornea that contains either calcium phosphate (associated with hypercalcemia) or noncalcified protein (*chronic actinic keratopathy* due to excessive ultraviolet light).

Corneal dystrophies are a heterogeneous group of hereditary, noninflammatory disease of the cornea that are classified as to the layer of cornea involved, including the epithelium, stroma, and endothelium. Epithelial dystrophies involve the formation of microcysts, defects in the basement membrane, or deposition of finely fibrillar substance in Bowman's layer. Stromal dystrophies result in characteristic forms of corneal opacification that results from the deposition of various substances (lipids, proteins, amyloid) within the stroma. Endothelial dystrophies involve abnormalities in the basement membrane of the corneal endothelium that result in corneal edema, and progressive visual loss.

Lens

Cataracts

Cataracts are one of the most common diseases of the lens. Cataracts are opacifications of the crystalline lens that may occur secondary to a variety of causes, including diabetes, tryptophan deficiency, corticosteroids, ultraviolet light, and trauma, among other causes. The most common cataract occurs with aging and begins when clefts accumulate between the lens fibers. Over time, degenerated lens material accumulates in these spaces and absorbs water, resulting in a swollen lens that may obstruct the pupil and cause glaucoma. In a mature cataract, the lens may degenerate and decrease in volume. Cataracts may be surgically removed.

Presbyopia

Presbyopia is an impairment of vision that occurs with aging in which the near point of vision becomes located farther from the eye. During aging the cuboidal subcapsular cells differentiate into elongated lens fibers, which cause the lens to lose its elasticity. Patients with presbyopia require spectacles for near vision.

Uvea

The uvea is composed of the choroid, which contains blood vessels and melanin, the ciliary bodies, which regulate the shape of the lens, and the iris. The choroid is situated deep to the retina and provides nutrient support for the overlying retina.

A variety of inflammatory conditions affect the uvea (uveitis), including inflammation of the iris (iritis), inflammation of the ciliary body (cyclitis), and iridocyclitis, a combination of the iritis and cyclitis). Iridocyclitis usually manifests as red eye, photophobia, pain, blurred vision, a pericorneal halo, and miosis. Adhesions may develop between various components, and include *posterior synechiae* between the iris and the lens and *peripheral anterior synechiae* between the peripheral iris and the anterior chamber angle.

Sympathetic ophthalmitis occurs in response to an injury in the opposite eye several weeks prior and is characterized by granulomatous inflammation involving the entire uvea. This disease may be complicated by vitiligo and graying of the eyelashes.

Sarcoidosis may affect the uvea in up to one-third of patients with this condition and is usually bilateral. Microscopically, the lesions are granulomatous and may be accompanied by calcific band keratopathy, cataracts, retinal vascularization, vitreous hemorrhage, and bilateral enlargement of the lacrimal and salivary glands (*Mikulicz syndrome*).

Retina

The retina is composed of the neural retina, which contains the rods and cones, and the retinal pigment epithelium (RPE), which is a single layer of cuboidal epithelium containing melanin. The fovea is the region of greatest visual acuity due to the highest concentration of photoreceptors and is located lateral to the optic disc. Surrounding the fovea is a yellow pigmented zone termed the macula lutea. Nerve fibers from the retina coalesce and exit the eye at the optic disc, which lacks photoreceptors and is therefore a physiological blind spot.

Retinal Hemorrhage

Retinal hemorrhages occur secondary to hypertension, diabetes mellitus, and central retinal vein occlusion. If the hemorrhage occurs within the nerve fiber layer, the axons spread apart, resulting in a flame-shaped appearance on funduscopy, whereas deeper hemorrhages tend to be rounded.

Vascular Occlusion

Vascular occlusion in the retina can result from thrombosis, embolism, stenosis, vascular compression, vasoconstriction, or intravascular sludging. If vascular occlusion is severe, ischemia may ensue, leading to swelling of axons and the formation of white fluffy patches that resemble cotton on funduscopy (cotton-wool spots). These lesions are reversible if the ischemia is corrected in time. Occlusion may affect the retinal artery or vein.

Central retinal artery occlusion occurs following thrombosis of the retinal artery, giant cell arteritis, or embolization and may result in blindness if the ischemia is not reversed. Intracellular edema, manifested by retinal pallor, occurs most prominently in the macula where the ganglion cells are most numerous. The fovea stands out in sharp contrast as a cherry-red spot. Small retinal emboli may result in transient unilateral blurred vision, termed *amaurosis fugax*.

Central retinal vein occlusion results in flame-shaped hemorrhages most prominent around the optic disc. Vision often recovers well, but may induce neovascularization of the iris and peripheral anterior synechiae. This results in closed-angle glaucoma with severe pain and repeated hemorrhages several months following occlusion.

Hypertensive Retinopathy

Hypertensive retinopathy occurs following long-standing hypertension and demonstrates characteristic findings, including:

- Arteriolar narrowing
- Flame-shaped hemorrhages in the retinal nerve fiber layer
- Exudates, including some that radiate from the center of the macula
- Cotton-wool spots in the superficial retina
- Microaneurysms

Arteriolosclerosis occurs in conjunction with long-standing hypertension and most commonly affects the retinal and choroidal vessels. By funduscopy, veins appear kinked where the arterioles cross over them (arteriovenous nicking), abnormal retinal arterioles appear as parallel white lines at sites of vascular crossings (arterial sheathing), and small superficial or deep retinal hemorrhages may occur.

Malignant hypertension is characterized by a necrotizing arteriolitis, with fibrinoid necrosis and thrombosis of the precapillary retinal arterioles.

Diabetic Retinopathy

Ocular symptoms occur in 20% to 40% of diabetics and affect almost all patients with type 1 diabetes. Diabetic retinopathy occurs in two stages. The first stage is termed background (nonproliferative) diabetic retinopathy, which occurs during earlier stages of the disease. This stage exhibits venous engorgement with sausage-shaped distentions, small hemorrhages (dot and blot hemorrhages), capillary microaneurysms, and waxy exudates. The retinopathy begins in the posterior pole of the retina, but ultimately may involve the entire retina.

Proliferative Retinopathy

Proliferative retinopathy occurs after approximately 10 years of diabetes and correlates inversely with the degree of glycemic control. This stage is characterized by the growth of delicate new blood vessels, fibrous tissue, and glial tissue toward the vitreous body. These vessels bleed easily and can result in vitreal hemorrhages. The fibrovascular and glial tissue may contract, causing retinal detachment and blindness. In addition to these changes, patients with diabetes may also demonstrate associated vascular disease of the retina.

Diabetic Iridopathy

Diabetic iridopathy occurs when a fibrovascular layer grows along the anterior surface of the iris and in the anterior chamber angle. This growth can lead to peripheral anterior synechiae, posterior synechiae, and hemorrhage within the anterior chamber (hyphema).

Diabetic Cataracts

Diabetic cataracts consist of a blanket of white needle-shaped opacities in the lens immediately beneath the anterior and posterior lens capsule, which are often bilateral and may demonstrate a "snowflake" appearance. In addition, age-related cataracts occur in diabetics at an earlier age than in the general population.

Retinal Detachment

During fetal development, the space between the sensory retina and the retinal pigment epithelium is obliterated when these two layers become apposed. However, when fluid (blood, exudates, liquid vitreous) accumulates within the potential space between these layers, the sensory retina may readily detach. Retinal detachment may also occur with aging, when vitreous body shrinks in size and pulls away from the neural retina, resulting in retinal tears and detachment. Additional factors leading to *retinal detachment* include retinal defects, diminished pressure on the retina (after vitreous loss), and weakening of the fixation of the retina. Retinal detachment results in degeneration of the photoreceptors, after which cystlike extracellular spaces appear within the retina.

Retinitis Pigmentosa

Retinitis pigmentosa refers to a variety of bilateral, progressive, degenerative retinopathies characterized clinically by night blindness and constriction of peripheral visual fields. In this disease, loss of rods and cones is followed by migration of retinal pigment epithelial cells into the sensory retina, and melanin appears within slender processes of spidery cells and accumulates around small branching retinal blood vessels. The clinical features are variable, but may eventually lead to contraction of the visual fields and tunnel vision. Central vision is usually preserved until late in the disease.

Macular Degeneration

The fovea is the central portion of the macula that contains the highest concentration of cones and is the point of greatest visual acuity. Degeneration of this region may occur with aging, certain drug toxicities (chloroquine), and certain inherited disorders. *Age-related macular degeneration* (ARMD) is the most common cause of blindness in the elderly and is classified as wet or dry. *Dry ARMD* results from degeneration of macula lutea, thickening of Bruch's membrane (between the choroid and the RPE) to form "drusen," atrophy and depigmentation of the RPE, and loss of choroidal capillaries. The overlying retina is compromised and the formation of blind spots occurs. As the drusen become revascularized, leakage from the new vessels leads to exudates and hemorrhages below the retina (*wet ARMD*). As macular degeneration progresses, central vision is impaired. Occasionally, this disease may be accompanied by bleeding into the subretinal space (hemorrhagic macular degeneration), which may be treated with laser photocoagulation.

Cherry-red Macular Spots

A cherry-red spot at the macula can result from central retinal artery occlusion or lysosomal storage diseases, such as the gangliosidoses.

Angioid Streaks

Angioid streaks refer to the vessel like appearance of fractures in Bruch's membrane in a number of systemic diseases.

Retinopathy of Prematurity

Retinopathy of prematurity (ROP) is a bilateral, iatrogenic disorder that occurs in premature infants who have been treated with oxygen after birth. High amounts of oxygen result in the obliteration of retinal blood vessels and lack of vascularization of the peripheral retina. When the infant returns to ambient air, the vascular endothelium and glial cells proliferate at the junction of the avascular and vascularized portions of the retina. In 25% of cases, ROP progresses to a cicatricial phase with retinal detachment, a fibrovascular mass behind the lens, and blindness.

Optic Nerve

Optic disc edema (papilledema) refers to a swelling of the optic nerve head where it enters the globe (optic papilla) and may occur secondary to a variety of causes, including increased intracranial pressure. Additional causes of papilledema include obstruction to the venous drainage of the eye, an infarct of the optic nerve, inflammation of the optic nerve, and multiple sclerosis. By funduscopy, the optic disc appears swollen with blurred margins and dilated vessels. Often, hemorrhages, exudates, and cotton-wool spots are present. If uncorrected, the normal blind spot enlarges over time and atrophic changes may lead to a loss of visual acuity.

Optic nerve atrophy is a thinning of the optic nerve caused by a loss of axons. Causes of optic nerve atrophy include long-standing edema of the optic nerve head, optic neuritis, optic nerve compression, glaucoma, retinal degeneration, and genetic mutations (*OPA1*, *OPA3*, and *WFS1* genes).

Glaucoma

Glaucoma is a collection of disorders characterized by excavation of the optic disc and a progressive loss of visual field sensitivity, often caused by increased intraocular pressure (ocular hypertension). Increased intraocular pressure occurs when the balance of aqueous humor production and drainage is upset, and can lead to pressure-induced degenerative changes in the retina and optic nerve head. Under normal conditions, the aqueous humor is produced by the ciliary body, and flows from the posterior chamber through the pupil to the anterior chamber, after which it drains into veins by way of the trabecular meshwork and canal of Schlemm. Glaucoma most often occurs with a congenital or acquired lesion of the anterior segment of the eye that mechanically obstructs the aqueous drainage. Patients with glaucoma commonly present with blurred vision and report the appearance of halos around lights. Over time, increased intraocular pressure may result in various findings, including:

- Cupped excavation of the optic nerve head
- Bulging of the cornea or sclera at weak points
- Optic nerve atrophy
- Degeneration of the ganglion cell layer of the retina with impaired vision
- Buphthalmos (extensively enlarged eye) if the increased pressure occurs before the age of 3 years when the eye is still pliable

Treatment of glaucoma is directed toward lowering intraocular pressure, and include correction of the underlying structural disorder, reducing the production of aqueous humor (i.e., by carbonic anhydrase inhibitors), or using ocular hypotensive agents in emergent cases.

Congenital Glaucoma

Congenital glaucoma is caused by developmental anomalies that lead to obstruction to the aqueous drainage. The majority of cases are X-linked recessive and commonly manifest in boys during infancy or early childhood. The disease usually involves both eyes and is associated with a deep anterior chamber, corneal cloudiness, sensitivity to bright light (photophobia), excessive tearing, and buphthalmos (enlarged eyes). Genes that have been implicated in congenital glaucoma include the cytochrome P4501B1 gene (*CYP1B1*), forkhead transcription factor gene (*FKHL7*), pituitary homeobox 2 gene (*PTX2*), and the paired box 6 gene (*PAX6*).

Primary Open-angle Glaucoma

Primary open-angle glaucoma occurs in patients without known underlying eye disease and occurs most commonly in the sixth decade. This is the most common form of glaucoma and is a major cause of blindness in the United States. In open-angle glaucoma, the anterior chamber angle is open and appears normal, although increased resistance to the outflow of the aqueous humor is present in the vicinity of the canal of Schlemm. The disease is commonly bilateral (although one eye may be more prominently affected) and may lead to retinal damage, optic nerve degeneration, and loss of peripheral vision. Patients with diabetes mellitus and myopia are at increased risk of primary open-angle glaucoma.

Primary Closed-angle Glaucoma

Primary closed-angle glaucoma occurs after age 40 years and affects persons without known underlying eye disorders. In closed-angle glaucoma, the anterior chamber is shallower than normal, and the angle is abnormally narrow. This disorder affects persons whose peripheral iris is displaced anteriorly toward the trabecular meshwork, which creates a narrow angle. When the pupil dilates (mydriasis), the iris obstructs the anterior chamber angle, impairing aqueous drainage and causing sudden episodes of intraocular hypertension. Ocular pain and halos or rings seen around lights accompany these episodes. Over time, closed-angle glaucoma can results in peripheral anterior synechiae (adhesions between the iris and the trabecular network) that further block the outflow of aqueous humor. *Acute closed-angle glaucoma* is an ocular emergency and ocular hypotensive treatment must be initiated within the first 24 to 48 hours to maintain vision.

Other Types of Glaucoma

Low-tension glaucoma demonstrates the characteristic visual-field defect and ophthalmoscopic features of chronic open-angle glaucoma without an increase in intraocular pressure. This condition most commonly affects the elderly.

Secondary glaucoma may occur with a variety of diseases, including inflammation, hemorrhage, adhesions, and neovascularization of the iris.

Myopia

Myopia is a refractive ocular abnormality in which light from the visualized object focuses at a point in front of the retina because of a longer than usual anteroposterior diameter of the eye. Myopia usually begins in young persons and varies in severity. Treatment involves corrective lenses or refractive surgery (LASIK).

Phthisis Bulbi

Phthisis bulbi is a nonspecific, end-stage eye that is small and soft, with a thickened, wrinkled sclera, detached sensory retina, displaced calcified lens, and shrunken, opaque cornea. Often, intraocular bone formation may occur. Overall, the eye appears disorganized and atrophic. Treatment is often enucleation.

Neoplasms

Metastatic lesions are the most common neoplasms that affect the eye. Of the neoplasms that arise within the eye, the majority arises from immature retinal neurons (retinoblastoma) and uveal melanocytes (melanoma).

Malignant Melanoma

Malignant melanoma represents the most common primary intra-ocular malignancy and originates from melanocytes or nevi in the uvea. These lesions often appear circumscribed and invade Bruch's membrane, forming a mushroom-shaped mass. Microscopically, these melanomas may contain spindle-shaped cells without nucleoli (spindle A cells), spindle-shaped cells with nucleoli (spindle B cells) or polygonal cells with distinct cell borders and prominent nucleoli (epithelioid cells). Variable amounts of necrosis are present. Melanomas that arise in the ciliary body and iris may extend circumferentially around the globe and are termed *ring melanomas*.

Because the eye does not contain lymphatics, spread of melanoma occurs via extension through the sclera and hematogenous spread. Treatment often involves enucleation of the eye, but radiotherapy or local excision may be of use. Over half of all patients with melanoma may survive for 15 years.

Retinoblastoma

Retinoblastoma is the most common intraocular malignant neoplasm of childhood and arises from immature neurons of the retina. Although the majority of retinoblastomas are unilateral and sporadic, approximately 6% of retinoblastomas are inherited and more commonly bilateral. These tumors arise from spontaneous or inherited mutations of the retinoblastoma (*Rb*) gene on 13q14.

Grossly, retinoblastomas are cream-colored tumors that contain scattered, chalky white, calcified flecks within yellow necrotic zones. Microscopically, these lesions are cellular and a variety of patterns may be present, including sheets of round cells with hyperchromatic nuclei and scant cytoplasm, or cells arranged around a central cavity (Flexner-Wintersteiner rosettes). Necrosis and calcification may be seen. Spread of retinoblastomas occurs by way of direct extension along the optic nerve to the brain or by hematogenous spread, often to the bone marrow.

Patients present with a white pupil (leukocoria), squint, poor vision, spontaneous hyphema, or a red, painful eye. Secondary glaucoma may occur. Some retinoblastomas grow toward the vitreous body (endophytic retinoblastoma), whereas others growth between the sensory retina and the retinal pigment epithelium, detaching the retina (exophytic retinoblastoma). Early diagnosis and treatment results in a high survival rate, although these patients are at risk for other malignancies, including osteogenic sarcoma, Ewing sarcoma, and pinealoblastoma.

Index

Page numbers in *italics* indicate figures. Those followed by "t" indicate tables.